INNOVATION IN
HEALTHY AND
FUNCTIONAL
FOODS

INNOVATION IN HEALTHY AND FUNCTIONAL FOODS

Edited by

**DILIP GHOSH • SHANTANU DAS
DEBASIS BAGCHI • R.B. SMARTA**

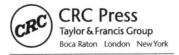

CRC Press
Taylor & Francis Group
Boca Raton   London   New York

CRC Press is an imprint of the
Taylor & Francis Group, an **informa** business

CRC Press
Taylor & Francis Group
6000 Broken Sound Parkway NW, Suite 300
Boca Raton, FL 33487-2742

© 2013 by Taylor & Francis Group, LLC
CRC Press is an imprint of Taylor & Francis Group, an Informa business

No claim to original U.S. Government works

Printed in the United States of America on acid-free paper
Version Date: 20120813

International Standard Book Number: 978-1-4398-6267-4 (Hardback)

Library of Congress Cataloging-in-Publication Data

Innovation in healthy and functional foods / editors Dilip Ghosh ... [et al.].
    p. cm.
    Summary: "Functional food developers are faced with challenges and opportunities in bringing these food products into the marketplace. This book addresses the latest innovation models, the regulatory framework around innovation, and social issues related to consumer perspectives on innovation versus the need for functional food products. Presented by professionals directly involved in the process, chapters cover food safety, packaging, and regulations; drivers and barriers in innovation; the marketing of functional foods globally; the changing dynamics of food consumption in developing countries; product innovation; technological development; functional food ingredients; and future trends"-- Provided by publisher.
    Includes bibliographical references and index.
    ISBN 978-1-4398-6267-4 (hardback)
    1. Food industry and trade--Technological innovations. 2. Natural foods industry--Technological innovations. 3. Natural foods--Processing. 4. Functional foods. 5. Agricultural innovations. I. Ghosh, Dilip K.

TP370.I566 2012
641.3'02--dc23
                                      2012009138

Visit the Taylor & Francis Web site at
http://www.taylorandfrancis.com

and the CRC Press Web site at
http://www.crcpress.com

Dedicated to those people who made this world beautiful through their innovations

Dilip Ghosh

Dedicated to my beloved teacher, Professor Mihir N. Das, DSc, Jadavpur University

Debasis Bagchi

Dedicated to my beloved family

Shantanu Das

Dedicated to my beloved mother, who allowed me to explore new avenues in life

R.B. Smarta

Contents

SECTION I   Introduction

SECTION II   Market and Trends

SECTION III   Consumer Perspective on Innovation versus Need

SECTION IV   Technological Development on Healthy and Functional Foods

SECTION V   Innovation in Functional Food Ingredients

SECTION VI   Market to Innovative Products

SECTION VII   Future Trends

Preface

Our new book *Innovation in Healthy and Functional Foods* endeavors to integrate two key contemporary concepts "innovation" and "functional and healthy foods," the major thrust in the world of food, nutrition, and nutraceuticals.

This book includes topics that have been researched in academia but have the potential to be applied in the food industry. The question arises in mind as to which step in the innovation process would be ideal for academia–industry collaboration. The collaboration may take place at any step in the innovation process, that is, ideation, feasibility, development, commercialization, and launch. However, we think the most ideal point is at stage zero, that is, even before a particular project has been conceived. At this stage, as the industry scans the consumers' needs and desires it can also scan the new technologies, solutions, and capabilities available within academia. It is always hard to decide when to adopt a technology from academic research into industrial development. Though there is no strict rule yet it can be said that an organization with strong R&D may adopt a technology in its initial stage and develop it further. On the other hand for a market-driven organization it is more convenient to adopt a mature technology. All these innovation concepts, though based on studies in multiple industries, can be successfully applied to the food industry.

The focus on food science and technology has transformed over centuries. In the past, the focus of food science and technology was food security. This resulted in rapid improvement in agricultural production techniques. Then the focus shifted to food safety and as a result a range of food preservation techniques were developed. Once the food was proven safe, the taste, flavor, texture, appearance, and other sensorial attributes of the food became the priority of the food industry to satisfy consumer acceptance. After the development of safe and tasty foods, the focus of food science and technology shifted toward healthy and functional foods. Functional food is defined as food capable of providing health benefits beyond basic nutrition. Today, consumers desire foods that are capable of playing not only a "health-promoting" but also a "disease-preventing" role, over and above their routine function of supporting growth and maintenance.

A functional food may be of four types: (1) a natural food in which one of the components has been naturally present at relatively high concentrations; (2) a food to which a component has been added to provide benefits; (3) a food from which a component has been removed so that the food has less adverse health effects; and (4) a food in which the absorption of one or more components has been increased to prove a beneficial effect. This book focuses mainly on the type 2 functional food and conducts a fairly detail exploration into the functional ingredients (e.g., omega-3, probiotics, protein, iron, etc.) and their delivery techniques into consumer foods.

Innovation in functional and healthy foods can be carried out successfully only by a cross-functional team as expertise in various subjects is required to be integrated. To be able to deliver the innovation process to the food industry, the contributors of this book have been identified carefully to make sure that they bring various skills and experiences including biological science, food science, engineering, marketing, regulatory, legal, financial, sustainability, and management. In an era of open innovation, all these skills do not need to be situated in one organization, Various organizations, commercial businesses, and research institutions can work together to lead to innovation. In the spirit of open innovation, our book brings together experts from both industry and academia.

This book puts together various aspects of innovation processes, consumer insights and trends in developed and developing markets for functional and healthy foods as well as a range of technological developments in functional foods and ingredients. Also, this book addresses three key drivers of future innovations in the food industry. These drivers are affordability, sustainability, and tightening of government regulation. A total of 34 chapters have been written by renowned experts from around the world and edited by our team.

Section I gives an overview of innovation in the food industry, focusing on safe, healthy, and functional foods.

Sections II and III discuss various aspects of the opportunities and scope in different markets for functional foods. Section II provides characteristics of the markets in different continents (the United States, Europe, Asia, and around the world) in terms of functional and healthy foods. Section III provides some insights in consumer perception of functional foods and ingredients.

Sections IV and V discuss various technological aspects associated with innovations in the food industry. Section IV focuses on innovations in food processing, packaging, and functional ingredient delivery technology, whereas Section V focuses on various functional and nutritional food ingredients.

Section VI deals with the connection between innovation and other parts of the business, such as marketing, sales, regulatory and finance, and analyzes commercial feasibility.

Section VII provides some insights into future trends such as food tourism, nanotechnology, sustainability, and globalization.

This book is intended for a broad audience associated with food and allied industries, with the intention of an overview of the contemporary food innovation. This book will be useful for professionals working in universities and research institutions, food, nutraceutical and pharmaceutical industries as well as for the students studying food technology and food business. Also, this book can be a good resource for the entrepreneurs looking for opportunities in food and nutrition industries.

Editors

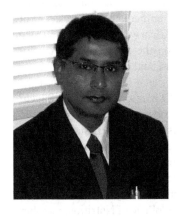

Dilip Ghosh received his PhD in biomedical science from University of Calcutta, India. Previously, he held positions in Organon (India) Ltd., a division of Organon International, BV and AKZO-NOBEL, the Netherlands; HortResearch, New Zealand; USDA-ARS, HNRCA at Tufts University, Boston, Massachusetts; The Smart Foods Centre, University of Wollongong, and Neptune Bio-Innovation Pty Ltd, Sydney, Australia. He has been involved for a long time in drug development (both synthetic and herbal) and functional food research and development both in academic and industry domains. He is a fellow of the American College of Nutrition and is also on the editorial board of several journals. Currently, Dr. Ghosh is a director, Nutriconnect, Sydney; Honorary Ambassador, Global Harmonization Initiative (GHI).

Dr. Ghosh has published more than 70 papers in peer-reviewed journals, numerous articles in food and nutrition magazines and books. His recent book, *Biotechnology in Functional Foods and Nutraceuticals*, was published by CRC Press in 2010. Dr. Ghosh is the review editor of *Frontiers in Nutrigenomics*; editorial board member, *Panacea E-Newsletter, India*; guest columnist of *NutraScope, India*; and associate editor and member, *Toxicology Mechanisms and Methods*, Taylor & Francis, USA (2006–2007). He can be reached at: dilipghosh@nutriconnect.com.au; dghosh@optusnet.com.au

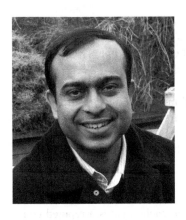

Shantanu Das works as product development manager at Riddet Institute (Centre for Research Excellence in Food and Nutrition), Massey University, New Zealand. In his current role, he is responsible for developing new technologies for commercial application in the food and nutrition industry. Dr. Das and his team undertake R&D projects in various areas related to functional foods, especially delivery systems of functional ingredients. His recent achievement is development of a patented technology for delivering probiotic bacteria at high concentration through shelf-stable foods, which received the "Food Industry Innovation Excellence Award 2011" from the New Zealand Institute of Food Scientists and Technologists. In his current role, Dr. Das has led a number of projects sponsored by domestic and international food industry.

Dr. Das completed his masters in dairy technology from National Dairy Research Institute, India. He completed his PhD in food technology and post graduate diploma in business management in New Zealand.

He has worked in the food industry for over 12 years, both in manufacturing and in R&D. He received the "PepsiCo Global Research & Development Award" in 2006 while working for PepsiCo Asia R&D.

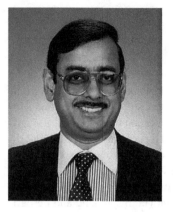

Debasis Bagchi received his PhD in medicinal chemistry in 1982. He is a professor in the Department of Pharmacological and Pharmaceutical Sciences at the University of Houston, Houston, Texas. Dr. Bagchi is also the director of Innovation & Clinical Affairs of Iovate Health Sciences International Inc., Oakville, Ontario, Canada. Dr. Bagchi is the immediate past president of the American College of Nutrition, Clearwater, Florida, and also serves as a distinguished advisor on the Japanese Institute for Health Food Standards, Tokyo, Japan, and immediate past chairman of the Nutraceuticals and Functional Foods Division of the Institutes of Food Technologists, Chicago, Illinois. Dr. Bagchi received the Master of American College of Nutrition Award in October 2010. His research interests include free radicals, human diseases, carcinogenesis, pathophysiology, mechanistic aspects of cytoprotection by antioxidants, regulatory pathways in obesity, diabetes, and gene expression.

Dr. Bagchi has 288 papers in peer-reviewed journals, 15 books, and 16 patents. He has delivered invited lectures in various national and international scientific conferences, organized workshops, and group discussion sessions. Dr. Bagchi is a Fellow of the American College of Nutrition, member of the Society of Toxicology, member of the New York Academy of Sciences, Fellow of the Nutrition Research Academy, and member of the TCE stakeholder Committee of the Wright Patterson Air Force Base, Ohio. Dr. Bagchi is a member of the Study Section and Peer Review Committee of the National Institutes of Health, Bethesda, Maryland. Dr. Bagchi is the associate editor of the *Journal of Functional Foods* and *Journal of the American College of Nutrition*, and also serving as editorial board member of numerous peer-reviewed journals including *Antioxidants and Redox Signaling*, *Cancer Letters*, *Toxicology Mechanisms and Methods*, and other scientific and medical journals. He is also a consulting editor of the CRC Press/Taylor & Francis.

Dr. Bagchi has received funding from various institutions and agencies including the U.S. Air Force Office of Scientific Research, Nebraska State Department of Health, Biomedical Research Support Grant from National Institutes of Health (NIH), National Cancer Institute (NCI), Health Future Foundation, The Procter & Gamble Company and Abbott Laboratories.

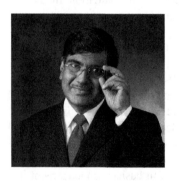

R.B. Smarta is the founder and managing director of Interlink Marketing Consulting Pvt. Ltd. He obtained an MSc in organic chemistry (drugs) from the University of Nagpur (1967), MMS from JBIMS University of Mumbai (1972), and a PhD in management sciences from the University of East Georgia (1982). Dr. Smarta is an FRSA (Fellow of the Royal Society of Arts) conferred by RSA, UK; CMC (Certified Member of Consultants) by IMCI; corporate trainer; and a teacher. He is a reputed consultant and mentor for corporations in the pharma, nutra, wellness, healthcare and lifescience industry, as well as a corporate trainer. He is faculty in leading management institutions such as JBIMS (Bajaj Institute of Management Studies), NMIMS (Narsee Monjee Institute of Management Studies), IIM (Indian Institute of Management), Indore, Pharmacy College, Manipal, and a guide to PhD students. Dr. Smarta is a board member of HADSA (part of IADSA (International Alliance Dietary/Food Supplement Associations)) and also an editor of *Nutrascope* (a HADSA Publication). He has authored two research books, namely, *Strategic Pharmaceutical Marketing* and *Revitalizing the Pharmaceutical Business*. He has coauthored one book namely (Mega) *Market in German and English*.

Dr. Smarta has published articles in journals and news magazines such as *Pharma Pulse*, *Modern Pharmaceuticals*, *Pharmabiz*, *Hindu*, *Business Today*, *Outline Today*.

Contributors

Leena Aarikka-Stenroos
Turku School of Economics
University of Turku
Turku, Finland

Philip E. Apong
Innovation & Clinical Affairs
Iovate Health Sciences International Inc.
Oakville, Ontario, Canada

Debasis Bagchi
Department of Pharmacological and
    Pharmaceutical Sciences
University of Houston College
    of Pharmacy
Houston, Texas

and

Innovation & Clinical Affairs
Iovate Health Sciences International Inc.
Oakville, Ontario, Canada

Virender K. Batish
Dairy Microbiology Division
National Dairy Research Institute
Haryana, India

Abhijit Bhattacharya
OmniActive Health Technologies Ltd.
Maharashtra, India

Alistair Carr
Institute of Food, Nutrition and
    Human Health
Massey University
Palmerston North, New Zealand

Dennis Chang
Centre for Complementary
    Medicine Research
and
School of Biomedical and Health Sciences
University of Western Sydney
New South Wales, Australia

Srikanta Chatterjee
School of Economics and Finance
Massey University
Palmerston North, New Zealand

Kerrie Close
Goodman Fielder Limited
New South Wales, Australia

Patrick Coppens
International Food and Health Law and
    Scientific Affairs
European Advisory Services
Brussels, Belgium

Shantanu Das
Riddet Institute
Massey University
Palmerston North, New Zealand

Jayant Deshpande
OmniActive Health Technologies Ltd.
Maharashtra, India

Mark L. Dreher
Nutrition Science Solutions
Wimberley, Texas

Ruth D'Souza
Interlink Marketing Consultancy Pvt. Ltd.
Maharashtra, India

C.P. Dunne
Combat Feeding Innovative Science
    Team
U.S. Army Research, Development, and
    Engineering Command
Natick, Massachusetts

Ashling Ellis
Riddet Institute
Massey University
Palmerston North, New Zealand

Melissa Fry
School of Biomedical Sciences and
    Pharmacy
University of Newcastle
New South Wales, Australia

Kata Galić
Faculty of Food Technology and
    Biotechnology
University of Zagreb
Zagreb, Croatia

Manohar L. Garg
School of Biomedical Sciences and
    Pharmacy
University of Newcastle
New South Wales, Australia

Dilip Ghosh
Nutriconnect
and
Global Harmonization Initiative
New South Wales, Australia

Sumita Ghosh
School of Built Environment
University of Technology
New South Wales, Australia

Suzanne Grant
Centre for Complementary Medicine Research
University of Western Sydney
New South Wales, Australia

Sunita Grover
Dairy Microbiology Division
National Dairy Research Institute
Haryana, India

Klaus G. Grunert
MAPP Centre for Research on Customer
    Relations in the Food Sector
Aarhus University
Aarhus, Denmark

L.M. Hallberg
Combat Feeding Innovative Science Team
U.S. Army Natick Combat
    Feeding Program
Natick, Massachusetts

Manki Ho
Cantox Health Sciences International
Mississauga, Ontario, Canada

Tin-Chung Huang
Institute of Health Industry Management
Ching-Kuo Institute of Management
    and Health
Taipei, Taiwan

Thom Huppertz
NIZO Food Research BV
Ede, the Netherlands

Girish P. Jakhotiya
Jakhotiya & Associates
Management Consultants
Maharashtra, India

Alex Kocenas
Cantox Health Sciences International
Mississauga, Ontario, Canada

Fanbin Kong
Department of Biological and Agricultural
    Engineering
University of California
Davis, California

Ashwani Kumar
Department of Biotechnology
Seth Jai Parkash Mukand Lal Institute
    of Engineering and Technology
Haryana, India

Parigi Ramesh Kumar
Central Food Technological Research
    Institute
Karnataka, India

Lisa Lähteenmäki
MAPP Centre for Research on Customer
    Relations in the Food Sector
Aarhus University
Aarhus, Denmark

Kuan-Huei Lee
School of Tourism
University of Queensland
Queensland, Australia

Timothy J. Lee
Tourism & Hospitality Management
Ritsumeikan Asia Pacific University
Beppu, Japan

K. Luechapattanaporn
PepsiCo Asia Pacific R&D
Bangkok, Thailand

Karen Ly
Cantox Health Sciences International
Mississauga, Ontario, Canada

Kristen Lyons
School of Social Science
University of Queensland
Queensland, Australia

Rekha R. Malia
Biosix Peptides India Pvt. Ltd.
National Incubation Center
Kerala, India

Larry McGirr
Cantox Health Sciences International
Mississauga, Ontario, Canada

Vikas Mittal
Riddet Institute
Massey University
Palmerston North, New Zealand

Arup Nag
Riddet Institute
Massey University
Palmerston North, New Zealand

Srinivas Nammi
School of Biomedical and Health Sciences
University of Western Sydney
New South Wales, Australia

D.B. Anantha Narayana
(retired)
Foods, Home & Personal Care
Unilever Research India
Karnataka, India

M.G. Parameswaran
Draftfcb Ulka Advertising
Maharashtra, India

Hashmukh Patel
Department of Dairy Science
South Dakota State University
Brookings, South Dakota

Lina Paulionis
Cantox Health Sciences International
Mississauga, Ontario, Canada

Melinda Phang
School of Biomedical Sciences and Pharmacy
University of Newcastle
New South Wales, Australia

Ilana Platt
Cantox Health Sciences International
Mississauga, Ontario, Canada

Devastotra Poddar
Riddet Institute
Massey University
Palmerston North, New Zealand

Kalpagam Polasa
Food and Drug Toxicology Research Centre
National Institute of Nutrition
Andhra Pradesh, India

V. Prakash
Research, Innovation, and Development
JSS Technical Instiution Campus
Karnataka, India

Munish Puri
Institute for Technology and Research
    Innovation
Deakin University
Victoria, Australia

Rajshri Roy
School of Molecular Bioscience
The University of Sydney
New South Wales, Australia

Birgitta Sandberg
Turku School of Economics
University of Turku
Turku, Finland

Raka Saxena
National Dairy Research Institute
Haryana, India

Gyorgy Scrinis
School of Historical and Philosophical Studies
University of Melbourne
Victoria, Australia

B. Sesikeran
Food and Drug Toxicology Research Centre
National Institute of Nutrition
Andhra Pradesh, India

M.L. Shankaranarayana
OmniActive Health Technologies Ltd.
Maharashtra, India

A.K. Singh
National Dairy Research Institute
Haryana, India

Harjinder Singh
Riddet Institute
Massey University
Palmerston North, New Zealand

R. Paul Singh
Department of Biological and
    Agricultural Engineering
University of California
Davis, California

R.B. Smarta
Interlink Marketing Consultancy Pvt. Ltd.
Maharashtra, India

A.K. Srivastava
National Dairy Research Institute
Haryana, India

Maya Sugiarto
Riddet Institute
Massey University
Palmerston North, New Zealand

J. Tang
Department of Biological Systems
    Engineering
Washington State University
Pullman, Washington

Ashok Vaidya
ICMR Advanced Centre of Reverse
    Pharmacology
Kasturba Health Society
Maharashtra, India

Madan Lal Verma
Institute for Technology and Research
    Innovation
Deakin University
Victoria, Australia

J. Wang
Department of Biological Systems
    Engineering
Washington State University
Pullman, Washington

Y. Wang
Department of Biosystem
    Engineering
Auburn University
Auburn, Alabama

Section I

Introduction

1 Innovation Journey
How to Improve R&D Leverage and Speed to Market

Dilip Ghosh, Shantanu Das, Debasis Bagchi, and R.B. Smarta

CONTENTS

1.1 INTRODUCTION

The eminent twentieth-century Nobel laureate scientist and humanitarian, Dr. Linus Pauling, says the following in relation to innovation: "The best way to have a good idea is to have a lot of ideas."

Each year, over a million companies are started in the United States but only about 10% of budding entrepreneurs can exist over the next 12–18 months (Mehta, 2004). Turning ideas into successful business ventures is tricky. A successful entrepreneurship encompasses an entrepreneur's knowledge, limitations, and strengths, which may be able to avoid some common pitfalls in starting up a biotech company. Introducing a new product to the market requires a chain of activities such as creating market demand and delivery channels and putting resources behind these ideas (Harrison and Waluszewski, 2008). Clearly, a successful beginning for a life sciences start-up and subsequent commercialization would be to build a team of people, bringing all aspects of these two distinct approaches together as soon as possible so that all the stakeholders in the new venture benefit from the best marriage of business and technology (Aarikka-Stenroos and Sandberg, 2011).

1.2 INNOVATION: A VERSATILE TOOL

Innovation is the process of creating and delivering new customer value in the marketplace and comes about through the successful combination of novel innovation and invention, and unique business opportunities (Dahlander and Gann, 2010). Innovation can emerge from anywhere that creates the right environment. In the traditional innovation processes, all the stages, that is, from concept to launch, are carried out within the organizational boundary. This traditional process is described as "closed" innovation because of its confinement within the organization. However, industry, including the food industry, is moving from "closed" to an "open" innovation paradigm. In an open innovation, a company uses its internal, as well as external, inputs for their innovation, and commercializes through their own business or external channels, as necessary.

Open innovation is leading to unprecedented inflows and outflows of information between research institutions and industry around the world. What is so powerful is that the information flow

3

is two-way. Scientists, technologists, health professionals, and engineers are getting more of an in-depth view of the market and its commercial realities, while resource managers and strategists within companies get to understand at the earliest stage (precompetitive stage) of the real potential of emerging knowledge. This leads to better problem definition and consequently better technology or product solutions being developed (find out "why," then you will know "how"). The transition of the food industry from closed to open innovation has created huge opportunities for research organizations to collaborate with industry partners. Nevertheless, the open innovation is currently one of the most debated topics in the management portfolio. Two issues require further investigation: (i) understanding the relevance of open innovation beyond high-tech industries and (ii) studying how firms implement open innovation in practice. The downsides of openness can result in resources being made available for others to exploit, with intellectual property being difficult to protect and benefits from innovation difficult to appropriate.

1.3   RADICAL CHALLENGES

In most cases, using existing methods and technology will generate the required minor improvements. A radical challenge should immediately push an organization into looking outside because inside knowledge will not be enough to solve the problem. A radical innovation will take an entirely novel approach to achieve a breakthrough. Since it is a radical change of mindset outside the traditional thinking, step-changing your solutions will necessitate a higher-risk approach but will result in higher reward and creation of value (Isherwood, 2009).

Due to the rapid changeover of technologies and manufacturing processes, there are several key challenges facing the healthy and functional food industry over the next few years, including

- Balancing technology-led versus consumer-led innovation to achieve successful R&D optimization
- Managing increasing regulatory burdens while finding opportunities for growth
- Despite economic downfall, strategic step for implementing radical innovation

1.4   ULTIMATE IMPLEMENTATION

To overcome these challenges, the following strategies will need to be assessed and implemented:

- Streamline in-house R&D structure for better delivery of more challenging projects to the business
- Strategic partnerships with key suppliers and universities
- Linkages with competitors (or joint ventures)
- Efficient customer relationship management system

REFERENCES

Aarikka-Stenroos, L. and Sandberg, B. 2011. From new-product development to commercialization through networks. *J. Business Res.*, 65: 207–209.

Dahlander, L. and Gann, D.M. 2010. How open is innovation? *Res. Policy*, 39: 699–709.

Harrison, D. and Waluszewski, A. 2008. The development of a user network as a way to re-launch an unwanted product. *Res. Policy*, 37: 115–130.

Isherwood, P. 2009. Accelerating innovation through external partnerships. *Food Sci. Tech.*, 22: 46–48.

Mehta, S. 2004. Paths to entrepreneurship in life sciences. *Nat. Biotech.*, 22: 1609–1612.

2 Innovations in Functional Food Industry for Health and Wellness

Parigi Ramesh Kumar and V. Prakash

CONTENTS

Specific dietary supplements and lifestyle changes in food habits can influence the way we eat food and create the need from our meals more in terms of assimilable nutrition leading to prevention of diseases both physical and mental to make tomorrow's 80s look like 60 years! The regulatory considerations of some of the supplements and complements on the label declaration would have a clear distinction on agricultural resources of the country to that of traditional foods related to public health, ethics, and the food security bowl built upon not only addressing noncommunicable diseases, but also the mechanism of action of functional foods from a holistic approach. The herbal supplements will strongly dominate this area challenging the food technologists for retaining the bioactive principles even after processing conditions of temperature, pressure, pH, other physical parameters, and ingredient technologies.

Health and desire for longevity have been inherent features in all social orders and at every stage, all human races have endeavored to achieve these goals. Only sustainable efforts are percolated through generations, even to the modern day. Ayurveda is one such inherited tradition of health and longevity. More interestingly, it has been sustaining itself, through many constraints of cultural, political, and technological invasions. This phenomenal rate of sustainability itself is a credential for Ayurveda. Health of our society ultimately rests upon the effective revival of Ayurveda in its full dignity (Govindarajan et al., 2005; Vaidya, 2006). The role of special ingredients in functional foods, such as what is now termed as *nutraceuticals*, is not new. Many of these claims are very clearly embedded in traditional and ethnic foods, the knowledge of which is transmitted from generation to generation especially the benefits of certain ingredients. The trend of functional foods, nutraceuticals, healthful foods, fortified foods have all become a very important area to address from a very firm scientific angle (Kuhn, 2008). In this context when we look at some of the bioactivities in foods and their potential, be it from vegetables or fruits, or from grains, all are trying to rediscover the functionality by addressing a number of health concerns from a food-based approach. When we look at this problem, it is also important from a basic and fundamental angle to look at the synergy of high science and high technology of how it could deliver nutritious foods which can make a difference at an affordable cost to the needy. It is not just the nutrition label but also the nutraceutical bioavailability and their functionality which is important. Therefore, the issue pertains to value addition to processed functional foods in such a way that the price difference that happens as a result of value addition should be in addition to the benefit that the consumer gets in terms of micro- and macronutrients along with nutraceuticals with a clear scientific validation of the claims and benefits of these functional foods along with the issues of food safety. One should also address the extent of food fortification as well as those novel ingredients using not only the traditional knowledgebase, but also some of the newer insights into peptides, functional carbohydrates, and other novel ingredients that can bring about a big change with their synergistic effect for better health and nutrition (Arvanitoyannis and Van Houwelingen-Koukaliaroglou, 2005).

The nutraceutical and functional food industry is a very vibrant industry today with the claims and clear mandate of health, wellness, and prevention of diseases as one of its main goals by using the present-day Knowledgebase cutting across various boundaries of science and technology. It has become a very important area with huge investments crossing over several billion dollars and has carved a niche with attractive propositions both for industrialists and manufacturers. The interest in nutraceuticals and functional foods are leveraged by market growth, market size, and of course customer-driven health agenda. Today, what a consumer really worries about is health and how the health care is managed, administered, and priced. Many a time, the nutraceutical and functional food informatics does emerge from traditional knowledgebase. The bioactive and nutritious ingredients in these foods and a combination of foods may open up new doors for Research & Development. One must partner and network with the knowledgebase around the world to leverage the nutraceutical information and merge into it the technology for benchmarking quality products for reaching out with clear validated claims and there is a huge potential in this area which needs to be explored fully and opportunities are unlimited (Prakash, 2008a,b).

2.1 TRADITIONAL MEDICINE AND FUNCTIONAL FOODS

India occupies a premier position in the use of herbal drugs. According to Narayana, "Ayurveda is understood to have been systematically documented in 1000 BC in the form of Charaka Samhita and Sushruta Samhita and later many other texts were added to it. While some of the texts have been lost, a number of them are available even today. Drugs and Cosmetics Act of India recognizes 57 such books, which collectively contain about 35,000 recipes and processes to make them" (Narayana, 2010, p. 245). In fact, India is one of the pioneers in the development and practice of the well-docu-mented indigenous systems of medicine the most notable being "Ayurveda" and "Unani." The *Materia Medica* of these systems contains a rich heritage of indigenous practices that have helped to sustain the health of rural people in India. India has a well-developed prosperous medicinal plant industry. Many recipes have been documented after several years of hard work and distilled knowl-edge in the traditional medicine with a focus on preventive and most of the times curative from a food-based approach (Valiathan, 2006). This is where the gut health and wellness have a very strong foothold in the area of nutraceuticals and functional foods with the platform of used knowledge with built-in evidence-based claims in many of the preparations (Patwardhan et al., 2004; Patwardhan, 2005; Mukherjee and Wahile, 2006; Vaidya, 2006; Vaidya and Devasagayam, 2007; Narayana, 2010).

Healthy functional foods play a significant role in the general health of infants, growing children, expectant mother, men, women, diabetics, and the aged. The right foods do have the power to prevent and have a rather soothing and healing effect keeping good health of body functions, aging, rejuve-nating, immuno-modulating, and prevention of many diseases. The environmental and dietary factors, that is, malnutrition and growing demand of nutraceuticals need tailoring practices through value addition to optimize the concentration and bioavailability of the desired food components, are some critical issues today. The present situation demands to screen the herbs, medicinal plants, unde-rutilized parts from herbal industries, agricultural waste for their phytonutrients/phytochemicals and nutraceuticals potential in order to identify the low-cost basic raw material and also development of processes for the preparation of custom-made herbal health protective nutraceuticals suitable for cottage, small scale, and or industrial-level production underpinning food safety. Nutraceutical/functional foods have the potential to be used as food supplements and, as growing evidence suggests, prevent aspects of certain diseases for well being. Certain biodynamic compounds or compound complexes derived from selected herbs and medicinal plants may have the ability to modulate the expression of gene(s) to achieve a desired positive effect or alleviation, and management of certain diseases. Serious efforts are needed in addressing the economically lower segment of the society to reach out nutraceuticals/functional foods for the eyes, liver, muscles, digestive system, skin, hypertension, as antioxidants, reduction of cholesterol, malnutrition issues of pregnant women, lactating mothers, growing children, and diabetics with specific attention for the optimal development of brain, growth and mental and functional abilities, and general health care of the society (Prakash, 2009).

2.2 ROLE OF TRADITIONAL FOODS AND FUNCTIONAL FOODS

The Food and Agricultural Organization of United Nations Report of 2004 (FAO Corporate Document Repository) of the Regional Expert Consultation of the Asia-Pacific network for Food and Nutrition on Functional Foods and their Implications in the Daily Diet (FAO, 2004) has defined that "It is vital that all traditional food be authentic, assure health, provide rich taste and has a background of mother/wife/husband in its originality especially when health claims are put on labels. It also has a charisma and is based on the availability of region-specific culinary practice and, of course, its acceptance depends on how hungry one is at the time of consuming the food! Food is regional, so also food technology as applied to traditional foods. When one looks at the three major aspects of factors that affect food selection and intake, it boils down to personal choice, economic factors, and social aspect. These things are related to physiological factors, additives, sensory properties, aroma, taste, texture, mood, beliefs, experience and, of course, the nutritional properties which also include the health aspects of foods. If one looks at the safety issues, one cannot forget the microbiology, the nutrition, the natural toxicants (if any present), the environmental contamination, the pesticide residue, the food additives, and food allergy" (FAO, 2004, p. 23). The author was a part of this FAO team in formulating the above guidelines and definitions.

There are several forces that shape health and nutritional formulations and its role in prevention of diseases as well as the well being of humans. The various parameters could be region-agri materials, the market forces, the economic imperatives, the financial policies, the human resource elements, the trade and economic complexities, and perhaps most importantly the cost-effectiveness and the local sustainability. When we look at such a complex socioeconomic pattern, the research and development in the national context reaches a higher pedestal by the network of government with people integrated with research and development on the one side and the market on the other, and in between the production units linking up the supply to the demand (Fogliano and Vitaglione, 2005).

The power of traditional food formulations for health is simply phenomenal but the question is, have we capitalized it fully? What about the health aspects of traditional foods, the marketing, and consumer preferences? Are we adapting the energy-saving processing equipments? Are we fully geared to the changing food laws? The treasure of informatics of Ethics and Traditional Foods (e.g., India and China along with other countries) need to be capitalized today, if we have to go in the right direction of processed foods with focus on nutrition with an emphasis on nutraceuticals. However scientific support to traditional documentation would support by reassuring the proven in this world of evidence-based documentation. Some examples that can be quoted in terms of the nutrition being forgotten which once upon a time perhaps was a symbol of health is *Rice Bran*. Since brown rice is no longer used frequently, we have lost a good quality protein in our diet in addition to edible dietary fiber, lecithin, oryzanol, vitamin E, and other phytosterols and of course a good percentage of rice bran oil. Another example is seaweed which makes a lot of difference in terms of its nutritional angle especially from the point of view of nutraceuticals where claims of its properties are enormous.

Therefore, the research trend in healthful foods today has linked up itself into preventive and perhaps curative aspects in terms of allergies, heart diseases, bone health, brain performance even eye health, gut health, as well as bone health. A personalized diet may someday be developed based on an individual's genetic code! This diet can then lessen the risk of certain diseases which that individual may be susceptible to. Studies focusing on the health benefits of ingredients may help pave the way for this new approach called nutrigenomics (Prakash, 2009).

In this context, the nutritional and processed food formulations play a very vital role and consumers are deeply concerned about how their health care is managed, administered, and priced. Many are frustrated with the expensive, high-tech, disease-treatment approach predominant in modern medicine. The consumer is seeking complementary or alternative beneficial products. Therefore it is time to address the functional foods and nutraceuticals from a different perspective. What do the terms functional foods and nutraceuticals mean in a larger sense? Why does this subject conjure up so much excitement for the future? Are we talking only about herbs and oils? Why are doctors and nutritionists looking at this area so intently? These are the very reasons why we should examine, explore, and study the topic. Consumers say that they strongly believe in the health-promoting benefits of functional foods. Much of this is due to a consumer base with long experience for a safe, high-quality food production in this country, as well as a trust in the pharmaceutical world, and a belief that medicine leads to improved health and quality of life. Consumers are adamant that we in the profession seek crucial links between diet and health. They are hungry to learn about foods that can help them live healthier and longer lives. Functional foods area of research includes the search for bioactive components that may through inclusion in the diet improve our health beyond what may typically be expected. These claims typically relate to structure–function relationships describing the effects on the body (Prakash, 2004).

2.3 INGREDIENTS AND FUNCTIONAL FOODS

Nutraceuticals are the focus on traditional food components of food that provide medical health benefits including the prevention and/or treatment of diseases. Functional foods provide specific benefits; medical foods are developed for use under medical supervision to treat or manage particular disease or nutritional deficiency. Nutraceuticals and functional foods are a hybrid of both the traditionally defined food and drug arenas. Food and health security are the fundamental requirements to ensure stability, security, and economic well being of the nation. It is the collective responsibility of individuals in general, and researchers and policy makers in particular to ensure the health and food and nutritional security in a nation (Prakash, 2009).

2.4 VALUE ADDITION AS A RESULT OF FUNCTIONAL FOODS

Value addition to foods which are tomorrow's need perhaps will be geared on through bioactive substances with a mandate of health and functional foods emerging toward well being and ultimately the nutritional aspects. Functional foods with bioactive substances especially with herbal formulations will perhaps dominate a large portion of that health food segment. When we talk about better knowledge of the impact of foods on health, perhaps we are looking at the beginning of functional foods. In a sense discovering that a particular compound is beneficial to the health is perhaps just the beginning of the development of marketable healthy foods. Of course, the substance must then be separated and put into a form in which it can be suitably protected and then released and absorbed once consumed with a clear mandate of safety. The new innovations in foods would include such innovative methods as encapsulation techniques for bioactive and ultimate incorporation into health-promoting foods (Herbert, 2004; Weiss et al., 2006). There are several kinds of foods that one sees in the market such as dietary supplements, medical foods, foods for special dietary uses, fortified or enriched foods, and functional foods. The addition of one or more essential nutrients to a food whether or not it is normally contained in the food for the purpose of preventing or correcting a demonstrated deficiency of one or more nutrients in the population or specific population groups is well documented (Weststrate et al., 2002; Prakash, 2004).

These are days of ohmics and biotechnology wherein genomics, proteomics, and toxicogenomics all become very important in terms of our understanding and reach out. The coming together of biotechnology and informatics is paying rich dividends. Genome projects, drug design, and molecular taxonomy are all becoming increasingly dependent on informatics. The scientific discipline that contributes to nutrigenomics as we march forward in the nutritional science and biotechnology perhaps is molecular medicine and pharmacogenomics. A blend of nutrigenomics and ethnic food composition will be a novel approach to offer nutritionally rich food and food products linking nutraceuticals with tradition. Such an approach may redefine a few model systems and the approach to be employed for the objectives defined. Also, the available information in ancient databases and various associated components needs to be digitized in order to understand global scenario on the subject in a comprehensive way and to identify targets for healthful foods firmly based on knowledge. The key element that distinguishes nutrigenomics from nutrition research is that the observable response to diet, or phenotype, is analyzed and/or compared in different individuals (or genotypes). Classical nutrition research essentially treats everyone as genetically identical, even while realizing that some individuals require more or less specific nutrients and the role of bioavailability of the nutrients (Kleerebezem, 2006; Prakash, 2009; Getz et al., 2010).

Therefore, ultimately the consumer is the key who determines what one wants and one's suggestion of course is given the basic importance for any product to reach the market and sustain. It is here that innovation stands as an excellent challenge and also the future depends upon such innovations (Ramesh Kumar and Prakash, 2005; Broring et al., 2006; Hsieh and Ofori, 2007). Today we need to look at a different ambience and atmosphere and we have to learn the new ways of thinking together with multi-institutional role and at the same time from the networking of such systems one can expect greater dividends than ever before. All this is possible provided the high science and technology is converted into adaptable technologies both in rural, semirural, and semi-urban to reach out to people who cannot afford a square meal but at the same time this reach out must ensure the cost-effectiveness of the product and at the same time respect the local and traditional habits of people for better food loaded with high nutrition and with the hygienic and safe food that can reach the needy. That is the true science of food technology as we march ahead with our knowledge in the area of functional foods.

2.5 NUTRACEUTICALS AND FUNCTIONAL FOODS

Screening and selection of underutilized plants, parts of herbs/medicinal plants for phytonutrients/phytochemicals, antioxidant activity, nutritional composition, and functional attributes will form the basis to develop custom-made health protective, promotive and disease-preventive nutraceuticals and functional food formulations with optimum nutrition, and specific functional attributes. Scientific validation and standardization of the formulations will provide safe, efficacious nutraceutical products of optimal quality. The present situation demands to screen, the herbs/medicinal plants, underutilized parts from herbal and spices in general and agricultural wastes and so on, for their phytonutrients/phytochemicals, antioxidant activity, unique nutritional composition, nutraceutical potential, and functional attributes to identify the low-cost basic raw material. The anticipated products include the development of nutraceutical/functional foods fortified with suitable phytonutrients/phytochemicals for cottage/small scale and/or large industrial level production focused clearly on food safety too in the chain. The nutraceuticals are capable of modulating the mechanism in which many nutrients are absorbed and delivered to the body better. The active ingredient(s) identified as phytonutrients/phytochemicals by screening could be incorporated into the food products for the prevention or treatment of particular disease or to improve the health condition. Nutraceuticals have potential as preventive medicine ultimately leading to a healthy society, and providing a mass gain in employment through cultivation, processing, and establishment of cottage, small- or large-scale industrial production in the entire food chain of tertiary value addition (Prakash, 2004).

2.6 HEALTH CLAIMS, FOOD CATEGORIES, AND FUNCTIONAL FOODS

For example the multiethnic population of Asia is known for diverse traditional and cultural practices and food habits. The forces that shape agri-business and food processing in Asian region are the indigenous raw material available for processing, the energy resources, socioeconomic status of nation as well as people. Increasing investments in food-processing sector and the purchasing power, the internal and export market outlets available, the fiscal policies, the skilled and unskilled human resource at the disposal of industry, trade and economic blocks, cost effectiveness, and local sustainability (Prakash, 2003). In the processed food sector, the emphasis is on the production of health foods with bioactive substances or better called as functional foods. Some terms commonly used in this context are (i) *Medical food*—a category of food for special dietary usage which are specially processed or formulated and presented for the dietary management of patients and may be used only under medical supervision, (ii) *Fortified or enriched foods*—the addition of one or more essential nutrients to a food whether or not it is normally contained in the food for the purpose of preventing or correcting a demonstrated deficiency of one or more nutrients in the population or specific population groups, (iii) *Nutraceuticals*—a food or parts of foods that provide medical health benefits including the prevention and/or treatment of diseases. Such products may range from isolated nutrients, dietary supplements and diets to genetically engineered designer foods, functional foods, herbal product, and processed foods such as cereals, soups, and beverages even though a strict definition always limits the application of nutraceuticals, and (iv) *Novel foods*—foods or food ingredients which have not hitherto been used for human consumption to a significant degree within the community (Prakash, 2003).

Functional foods can be designed to "eliminate" a component known or identified as causing deleterious effect to the consumer (e.g., an allergenic protein), to "*increase*" the concentration of a component naturally present in foods (for beneficial effect), to "add" a component which is not normally present in most foods (for beneficial effect), to "replace" a component, usually a macro- or micronutrient, the intake of which is usually excessive for which beneficial effects have been demonstrated. Some of the clinically proven relationships between specific nutrients/foods and health are calcium and osteoporosis, sodium and hypertension, dietary fat and cancer risk, dietary saturated fat and cholesterol and risk of coronary heart disease, beneficial effects of fiber-containing grain products, fruits and vegetables for cancer, soluble fiber, soy proteins, plant sterols, plant stenol esters for coronary heart disease, folate and neural tube defects, dietary sugar and dental caries, and so on. There are many more novel ones added to this category continuously such as bioactive peptides from milk, soy isoflavones, nuts, prunes, and so on and is a dynamic process (Prakash, 2003; Clydesdale, 2004; Ohama et al., 2006).

2.7 FOOD SAFETY ISSUES AND FUNCTIONAL FOODS

Food safety is another aspect of quality which cannot be ignored when development of new and traditional foods are targeted. The various aspects involved are mycotoxins, pesticide residue monitoring, food safety through biotechnological approach, food irradiation and its awareness, improved analytical techniques for detection of any deleterious components, GM food analysis, organic foods and the overall knowledge of food analysis, and of course recommendations from the *Codex alimentarious* as a guiding principle in bench-marking food safety parameters. Need for value addition to agro-based raw material through appropriate technology is a must in functional foods production. The need of the hour is to promote the establishment of agro-processing units in the producing areas to reduce wastage, increase value addition, and create farm employment in rural areas. Small-scale industries and women entrepreneurs can play a major role in sustainable rural technologies. Convergence of technologies and emergence of products and processes by interfacing and networking with other institutions in the nation are the need of the hour in the developing countries. This can be done with partnership and alliances between scientists, academia, industries, and entrepreneurs. A constant and continuous effort in training the trainers is also required for sustainability of the quality is more relevant at this juncture (Coppens et al., 2006; Prakash, 2008a,b; Prakash and van Boekel, 2010).

In conclusion, the current perspective of ethnopharmacology and drug discovery along with many of the disease management and role of Rasayana and herbs in traditional Indian medicine of Ayurveda and the role of reverse pharmacology and its importance of functional materials constituting the functional foods through functional ingredients and bioactive molecules and even demanding today's knowledge of nanotechnology is very critical. Functional food design and health and providing adequate scientific support for health claims have become important from the point of both regulatory and new innovations in functional foods. The point of safety and functionality relying upon clinically certifying health benefits on one side and epidemiologically documented food on the other has a very major role to play in today's efficacy trial and data of functional foods. The individual health through functional foods becomes a reflection of nation's health. Tradition, culture, and customs in a society have all played a major role in today's functional food products in the market.

The molecular advances and novel biotechnological innovations are pushing the functional foods into the realm of health and wellness orbit through nutridynamics and related framework on a firm food safety basis and the scientific fraternity must ensure greater responsibility for communication of risk, detailed risk assessment and analysis, and risk management. The public health and ethical issues and functional foods shall remain as a point of mainstream discussion as new science emerges with greater emphasis on bioinformatics, human intervention studies, bioavailability studies, *in vitro* and *in vivo* screening through biomarkers, and the functional food technology engulfing with consumer understanding will play a major role (Schroeder, 2007). Therefore, the evidence-based claims of nutraceuticals and ingredients will play a critical role in improving the success, opportunity, and challenges of functional foods for health and wellness through front-end innovations and convergence of food technology with medical fraternity and the role played by nutrigenomics in individual and public health will dominate the issue of the strength of functional foods which perhaps depends strongly in reverse pharmacological work in depth. A broader question also perhaps is "Which food is not a functional food"?

REFERENCES

Arvanitoyannis, I.S. and Van Houwelingen-Koukaliaroglou, M. 2005. Functional foods: A survey of health claims, pros and cons, and current legislation. *Critical Reviews in Food Science and Nutrition*, **45**, 385–404.

Broring, S., Cloutier, L.M., and Leker, J. 2006. The front end of innovation in an era of industry convergence: Evidence from nutraceuticals and functional foods. *R&D Management*, **36**, 487–498.

Coppens, P., Fernandes da Silva, M., and Pettman, S. 2006. European regulations on nutraceuticals, dietary supplements and functional foods: A framework based on safety. *Toxicology*, **221**, 59–74.

Clydesdale, F. 2004. Functional foods: Opportunities & challenges. *Food Technology*, **58**, 35–40.

Fogliano, V. and Vitaglione, P. 2005. Functional foods: Planning and development. *Molecular Nutrition & Food Research*, **49**, 256–262.

Getz, J, Adhikari, K., and Medeiros, D. 2010. Nutrigenomics and public health. *Food Technology*, **1**, 29–33.

Govindarajan, R., Vijayakumar, M., and Pushpangadan, P. 2005. Antioxidant approach to disease management and the role of "Rasayana" herbs of Ayurveda. *Journal of Ethnopharmacology*, **99**, 165–178.

Herbert, C.M. 2004. Innovation of a new product category—Functional foods. *Technovation*, **24**, 713–719.

Hsieh, Y. P. and Ofori, J.A. 2007. Innovations in food technology for health. *Asia Pacific Journal of Clinical Nutrition*, **16**(Suppl. 1), 65–73.

Kleerebezem, M. 2006. Molecular advances and novel directions in food biotechnology innovation. *Current Opinion in Biotechnology*, **17**, 179–182.

Kuhn, M.E. 2008. Making sense of health claim regulations. *Food Technology*, **6**, 70–73.

Mukherjee, P.K. and Wahile, A. 2006. Integrated approaches towards drug development from Ayurveda and other Indian system of medicines. *Journal of Ethnopharmacology*, **103**, 25–35.

Narayana, D.B.A. 2010. Reverse pharmacology for developing functional foods/herbal supplements; approaches, framework and case studies. In: *Functional Food Product Development* (Eds. J. Smith and E. Charter). Wiley-Blackwell, Oxford, UK. doi: 10.1002/9781444323351. Chapter 12, pp. 244–256.

Ohama, H, Ikeda, H., and Moriyama, H. 2006. Health foods and foods with health claims in Japan. *Toxicology*, **221**, 95–111.

Patwardhan, B. 2005. Ethnopharmacology and drug discovery. *Journal of Ethnopharmacology*, **100**, 50–52.

Patwardhan, B., Vaidya, A.D.B., and Chorghade, M. 2004. Ayurveda and natural products drug discovery. *Current Science*, **86**, 789–799.

Prakash, V. 2003. The role of nutraceuticals and quality food parameters for better nutrition and better health. *Proceedings of the IX Asian Congress of Nutrition, Nutrition Goals for Asia—Vision 2020*. Chapter 33. Nutrition Foundation of India, New Delhi, pp. 591–593.

Prakash, V. 2004. Report of the regional expert consultation of the Asia-Pacific network for food and nutrition on functional foods and their implications in the daily diet. *FAO Corporate Document Repository*. Food and Agriculture Organization of the United Nations regional Office for Asia and the Pacific, Bangkok, Thailand.

Prakash, V. 2004. Food technology, nutrition & health foods. *Prof. A.N. Bose Memorial lecture*. Association of Food Scientists and Technologists, India, Kolkata, India.

Prakash, V. 2008a. A new paradigm shift of food safety aspects in India. *The World of Food Science*. Vol. 5. (Global Developments in Food Standards and Regulations). IUFoST, Ontario, Canada-IFT, Chicago, IL, USA.

Prakash, V. 2008b. Nutraceuticals and functional foods—What the future holds? *Invited Lecture, 14th World Congress of Food Science and Technology*, International Union of Food Science and Technology (IUFoST), Shanghai, China.

Prakash, V. 2009. Nutrition, health and wellness—Ethnic & traditional foods. *Special Lecture, 19th International Congress of Nutrition (ICN 2009)*, Bangkok, Thailand.

Prakash, V. and van Boekel, M.A.J.S. 2010. Nutraceuticals: Possible future ingredients and food safety aspects. In: *Ensuring Global Food Safety* (Eds. C.E. Boisrobert, A. Stjepanovic, S. Oh, and Huub, L.M. Lelieveld). Academic Press, Oxford, pp. 333–338.

Ramesh Kumar, P. and Prakash, V. 2005. Value addition to agricultural resources—The IPR angle. *Journal of Intellectual Property Rights*, **10**, 434–440.

Schroeder, D. 2007. Public health, ethics, and functional foods. *Journal of Agricultural and Environmental Ethics*, **20**, 247–259.

Vaidya, A.D.B. 2006. Reverse pharmacological correlates of Ayurvedic drug actions. *Indian Journal of Pharmacology,* **38**, 311–315.

Vaidya, A.D.B. and Devasagayam, T.P.A. 2007. Current status of herbal drugs in India: An overview. *Journal of Clinical Biochemistry and Nutrition*, **41**, 1–11.

Valiathan, M.S. 2006. *Towards Ayurvedic Biology, a Decadal Vision Document*. Indian Academy of Sciences, Bangalore, India.

Weiss, J., Takhistov, P., and McClements, J. 2006. Functional materials in food nanotechnology. *Journal of Food Science*, **71**, R107–R116.

Weststrate, J.A., van Poppel, G., and Verschuren, P.M. 2002. Functional foods, trends and future. *British Journal of Nutrition*, **88** (Suppl. 2), S233–S235.

3 Developments and Innovations in Dietary Supplements and Functional Foods

M.L. Shankaranarayana, Jayant Deshpande, and Abhijit Bhattacharya

CONTENTS

Traditionally, food products have been developed for aroma, taste, texture, appearance, and convenience for the consumer. The development of products to specifically deliver a health benefit is relatively a new trend, and recognizes the growing acceptance of the supportive and protective role of diet in prevention of disease and treatment. This link has influenced in the recent years with the emergence of dietary supplements and functional foods. This change in motivation and innovative approach for dietary supplements and functional foods has moved in formulating foods for health benefits and gaining entry into new areas of understanding like high-quality products, specialized delivery systems for nutrients, high level of emphasis on safety and toxicological evaluation even though these nutrients may be from food and plant origin, evidence of absorption, impact on metabolism or on structure and function, and placing the consumption and communication of such nutrients within a framework of various local and international health regulations.

3.1 DEVELOPMENT OF TERMINOLOGY, DEFINITIONS, AND REGULATORY FRAMEWORK

Dietary supplements are designed for those who seek to compensate the essential nutrients that they lack due to poor daily diet, medical conditions, or eating habits. It is generally believed that dietary supplements help maintain a proper health balance. Dietary supplements also help our immune system. The stronger the immune system, the more resistant body can be against disease. By and large, dietary supplements are not intended to treat, diagnose, or cure and may be largely to reduce the risk of certain diseases and protection of health. The health claims have to be based on genuine scientific evidence which will help in the development and growth of dietary supplements and functional foods. Legislation in respect of the nutrient content and health to protect the consumer should not be considered as barriers of product development and economic growth, though certain difficulties are encountered in the initial stages. Evidence of health benefits of limited dietary supplements and functional foods is well established but there are many products with limited or no sufficient scientific evidence of health benefits, which needs to be strengthened. Thus dietary supplements have a great potential to benefit health, quality of life, healthy aging, and will significantly contribute to improved physical and mental fitness.

In most countries, the sale and promotion of foods and drugs are governed by government regulations. In some countries, the act is for both food and drugs, as in the Food and Drugs Act and Regulations in Canada or the Federal Food, Drug and Food, and Cosmetic Act in the United States. In other countries, there are separate acts for foods and drugs. In the United Kingdom, the foods are regulated by the Ministry of Agriculture, Fisheries and Food (MAFF), in conjunction with the Department of Health (DH) while drugs are regulated by the Medicines Control Agency (MCA).

A drug is a substance manufactured, sold, or prescribed for use in the diagnosis, treatment, mitigate or prevention of disease or restoring, correcting or modifying organic functions in man or animal. In the recent years, the existing definitions of food and drug are debated and questioned because of the better understanding of the role/function of foods and constituent of foods, natural products, herbal products, botanicals and dietary supplements in the promotion of health and reduce the risk or treat disease. There is a trend for consumer demand for health-promoting ingredients from foods/herbs as it is considered a safe and cost-effective alternative to drugs or other traditional therapies.

A dietary supplement also known as nutritional supplement or food supplement is a preparation intended to supplement the diet and provide nutrients such as vitamin, minerals, fibers, fatty acids, or amino acids that may be missing or may not be consumed in sufficient quantity in a person's diet. They are considered as foods, natural health products, or drugs also. Supplements containing vitamins and minerals are included as a category of food (*Codex Alimentarius*).

There are a number of terms used for natural products such as nutraceuticals, functional food, medical food, phytochemical/phytonutrient, herbal products, and botanicals. The term nutraceutical is derived from nutrition and pharmaceutical. It is described as any substance that may be considered a food or part of food that provides medical/health benefits, including the prevention and treatment of disease. Such products may range from isolated nutrients, dietary supplements and diets to herbal products. Functional foods are those that, by virtue of the presence of physiologically active food components, provide health benefits beyond basic nutrition. It is also a food fortified with added or concentrated ingredients to functional levels which improves health or performance (Health Canada).

Functional foods include enriched cereals, breads, sport drinks, bars, and fortified snack for prepared meals, baby foods, and many more. The potential functions of nutraceuticals/functional food ingredients are generally related to maintenance or improvement of health. In the United States, the terms functional foods and nutraceuticals have been used interchangeably. A clear demarcation is required between these products because they are sold and consumed as foods versus products where a particular component has been isolated from a food and is sold in the form of a tablet, capsule, powder, or other concentrated form. According to Health Protection Branch of Health Canada, "A functional food is similar in appearance to conventional foods, is consumed as part of a usual diet and has demonstrated physiological benefits and or reduces the risk of chronic disease beyond basic nutritional function." A nutraceutical is a product produced from foods but sold in pills, powders, and other medicinal forms not generally associated with food and demonstrated to have a physiological benefit or provides protection against chronic disease (Scott et al., 1996, Recommendations for defining functional foods, A discussion paper, Bureau of Nutritional Sciences, Food Directorate, Ottawa, Health Canada). Nutraceutical substances are found in plants, animals, and sometimes in microbes, example choline and phospholidylcholine. Nonfood sources of nutraceutical substances have been obtained from fermentation methods, for example amino acids and eicopentaenoic acid (EPA) by bacteria. There are several nutraceutical substances which are found in higher concentrations in specific foods such as lutein in spinach/kale; lycopene in tomato; catechins in green tea; isoflavone in soy bean; capsaicinoids in red pepper fruits; EPA and docosahexaenoic acid (DHA) in fish oil and many others. By their mechanism of action, nutraceuticals are classified under antioxidant, anti-inflammatory, osteoprotective, anticataract, anticarcinogenic, and so on.

There are foods specifically designed for nutrition-related disorders which consist of two types called medical foods and foods for special dietary use. Medical foods are specially formulated and processed to be consumed under the direction of a physician, intended for a specific dietary management of a patient who has limited or impaired capacity to ingest, digest, absorb, or metabolize ordinary foodstuffs. This food product has distinctive nutritional composition not available in normal diet meant for healthy people. The foods for special dietary use are formulated for specific purposes like food allergy and the nutrient composition is the same as for healthy people. Because of the very specific use, the medical foods are exempted from nutrition labeling requirements of Nutrition Labeling and Education Act of 1990 (NLEA) in the United States. However, under the regulations of FDA, the medical foods conform to stricter preparation and quality control as well as evaluation procedures as these products are intended for sick people (Department of Health and human Services, Food and Drug Administration, 1996).

A new dietary ingredient (NDI) means a dietary ingredient that was not marketed in the United States before 1994. Old dietary ingredient means a dietary ingredient that was marketed in the United States before October 1994. In case of NDI, premarketing notification is required. Dietary supplement with NDI can only reach the market after 75 days of notification procedure. In 1997, FDA published in Federal Register a final rule that established safety regulation.

Phytonutrients are plant food components other than macronutrients, vitamins, or minerals that have some scientific data supporting a health benefit for humans. Examples include antioxidants from lycopene from tomato, grape seed extract, and sterol esters from vegetable oil that can decrease moderately cholesterol level. Phytonutrients can be used as either dietary ingredient or as dietary supplement or food ingredients in functional foods, as long as they meet the appropriate regulatory requirements.

A glance of the market situation shows that there are many different types of products coming under the umbrella of natural products with health benefits causing confusion regarding what these products should be called, how they should be regulated, safety level, and the scientific strength of health claims. As dietary supplement's use becomes more widespread, there are growing concerns about safety which are receiving attention by health regulations. These issues have caused concerns for governments, industry, and the academics around the world, particularly in the developed countries, wherein there is greater consumer interest. It is important and necessary to understand the scenario of the situation in some of the key countries.

Food supplement means food stuffs. The purpose of which is to supplement the normal diet and which are concentrated sources of nutrients or other substances with a nutritional or physiological effect, alone or in combination, marketed in dose form namely capsules, tablets, pills, and other similar forms. The supplements may be used to correct nutritional deficiencies or maintain an adequate intake of certain nutrients. Since large intake doses of certain nutrients such as vitamins and minerals may be harmful, maximum levels are necessary to ensure safety in the use of food supplements. As a first stage in the European Union, there are specific rules pertaining to vitamins and minerals as ingredients in foodstuffs (EU Food Supplement Directive, 2002/46/EC, p. 6, *Off. J. Eur. Commun.*).

In the United States, a dietary supplement is defined under Dietary Supplement Health and Education Act, 1994 (DSHEA), as a product taken by the mouth intended to supplement the diet and contains any of the following dietary ingredients, a vitamin (except pyridoxine), a mineral, a herb (excluding Ma Huang/ephedrine, tobacco) or amino acid, a concentrate, metabolite, constituent extract, or combination of any of the above. In addition, it has to conform to the following: in the form pill, capsule, tablet, powder or liquid form; not as a replacement for a conventional food, or as a sole item of meal/diet. Dietary supplements are placed in a special category under the general umbrella of foods and not drugs and labeled as dietary supplements.

The DSHEA distinguishes dietary supplements from both foods and drugs and provides separate regulations for these preparations and products. Whereas the health claims permitted for nutrients have to be in accordance with approved wordings/statement, regulations for supplements are less rigid in terms of wording but with no relationship to a disease. Most of the countries, other than the United States, have not created a special category for dietary supplements and further there are considerable differences in the regulatory aspects. The FDA regulates dietary supplements as a category of foods and not as drugs. The level of scientific information available among the various dietary ingredients varies markedly. This is because for many dietary supplements/ingredients the chemistry and physiology, preclinical, clinical information, and mechanism of action are well known. For others, by contrast, much of information is missing. The content and concentration preparation of some commercial products is of high quality and follows good agricultural, laboratory, and manufacturing practices. Again by contrast, the preparations may not be reliable making them subject to high variability in the content of the active ingredients. In 2007, the FDA has implemented a current Good Manufacturing Practices (CGMP) policy to ensure dietary supplements are produced in strict quality conditions, free of contaminants/impurities, and are labeled accurately following high standards of manufacturing, packaging, storage, quality control, plants/facility, testing, record keeping, and satisfying the customers, complaints (US FDA, 2007, Dietary Supplements Final Rule). Further, manufacturers are required to evaluate the identity, purity, strength, and composition of the dietary supplements.

The information such as ingredients and claims such as nutrient content, structure/function, and health relationship are provided on the label of food/dietary supplements. Manufacturers are solely responsible for the claims which should be truthful and not misleading. Nutrient information is compulsory in many countries such as in the United States and others. Nutrient content claims on the package indicate the content of a particular nutrient that the manufacturer wants to promote for health reasons, though there may be no connection with health. The examples are low fat, high fiber, cholesterol-free, and others. Consumers need a prior knowledge of the necessity of why they should buy a product with low fat or high fiber.

A health claim has two components, namely, a substance (food/dietary supplement/food component/dietary ingredient) and a disease or health-related condition. Health claims describe a relationship between a dietary supplement/ingredient and reducing the risk of a disease or health-related condition. To secure a health claim, clinical evidence substantiating the relationship to FDA's satisfaction must be presented to the agency as part of a formal petition process. Currently, health claims are subject to an evidence-based ranking system (A = highest; D = lowest). Unqualified health claims are those with clinical substantiation that meets FDA's significant scientific agreement standard and are awarded the highest ranking "A." Qualified health claims are those that have less substantiating data than required by significant scientific agreement and they are ranked from "B" to "D." Rank "D" indicates the FDA conclusion that there is little scientific evidence to support the claim. There are three ways of making claims on the label or in labeling a dietary supplement:

1. Nutrition Labeling and Education Act 1990 (NLEA) and DSHEA (1994) provide for FDA to issue regulations authorizing health claims for foods and dietary supplements, after FDA's careful review of the scientific evidence submitted. NLEA permits the use of label claims that characterizes the level of structure/function claim. This claim describes that a dietary supplement/nutrient plays a role in a particular biological process. Examples of such claims are: high fiber maintains bowel regularity; calcium builds strong bones; iron is important for the functioning of red blood cells. These are not preapproved by FDA, therefore a disclaimer on the label is required stating not evaluated by FDA and also the product not intended to diagnose, treat, cure, or prevent any disease.
2. Food and Drug Administration Modernization Act, 1997 (FDAMA) provides for health claims based on authoritative statement of a scientific body of the US government/National Academy Sciences. Dietary supplements are not included in this category.
3. Structure—function claims are used for dietary supplements and rarely for food products. Most structure—function claims describe the role that a nutrient or dietary ingredient has on the structure or function of the body, for example, calcium builds strong bones. Although no formal approval is required from FDA, there is an indication that they will accept.

Generally, health claims may relate to components of foods or foods themselves. We can recognize three types of claims:

1. Generic health claims are related to a nutrient(s), in the context of a total diet, to a specific disease or condition. As earlier mentioned, diets low in saturated fat and cholesterol and rich in fruits, vegetable, and grain products containing particularly soluble fiber may reduce the risk of cardiovascular disease. The claim is specific and related to the nutrients and not to the product. The basis of the claim is dependent on the adequate scientific evidence furnished demonstrating the beneficial effect of the nutrient in the prevention or treatment of the disease condition.
2. Commodity/ingredient health claims are related to specific ingredient/commodities present in a product such as diets high in oat bran/oatmeal and low in saturated fat and cholesterol may reduce the risk of heart disease. Similar to the generic claims, the basis of permitting such claims is dependent on the sufficient scientific data supporting the beneficial effect of the commodity/ingredient in the prevention or treatment of the disease condition (Department of Health and Human Services, FDA, 1997).
3. Product-specific claim describes that the individual product bearing the claim has a protective effect against a disease, that it either reduces the risk of the occurring or its useful in treating or reducing the symptoms of a preexisting condition. Extensive studies such as experimental, observational/epidemiological, human interventional, and proper evaluation are required. Approved qualified health claims are available subject to enforced discretion. The examples are fish oil to improve brain, green tea and tomato for cancer risk, cranberry juice for urinary tract health maintenance. The average consumer is unlikely to understand the distinction between using the product for preventing and using it to treat an infection (not much supporting evidence). This requires the product to be evaluated in accordance as per the guidelines adopted for drugs. However, product-specific health claims for foods are not allowed in the United States. Due to this, qualified claims are open to be used by

companies manufacturing similar products though there is variation in the bioactive content in the product.

The health claims permitted under NLEA for foods in the United States are essentially generic and product-specific. Presently, functional foods also have to be regulated under these guidelines. Dietary supplements cannot be declared to be protective against or treat a disease. Any purified products for which a relationship of disease is mentioned in a claim are considered drugs. Addition of new products is filling the pipeline worldwide to respond to the challenges of the dynamic nutraceutical market.

A prudent vision is to bring potential products that have excellent and proven performance of reducing the important risk factors so as to improve and benefit human health.

The U.S. office of dietary supplements has a 5-year mission program with a focus on objectives such as

1. Providing intellectual leadership in the role of dietary supplements in promoting health and reducing the risk of disease
2. Funding new research and training to expand the general knowledge on dietary supplements
3. Supporting the development of research tools for the study of dietary supplements
4. Compiling and updating scientific knowledge and information available from research publications (Shane Starling, Nutrition Ingredients—usa.com, Office of Dietary Supplements, Outlines of 5 year Plan)

In Japan, in addition to regular food, there is a category called "Foods for Special Dietary Use (FOSHU)" which refers to foods that are approved/permitted for specific groups. In this are included formulas for pregnant women, infant formulas, elderly people with difficulty in masticating/swallowing, medical foods for sick, and foods with health claims. Another category for foods with health claims, that is, "Foods with Nutrient Functions Claims (FNFC)" deals with 12 vitamins and 5 minerals specified by Ministry of Health, Labor, and Welfare (MHLW). The other category of foods with health claims is defined as "Foods for Specified Health Use (FOSHU)" under the same ministry.

FOSHU refers to foods containing ingredient with functions for health and officially approved to claim its physiological effect on the human body. FOSHU is intended to be consumed for the maintenance/promotion of health or special health uses by people who wish to control health condition, including blood pressure, blood cholesterol. In order to sell a food as FOSHU, the assessment for the safety of the food and effective functions for health is required and the claim must be approved by MHLW. This legislation/regulation came into effect in 1991 and the FOSHU market started from 1994. New FOSHU started capsules and pills approved in 2001 and new FOSHU category created in 2005. So far, 600 products have been approved. The ministry has an organized approval system which involves academics and the Health and Nutrition Research Laboratory. The food has to satisfy the criteria such as

1. Improvement of dietary habits and enhancement of health.
2. Health benefits of the food/ingredients should have clear medical and nutritional functions.
3. Defined amounts of food/its constituents should be indicated.
4. Food and its constituents should be proven safe.
5. Test methods for the physicochemical properties, the qualitative and quantitative determination of the constituents should be well defined.
6. The nutritional composition of the product should be closer to the similar foods.
7. The food is meant for daily use and not occasionally.
8. The product should be like an ordinary food and not as capsules, pill, powder, or liquid concentrate.

After approval, the health benefits may be stated on the label without any exaggeration. The label will have both nutrition facts and health claims.

Foods with nutrients such as vitamins and minerals will have labels indicating nutrient function claims specified by MHLW, conforming to standards and specifications, recommended daily intake within the specification range, nutrient formulation and warning, if any, like excess neither cures nor promotes health. The vitamins included are vitamins A, B1, B2, B6, B12, C, D, E, niacin, biotin, pantothenic acid, and folic acid; minerals such as calcium, copper, iron, magnesium, and zinc.

The approved FOSHU foods deal with specific health issues such as gastrointestinal condition, blood pressure, blood cholesterol, blood sugar, dental health and hygiene, mineral absorption, bone health, and accumulation of body fat. The product contains the relevant ingredient exhibiting the required specific health function and the approved health claim is declared on the label. Examples of claim help to maintain good gastrointestinal condition, maintain blood pressure at normal level, maintain cholesterol at normal level, and keep blood glucose level normal, maintain strong and healthy teeth, promote absorption of calcium/iron, maintain bone health, and help in reducing the body fat accumulation.

In addition to regular FOSHU, there are three types of FOSHU: (1) qualified FOSHU wherein food with health function not sufficiently substantiated with scientific evidence or meeting the level of FOSHU, (2) standardized FOSHU which has established standards and specifications with sufficient FOSHU after accumulation of scientific evidence, and (3) reduction of disease risk FOSHU, example, proper amount of calcium helps young women reduce the risk of osteoporosis. Reduction of risk claim is permitted with nutritional and clinical data provided for the ingredient. Food items approved in Japan are eligible to display FOSHU label after establishing the presence of physiologically active components that are stable in food materials and have been preserved using standard scientific procedures including human trials to be effective against specific diseases as hypertension, allergy, and raised blood cholesterol.

During the initial period of formation of European Community, the entire field of nutraceuticals and functional foods was fragmented and each member country having its own direction. The research studies of functional ingredients started showing promising prospects for the use of such ingredients in food products, resulted in value addition to manufacturers and benefits to consumer health. In 2002, a General Food Law called Regulation (EC) No. 178/2002 laid down the general principles and requirements of food law and created an independent Food Authority (European Food Safety Authority) endowed with the task of giving scientific advice on issues based on risk analysis comprising of scientific risk assessment, risk management, and risk communication. The law prohibits the attribution to a food the property of preventing, treating, or curing a human disease or any reference to such properties.

European food law recognized five framework directives: food labeling, food additives, materials in contact with food, official control on foodstuffs, and foods for particular nutritional uses (PARNUTS). These framework directives formed the basis for a later harmonized system of food law. Under EC Regulation (no. 178/2002), food or foodstuff as meaning any substance or product processed or unprocessed intended for ingestion by humans. Herbs could be regulated as dietary supplements or foodstuffs. As the regulation applies to all foodstuffs, its general principles also covers foods with added functional properties such as food supplements which include functional foods, nutraceuticals, and dietetic foods/dietary foods. Food supplements are foodstuffs. The purpose of which is to supplement the normal diet and which are concentrated sources of nutrients or other substances with a nutritional or physiological effect, alone or in combination, marketed in dose form like capsules, tablets, and in liquid or similar form. The approaches on foods with health effects were on two lines: (1) foods for particular nutritional uses (PARNUTS) and (2) functional foods, referred as Functional Food Science in Europe, a concept initiated and supported by International Life Science Institute (ILSI) Europe. PARNUTS or dietetic foods are specially manufactured products intended to satisfy the particular nutritional requirements of specific groups of people with disturbed metabolism or physiological conditions. These are baby foods, foods for people suffering from gluten or lactose-intolerance, foods for special medical purposes. The object of functional food science in Europe was to provide opportunity for functional foods to improve its industrial competitiveness in the context of a growing world market and to help establishing a multidisciplinary discussion forum for the growth of this industry.

The European community has established harmonized rules to help ensure that food supplements are safe and properly labeled. In the European Union, food supplements are regulated as foods and in the first instance the focus is on vitamins and minerals as ingredients of food supplements and later extended to other active substances commonly used in supplements such as amino acids, fatty acids, and plant extracts. Food supplements containing vitamins and minerals have to conform to the regulation regarding the upper tolerable safe intake levels of vitamins and minerals. It must be noted that the legislation does not consider functional foods or nutraceuticals as specific food categories.

Presently, the nutritional substances that can be added are controlled through positive lists included in the five directives and one regulation. Directives 2001/15/EC and 2009/39/EC permit the use of substances for specific nutritional purposes in foodstuffs, and dietetic foods/special medical purposes. The lists include the nutrients such as vitamins, mineral substances, and other nitrogen-containing compounds such as choline and inositol. The Directives 2002/46/EC and Regulation EC1925/2006 permit the use of vitamins, minerals, and other substances to foods and food supplements. Directives 2006/141/EC, 2006/125/EC, and Regulation EC 1925/2006 permit the use of various nutritional substances and certain substances to infant formula, processed cereal-based foods, baby foods for infants, and young children aged up to 3 years (European Commission Administrative Guidance on Submission for Safety Evaluation of Substances Added for Special Nutritional Purposes in the Manufacture of Foods, September, 2009, Food Law, Nutrition and Labeling Unit). A technical dossier is required to be prepared according to the guidelines and procedure to the European Commission, Brussels, Belgium for approval.

European Regulation on nutrition and health claims has come into effect from July 2007. This has created numerous complex challenges and issues regarding scientific, regulatory, and consumer aspects which remain to be solved. The new regulations of nutritional and health claims are expected to bring value and clarity to the European functional foods market. There are many companies already manufacturing and marketing functional foods using health-related claims for years. This has caused some temporary problems. The legislation is modular with basic framework and adequate provision to fill the gaps in the coming years.

The scope of regulation is broad covering labeling, presentation, and advertising of the foodstuffs. A nutrition claim suggests that a food has particular beneficial nutritional properties, for example: low fat and high fiber. It may indicate the energy value of a food and the information on other nutrients such as protein, carbohydrates, fat, fiber, sodium vitamins, and minerals. It is mentioned that the data of the nutrients alone do not constitute a nutrition claim. The claim should be substantiated by scientific evidence. Further, the foods bearing nutrition and health claims must also meet certain nutritional requirements also called nutrient profiles which will be prepared by a panel of experts under the guidance of European Food Safety Authority. Nutrient profile is a complex and highly debated issue and is included in the interest of the consumers. The profile will help the consumers in the diet choice and ensuring benefit to those who utilize the claims to good health. The main purpose is to prevent the nutritional health claim on foods of unhealthy composition.

Health claims are defined as any claim that suggests or implies that a relationship exists between a food category, a food, or one of its constituents and health in accordance with Article 13(1) health claims. The regulation makes scientific data compulsory for health claims on food products. There are two types of health claims relevant to functional foods:

1. Enhanced functional claims referring to specific physiological, psychological functions, and biological activity beyond their established role in growth, development, and other normal functions of the body

2. Reduction of disease risk that relate to consumption of a food/food component that might help reduce the risk of a specific disease or condition due to specific nutrients or nonnutrients contained within, for example sufficient calcium intake may help to reduce the risk of osteoporosis in later years

In the process of establishing a health claim, a collaborative and concerted approach of a team consisting of researchers, industry representatives, and regulators is required to work together for assessing and evaluation of the scientific basis of the claim. EFSA tasks include

1. Drawing up a positive list of many well-established general functional health claims
2. Giving opinion on individual applications for health claims, new functional health claims for a specific food
3. Evaluation of claims regarding risk reduction and child development
4. Providing guidance on preparation of applications for the authorization of health claims
5. Giving scientific advice on nutrient profiles

EFSA has guidelines on how applicants can submit health claims. EFSA is responsible for verifying the scientific substantiation of claims through a standing committee. The list of permitted health claims shall be based on generally accepted science evidence. The data should demonstrate the claimed effect beneficial for human health and further cause and effect relationship between consumption of the food item and claimed effect. The experimental study should have all details such as dose response, good clinical trials, multicentral studies, qualified, trained and professional team, specificity, biological role, quantity required for consumption versus claimed effect. In addition, the beneficial effect has to be demonstrated being relevant for health both from nutrition and physiologic function. The wording used to make health claim should be truthful, clear, reliable, and useful to the consumer in choosing a healthy diet. In spite of all this, there appears to be some confusion over what exactly is needed in the way of scientific data to support claims. Probably, they are not sure what evidence is required and how much is enough. The claims on foods labeling presentation or marketing in the EU are clear, accurate, and based on the evidence accepted by the whole scientific community. EFSA has published in their final list 4637 General function health claims after consolidation process of examination of 44,000 claims submitted from member states.

3.2 DEVELOPMENTS IN THE FIELD OF NUTRITIONAL SUPPLEMENTATION INGREDIENTS

3.2.1 Vitamins

Vitamins are essential micronutrients for life and well-being of man. Vitamins are differentiated from the essential organic macronutrients, namely, proteins, carbohydrates, and fats by quantities required, individual vitamins required in the range of several micrograms to nearly 100 mg. Normally they are ingested by man as constituents of foods. There are special situations like pregnancy and lactation, infections, postsurgery periods, and other medical conditions during which time vitamin intake may have to be increased. Vitamin D is synthesized in skin of man and animals under the influence of ultraviolet light. On occasions where foods do not supply sufficient vitamin intake, dietary supplements, or pharmaceutical preparations may provide the need. Vitamin deficiencies have been a major cause of diseases such as blindness, rickets, decreased clotting, beriberi, pellagra, nervous disorders, dermatitis, anemia, scurvy, and others. Administration of vitamins in the advanced deficiency conditions will usually reverse the most of the clinical changes with an exception. An example of adequate amounts of vitamin A will not reverse the pathological state of blindness in man because the clinical signs are the end result of the deficiency. With vitamin A, 11-*cis*-retinal is the active compound in vision. Vitamin E functions as a biological antioxidant, and maintains stability and integrity of biological membranes. Vitamin K is required for the synthesis of four blood proteins in the coagulation system.

Vitamins may be classified into two groups: (1) fat soluble represented by vitamins A (retinol), D (calciferol), E (α-tocopherol), and K (phylloquinone) and (2) water soluble which includes thiamin (B1), riboflavin (B2), pyridoxine (B6), cobalamin (B12), niacin (nicotinic acid), pantothenate (pantothenic acid), folate/folacin (folic acid), and vitamin C (ascorbic acid). Excess intake of water-soluble vitamins beyond the body's ability to absorb them is generally excreted. Excess dosage of vitamin A and D can lead to storage with some undesirable effects which result not from food sources but from self-medication of vitamin concentrates. The evolution of man's food supply can be seen as occurring in three developmental periods: (1) natural/whole food, (2) processed and refined food, and (3) convenience (ready to eat) and fabricated food. The various processing steps destroy or remove certain vitamins and therefore there is a need for addition of vitamins in selected foods, vitamin C in fruit beverages, vitamins A and D in milk and fats.

Vitamin A is the isoprenoid polyene alcohol also called retinol or axerophthol. Retinol complexed with a protein (retinol-binding protein) is the principal form of transport of the vitamin in blood from the liver. Retinol esters, vitamin A palmitate, or acetate in all-trans isomeric form are manufactured by chemical synthesis and these are usually used in food applications. Vitamin A in the human diet is derived from preformed vitamin A (retinol) and from provitamin A carotenoids which vary in content in natural foods. The better sources are butter, egg, fish oil, and so on. Biosynthesis of vitamin A from the carotenoid vitamin A precursors such as β-carotene takes place mainly in the intestinal mucosa first forming retinal and then retinol transported to liver for storage. The metabolism of vitamin A is quite clearly understood as it is related to vision. Vitamin A plays an important role in the growth, synthesis of glycoproteins, and maintenance of mucus-secreting cells of epithelia. Deficiency symptoms of the vitamin lead to xerophthalmia and night blindness. Depletion of carrier protein and the resultant poor transport of vitamin may lead to hypovitaminosis. Long period daily intake of high levels of excess vitamin A can cause head ache, nausea, and in more severe conditions joint pain and loss of hair. The term retinol is used and 1 retinol equivalent = 1 μg retinol = 6 μg β-carotene = 10 IU vitamin A activity from β-carotene = 3.33 IU vitamin A activity. Vitamin A has been successfully added to several dairy-based food products.

Vitamin D is fat soluble and occurs in two forms D2 (calciferol) and D3 (cholecalciferol). These are formed from the irradiation process of appropriate sterol followed by purification steps. Vitamin D3 is biologically active and it is produced in human skin by exposing the body to direct sunlight. Vitamin D3 could be considered also as hormone. It is converted into more polar metabolites before it could function. The first metabolite is 25-OH-cholecalciferol (25-OH-D3) produced in liver and it is later converted in kidney to form 1,25 $(OH)_2$ D3 (calcitriol) which is metabolically active and stimulates intestinal calcium transport and bone calcium mobilization. The importance of vitamin D3 in human nutrition resides in its role as a regulator of the metabolism of calcium and phosphate. The 25-OH-cholecalciferol is the main circulating form of the vitamin and measures of its level in blood are used as a biochemical indicator of vitamin D status.

The principal use of vitamin D is in the prophylaxis and treatment of disorders of calcium–phosphorus metabolism. Acute deficiency of vitamin D leads to a condition called as rickets in children and osteomalacia in adult. Prolonged vitamin D deficiency and the compensatory increase in parathyroid hormone which releases calcium from bone to maintain to blood levels may be a possible etiological factor in the genesis of osteoporosis. Senile osteoporosis may be due to lack of vitamin D and therefore elderly persons should continue to take an adequate intake. Intake of higher amounts than recommended can cause calcification of soft tissues, kidney, arteries, and other organs. Most of the pasteurized fluid milk, cereal products, margarine, and so on are nitrified with vitamin D.

Vitamin E is a generic name for a series of lipid-soluble tocol and trienol compounds of which α-tocopherol is of major importance. There are four forms of tocopherol: alpha, beta, gamma, and delta formed from tocol structure bearing a saturated isoprenoid C16-side chain and similarly four forms of tocotrienol: alpha, beta, gamma, and delta formed from trienol structure bearing three double bonds in the C16-side chain. There are three methyl groups in 5,7, and 8 in alpha, two methyl groups in 5 and 8 position in beta, two methyl groups in 5,8 position in gamma, and one methyl group in delta both in tocopherols and tocotrienols. Vitamin E is an essential nutrient not synthesized in human body and the source is from plant foods, particularly vegetable oils. Vitamin E is a natural oxidant which helps to prevent the oxidation of polyunsaturated fatty acid residues in membrane phospholipids by oxygen-free radicals. The absorption of vitamin E is similar to other fat-soluble vitamins linked to fat absorption and facilitated by the presence of bile salts. The α-tocopherol is associated mainly with low-density lipoproteins (LDLs). Oral administration of iron interferes with intestinal absorption of vitamin E. α-Tocopherol supplementation helps in better absorption of fat, needed in special cases. Vitamin E protects against atherosclerosis by preventing the oxidation of LDL. Tocopherols are viscous, pale yellow liquids freely soluble in vegetable oils. In the presence of iron salts, they undergo oxidation forming quinines. Tocopherols have been used as antioxidant in stability studies of vegetable oils and processed foods.

Vitamin K consists of three compounds related to 2-methyl-1,4-naphthoquinone called vitamin K1 (phylloquinone), K2 (menaquinone-4/6/7), and K3 (menadione). Natural dietary vitamin K1 is of plant origin and vitamins K2 produced in the intestinal bacteria contribute to total vitamin K intake. The two water-soluble synthetic forms of vitamin K are menadione (K3) and menadiol (K4), which are used as dietary ingredients in multiple supplements. There is evidence suggesting that vitamin K plays an important role in bone metabolism and that perhaps vitamin K insufficiency may be a contributory factor in osteoporosis (Ball, 2004). Vitamin K deficiency is rare and is indispensable for the function of the blood coagulation system. Vitamin K is required for the synthesis of four blood clotting proteins, namely prothrombin.

Thiamin (vitamin B1) is one of the vitamins of so-called B complex comprising of two other essentials such as B2 (riboflavin) and B3 (niacin). Thiamin is a complex organic molecule containing a pyrimidine and a thiazole nucleus joined by a methylene bridge. One of the main functions of thiamin is energy metabolism of carbohydrate. Thiamin in the form of its pyrophosphate ester (cocarboxylase) participates in the normal metabolic process. It is essential for life and is present in almost all living cells. It is present as in free form as mono-, di-, and triphosphoric esters. Thiamin deficiency causes beriberi, which results in disorders in the function of the organs and tissues involved in the metabolism of carbohydrates, nervous system, the heart, the liver, gastrointestinal tract, and muscle tissue. Further, the deficiency can also lead to depression and failure to concentrate. Thiamin is found in whole grain cereals, nuts, and nut products. Thiamin is rapidly and actively absorbed from the small intestine and transformed by phosphorylation within the body into active coenzyme thiamin pyrophosphate (cocarboxylase). Riboflavin is eliminated in the urine.

Vitamin B2 (Riboflavin) is a yellow–orange pigment containing an isoalloxazine nucleus and a ribose side chain. Riboflavin occurs in a free state but most usually in the form of a di-nucleotide or a phosphate ester. It may be bound to a protein. It is widely distributed in foods with dairy products, meat, fish, egg, and green vegetables being good dietary sources. Prolonged exposure to light destroys riboflavin. If high doses of riboflavin are consumed, it is excreted unchanged in urine. At low intakes, riboflavin is efficiently absorbed but this active absorption process has a limitation in capacity. Generally, supplements may provide 3 mg/day.

Vitamin B3 (niacin, niacinamide) is also called antipellagra vitamin and is pyridine-3-carboxylic acid. It is both an amine/amide and a carboxylic acid. Niacin is used in food supplements while niacinamide in pharmaceutical preparations. Pellagra occurs in maize-eating populations. Maize contains niacin in bound form and hence not available. Niacin and niacinamide are found in foods in combined forms as nicotinamide adenine dinucleotide (NAD) and nicotinamide adenine dinucleotide phosphate (NADP). Niacin can be obtained from the diet or it can be synthesized in the body from tryptophan present in dietary protein. The symptoms of pellagra are coarse skin with lesions turning dark color in the body. In acute cases, the disease leads to dermatitis, diarrhea, dementia, and death. Many multivitamin preparations contain up to 100 mg/day.

Vitamin B5 (pantothenic acid, pantothenate) is a precursor of coenzyme A and also an anti-gray factor. Though there are no established requirements reported, the safe intake level dosage is 3–7 mg/day. Free pantothenic acid is unstable and hence calcium pantothenate is in practical applications.

Vitamin B6 (pyridoxine) is a generic term covering three biologically active substances such as pyridoxine, pyridoxal, and pyridoxamine (alcohol, aldehyde, and amine) as well as their phosphorylated derivatives. It is an essential nutrient and necessary component in the diet of man. Vitamin B6 occurs in milk in the form pyridoxal or pyridoxamine. Pyridoxine is present in many food supplements and multivitamin preparations, generally containing doses of up to 10 mg/day. These are readily absorbed from the intestinal tract and are rapidly metabolized.

Vitamin H (biotin), a mono-carboxylic acid containing cyclic urea with sulfurs, is dextro-rotatory and plays an important role in fatty acid synthesis. It is present in good amounts in whole grain, egg yolk, and so on. Biotin deficiency causes dermatitis. Biotin therapy is an accepted treatment for genital defects in biotin-associated enzymes and it appears to be helpful in the treatment of brittle nails and abnormal glucose tolerance. Biotin is a cofactor of several carboxylase enzymes which are associated with gluconeogenesis and fatty acid synthesis.

Vitamin C (L-ascorbic acid) is important in human nutrition and its deficiency causes scurvy causing general damage of connective tissue, bleeding gums, and loose teeth. Vitamin C occurs as ascorbic acid and its reversibly oxidized form dehydroascorbic acid, both of which are biologically active in all living tissues. Vitamin C is present in fruits and vegetables. It is an antioxidant and helps to protect tissues from damaging effects of free radicals. Vitamin C acts cofactor in the synthesis of carnitine and the synthesis of several nerve transmitters, peptide hormones, and noradrenaline. The presence of vitamin C in gut increases the non-hemeiron. Ingested ascorbic acid is readily absorbed from the intestinal tract.

Ascorbic acid is important in the metabolism of amino acids, particularly in the oxidation of phenylalanine and tyrosine. The intake of vitamin C supplement may vary from 65 mg to 500 mg/day.

Folic acid (folate, folacin) was referred as antianemia factor and the term folate covers several derivatives of the parent folic acid (pteroylmonoglutamic), a pteridine linked to p-aminobenzoic acid and glutamic acid. The name folacin is most widely used and it is present in many natural foods. Women who are pregnant or planning a pregnancy are advised to take supplemental dose of folic acid which helps in reducing the risk of the baby developing a neural tube defect. The defect covers several developmental defects in which the brain, spinal cord, skull, and vertebral column fail to develop normally. The deficiency of folacin may be due to reduced dietary levels, impaired absorption, and interference with sulfonamides or antibiotics. The average intake of folate from food may vary and generally around 200 µg/day.

Vitamin B12 (cobalamin, cyanocobalamin) is comprised of several, complex cobalt-containing compounds. The vitamin is foods in all foods of animal origin. The occurrence of vitamin B12 in nature is primarily the result of microbial synthesis. The inorganic element cobalt must be present for the microorganism to synthesize vitamin B12. Five forms of vitamin B12 have been observed in foods, namely, adenosylcobalamin, hydroxocobalamin, methylcobalamin, cyanocobalamin, and sulfitocobalamin. The absorption of vitamin B12 from the gastrointestinal tract is dependent on constituent of gastric juice called intrinsic factor. The intrinsic factor interacts with vitamin B12 in the presence of calcium ions and protects it during the transit to the ileum where absorption of vitamin B12 takes place. The vast majority of cases of vitamin B12 deficiency is due to its inadequate absorption from the gastrointestinal tract resulting from a breakdown in the complicated absorption. Vitamin B12 treatment is specifically for Addisonian pernicious anemia. Prolonged B12 deficiency causes irreversible damage to the spinal cord. Boiling milk with tea depletes Vitamin B12. The synthetic form cyanocobalamin is widely used in vitamin supplements.

3.2.2 MINERALS

The term mineral or mineral nutrient refers to those elements other than carbon, hydrogen, oxygen, sulfur, and nitrogen which are present in foods and in the diet.

Minerals may be classified into two groups depending on the level required in the diet:

1. The macro or major elements which are required at 100 mg or more—these include calcium, phosphorus, magnesium, sodium, potassium, and chloride.
2. The micro or trace elements which are required at less than a few milligrams and particularly chromium, iodine, molybdenum, and selenium in micrograms per day. The trace elements include iron, zinc, copper, iodine, manganese, chromium, cobalt, molybdenum, selenium, boron, and others.

Definitive effects from deficiencies of the macroelements and trace elements iron, copper, zinc, copper, iodine, manganese, chromium, and cobalt have been demonstrated in humans.

Minerals in general serve a wide range of physiological functions: as structural components of bone and other tissues, as enzyme cofactors, in maintenance of ionic strength composition of body fluids, as components of biologically active molecules, and as necessary constituents of metalloprotein.

Calcium is required for formation of bone. An adult human body contains more than a kilogram of calcium and almost all of it is concentrated in the mineral component of the skeleton as the calcium phosphate compound hydroxyapatite. Bone mineral gives mechanical strength to bones and teeth. Calcium of 1% or so is also required outside the skeleton for a number of functions such as intracellular regulator, release of nerve transmitters and hormones, cofactor for some enzymes including blood clotting, electrical excitation and contraction of muscles, and in nerve and heart function. Dietary deficiency in the child results can result in rickets syndrome. The average calcium intakes from food may range from 700 to 800 mg/day.

Iron is present in the hemeportion of hemoglobin, myoglobin, and the oxidation–reduction hemoproteins. The dietary source of iron is the organic heme in meat and fish and fruits and vegetables. Iron is stored in liver and bone marrow as ferritin and hemosiderin. Dietary iron deficiency depletes the iron stored as iron is required for formation of iron proteins and further deficiency lowers the blood hemoglobin level to the point of anemia, with decrease in oxygen-carrying capacity.

Most of the inorganic iron in food is in ferric state and inorganic iron is poorly absorbed than organic heme iron. Therefore, ferrous iron is used in supplements for better absorption. Substances in food such as vitamin C and alcohol can increase inorganic iron absorption while phytate, fiber, and tannin can inhibit inorganic iron absorption.

Copper is clearly established as an essential mineral. Nuts and shellfish have higher concentrations of copper. Drinking water may also contain significant amounts of copper.

There are several copper-containing enzymes and proteins in the body such as ceruloplasmin in hemoglobin synthesis, tyrosinase and dopamine hydroxylase in the synthesis of pigment melanin and catecholamine nerve transmitters, and copper as a cofactor for certain types of superoxide-dismutase as antioxidant nutrient in some reactions.

Magnesium is a major intracellular cation involved as an enzyme cofactor, particularly in the reactions in which phosphate or phosphorylated compound is involved. The plasma level of ionic magnesium is important for regulation of neuromuscular irritability. Several enzyme reactions in the cell are magnesium dependent for example, magnesium binds to the substrate and so increases its affinity for the enzymes as in kinase binding to adenosine triphosphate (ATP) in magnesium complex-ATP; magnesium binds directly to the enzyme to make it active as in RNA and DNA polymerase. Magnesium is mainly located in bones and hypocalcemia is a manifestation of magnesium deficiency. Magnesium is required for both the secretion of parathyroid hormone and its effects on target tissues and also for hydroxylation of vitamin D to 25-hydroxy-vitamin in the liver. Magnesium is present in many multinutrient supplements and in combination with calcium and vitamin D.

Zinc is clearly established as an essential nutrient. It is best absorbed from meat and fish and the other sources are cereals and pulses. Zinc is important in cell division and there are several zinc-containing enzymes involved in DNA synthesis. Zinc supplements have been investigated for their potential value in conditions such as treating anorexia nervosa, promotion of wound healing, and reducing symptoms of common cold and enhancing immune function.

Vitamins and minerals are essential nutrients required in small amounts compared with the total weight of food consumed. That is why they are collectively termed micronutrients. It was the initial discovery of the observation of the essentiality of these micronutrients based on certain deficiency diseases caused by their absence in the diet leading to the concept of dietary supplements food fortification. Clinical signs as indicators of micronutrient status tend to be nonspecific and invisible for a long period. However, there are some examples wherein the clinical signs may be associated with a particular nutrient deficiency: swollen thyroid gland an indication of dietary iodine deficiency; pale pink conjunctiva indicating iron deficiency anemia; spongy lesions at the corners of mouth indicating riboflavin (vitamin 12) deficiency; night blindness may be an early indication of vitamin A deficiency. Biochemical tests of micronutrient status in the body are specific and reliable. The examples are blood hemoglobin levels and ferritin concentrations in serum to assess iron status, total tocopherol level in serum for vitamin E, and vitamin C, folic acid level in serum.

The exact mechanism of mineral absorption by the intestine is unknown. The efficiency of absorption from the intestinal lumen and subsequent utilization vary considerably among the different elements and the problem of biological availability or biological utilization is a significant factor in mineral nutrition. The two basic factors determining the biological availability are the chemical form of the mineral nutrient in the food and the other forming a complex of the mineral with other compounds in the food. Selenium is present both in free and bound form, seleno-amino acids. Zinc, copper, and molybdenum metalloproteins also occur in foods. Other diet constituents influence biological availability mainly through relative binding potential and solubility. The organic acids such as citric, malic, and tartaric naturally present may form soluble complexes with the different metal ions. These soluble complexes are generally better absorbed.

The two vitamins, ascorbic acid and vitamin D help in better utilization of non-heme iron and calcium utilization respectively from the diets.

3.2.3 CAROTENOIDS

Carotenoids are a large group of fat-soluble tetra-terpenoids (C-40) plant pigments widely distributed in nature possessing a common chemical feature, a polyisoprenoid structure, a long-conjugated chain of double bonds in the central portion of the molecule, and near symmetry around the central double bond. The basic structure can be modified in a variety of ways such as cyclization of the end groups and introduction of oxygen functions to yield a large family of greater than 600 compounds, exclusive of *cis-trans*-isomers. Fruits and vegetables of green, orange, and red color are the most sources of carotenoids in the human diet. Carotenoids are classified into hydrocarbon carotenoids, with β-carotene and lycopene being the important members, and oxycarotenoids (xanthophylls), to which belong β-cryptoxanthin, lutein, zeaxanthin, and astaxanthin (Straub, 1987).

Carotenoids are also present in animals and microorganisms. The characteristic yellow, orange, and red color of carotenoids play an important role in photosynthesis, provitamin A activity, and physiological reactions in human body. Their presence in the diet may reduce the risk of cardiovascular disease, lung cancer, cervical dysplasia, and age-related macular disease (Prasad and Edwards-Prasad, 1990; Matthews-Roth, 1991; Snodderly, 1995; Olson, 1996; Kritchevsky, 1999).

3.2.3.1 β-Carotene

β-Carotene is a fat-soluble pigment made up of eight isoprene units cyclized at both the ends. In humans, the β-carotene is converted into vitamin A activity as retinal, retinol, and retinoic acid. It has also antioxidant activity and in the skin gives protection against solar radiation damage.

β-Carotene being fat soluble follows the same intestinal absorption pathway as dietary fat. After absorption by the small intestine mucosa, β-carotene in triacyl–glycerol matrix in chylomicrons undergoes partial conversion into vitamin A by reaction with β-carotene 15, 15'-oxygenase and then secreted into lymph for transport to liver and other parts of the body.

It is incorrect to assume that all natural components in the diet are inherently safe. β-Carotene is an example of controversy wherein the different studies have shown conflicting results. Probably, the reasons may be improper designed studies and commercial interest of interpreting and highlighting the positive results. The epidemiologic observations of possible protective effects of high β-carotene intakes from colored fruits and vegetables have a reduced risk of dying prematurely from cancer and heart disease. This prompted for a number of large-scale studies of β-carotene-containing supplements. A Cancer Prevention Study in China (Linxian) showed that subjects given a combination of β-carotene (15 mg), vitamin E, and selenium for a period of 5 years had significantly lower cancer and total mortality than those not receiving it (Blot et al., 1993). The study had drawbacks such as combined supplement, beneficial role of β-carotene as vitamin A provider. Subsequent controlled studies by others failed to reproduce the benefit seen in the Chinese study. The trials of ATBC and CARET showed possible evidence of harm from β-carotene supplements in relation to cancer among high-risk individuals such as smokers and asbestos workers (Group, 1994; Omenn et al., 1996; Hennekens et al., 1996; Rapala et al., 1997) reported increased death rates from coronary heart disease in the smokers group who were administered β-carotene supplements compared with those receiving either the placebo or vitamin E supplements. In a meta-analysis of eight trials β-carotene supplements involving 138,113 subjects, a dose range of 15–50 mg/day and follow-up range from 15 to 144 months, suggested a small but statistically significant increase in all-cause mortality and cardiovascular deaths (Vivekanathan et al., 2003). In view of the above evidence of potential harm from β-carotene, Food Standards Agency has suggested a safe upper level for supplements of only 7 mg/day compared with 15–50 mg/day (FSA, 2003).

In spite of some disturbing indications that β-carotene might increase risks slightly, at least for some sections of people, still the β-carotene supplements continue to be sold.

It is argued that balanced mixtures of natural carotenoids from a diet high in fruits and vegetables are safe because of the possible presence of many putative anticarcinogenic substances.

3.2.3.2 Lycopene

Lycopene is the main carotenoid responsible for the red color of tomato and tomato products and has been suggested as the main phytochemical responsible for the beneficial effects of tomatoes. It is also present in small amounts in papaya, water melon, and guava (Mangels et al., 1993; Scott and Hart, 1995). It has attracted considerable interest and attention because of the epidemiologic literature showing increased evidence demonstrating an inverse correlation between consumption of tomato products rich in lycopene and the risk of several types of cancer and cardiovascular diseases (Giovannucci, 1999; Sesso et al., 2003). The ability of lycopene to act as a potent antioxidant is believed to be responsible for protecting cells against oxidative damage and thereby reducing the risk of chronic disease, substantiated by human cell cultures and animals (Levy et al., 1995; Nagasawa et al., 1995; Stahl and Sies, 1996; Sies and Stahl, 1998).

Lycopene is a 40-carbon ($C_{40} H_{56}$) aliphatic acyclic hydrocarbon with 11 linearly arranged conjugated carbon–carbon double bonds. As a result of the highly conjugated nature of lycopene, it is susceptible to oxidative degradation and isomerization. Lycopene can theoretically exist in a large number of geometrical isomeric configurations. It is present in plant sources mainly in trans-isomeric form. Lycopene is symmetrical planar and has no vitamin A activity. Lycopene is quite stable in its in natural form within tomato tissue. However, prolonged physical and thermal-processing results in disruption of cell wall constituents exposing lycopene to degradation reactions.

The human body does not synthesize carotenoids and therefore diet is the only source of these components in blood and tissues. About 85% of the dietary lycopene comes from tomato fruit and tomato products and the remaining from other fruits such as papaya, water melon, guava, and others

(Bohm et al., 2001). A higher percentage of *cis*-lycopene is present in tissues than *trans*-lycopene (Stahl and Sies, 1992). This may be due to *cis*-lycopene being better absorbed, *in vivo* isomerization, or increased tissue uptake. The dietary lycopene in the form of tomato paste increased the serum lycopene 2.5-fold compared against an equivalent amount of lycopene provided in the form of fresh tomatoes. This improved bioavailability of lycopene from heat-processed foods may be ascribed to its release from the plant tissue matrix, weakening the formation of lycopene–protein complex, and heat-induced conversion of *trans*- to *cis*-isomers (Erdman et al., 1993, 1988; Clinton, 1998; Agarwal et al., 2001). The percentage of *cis:trans* lycopene in plasma has been shown to increase from 58:42 to 62:38 after 1 week consumption of processed tomato products (Hadley et al., 2003). Lycopene has been shown to be present in more than 15 different geometrical configurations in human prostrate tissue, where the *cis*-isomer content is higher in the range 80–90% than that observed in serum (Stahl and Sies, 1992).

Tomatoes are a common vegetable most widely consumed both in fresh and processed form. The estimated average daily intake of lycopene reported among Canadian population is 25 mg, Americans 5–8 mg, British elderly ladies 1 mg, and Germans 1.3 mg (Scott et al., 1996; Pelz et al., 1998; Rao et al., 1998; Matulka et al., 2004). Generally, lycopene is the most prominent in testes, adrenal glands, liver, and prostate tissues while present in relatively small amounts in kidneys, lungs, and ovary tissues (Kaplan et al., 1990; Schmitz et al., 1991; Gann et al., 1999; Van Breemen et al., 2002).

Several epidemiological studies and reviews have been carried out describing the role of lycopene in association with the prevention of prostate cancer (Nguyen and Schwartz, 2000; Hadley and Schwartz, 2005; Kun et al., 2006). Giovannucci conducted a study and reported an inverse relationship between the consumption of tomato and tomato products, blood lycopene, and the risk of prostate, lung, and colon cancer (Giovannucci, 1999). A case control study of 65 prostate cancer patients and 132 cancer-free controls showed significant inverse association of prostate cancer with plasma content of lycopene (Lu et al., 2001). A comparison of normal versus malignant human prostate tissue showed mainly prostate to have higher concentrations of lycopene (Clinton et al., 1996).

In a study of prostate cancer prevention trial of examination of 9559 participants, it was found that there was no association of a single nutrient like lycopene or set of nutrients with risk of prostate cancer (Kristal et al., 2010). FDA research examination of 81 studies on lycopene and tomato consumption observed that no evidence was to support a relationship between consumption and the risk of prostate cancer (Kavanaugh et al., 2007).

Lycopene lowers the oxidation of LDL cholesterol and may thereby reduce the risk of cardiovascular diseases (Diaz et al., 1997; Gerster, 1997). Several studies have shown a direct correlation between tomato and tomato products consumption and a reduced risk for coronary heart disease (Agarwal and Rao, 1998). Further, as the level of lycopene increases in the serum, there is a reduction in the levels of oxidized LDL.

The evidence in support of the role of lycopene in the prevention of cardiovascular disease stems primarily from the epidemiological observation of normal and at risk populations. The EURAMIC study employed subjects from 10 countries and, after evaluation for a relationship between antioxidant status and acute myocardial infarctions, found lycopene levels were found to be protective (Kohlmeir et al., 1997). This observation was confirmed in a later Rotterdam study (Klipstein-Grobusch et al., 2000).

3.2.3.3 Xanthophylls

These are oxycarotenoids having ring structures at the end of the conjugated double bond chain with polar functions like hydroxyl group. The examples for xanthophylls include lutein, zeaxanthin, β-cryptoxanthin, and so on. Mammalian species do not synthesize carotenoids and therefore these have to be obtained from dietary sources such as fruits, vegetables, and egg yolks. Lutein and zeaxanthin contribute to yellow and orange–yellow colors, respectively. Lutein and zeaxanthin can be present in plant material in the free form and also in ester form. Lutein is present in green leafy vegetables such as spinach, kale, and broccoli in the free form; fruits such as mango, orange, and papaya; red paprika, algae, yellow corn contain lutein in the form of its esters. It is also present in the blood stream and various tissues in human body and particularly in the macula, lens, and retina of the eye. Meso-zeaxanthin is an optical isomer of zeaxanthin and is normally present in certain sea foods and egg yolk.

Together lutein, zeaxanthin, and meso-zeaxanthin form macular pigment located in the center of retina, directly behind the lens in the eye. The macular pigment acts as antioxidant protecting the retina from oxidative degradation and also blocking the damaging effect of ultraviolet rays on the retinal fluid composition, particularly lipids. A life time slow and steady damage of the macula can lead to age-related macular degeneration and cataract.

As already mentioned, the macular pigment of the eye is composed primarily of three xanthophylls pigments, namely, (3R,3′R,6′R)-lutein, (3R,3′R)-zeaxanthin, and (3R,3′S)-zeaxanthin in the order 36%, 18%, and 18% of the total carotenoid content of the retina along with the remaining 20% consisting of minor carotenoids such as oxo-lutein, epi-lutein, and β-,-β-carotene 3,3′-dione (Landrum and Bone, 2001). Although these xanthophylls pigments are found throughout the tissues of the eye, the highest concentration is seen in the macula lutea region of the retina, including a central depression in the retina called fovea. The concentration of xanthophylls pigments increases progressively toward the center of the macula and in the fovea, the concentration of these xanthophylls pigments are approximately thousandfold higher than in other human tissues (Landrum et al., 1992). The fovea is a relatively small area within the macula, in which the cone photoreceptors reach their maximal concentration. About 50% of the total amounts of the xanthophylls are concentrated in the macula where zeaxanthin dominates over lutein by ratio of 2:1 (Handleman et al., 1992; Billsten et al., 2003). At the center of the retinal fovea, zeaxanthin is 50:50 mixture of (trans-3R,3′R)-zeaxanthin and (trans-3R,3′S)-zeaxanthin along with small quantity of (3S,3′S)-zeaxanthin (Landrum and Bone, 2001).

The ability to increase the amount of macular pigment by dietary supplementation with lutein has been demonstrated (Landrum et al., 1996). The reduced vision function due to cataract and the adult blindness due to age-related macular degeneration (AMD) can be substantially controlled by consuming fruits and vegetables and dietary supplements containing lutein and (R,R)-zeaxanthin and (R,S)-zeaxanthin available from sea foods denying the vegetarian population. Although (R,S)-zeaxanthin present in eye is considered a metabolic product originating from lutein, the need for dietary supplementation of (R,S)-zeaxanthin is now recognized to improve the macular pigment density (Landrum and Bone, 2001). Similarly, the study has shown that (R,R)-zeaxanthin gains entry to blood and finally to macula (Breithaupt et al., 2004). Lutein and zeaxanthin dietary supplements in human trials have shown to raise the macular pigment density and serum concentrations of these carotenoids (Bone et al., 2003).

To date, little is known about the mechanism of formation, uptake, and deposition of meso-zeaxanthin in the retina of the eye. Khachik et al. (1999) have reported the presence of 2–3% of (3R,3′S), meso-zeaxanthin in 20 normal human plasma samples and proposed the metabolic pathways of its formation from dietary lutein and zeaxanthin. There is evidence and reasons supporting the hypothesis that the carotenoids lutein, zeaxanthin, and meso-zeaxanthin are readily bio-available and consequently increase macular pigment levels (Bone et al., 2006; Landrum and Bone, 2007; Thurnham et al., 2007, 2008).

In present days, there is high demand for xanthophyll crystals containing high amounts of *trans*-lutein and/or zeaxanthin for its use as antioxidants, prevention of cataract, and macular degeneration, as lung cancer-preventive agent, as agents for the absorption of harmful ultraviolet light from sun rays and quencher of photo-induced free radical and reactive oxygen species, and so on. A number of commercial products from natural source are now available to facilitate the formulation of industrial and commercial products with lutein or (R,R)-zeaxanthin. Xanthophylls composition containing all the essential macular xanthophylls and high concentrations of particularly trans-lutein at least 85% and balance comprising of (R,R)-zeaxanthin and (R,S)-zeaxanthin in equal or higher ratios derived from the same natural source (marigold flower petals) as commercial lutein or zeaxanthin are now available. Evidence of the protective role of *trans*-lutein, (*R,R*)-zeaxanthin, and (*R,S*)-zeaxanthin in maintaining eye health has been found based on correlation between dietary supplements versus serum levels and the macular pigment density (Bone et al., 2007; Thurnham et al., 2008). Under the circumstances explained above, it is desirable and useful for industry and nutritional product formulators to have a xanthophylls concentrate consisting of all the macular xanthophylls obtained from a commercially scalable process, and made from natural source material same as that which is already accepted by the market for lutein, (*R,R*)-zeaxanthin and (*R,S*)-zeaxanthin. The product prepared should have 5:1 lutein:zeaxanthin ratio, as found in regular diet and in plasma. The product so prepared should also be made from safe solvents (GRAS) for producing dietary supplements suitable for human consumption, with minimum solvent residues, and specifications of lutein and zeaxanthin isomers keeping in mind visual function and market requirements.

3.2.4 POLYUNSATURATED FATS

3.2.4.1 Polyunsaturated Fatty Acids

Fat is one of the classes of nutrients. The other two are protein and carbohydrates. The main function of fat is to produce energy for the body. There are three types of fat: triglyceride, cholesterol, and phospholipids. Triacylglycerol is the principal component of dietary fats and oils and is made up of three fatty acids attached by ester linkages. All dietary fats contain a mixture of saturated, mono-unsaturated, and polyunsaturated fatty acids (PUFA) but their relative proportions vary enormously. Fatty acids are composed of a hydrocarbon chain of variable length and carboxyl group at one end. Fatty acids having a double bond in the hydrocarbon chain are termed unsaturated fatty acids and with just one double bond, monounsaturated and with more than one as polyunsaturated acids. Fats from milk, meat, and tropical oils such as palm oil and coconut oil tend to be rich in saturates and monounsaturates but low in polyunsaturated fatty acids; fat from ruminating animals is particularly low in polyunsaturated fatty acids. There are two groups of fatty acids, called essential fatty acids, based on linoleic acid (omega-6-group which includes gamma linolenic acid/GLA) and α-linolenic acid/ALA (omega-3-group, which includes eicosapentaenoic acid/EPA, and docosahexaenoic acid/DHA) which cannot be synthesized in the human body and must be obtained from the diet. Generally, vegetable oils such as sunflower oil, corn oil, and safflower oil tend to be rich in the linoleic acid and omega-6-series of polyunsaturated fatty acids while fish and other marine oils tend to be rich in the omega-3-series and are the only substantial dietary source of the long-chain PUFA such as EPA and DHA.

In recent years our understanding of the relationship between plasma cholesterol concentration and atherosclerosis has become confusing and complicated. Lipids including cholesterol are transported in water-based plasma as soluble protein–lipid complexes (lipoproteins). The dietary fat after absorption in the intestine gains entry into the bloodstream in the form of protein-coated droplets called chylomicrons which are later assimilated and removed from the plasma. Finally, high-, low-, and very low-density lipoproteins remain in plasma and can be separated by centrifugation method. LDL is a cholesterol-rich fraction which accounts for about 70% of the total plasma cholesterol. With increasing concentration of LDL in blood it tends to be deposited in artery walls resulting in cardiovascular diseases. This cholesterol present in LDL is referred as bad cholesterol and the cholesterol in high-density lipoproteins (HDL) as good cholesterol. The HDL-cholesterol concentration is negatively correlated with the risk of coronary disease. It is desirable to increase the HDL concentration in blood while reducing the LDL concentration. Very-low-density lipoprotein (VLDL) is a triacylglycerol-rich lipoprotein fraction which is the main carrier of endogenously produced triacylglycerol from the liver to adipose tissue. The level of VLDL is low in fasting blood of healthy people. A high VLDL is found in conditions such as diabetic and obesity and may be associated with an increased risk of coronary disease.

The primary source of omega-3 fatty acid is fish and fish oil supplements. Higher fat-fish such as salmon, mackerel, tuna, herring, and sardines are excellent sources of EPA and DHA. Efforts to increase the omega-3 fatty acids content in traditional foods have included feeding fish oils or flax seed oil to pigs and chickens (Howe et al., 2002). Omega-3 fatty acids have been a part of the human diet for several centuries and no reported toxicity. Fish oil (menhaden oil) has the GRAS status by U.S. FDA in 1997 and suggested the intakes up to 3 g/day of marine omega-3 fatty acid as safe in the diet. A number of expert groups from various countries have recommended intakes of 200–800 mg/day of EPA plus DHA (Simopoulos et al., 2000). The American Heart Association has recommended that persons with known coronary heart disease should have an intake of about 1 g of EPA plus DHA per day (Kris-Etherton et al., 2002). One of the problems of fish oil is fishy smell which is removed or minimized by processing under vacuum and nitrogen atmosphere. The fishy belch can be minimized by bedtime consumption or enteric coating. Omega-3 fatty acids, derived from microbial sources, are free of fishy flavors characteristic of most fish oil supplements. This involves extraction using organic solvents and due to high cost very limited of demand.

Modern diets tend to have a much higher ratio of omega-6 to omega-3 fatty acids than has in the past. The omega-6 rich diets would be expected to lead to reduced production of the long-chain omega-3 fatty acids such as EPA and DHA and consequently minimal content in membrane phospholipids. The increased use of vegetable oils and margarine has greatly increased the ratio of omega-6 to omega-3 polyunsaturated fatty acids in many countries. The realization of decreasing levels of omega-3 fatty acids and increasing levels of omega-6 fatty acids in our diets has prompted to modify existing foods to help correct this imbalance (Lewis et al., 2000; Metcalf et al., 2003). The desirable ratio suggested is 4–5:1 (Jones and Krubow, 1999).

3.2.4.2 Flax Seed Oil

Flax seed oil is derived from the seeds of the flax plant (*Linum usitatissimum*), native of the Middle East. The oil is also called linseed oil used in paints and varnishes. Flax seed oil is marketed as a dietary supplement based on its high content of α-linolenic acid, the precursor of omega-3- series of fatty acids. It is considered as a vegetarian alternative to fish oil being a source of EPA and DHA. However, in human studies it has shown poor conversion into EPA and DHA, thereby establishing not a good source of long-chain omega-3-fatty acids

For general health, both omega-6 and omega-3 fatty acids are required but they should be in a desirable ratio range such as 2:1–4:1. They play a crucial role in brain function as well as normal growth and development. They also help stimulate skin, hair growth, maintain bone health, regulate metabolism, and maintain the reproductive system. For various reasons such as consumption of corn, safflower, and sunflower oils which contain high linoleic acid and GLA from supplements lead to excess omega-6 fatty acids which has deleterious health consequences including cardiovascular deaths. Harmful effects can be minimized by reducing the excessive intake of omega-6 fatty acids and increasing the dietary intake of omega-3 fatty acids such as EPA and DHA, the fish oil fatty acids.

A Danish study reported that acute myocardial infarction rates were significantly lower in Greenland Eskimos compared to similar age and sex-matched. Danes attributed to high fish consumption and indicating a link between omega-3 fatty acids and cardio-protective effect (Bang and Dyerberg, 1980). Similarly, the inhabitants of the Japanese island Okinawa also showed low cardiovascular mortality rates, indicating association with high fish consumption (Kagawa et al., 1982). In three separate studies, a relationship between a blood measure of omega-3 fatty acids and risk for coronary heart disease was reported (Siscovick et al., 1995; Lemaitre et al., 2002).

Omega-3 fatty acids found in fish oils and flaxseed oil are useful in a wide variety of conditions and chronic diseases. There are several studies where the intake of omega-3 fatty acids have shown reduction in oxidant stress (Mori et al., 2000), suppression of the production of pro-inflammatory compounds in the body and thereby helping conditions such as arthritis (Belluzi et al., 2000; Adam et al., 2003), improvement in serum lipids and provide cardiovascular protection (Jacobson, 2007), and increase bone density in young men (Hogstrom et al., 2007).

3.2.5 SOY FOODS AND ISOFLAVONES

Isoflavones are a subclass of flavonoids and are present in food plants such as soy, red clover (*Trifolium pratense*), and alfaalfa. The main dietary sources are soybeans and soy foods. The well-known isoflavones are genistein (4′,5,7-trihydroxyisoflavone), daidzein (4′,7-dihydroxyisoflavone), and glycitein (4′,7-dihydroxy-6-methoxy isoflavone). The corresponding glycosides are genistin, daidzin, and glycitin, respectively. They can also be present as glucosides each esterified with either acetic or malonic acid. The isoflavones present in red clover are methylated and they are formononetin (4′-methoxy-7-hydroxyisoflavone) and biochanin-A (4′-methoxy-5,7-hydroxyisoflavone). The carbohydrate part is removed by fermentation or during digestion in the gastrointestinal tract. Plasma isoflavone levels increase proportionately in relation to the amount ingested. Isoflavones circulate in plasma mostly in the conjugated form, bound to glucuronic acid. The glycosides undergo hydrolysis *in vivo* and the liberated aglycone as well as the free isoflavones from the diet are absorbed in the intestine (Setchell et al., 2002). It is the aglycone part which is responsible for the effects of isoflavones in the human body. This aglycone part corresponds to 60% of the glycoside. That is 100 mg of isoflavone glycoside correspond to 60 mg of isoflavone aglycone.

Miso soup is an important constituent of the Japanese nutrition and is usually consumed for breakfast. Miso, natto, or tofu is the basic diet and these contain soy-based nutrition with isoflavones. In addition, soy product is also used as excipients or protein source in food manufacturing. Typical soy consumption is approximately 65 g/day corresponding to 25–55 mg isoflavones with higher values in Japan, less in Hong Kong, Singapore, and in certain regions of China. A study shows a correlation of 75 mg isoflavone consumption from diet and a reduced risk of prostate cancer in certain regions of China. Based on a study of soy and isoflavone consumption in relation to prostate cancer risk in China, a range of up to 100 mg of isoflavones daily has been considered safe by experience and in addition beneficial to health. Soy food does not play an important role in European dietary habits and hence exposure to isoflavones is low. However, small amounts of nutritional isoflavones come from milk products with the animals grazing pastures with red clover (Antignac et al., 2003).

Soy foods have antioxidant properties which protect the cardiovascular system from oxidation of LDL cholesterol. The oxidized LDL accumulates in the arteries as patches of fatty build up which blocks the flow of blood resulting in atherosclerosis. Genistein inhibits the growth of that from this artery-clogging plaque. Arteries damaged by atherosclerosis usually form blood clots (Zhang et al., 2003). Dietary soy products because of their estrogen-like effects showed low frequency of hot flashes among Japanese and South East Asian women (Adlercreutz et al., 1992; Nagata et al., 1999, 2001). Soy extracts or soy foods adjusted to a defined content of isoflavones yielded a substantial reduction in the menopausal complaints and in the severity and frequency of hot flashes in different studies (Drapier et al., 2002; Colacurci et al., 2004; Cheng et al., 2007). During menopause period, the decreased estrogen levels prevent calcium absorption causing bone loss and possibly osteoporosis. Isoflavones are reported to provide protection against bone loss. A double-blind, placebo-controlled, randomized trial with about 200 postmenopausal Chinese women administering isoflavones (80 mg + calcium 500 mg) showed a moderate but significant effect on the maintenance of hip bone mineral density with low initial bone mass (Chen et al., 2003). Another randomized, placebo-controlled, double blind (3 years) providing 80–120 mg isoflavone supplement to postmenopausal women showed modest beneficial bone health (Alekael, 2010).

3.2.6 PHYTOSTEROLS

Phytosterols, also called plant sterols, are natural components of all plant cells. They act as a structural component in the cell membrane. Sterols are high-melting alcohols with a structure based on cholestane (having the same sterol ring structure as cholesterol but lacking the β-hydroxyl group). Most natural phytosterols contain one or two carbon–carbon double bonds and are considered unsaturated while phytostanols are completely saturated molecules, with no carbon–carbon double bonds. Sterols are classified into three main groups based on the presence or absence of methyl moieties at the 4-position in the A ring: (1) 4-des-methyl sterols/stanols: campesterol, sitosterol, campestanol, and sitostanol, (2) 4-mono-methyl sterols: cycloeucalenol and obtusifoliolo, and (3) 4,4′- dimethyl sterols: cycloartenol, butyrospermol.

The commonly occurring natural plant sterols are the des-methyl sterols, sitosterol, campesterol, and stigmasterol. Dietary intake ranges from 250 to 500 mg/day with a composition of about 65% sitosterol, 30% campesterol, and 5% stigmasterol and trace amounts of other sterols (Salen et al., 1970; Ling et al., 1995).

Phytosterols have been known to lower cholesterol in humans since more than five decades, a finding that has resulted in the development of various food products enriched with these compounds. The serum cholesterol-lowering effect of phytosterols, when consumed at levels of 1.5–2 g/day, has led to great interest in phytosterol-enriched foods and their development. By providing a strict uncooked vegan diet containing 732 mg/day of total phytosterols to patients with rheumatoid arthritis, a significant decrease was found in both total and LDL cholesterol levels in the serum (Agren et al., 2001). A comparative study of commercial corn oil containing naturally present phytosterols against a purified corn oil free from sterols showed that cholesterol absorption was significantly higher in the case of purified oil free from phytosterols (Ostlund et al., 2002).

The major sources of phytosterols for dietary supplements and functional foods are tall oil and vegetable oil deodorizer distillate. Stanols obtained from tall oil soap/pitch contain primarily sitostanol and campestanol in a ratio of about 92:8. Stanols derived from soy oil have a sitostanol/campestanol ratio of about 68:32. The first phytosterol product was a cholesterol-lowering pharmaceutical, cytellin, containing sitosterol in free form (Moreau et al., 2002). The first phytosterol functional food was Benecol spread launched in Finland, containing phytostanols esterified to natural fatty acids from vegetable oils. Presently, there are several phytosterol and phytostanol products marketed in many EU countries, Japan, Australia, the United States, and others (Dutta, 2004).

3.3   SPICE-BASED ANTIOXIDANTS AND NUTRIENTS

3.3.1   PIPERINE

Piperine is classified as an alkaloid present in black pepper. Although black pepper is used as a spice for its pungency in foods, it is widely used in many parts of the world for therapeutic and medicinal properties. Piperine is isolated from black pepper oleoresin. Piperine has thermogenic activity and helps in boosting the body's metabolic rate and consequently leading to weight loss. It has anti-inflammatory properties and also in production of serotonin in brain helping in relief of pain.

Piperine is established as a bioavailability enhancer of various structurally and therapeutically diverse drugs and other substances (Shoba et al., 1998; Badmev et al., 2000). The bioavailability of drugs in it is of great clinical significance. The mechanism responsible for the bioavailability enhancing action of piperine is poorly understood (Atal et al., 1985).

3.3.2   CURCUMIN

Curcumin is obtained by the solvent extraction of the ground rhizomes of *Curcuma longa* L. with the subsequent purification of the resultant extract. Curcumin consists essentially of three different polyphenolic pigment components together referred as curcuminoids: curcumin being the major and demethoxycurcumin (DMC) and bis-demethoxycurcumin (BDMC) in minor concentrations. The importance of turmeric in medicine is attributed to phenolic groups which are known to possess anti-inflammatory, antioxidant, antimutagenic, antitumor, and antidiabetics effects in biologic systems (Aggarwal et al., 2003; Joe et al., 2004; Antony and Shankaranarayana, 2001).

Almost 2500 preclinical studies *in vitro* and *in vivo* have prompted various clinical trials in human subjects. Almost 40 different clinical trials comprising of 25–30 human subjects have been completed (Goel et al., 2008; Strimpakos and Sharma, 2008). Three different phase-1 clinical trials performed for determining safety have shown that curcumin administered at doses as high as 15 mg/day orally for 3 months is safe. Based on extensive research data of a 2-year period, it has been shown that curcumin mediates its anti-inflammatory effects through the downregulation of inflammatory transcription factors, enzymes. Because of the crucial role of inflammation in most chronic diseases, the potential of curcumin has been examined in neophase, neurological, cardiovascular, pulmonary, and metabolic diseases (Aggarwal and Sung, 2008).

3.3.3 CAPSAICIN

The lipophilic alkaloid capsaicinoids are the major pungent principle in chillies (*Capsicum annuum*) chiefly comprising of capsaicin, dihydro-capsaicin, and nor-dihydro-capsaicin. The daily intake of capsaicin varies widely, 1.5 mg in Europe, 25–200 mg in countries such as Thailand, Mexico, and India (Kozuke et al., 2005). *Capsaicin* has been reported to increase thermogenesis by enhancing catecholamine secretion from the adrenal medulla. Increase in thermogenesis induces is attributed to β-adrenergic stimulation. The capsaicin-induced energy metabolism seems to be mediated by catachol energy metabolism from the sympathetic activation of nerves. Capsaicin is known to reduce appetite levels, reduction in body mass (fat), and desirable reduction in levels of critical markers of weight maintenance such as blood glucose, insulin, triglyceride, and leptin. Microencapsulation techniques are now available to release the capsaicin into intestine, avoiding the burning and irritation in stomach. Certain varieties of sweet chillies containing nonpungent substances called capsiates are known to cause weight loss.

The requirements of sport supplements are (1) need to have direct effect on performance, on strength and power, (2) promoting and enhancing body recovery, (3) possessing effective immune function, and (4) providing energy for the work out. In the following section, selected key supplements which have performed well by evidence of research supplements are discussed.

3.3.4 CREATINE

Creatine has been in supplements market for more than a decade and is a naturally occurring amino acid derived from glycine, arginine, and methionine. The source of this is mainly from meat and fish (Balsom et al., 1994). Creatine has been proven to increase strength, muscle mass, and sprint performance and recovery. Creatine has been researched more than any other nutritional supplement on the market today. Creatine is a nitrogenous organic compound obtained predominantly from the ingestion of meat or fish, although it is also synthesized endogenously in the kidney, liver, and pancreas. When creatine enters the muscle cell, it accepts a high-energy phosphate and forms phosphocreatine (PC). PC is the storage form of high-energy phosphate, which is used by the skeletal muscle cell to regenerate ATP rapidly during bouts of maximum muscular contraction (Hirovonen et al., 1987). The conversion of ATP into adenosine diphosphate (ADP) and a phosphate group generates the energy needed by the muscles during short-term, high-intensity exercise. PC availability in the muscles is vitally important for energy production, as ATP cannot be stored in excessive amounts in muscle and is rapidly depleted during bouts of exhaustive exercise. Oral creatine monohydrate supplementation has been reported to increase muscle creatine and PC content by 15–40%, enhance the cellular bioenergetics of the phosphagen system, improve the shuttling of high-energy phosphates between the mitochondria and cytosol via the creatine phosphate shuttle, and enhance the activity of various metabolic pathways.

Scientific studies indicate that creatine supplementation is an effective, safe nutritional strategy to promote gains in strength and muscle mass during resistance training (Greenwood et al., 2003).

Creatine has become one of the most popular nutritional supplements for resistance-trained athletes and bodybuilders.

3.3.5 PROTEIN AND AMINO ACIDS

Protein is the main component of muscles, organs, and hormones. The cells of muscles, tendons, and ligaments are maintained, repaired, and enhanced with proteins. Skeletal muscle growth is possible only when muscle protein synthesis exceeds muscle breakdown, thus adequate dietary protein postworkout of protein supplements has shown increase in protein synthesis and muscle mass. The recent trend is to supplement branched-chain amino acids (BCAAs). The BCAAs include leucine, isoleucine, and valine. BCAAs are the only amino acids that are used exclusively for the synthesis of tissue protein and not for other hormones. The BCAAs cannot be broken down in the liver like the other AAs. Ingestion of AAs after resistance exercise has been shown at many time points in several studies to stimulate increases in muscle protein synthesis, cause minimal changes in protein breakdown, and increase overall protein balance.

3.3.6 CARNOSINE AND β-ALANINE

Amino acids are organic compounds that combine to form proteins. When proteins are degraded, amino acids are left. The human body requires a number of amino acids to facilitate skeletal muscle growth and repair and for the hormonal development that is necessary for adaptation to stress. Amino acids supplementation has undergone extensive research with a suggestion that pre- and postworkout amino acid supplementation can increase protein synthesis and slow down degradation.

Carnosine, a dipeptide comprised of the amino acids histidine and β-alanine, occurs naturally in brain, cardiac muscle, kidney, and stomach and in large amounts in skeletal muscles. Carnosine has been widely studied for its contribution to improved wound healing, its antioxidant activity, and its anti-aging properties. Carnosine is found in high concentrations in skeletal muscle, primarily type II muscle fibers, which are the fast-twitch muscle fibers used during explosive movements such as weight training and sprinting. It has also been concluded that carnosine levels are found in higher concentrations in athletes whose performance demands serious anerobic output. However, carnosine is rapidly degraded into β-alanine and histidine as soon as it enters the blood by the activity of enzyme carnosinase. Thus, β-alanine is believed to be the answer to increasing carnosine in skeletal muscle. Recent studies have demonstrated that taking β-alanine orally is effective at increasing carnosine levels. Individuals who take oral β-alanine on a regular basis can expect to increase their muscles' synthesis of carnosine by up to 64% (Harris et al., 1998).

3.3.7 ARGININE

Arginine is one of the amino acids produced in the human body during the digestion or hydrolysis of proteins. Arginine can also be produced synthetically. Because it is produced in the body, it is referred to as nonessential, meaning that no food or supplements are necessary for humans. Arginine compounds can be used to treat people with liver dysfunction because of its role in promoting liver regeneration.

Arginine has several roles in the body: it assists wound healing, helps remove excess ammonia from the body, stimulates immune function, and promotes secretion of several hormones, including glucagon, insulin, and growth hormone. NO_2 is a compound produced from arginine that elicits arteriole vasodilation and assists in nutrient transport/recovery in muscle. This action has been proposed to cause a perpetual muscle pump in users and promote gains in muscle. It is important to discuss arginine as a nutritional supplement. Arginine or NO_2 has been one of the hottest supplements over the last few years. There is a belief that there are tons of anecdotal evidences that suggest that arginine is a powerful modulator of strength and performance.

3.3.8 GLUTAMINE

This is the most abundant amino acid in the body, representing about 60% of the amino acid pool in muscles. In a healthy person, the concentration of glutamine in the blood is three to four times greater than all other amino acids. Glutamine serves a variety of functions in the body including cell growth, immune function, and recovery from stress (Candow et al., 2001). Glutamine also contributes to the prevention of muscle breakdown, increase in growth hormone, protein synthesis, improved intestinal health, decrease in the risk of overtraining, and improved immune system function.

Glutamine is also believed to play a large role in enhancement of the immune system. Intense physical training may have a negative effect on the immune system by causing transient suppression of the entire system. The demands on muscle and other organs are so high during intense physical training that the immune system may suffer from a lack of glutamine that temporarily affects its function. It has been suggested that because skeletal muscle is the major tissue involved in glutamine production skeletal muscle must thus play a vital role in the process of glutamine utilization in the immune cells.

3.3.9 WHEY PROTEIN

This is marketed to those wishing to gain muscle mass and strength. Whey protein is a combination of β-lactalbumin, α-lactalbumin, blood protein, lactose, and minerals. Whey protein contains the highest concentration of the branched chain amino acids isoleucine, leucine, and valine of common dietary proteins. Many believe supplementation of these branched chain amino acids reduce the breakdown of muscle tissue and must be present in muscle cells for protein synthesis (Walzem et al., 2002).

3.4 CONCLUSION

Originally, foods had a nutritive property to provide health and prevention of disease. Today, the food and beverages available have a compromised nutritive value due to industrial-processing conditions. The refined foods contain less and often miniscule amounts of vitamins and minerals and other compounds which the plants provide for us. In nature, phytochemicals are present as a mixture. There is a realization of gradual shift from one active principle hypothesis to heterogeneous composition of extracts. The functional performances of the extracts are not reproduced by any single component or even a mixture of few select ingredients. Today, we see nutritional supplements for eye health, bone health, heart health, skin health, and so on. Thus, dietary ingredients from plant, animals, and microbes play a major role in regulating human health and disease.

Dietary supplements and functional foods are a natural choice to offset the prevalent limitations in our daily lives. The concept of functional food was conceived in the context of nutrition during space travel. The modern concept of dietary supplements and functional foods for the general population is a recent development among most countries mainly due to well-researched nutrients from both plants and animals.

In the recent years, there have been several innovations in the areas of extraction, isolation, and purification, analysis, delivery system, safety evaluation, bioavailability and absorption, and clinical research. However, unlike pharmaceutical industry which deals with purified molecules, the situation is different in dietary supplements due to lack of standard preparations for various reasons. Many firms are able to get GRAS status before launching the products into market because of the fairly simplified protocol, if adequate safety data are furnished. Similarly, the safety decisions are governed by European Food Safety Act based on rigorous science-based evidences.

Most of the countries have their own legislation for nutritional supplements and functional foods. Decisions and policies from regulatory bodies such as Codex Alimentarius, World Health Organization (WHO), and the Food and Agriculture Organization (FAO) have become increasingly important for dietary supplement companies. In this context, the International Alliance of Dietary Food Supplementation Association works closely with these international bodies to ensure the views of the dietary supplementation industry are taken into account in the formulation of policy.

REFERENCES

Adam, O., Beringer, C., Kless. T. et al. 2003. Anti-inflammatory effects of a low arachidonic acid diet and fish oil in patients with rheumatoid arthritis. *Rheumatol. Int.*, 23: 27–36.

Adlercreutz, H., Hamalainen, E., Gorbach. S., and Goldin, B. 1992. Dietary phyto-estrogens and the menopause in Japan. *Lancet*, 339: 1233.

Agarwal, S. and Rao, A.V. 1998. Tomato lycopene and low-density lipoprotein oxidation: A human dietary intervention study. *Lipids*, 33: 081–984.

Aggarwal, B.B. and Sung, B. 2008. Pharmacological basis for the role of curcumin in chronic diseases: An age old spice with modern gadgets. *Trends in Pharmacol. Sci.*, 30: 85–94.

Agarwal, A., Shen, H., Agarwal, S., and Rao, A.V. 2001. Lycopene content in tomato products: Its stability and *in vivo* antioxidant properties. *J. Medicinal Food*, 4: 9–15.

Aggarwal, B.B., Kumar, A., and Bharti, A.C. 2003. Anti cancer potential of curcumin: Pre-clinical and clinical studies. *Anticancer Res.*, 23: 363–398.

Agren, J.J., Tvrzicka, E., Nenonen, M.T., Helve, T., and Hanninen, O. 2001. Divergent changes in serum sterols during a strict uncooked vegan diet in patients with rheumatoid arthritis. *Brit. J. Nutr.*, 85: 137–139.

Alekael, D.L., Van loan, M.D., Kochler, N., and Hanson, L.N. 2010. The soy isoflavones for reducing bone loss study: A 3 y randomized controlled trial in postmenopausal women. *Am. J. Clin. Nutr.*, 91: 218–230.

Antignac, J.P., Cariou, R., Le Bizea, B., Craveli, J.P., and Andres, F. 2003. Identification of phytoestrogen in bovine milk using LC tandem Mass spectrometry. *Rapid Commun Mass Spectrom.*, 17: 1256–1264.

Antony, J. and Shankaranarayana, M.L. 2001. Curcuminoids: Background and benefit. *Nutraceutical World*, 47–48.

Atal, C.K., Dubey, R.K., and Singh, J. 1985. Bio chemical basis of enhanced drug boavailability or piperine: Evidence that piperine is a potent inhibitor of drug metabolism. *Phartmacol. Exp. Ther.*, 235: 258–262.

Badmev, V.V., Majeed, M., and Prakash, L. 2000. Piperine derived from the black pepper increase the plasma levels of coenzymes Q10 following oral supplement. *J. Nutr. Biochem.*, 95: 109–113.

Ball, G.F.M, 2004. *Vitamins: Their Role in the Human Body*. Oxford: Blackwell.

Balsom, P.D., Soderlund, K., and Ekblom, B. 1994. Creatine in humans with special reference to creatine supplementation. *Sports Med.*, 18: 268–280.

Bang, H.O. and Dyerberg, J. 1980. Lipid metabolism and ischemic heart disease in Greenland Eskimos. *Adv. Nutr. Res.*, 3: 1–22.

Belluzi, A., Boschi, C., Munarini, A., Cariani, G., and Miglio, F. 2000. Polyunsaturated fatty acids and inflammatory bowel disease. *Am. J. Clin. Nutr.*, 71: 339s–342s.

Billsten, H.H., Bhosale, P., Yemelvanoy, A., Bernstein, P.S., and Polivka, T. 2003. Photophysical properties of xanthophylls in carotene proteins from human retina. *Photochem. Photobiol.*, 78: 138–145.

Bohm, F., Edge, R., Burke, M., and Truscott, T.G. 2001. Dietary uptake of lutein protects human cells from singlet oxygen and nitrogen dioxide. *J. Photochem. Photobiol. B: Biol.*, 64: 176–178.

Bone, R.A., Landrum, J.T., Guerra, L.H., and Ruiz, C.A. 2003. Lutein and Zeaxanthin dietary supplements raise macular pigment density and serum concentrations of these Carotenoids in human. *J. Nutr.*, 133: 992–998.

Bone, R.A., Landrum, J.T., Cao,Y., Howard, A.N., and Thurnham, D.I. 2006. Macular pigment response to a xanthophyll supplement of lutein, zeaxanthin and meso-zeaxanthin. *Proc. Nutr. Soc.*, 65: 105A.

Bone, R.A., Landrum, J.T., Cao,Y., Howard, A.N., and Alvarez-Caldron, F. 2007. Macular pigment response to a supplement containing meso-zeaxanthin. *Nutr. Metabol.*, 11: 1–8.

Blot, W.J., Lu, J.Y, Taylor, P.R. et.al. 1993. Nutrition intervention trials in Linxian. China: Supplementation with specific vitamin/mineral combinations, cancer incidence and disease specific mortality in the general population. *J. Natl. Cancer Inst.*, 66: 1191–1208.

Breithaupt, D.E., Weller, P., and Wolters, M. et al. 2004. Comparison of plasma responses in human subjects after the ingestion of (3R,3′R)-zeaxanthin dipalmitate from wolfberry (*Lycium barbarum*) and non-esterified (3R,3′R)-zeaxanthin using Chiral HPLC. *Brit. J. Nutr.*, 91: 707–713.

Candow, D.G., Chilibeck, P.D., Burke, D.G., Davison, K.S., and Smith-Palmer, T. 2001. Effect of glutamine supplementation combined with resistance training in young adults. *Eur. J. Appl. Physiol.*, 86: 142–149.

Chen, Y.M., Ho, S.C., Lam, S.S., and Woo, J.L. 2003. Soy isoflavones have a favorable effect on bone loss in Chinese postmenopausal women with lower bone mass: A double-blind, randomized, controlled trial. *J. Clin. Endocrinol. Metab.*, 88: 4740–4747.

Cheng, B., Warner, M., Wilczek, B., Warner, M., Gustaffson, J.A., and Landgren, M. 2007. Isoflavones treatment for acute menopausal symptoms. *Menopause*, 14: 468–473.

Clinton, S.K. 1998. Lycopene: Chemistry, biology and implications for human health and disease. *Nutr. Rev.*, 56: 35–51.

Clinton, S.K., Emenhiser, C., Schwartz, S.J. et al. 1996. Cis-trans lycopene isomers, carotenoids and retinal in the human prostate. *Cancer Epidemol. Biomarkers Prev.*, 5: 823–845.

Colacurci, N., Zarconone, R., Boretti, A. et. al. 2004. Effects of soy isoflavones on menopausal neurovegetative symptoms. *Minerva Ginecol.*, 56: 407–412.

Department of Health and human Services, FDA. 1996. Regulation of medical foods: Advance notice of proposed rulemaking. *Federal Register*, 61: 60661–606711.

Department of Health and Human Services, FDA. 1997. Food Labeling, health claims: Soluble fiber from whole oat and risk of coronary heart disease. *Federal Register*, 62: 15343–15344.

Diaz, M.N., Frei, B., Vita, J.A., and Keaney, J.F. 1997. Antioxidants and atherosclerotic heart disease. *N. Engl. J. Med.*, 337: 247–255.

Dietary Supplement, Health and Education Act. 1994 (DSHEA).

Drapier Faure, E., Chantre, P., and Mares, P. 2002. Effects of a standardized soy extract on hot flashes: Multi-centered, double blind, randomized, placebo-controlled study. *Menopause*, 9: 329–334.

Dutta, P. C. 2004. Plant sterols in functional foods. In: *Phytosterols as Functional Food Components and Nutraceuticals*. New York, NY: Marcel Dekker Inc. pp. 317–345.

Erdman, J.W., Bierer, S., and Guggar, E.T. 1993. Absorption and transport of carotenoids. *Ann. NY Acad. Sci.*, 691: 76–85.

Erdman, J.W., Poor, C.L., and Dietz, J.M. 1988. Factors affecting the bioavailability of vitamin A, carotenoids and vitamin E. *Food Technol.*, 42: 214–221.

European Commission Administrative Guidance on Submission for Safety Evaluation of Substances Added for Special Nutritional Purposes in the Manufacture of Foods, September, 2009, Food Law, Nutrition and Labeling Unit.

Food and Drug Administration Modernization Act. 1997 (FDAMA).

FSA, 2003. Safe upper levels for vitamins and minerals, Report of the expert group on vitamins and minerals,www.food.gov.uk/multimedia/vitamin 2003.pdf.

Gann, P.H., Ma, J., Giovannucci, W. et al. 1999. Lower prostate cancer risk in men with elevated plasma lycopene levels. Results of a prospective analysis. *Cancer Res.*, 59: 1225–1230.

Gerster, H. 1997. The potential role of lycopene for human health. *J. Am. Coll. Nutr.*, 16: 109–126.

Giovannucci, E. 1999. Tomatoes, tomato-based products, lycopene and cancer: Review of the epidemiologic literature. *J. Natl. Cancer Inst.*, 91: 317–331.

Goel, A., Kunnumakkara, A.B., and Aggarwal, B.B. 2008. Curcumin: From kitchen to clinic. *Biochem. Pharmacol.*, 75: 789–790.

Greenwood, M., Kreider, R.B., Greenwood, L., and Byars, A. 2003. Cramping and injury incidence in collegiate football players are reduced by creatine supplementation. *J. Ath. Train*, 38: 216–219.

Hadley, P. and Schwartz, S.J. 2005. Lycopene. In: *Encyclopedia of Dietary Supplements*, Eds. P. Coates, M. Blackman, G. Craig et al. New York, NY: Marcel Dekker, pp. 421–434.

Hadley, C.W., Schwartz, S.J., and Clinton, S.K., 2003. The consumption of processed tomato products enhances plasma lycopene concentrations in association with a reduced lipoprotein sensitivity to oxidative damage. *J. Nutr.*, 133: 727–732.

Handleman, J., Dratz, C.C., and Van Kujik. 1992. Measurements of carotenoids in human and monkey retinas. In: *Methods in Enzymology*, Ed. L. Packer. New York, NY: Academic Press, 213A, pp. 220–230.

Harris, R., Dunnett, M., and Greenhaf, F.1998. Carnosine and taurine contentsin individual fibres of human muscle. *J. Sports Sci.*, 16: 639–643.

Hennekens, C.H., Buring, J.F., Manson, J.F. et al. 1996. Lack of effect of long-term supplementation with beta carotene on the incidence of malignant neoplasms and cardiovascular disease. *N. Engl. J. Med.*, 334: 1145–1149.

Hirovonen, J., Arteaga, C., Risko, H., and Harkonen, K. 1987. Breakdown of high energy phosphate compounds and lactate accumulation during short supramaximal exercise. *Eur. J. Appl. Physiol.*, 285: 253–259.

Hogstrom, M., Nordstrom, P., and Nordstrom, A. 2007. Fatty acids are positively associated with peak bone mineral density and bone accrual in healthy men: The NO_2 study. *Am. J. Clin. Nutr.*, 85, 803–807.

Howe, P.R., Downing, J.A., Grenyer, B.F., Grigonis-Deane, E.M., and Bryden, W.L. 2002. Tuna fish-meal as a source of DHA for n-3 PUFA enrichment of pork, chicken and eggs. *Lipids*, 37: 1067–1076.

Jacobson, T.A. 2007. Beyond lipids: The role of omega-3 fatty acids from fish oil in the prevention of coronary heart disease. *Curr. Atheroscler. Report*, 9: 145–153.

Joe, B., Vijaykumar, M., and Lokesh B.R. 2004. Biological properties of curcumin—Cellular and molecular mechanism. *Crit. Rev. Food Sci. Nutr.*, 44: 97–111.

Jones, P.J.H. and Krubow, S. 1999. Lipids, sterols and their metabolites. In: *Modern Nutrition in Health and Disease*, Eds. M.E. Shils et al. 9th edn. Philadelphia: Lippincott, Williams and Wilkins, pp. 67–94.

Kagawa, Y., Nishizawa, M., and Suzuki, M. 1982. Eicosopolyenoic acid of serum lipids in Japanese islanders with low incidence of cardiovascular disease. *J. Nutr. Sci. Vitaminol.*, 28: 444–453.

Kaplan, L.A., Lau, J.M., and Stein, E.A. 1990. Carotenoid composition, concentration and relationships in various human organs, *Cell. Physiol. Biochem.*, 8: 1–10.

Kavanaugh, C.J., Trumbo, P.R., and Elwood, K.C. 2007. FDA'S evidence based review of qualified health claims: Tomatoes lycopene and cancer. *J. Natl. Cancer Inst.*, 99: 1074–1085.

Khachik, F., Bertram, J.S., Huang, M.T., Fahey, J.W., and Talalay, P. 1999. Dietary carotenoids and their metabolites as potentially useful chemo protective agents against cancer. In: *Antioxidant* Eds. *Food Supplement in Human Health*, Eds. L. Packer et al. London: Academic Press, pp. 203–29.

Klipstein-Grobusch, K., Launer, L.J., Geleijnse, J.M., Boeing, H., Hofman, A., and Witteman, J.C.M. 2000. Serum carotenoids and atherosclerosis, The Rotterdam study. *Atherosclerosis*, 148: 49–56.

Kohlmeir, I., Kark, J.D., Gomez-Gracia, E. et al. 1997. Lycopene and myocardial infarction risk in the EURAMIC study. *Am. J. Epidemiol.*, 146: 618–626.

Kozuke, N., Han, J.S., and Kozuke, E. et al. 2005. Analysis of eight capsaicinoids in peppers and pepper-containing foods. *J. Agr. Food Chem.*, 53: 9172–9181.

Kris-Etherton, P.M., Harris, W.S., and Appel, L.J. 2002. Fish consumption, fish oil, omega-3 fatty acids, and cardiovascular disease. *Circulation*, 106: 2747–2757.

Kristal, A.R., Arnold, K.B., Neuhouer, M.L. et al. 2010. Dietary supplements use and prostate risk: Results from the prostate cancer prevention trial. *Am. J. Epideiol.*, 172: 566–677.

Kritchevsky, S.B. 1999. Beta-carotene, carotenoids and the prevention of coronary heart disease. *J. Nutr.*, 129: 5–8.

Kun, Y., Lule, U.S, and Xiao-Lin, D. 2006. Lycopene: Its properties and relationship to human health. *Food Rev. Intl.*, 22: 309–333.

Landrum, J.T., Bone, R.A., Moore, L., and Gomez, C. 1992. Analysis of zeaxanthin distribution within individual human retinas. In: *Methods in Enzymology*, Ed. L. Packer, New York: Academic Press, 213A, pp. 457–467.

Landrum, J.T., Bone, R.A., Kilburn, M.D., Joa, H., and Gomez, C. 1996. Dietary lutein supplementation increases macular pigment. *FASEB. J.*, 10: A242.

Landrum, J.T. and Bone, R.A. 2001. Lutein, zeaxanthin and the macular pigment. *Arch. Biochem., Biophys.*, 385: 28–40.

Lemaitre, R.N., King, I.B., Mozaffarin, D., Kuller, L.H., Tracy, R.P., and Siscovick. D.S. 2002. N-3 polyunsaturated fatty acids, fatal ischemic heart disease and non-fatal myocardial infarction in older adults. The cardiovascular health study. *Am. J. Clin. Nutr.*, 76, 319–325.

Levy, J., Bosin, E., and Fedman, B. 1995. Lycopene is more potent inhibitor of human cancer cell proliferation than either alpha-carotene or beta-carotene. *Nutr. Cancer*, 24: 257–266.

Lewis, N.M., Seburg, S., and Flanagan, N.L. 2000. Enriched eggs as a source of n-3 polyunsaturated fatty acids for humans. *Poult. Sci.*, 79: 971–974.

Ling, W.H. and Jones, P.J.H. 1995. Dietary phytosterols: A review of metabolism, benefits and side effects. *Life Sci.*, 57: 195–206.

Lu, Q.Y., Hung, J.C., and Heber, D. 2001 Inverse associations between plasma lycopene and other carotenoids and prostate cancer. *Cancer Epidemiol. Biomarkers Prev.*, 10: 749–756.

Mangels, A.R., Holden, R., Beecher, G.R. et al. 1993. Carotenoid content of fruits and vegetables: An evaluation of analytical data. *J. Am. Diet. Assoc.*, 93: 284–296

Matthews-Roth, M.M. 1991. Recent progress in the medical application of carotenoids. *Pure and Appl. Chem.* 63: 147–156.

Matulka, R. A., Hood, A. M., and Griffths, J.C. 2004. Safety evaluation of natural tomato oleoresin extract derived from food-processing tomatoes. *Regul. Toxicol. Pharmacol.*, 39: 390–402.

Metcalf, R.G., James, M.J., Mantzioris, E., and Cleland, L.G. 2003. A practical approach to increasing intakes of n-3 polyunsaturated fatty acids: Use of novel foods enriched with n-3 fats. *Eur. J. Clin. Nutr.*, 57: 1605–1612.

Moreau, R.S., Whitaker, B.D., and Hicks, K.B. 2002. Phytosterols, phytostanols and their conjugates in foods: Structural diversity, quantitative analysis, and health promoting uses. *Prog. Lipid Res.*, 41: 457–500.

Mori, T.A., Puddey, I.B., Burke, V. et al. 2000. Effect of omega-3 fatty acids on oxidative stress in humans: GC-MS measurement of urinary F2-isoprostane excretion. *Redox. Rep.*, 5: 45–46.

Nagasawa, H., Mitamura, T., Sakamoto, S., and Yamamoto, K. 1995. Effects of lycopene on spontaneous mammary tumor development in SHN virgin mice. *Anticancer Res.*, 15: 1173–1178.

Nagata,C., Shimuzu, C., Takami,R., Takeda, N., and Yasuda, K. 1999. Hot flashes and other menopausal symptoms in relation to soy product intake in Japanese women. *Climacteric*, 2: 6–12.

Nagata, C., Takatsuka, N., Kawakami, N., and Shimizu, H. 2001. Soy product intake and hot flashes in Japanese women: Results from a community based prospective study. *Am. J. Epidemiol.*, 153: 790–793.

Nguyen, M.L. and Schwartz, S.J. 2000. Lycopene. In: *Natural Food Colorants*, Eds. G.L. Lauro, and F.J. Francis, New York: Marcel Dekker, pp. 153–192.

Nutrition Labeling and Education Act 1990 (NLEA) and DSHEA. 1994.

Olson, J. A. 1996. Benefits and liabilities of vitamin A and carotenoids. *J. Nutr.,* 126: 1208–1212.

Omenn, G.S., Goodman, G.E., Thornquist, M.D. et al. 1996. Combination of beta-carotene and vitamin A on lung cancer and cardiovascular disease. *N. Engl. J. Med.*, 334: 1150–1155.

Ostlund, R.E., Racette, S.B., Okeke, A., and Stenson, W.F. 2002. Phytosterols that are naturally present in commercial corn oil significantly reduce cholesterol absorption in humans. *Am. J. Clin. Nutr.*, 75: 1000–1004.

Pelz, R., Schmidt-Faber, B., and Heseker, H. 1998. Carotenoid intake in the German National Food Consumption Survey. *Z. Ernahrungswiss.*, 37: 319–327.

Prasad, K.N. and Edwards-Prasad, J. 1990. Experiments of some molecular cancer risk factors and their modification by vitamins. *J. Am. Coll. Nutr.*, 9: 28–34.

Rao, A.V., Waseem, Z., and Agarwal, S. 1998. Lycopene content of tomatoes and tomato products and their contribution to dietary lycopene, *Food Res. Int.*, 31: 737–741.

Rapala, J.M., Virtamo, J., Ripatti, S. et al. 1997. Randomized trial of alpha-tocopherol and beta-carotene supplements on incidence of major coronary event in men with previous myocardial infarction. *Lancet*, 349: 1715–1720.

Salen, G., Ahrens Jr., E.H., and Grundy, S.M. 1970. Metabolism of beta-sitosterol in man. *J. Clin. Invest.*, 49: 952–967.

Schmitz, H.H., Poor, C.L., Wellman, R. B., and Erdman, J.W. 1991. Concentrations of selected carotenoids and vitamin A in human liver, kidney and lung tissues. *J. Nutr.*, 121: 1613–1621.

Setchell, K.D., Brown, N.M., Zimmer-Nechemirs, L. et al. 2002. Evidence for lack of absorption of soy isoflavone glycosides in humans supporting the crucial role of intestinal metabolism for bioavailability. *Am. J. Clin. Nutr.* 76: 447–453.

Scott, K.J. and Hart, D.J. 1995. Development and evaluation of an HPLC method for the analysis of carotenoids in foods and the measurement of the carotenoid content of vegetables and fruits. *Food Chem.*, 54: 1101–1111.

Scott, K.J., Thurnhanm, D.I., Hart, D.J., Bingham, S.A., and Day, K. 1996. The correlation between the intake of lutein, lycopene and beta-carotene from vegetables and fruits and blood plasma concentrations in a group of women aged 50–65 years in the UK. *Br. J. Nutr.*, 75: 409–418.

Sesso, H.D., Liu, S., Gaziano, J.M., and Buring, J.E. 2003. Dietary lycopene, tomato-based food products and cardiovascular disease in women. *J. Nutr.*, 133: 2336–2341.

Shoba, G., Joy, D., Joseph, T., Majeed, M. et al. 1998. Influence of piperine on the pharmacokinetics of curcumin in animals and human volunteers. *Planta Med.*, 64: 353–356.

Sies, H. and Stahl, W. 1998. Lycopene: Antioxidant and biological effects and its bioavailability in humans. *Proc. Soc. Exp. Biol. Med.*, 218: 121–124.

Simopoulos, A.P., Leaf, A., and Salem, N. Jr. 2000. Workshop statement of the essentiality of and recommended dietary intakes for omega-6 and omega-3 fatty acids. *Prostag. Leuko. Ess. FAs.*, 63: 119–121.

Simopoulos. A.P. 1989. Summary of the NATO advanced research workshop on dietary omega-3 and omega-6 fatty acids: Biological effects and nutritional essentiality. *J. Nutr.*, 119: 521–528.

Siscovick, D.S., Raghunathan, T.E., King, I. et al. 1995. Dietary intake and cell membrane levels of long-chain n-3 polyunsaturated fatty acids and the risk of primary cardiac arrest. *J. Am. Med. Assoc.*, 274: 1363–1367.

Snodderly, D.M. 1995. Evidence for protection against age-related macular degeneration by carotenoids. *Am. J. Clin. Nutr.*, 62: 1448S–1461S.

Stahl, W. and Sies, H. 1992. Uptake of lycopene and its geometrical isomers is greater from heat-processed than from unprocessed tomato juice in humans. *J. Nutr.*, 122: 2161–2166.

Stahl, W. and Sies, H.1996. Lycopene: A biologically important carotenoid for humans. *Arch. Biochem. Biophys.*, 336: 1–9.

Straub, O. 1987. *Key to Carotenoids*, 2nd edn. Basel: Berkhauser Verlag.

Strimpakos, A.S. and Sharma, R.A. 2008. Curcumin: Preventive and therapeutic properties in Laboratory studies and clinical trials. *Antioxid. Redox. Signal*, 10: 511–545.

The Alpha-Tocopherol, Beta-Carotene Cancer Prevention Study Group. 1994 The effect of vitamin E and beta-carotene on the incidence of lung cancer and other cancer in male smokers. *N. Engl. J. Med.*, 330: 1029–1035.

Thurnham, D.I., Tremel, A., Howard, A.N. et al. 2007. Macular zeaxanthin and lutein—A review of dietary sources and bio-availability and some relationship with macular pigment optical density and age-related macular disease. *Nutr. Res. Rev.*, 20: 163–179.

Thurnham, D.I., Tremel, A., and Howard, A.N. 2008. A supplementation study in human subjects with a combination of meso-zeaxanthin, (3R,3′R)-Zeaxanthin and (3R,3′R,6′R)-Lutein. *Brit. J. Nutr.*, 100: 1307–1314.

Van Breemen, R.B., Xu, M.A., Viana, L., Chen, M., and Bowen, P.E. 2002. LC-MS of cis- and trans-lycopene in human serum and prostate tissue after dietary supplementation with tomato sauce. *J. Agr. Food Chem.*, 50: 2214–2219.

Vivekanathan, D.P., Penn, M.S., Sapp, S.K., Hsu, A., and Topol, E.J. 2003. Use of antioxidant vitamins for the prevention of cardiovascular disease: Meta-analysis of randomized trials. *Lancet*, 361: 2017–2023.

Walzem, R.L., Dillard, C.J., and German, J.B. 2002. Whey components: Millennia of evolution create functionalities for mammalian nutrition. *Crit. Rev. Food Sci. Nutr.*, 42: 353–375.

Zhang, X., Shu, X.O., Gao, Y.T. et al. 2003. Soy food consumption is associated with lower risk of coronary heart disease in Chinese women. *J. Nutr.*, 133: 2874–2878.

4 Innovation in Food Safety and Regulation

Kalpagam Polasa and B. Sesikeran

CONTENTS

As mankind has evolved from hunter gatherer to civilized *Homo sapiens* of this era, there has been steady change in his lifestyle including his occupation. The twenty-first century has witnessed transition from agriculture as main source of income to industry-based occupation. One of the booming industries of the modern era is the food industry particularly the food processing industry.

Food ranks topmost in the basic need of man. It is required for normal functioning of body and for healthy growth. Food which is composed of carbohydrates, water, fats, proteins, vitamins, and minerals is eaten or drunk for nutrition or pleasure.

Food safety concern deals with supply of food that is safe for the consumer. Rising liberalization of agro-industrial markets and the worldwide integration of food supply chains require new approaches and systems for assessing food safety. Food processors and retailers are sourcing their ingredients worldwide and it can be hard to track the source or produce of a particular ingredient. Retailers buy their produce from all over the globe. International trade in high-value food products (fresh and processed fruits and vegetables, fish, live animals and meat, nuts and spices) has expanded enormously in the last 25 years. Presently, concern for food safety is one of the topmost priorities of all the countries across the globe. This concern is ever increasing with every new report on unsafe food ingredient or food itself linking their consumption to animal or human adverse health effect (Arthur, 2002).

According to WHO (1984), food safety can be defined as the assurance that food will not cause harm to the consumer when it is prepared or eaten according to its intended use. The food safety encompasses safety of the food at every step in the food cycle from production, processing at farm level, storage, transportation, distribution, retail, and preparation of food at household or establishments (Robert [Skip] and Steward, 2003a).

4.1   IMPACT OF GLOBAL TRENDS ON FOOD SAFETY

Food business in the new economy is a global business. Food that is produced in one part of the world is being processed, distributed, and consumed in different parts of the world. This regional, national, and global food chain has required parallel changes in food science and technology including food preservation. Environmental changes like climate change also impact food safety by altering the microbial ecology of the environment accompanied with emergence of newer food pathogens, which are not contained within a single country (Lichtenberg, 2003). Increased food export and import as a result of globalization has compounded the safety problems.

4.2   FOOD SAFETY ISSUES

They are broadly classified as biological, chemical, and physical. The biological hazards are living microorganisms and parasites. The chemical hazards are naturally occurring poisons and other chemicals which include additives, colors, flavors, dry residues, fertilizers, pesticides, food contact material, and packaging materials. The physical contaminations are glass, hair, metal, stones, wood, plastic, bone, and so on. Heavy metals like lead, cadmium, arsenic, and pollutants resulting from human activity occur as contaminants in food (Robert [Skip] and Steward, 2003b).

4.3   FOOD SAFETY AND NUTRITION

Food is essential for sustenance of life and well being. The basic concepts of nutrition are undergoing transformation. The age-old idea of an "adequate diet" to provide enough nutrients to ensure survival of an individual has become obsolete. The current trend is to replace the concept of "adequate nutrition" with "optimum nutrition." The terms like "functional foods," "foods for specific health use," or "specific health-promoting foods" have been coined suggesting that foods may have a beneficial action on certain functions in the organisms that goes beyond their nutritional effects (Polasa and Sudershan Rao, 2009).

Nutrients are now being used not only to correct the nutrient deficiencies, but also for other functions. This has led to the development of products collectively called as "nutraceuticals." The Indian nutraceuticals market estimated at Rs. 440 crores which is <1% of world market estimated at Rs. 51,480 crores is in its infancy. However, the Indian nutraceuticals market is estimated to have grown 18% Cumulative Annual Growth Rate (CAGR) in last 3 years compared to the world market of 7% (CAGR) (Ernst and Young/FICCI, 2009). The nutritional needs are nutrition deficiency needs, disease or condition-specific needs, and achievement needs. Nutrition deficiency needs stem out of not getting proper nutrition (micro- and macronutrients) in the balanced proportion required for development of body and normal physiological functions. Malnutrition is quite a common phenomenon in India. Disease or condition-specific needs are due to disease or certain conditions. This may be due to the reason that either the body is not able to make nutrition available to the system to meet the normal requirement or the requirement itself has gone up. Achievement need is that excess nutrition is required under certain conditions (Polasa and Sudershan Rao, 2009).

4.4   NUTRACEUTICALS IN DEMAND

These may be categorized into three categories. They are functional foods, functional beverages, and dietary supplements. Functional food is a generic term that has been linked to health benefits. In India, functional food and functional beverages have started gaining momentum because of aggressive marketing by the fast-moving consumer goods players (Ernst and Young/FICCI, 2009). Some of nutraceuticals that are marked in India are products enriched with micronutrients and functional ingredients having therapeutic or medicinal value, dietary supplements in powder or liquid forms, functional ingredients in capsule form, ready to drink beverages, and so on (Ernst and Young/FICCI, 2009). The three important parameters which decide the salability of food product are consumers' taste preferences, health claims, and convenience (Gibson and Williams, 2003).

4.5   REGULATION

Functional foods do not possess clear cut legal definition and it is difficult to decide whether a new product should be labeled as food, supplement, or drug. These categories are regulated differently in different countries (Hasler, 2005).

The regulatory authorities face the challenge that has arisen from growing scientific understanding about the role of diet nutrients and bioactive non-nutrients in foods and the development of concept of optimum nutrition that would benefit an individual, including prevention of disease. The health claim is different from nutrient consent claim or nutrient functional claim and in many countries falls into the gray regulatory area between food and medicinal claims. Japan is the only country which has defined these foods under "Foods for Specified Health Uses (FOSHU)." The health claim can be of two types. A "generic" health claim is a claim that can be applied to a range of food stuffs, while a "product-specific" health claim applies to a single product or product range. The claim can be "direct," that is the food itself has some property or can be an indirect claim, that is, food having a particular ingredient has some beneficial property (Hasler, 2005).

4.6   INDIAN REGULATION

The concept of using foods as health supplements are clearly dealt in Ayurveda and many products are prescribed in Indian traditional medical practice. These are available to consumers directly as over the counter (OTC) drugs without medical prescription. Labeling and strict control over formulations and branding are not required for most products. The functional foods, nutraceuticals novel foods, and so on are dealt in Section 4.5 of the New Food Safety and Standard Act 2006.

These products will be approved by specific scientific panel. The framework for regulation is given in the new Act.

According to the Act, foods for special dietary uses or functional foods or nutraceuticals or health supplement means foods that are specifically processed to meet particular dietary requirement due to specified disease/disorder and the composition of this product may differ significantly from composition of ordinary food comparable by nature. These products cannot claim to cure or mitigate any disease or disorder in the label except for certain health benefit as may be permitted by the regulations made under this Act.

Different countries have made various approaches to use of health claims on functional foods. However, the central theme seems to be that any health claim can be made only on sound scientific substantiation and validation. The global consensus is that the regulatory authority must protect the consumer, promote fair trade, and encourage innovation in the food industry (Polasa and Sudershan Rao, 2009).

4.7 GENETICALLY MODIFIED FOODS

These are foods that are developed and marketed because there is some perceived advantage either to the producer or consumer of these foods. The objective is to produce food which will have lower price and greater benefit (in terms of nutrition or cultivation etc.). The aim was also to improve the crop protection. These plants are resistant to insects, pests, diseases, viruses, and or may be tolerant to herbicides.

4.8 SAFETY ASSESSMENT OF GM FOODS

Consumers are of the view that the traditional foods are safe, whereas the GM foods are viewed with caution. All the national authorities consider that specific assessments are necessary. Specific guidelines have been framed for rigorous evaluation of GM organisms and GM foods relative to both human/animal health and the environment. These types of testing are not performed for traditional foods (Kuiper et al., 2002). Hence there is a significant difference in the evaluation process prior to marketing for these two types of foods. One of the objectives of the WHO Food Safety Program (FAO/WHO, 1991; FAO, 2003) is to assist national authorities in the identification of foods that should be subject to risk assessment including GM foods, and to recommend correct assessments.

4.9 DETERMINATION OF POTENTIAL RISKS TO HUMAN HEALTH (FAO, 2003)

Some of the important points in determining the risks are

1. Direct health effects (toxicity)
2. Tendencies to induce allergic reaction (allergenicity)
3. Specific constituents that may have nutritional/toxic properties
4. Stability of inserted gene
5. Changes in nutrient composition associated with genetic modification
6. Any unintended effects due to genetic modification

4.10 RISK TO ENVIRONMENT (FAO, 2003)

Issues of concern are mainly on the capability of the genetically modified organisms (GMO) to escape and introduce the engineered genes into natural plants, persistence of the GMO, susceptibility of nontarget organisms to the gene product, stability of the gene, and loss of biodiversity.

4.11   SAFETY OF GM FOODS

GM foods are assessed for safe on case-to-case basis. The GM foods which are approved internally are being consumed in some countries and no adverse effects have been reported. Continuous use of risk assessments based on the codex principles and postmarket surveillance is mostly the basis for evaluating the safety of GM foods (Codex, 2003; FAO, 2003).

4.12   REGULATION INDIA

In India GM foods are regulated under the Environment Protection Act (1986) Rules. These rules are called the Rules for the Manufacture, Use, Import, Export, and Storage of Hazardous Microbes, Genetically Engineered Organisms. The Genetic Engineering Approval Committee (GEAC) has been authorized as the interministerial body under the Ministry of Environment and Forests to be the authority to permit any manufacture, use, import, export, and storage of hazardous microbes and GMOs. In practice, it is the Review Committee on Genetic Manipulation (RCGM) under the Department of Biotechnology that is currently permitting limited field trials and imports of GM material for research purposes. These are also guidelines that have been prepared for experimentation and release (FSSAI, 2010).

There are prescribed formats for import and use of GMO's which will be reviewed by the regulators. There are some GM crops namely GM potato, GM mustard, GM brinjal, and GM rice which are waiting for approvals at various stages.

4.13   ORGANIC FOODS

These foods refer to the plants that have been cultivated without using chemical fertilizers, pesticides and insecticides hormones, and antibiotics. Organic farming does not cause soil erosion or damage to the environment although the yield may be reduced. The labelings of foods as organic-specialized inspectors for the certification visit the farm annually and check the farm site and the records that have been maintained by the farm foods that are labeled as 100% organic must have only organically grown components except for added water and salt foods that are labeled organic need to have at least 95% organic ingredients except for added water and salt. Products that claim made with organic ingredients must contain at least 70% organic ingredients except for added water and salt (Codex, 1999).

4.14   SAFE FOOD MANUFACTURE

India is one of the important food producers in the world and Indian food-processing industry is one of the largest industries in the country. The Indian food industry is estimated to be of value of USD 200 billion and is expected to grow to USD 310 billion by 2015. The Indian food-processing industry is worth estimate if USD 70 billion (Ernst and Young/FICCI, 2009). The Ministry of Food Processing, Government of India has identified the following segments within the food-processing industry. They are (i) dairy, fruits and vegetable processing, (ii) grain processing, (iii) meat and poultry processing, (iv) fish cultivation, and (v) packaged foods, beverages, and packaged drinking water. The primary food processing (packed fruits and vegetables, flour, rice, tea, spices, milk, etc.) constitutes nearly 60% of processed foods. The dairy sector ranks first in terms of processed foods with several products namely dairy whitener, cheese, ice-cream, butter, and clarified butter. The market is expected to grow at 15–20% over the next 3 years (Annual Report, Ministry of Food Procuring, GOI, 2003–2004).

India produces the widest range of fruits and vegetables in the world. Major processed items are fruit pulps and juices, fruit-based beverages, canned fruits and vegetables, jams, squashes, pickles, and dehydrated products. Other processing industries are those pertaining to meat and poultry, marine products, grain and production of beer, and other alcoholic beverages (Annual Report, Ministry of Food Procuring, GOI, 2003–2004).

4.15 CONSUMER FOODS

Packaged ready to eat, ready to cook products constitute this segment. Packaged drinking water, aerated drinks, and alcoholic beverages also belong to this sector (Annual Report, Ministry of Food Procuring, GOI, 2003–2004).

4.16 DRIVERS OF GROWTH AND CONSTRAINTS TO INNOVATION

This sector will flourish in the years to come due to changing lifestyles, food habits, thrust on organized food retail, and urbanization. Due to changes in lifestyle habits, there has been progressive and notable change in consumption pattern in India. Presently the growth rates for fruits, vegetables, meats, and dairy have risen significantly. In developed nations, more of processed and convenience foods are in demand. There is also an increasing demand for organic, functional, and diet foods.

Some of the adversaries for growth of food-processing industry in India are poor infrastructure in terms of cold storage, warehousing, improper quality systems and testing facilities, inefficient supply chain and too many middle men in food chain, high cost of transportation and inventory carrying cost, religious taboos, cultural preferences, economics such as cost, tax, and so on.

4.17 CRITICAL FACTORS IN FOOD-PROCESSING INDUSTRY

Although the Indian food-processing industry's growth potential cannot be disputed, certain key factors will promote the expansion. Quality maintenance throughout the production cycle will improve yield as well as ensure long shelf life. In case of vegetables, fruits, and other perishables precooking facilities, controlled atmospheric storage and radiation facilities will ensure quality. In order to increase market penetration competitiveness and product innovation could be key factors. Innovation in production, packaging, and product usage are other desirable factors (Annual Report, Ministry of Food Procuring, GOI, 2003–2004).

4.18 FOOD SAFETY IN FOOD PROCESSING

Regulators all over the world are concerned with microbial contaminants such as *Escherichia coli 0157:H7, Listeria monocytogenes*, and other pathogens in foods. This has led to the development of Hazard Analysis Critical Control Points (HACCPs) system in food-processing units. This program is generally tailor made to each processing facility to ensure safety of a particular product by identifying, monitoring, verifying, and controlling critical-processing steps. Traditionally food safety control measures were to conduct microbiological testing of finished products and their ingredients. This system is now replaced with automated online control systems to monitor safety and hygiene as per a definite plan. The microbial evaluation of finished goods are carried out by using rapid monitoring methods using adenosine triphosphate (ATP) bioluminescence electrical monitoring, antibody-based assays, and DNA and RNA probes.

4.19 HAZARD ANALYSIS CRITICAL CONTROL POINT AND GOOD MANUFACTURING PRACTICE (CODEX, 2003)

HACCP is a management system in which food safety is addressed through the analysis and control of biological, chemical, and physical hazards from the time of raw materials production, procurement and handling to manufacturing distribution, and consumption of finished food. This system is an effective system to ensure food safety. Briefly this method follows the following steps (Codex, 2003):

1. Conduct the hazard analysis.
2. Determine the critical control points (CCPs).
3. Establish the critical limit for each step.
4. Establish a system to monitor control of each CCP.
5. Establish the corrective action to be taken when monitoring indicates that a particular CCP is not under control.
6. Establish the procedures for verification to confirm that the HACCP system is working effectively.
7. Establish the record keeping and documentation procedures.

4.20   PREREQUISITE PROGRAMS

The production of safe food requires that HACCP must be based on prerequisite programs. These provide the basic environmental and operating conditions required for production of safe food. The practices and basic conditions required for producing foods intended for international trade is given in the *Codex Alimentarius General Principles of Food Hygiene*. The industries adopt procedures that are specific to their operations of which some may be proprietary. The prerequisite programs also are concerned with ensuring the suitability and wholesomeness of the foods for consumption. These programs are assessed during the design and implementation of each HACCP plan and are documented, audited, and managed separately from the HACCP plan. Sometimes some aspects of prerequisite programs may be incorporated into the HACCP plan. Some of the examples of prerequisite plan are vendor evaluation, site plan, floor plan, designs of equipment, specification of packaging materials, ramification in production environment, personal hygiene and health of personals, training of all employees, and most of all the commitment of the top management to HACCP program (Codex, 2003).

Computer software is widely used to manage data and in food safety management. Computer-based HACCP development software can help in saving time, reducing documents, sharing information, keeping the HACCP data organized, and helping in giving technical inputs on food safety hazards, controlling measures monitoring, and verification procedures (Lund et al., 2000).

4.21   HACCP AND ISO

HACCP and ISO can be both followed by a unit. HACCP focuses on product safety while the ISO standards focus on the overall quality management system. Established ISO compliant quality management system can be of advantage to implement HACCP plan.

4.22   HACCP AND GMP

Undoubtedly HACCP programs are designed and implemented to produce safe food and are preventive plans. However, the HACCP programs cannot guarantee that all foods will be safe. The GMPs include all the conditions required for manufacturing, packaging, or maintaining food hygiene in the manufacturing unit with proper facility, machinery design, and maintenance. The Standard Operating Procedures (SOPs) recall procedures; traceability must be established prior to implementation of successful HACCP programs. Some of the key factors in GMP are use of good quality raw materials that are contaminant free, hygienically maintained equipment and their periodic sanitization, sterile air in environs of processing area, and training personnel to use safe food-handling practices (Codex, 2003).

4.23   PRODUCT RECALL, TRACEABILITY, AND SURVEILLANCE

Foodborne diseases are an important cause of morbidity and mortality. WHO is promoting laboratory-based surveillance of foodborne diseases in all countries. In cooperation with its member states, WHO is working to support the development of internationally agreed upon guidelines for data collection in countries (Codex, 2006).

In the United States, Centre for Disease Prevention Centre (CDC) is responsible for nationwide surveillance of outbreaks and tracking new and emerging pathogens. In India, foodborne diseases are not categorized separately in the Health Information of India. At present, the occurrence of food poisoning is reported to the food health authorities. Surveillance for foodborne illnesses would involve epidemiological investigation, environmental and laboratory analysis of incriminating food. In India systematic surveillance system has to be established along with an early warning system. Food net sites and networking are required for establishing rapid alert system. This exists in all developed nations. The food laboratories must be equipped with state-of-the-art technology including DNA finger printing to identify the infectious agents and to trace the source with the cooperation by epidemiologists and food safety scientists. Strict implementation of HACCP and preventive measures are to be made to address public health problems. These tasks would include inspection procedures, sampling, and analytical methods. In 2010, eggs worth several millions were recalled due to reported presence of *Salmonella* in the United States and presence of hepatitis A in frozen strawberries is another example (FDA, 2011).

4.24   TECHNOLOGICAL ADVANTAGES AND FOOD SAFETY

Newer packaging and processing techniques can be used to extend shelf life of many packaged foods. Packaging has undergone some innovative product developments to ensure food safety as certain components of packing such as printing inks, labels, colors, and seals can affect food quality. The deterioration of packaged food occurs through transfer of these components into foods. The atmosphere surrounding the food also influences its shelf life, for example, high temperatures, humidity, undesirable odor from environment may affect the food quality (Rupp, 2003).

Innovative packaging such as vacuum packaging, controlled atmosphere packaging (CAP), or modified atmosphere packaging (MAP) involves sealing package under vacuum or one time gas flushing and sealing. Three types of gases are used singly or in combination, namely, nitrogen, carbon dioxide, and oxygen (Rooney, 2003).

Active packaging includes additives capable of scavenging or absorbing oxygen, carbon dioxide, moisture, odor, and flavors. This may be in powder (of iron and calcium hydroxide) form in sachet. Intelligent packaging provides a means to monitor and relay information regarding the status of contents and verifies information. Food-packaging manufacturers have developed several innovative intelligent packages that include time, temperature indicators, antitheft, and use of radio-frequency identification (RFID) methods.

4.25   MIGRATION OF FOOD CONTACT MATERIALS

These may be from utensils or materials used during processing. The extent of migration of packaging material into food matrix depends on nature of material. The migration of chemicals from inks, plastics, and other materials such as cardboard, and so on, can import undesirable flavors and can be potentially toxic. In processing units, it could be the equipments, stainless steel drums, rubber, plastics, concrete, mesh belts, soft metals, and cheap quality ceramics with paint. Ceramics which are of poor quality may result in leaching of lead and other heavy metals particularly when in contact with acidic beverages such as fruit juices. Cans with lead-soldered seams are source of not only lead but also other metals such as tin, cadmium, and chromium.

4.26   FOOD LABELING

Codex Alimentarius has documented guidelines to be followed by food industry internationally. The label is supposed to describe the product, list all the ingredients, provide nutritional information, approved health claims, best before or use by date, storage conditions, place of origin, and instructions for use. There must be either bar code or batch identifier and standard specification especially for those of microbial heavy metals, pesticides preservatives, flavorings, and food colors limits (Codex, 1985, 1997).

Consumers must be able to make their choice of foods and buy according to their requirements. The regulatory agency of every country monitors food labels on packed foods in order to prevent mislabeling or misdescription of food. Although mislabeling may not cause safety issues, it is construed as fraud.

The FSSA Act 2006 of India defines labeling as "labeling includes any written, printed, or graphic matter that is present on the label accompanying the food." Regulation requires (i) every prepackaged food to carry a label, (ii) prepackaged food shall not be described or presented on any label in a manner that is false, misleading, or deceptive or is likely to create erroneous impression regarding its character in any respect, (iii) label in prepackaged food to be applied in such a manner that they will not be separated from the container, and (iv) contents of the label shall be clear, prominent, and legible. The Act also gives other details on distribution, sale, and packaging conditions.

In the USA, the nutritional labeling rules are given in Nutrition Labeling and Education Act (NLEA, 1990) for most of the foods except meat and poultry and authorizes the use of nutrient content claims based on FDA-approved health claims (FDA, 2009).

4.27   NUTRITION INFORMATION PANEL

Under the labels "Nutrition Facts" panel, manufacturers are required to provide information on certain nutrients. The orders in which they must appear are as per codex guidelines in most of the countries.

The label also gives Daily values in terms of percent and serving sizes. The daily values comprise of two sets of dietary standards; Daily Reference Values (DRVs) and Reference Daily Intakes (RDIs) (Codex, 1997; FSSAI, 2006).

4.28   INNOVATION IN ANALYSIS OF CONTAMINANTS IN FOODS

The development of quick methods to detect microbial pathogens in foods is to prevent foodborne illness and to meet the regulatory and quality standards like HACCP programs. Rapid microbial detection methods are also useful in the recall of contaminated foods. Automated diluters help in preparation of samples fast. Automated plating also aid in distributing liquid samples on to the surface of a rotating prepoured agar plate. Colony-counting systems are in use very widely and the data is fed into the computer. The hydrophobic grid membrane filter (HGMF) technique is a membrane filter to count even low numbers of microorganisms by filtration of large volumes. This can be used for detection of coliforms, *E. coli*, *E. coli* 0157:H7, and *Salmonella*. An example of this system is ISOGRID system (Neogen, Inc., Lansing, MI), which is an automated instrument that can count cells in seconds (Diez-Gonzalez and Karaibrahimoglu, 2005).

Rapid biochemical assays are also available, many of which are validated by AOAC international Immunoassays based on antigen antibody Precipitation, Enzyme Limited Immuno Sorbent Assay (ELISA), immunochromatography, automated immune assays and electro immunoassays, polymerase chain reaction (PCR), and other nuclear acid-based tests are available to detect pathogenic microbes in foods (Diez-Gonzalez and Karaibrahimoglu, 2005).

The PCR, nucleic acid-based techniques, and immune assays are also used to detect genetically modified foods and food allergens. Pesticide residues in foods are a global concern. The regulatory bodies all over the world have monitoring programs to check the residues. Food matrices vary widely in composition and pose challenge to the analyst. The analytical process involves sample preparation, homogenization, extraction, cleanup, concentration, and quantitation. GC, MS, LC/MS methods are used in detection. Efforts are on to develop cost-effective mobile mini lab devices to conduct analysis in the field. Presently QuECHERS method is used for sample preparation followed by automated GC/MS and LC MS–MS analysis (Lehotay and Mastovska, 2005). Other contaminants like polyaromatic compounds (PACs) are analyzed using high-resolution gas chromatography (HRGC), fast gas chromatography (GC), and multidimensional chromatography. Other sophisticated techniques used in food analysis are high-performance liquid chromatography (HPLC), supercritical fluid chromatography (SFC) where supercritical carbon dioxide is the mobile phase and GC or LC detector is used. Spectroscopic techniques based on ultraviolet (UV), visible (Vis), infrared (IR), nuclear magnetic resonance (NMR), atomic absorption and atomic emission (AAS) are used (Hayward, 2005; Tunick, 2005).

Several analytical techniques are available to test the foods and obtain quick and reliable results.

4.29   NANOTECHNOLOGY IN FOOD SAFETY

The word "Nano" is derived from the Greek for "dwarf." A nanometer is a one billionth of a meter (10^{-9} m). Nanoparticles have a size below 100 nm and have unique ability for novel applications and benefits (Dingman, 2008).

Many nanomaterials are used in different food applications. Titanium oxide which has a particle size of <100 nm is widely used as food additive and antimicrobial agent for food-packaging and storage containers. Silver nanoparticles are zinc and zinc oxide used as antimicrobial agents as well as nutritional additives.

Functionalized nanostructure materials are used as novel nanosensors, packaging materials, and for targeted nutrient delivery systems (Alfadul, 2010).

Silicon dioxide and carbon nanoparticles of few hundred nanometer in size are used as food additives and for food packaging. Silver, platinum, and gold nanowires are used as biosensors to improve the food analysis (Dingman, 2008).

4.30   NANOTECHNOLOGY IN FOOD APPLICATION AND PROCESSING

Nanotechnology can be applied to every step in the food cycle from farm to fork. Application of this technology can help in food production processing, packaging, and storage.

The four major areas in food industry that will find extensive nanotechnology application are (i) development of new functional foods, (ii) micro- and nanoscale processing, (iii) product development, and (iv) design of methods and instrumentation for food safety and biosecurity (Moraru et al., 2003).

Probiotics can be nano encapsulated and incorporated in yoghurt, fermented milk, cheese, and fruit-based drinks.

4.31   NANOSENSORS AND PATHOGEN DETECTION

Detection of small quantities of chemical or biological contaminant such as virus, bacteria, or toxin is one more potential use of nanotechnology. Biosensors play an important role in food safety particularly in food-processing system.

The nanoparticles can be tailor made to specifically attack any food pathogen. The advantage of biosensor is that thousands of nanoparticles can be placed on a single nanosensor to quickly and accurately detect the presence of many microbes. The application can be used to detect pathogens in food and water quickly and accurately (Dingman, 2008).

4.32 NANOFOODS

This denotes a food that has been cultivated, produced, processed, or packaged using nanotechnology or to which nanomaterials are added. It has potential applications in foods such as prevention of microbial spoilage, detection of contaminants, enriched or fortified foods, and so on (Dingman, 2008).

4.33 SAFETY OF NANOMATERIALS

Many countries have identified the potential application of nanotechnology in agrifood area. It is a nascent and growing field and market for novel foods with nanocomponents will increase. In this context, it is necessary to prove the safety of these materials on human health. The biological properties including the toxicological effects of nanomaterials are largely dependent on their physicochemical properties, size, shape, and structure. Occupational health risks to people who are involved in handling, manufacture, package, transport of foods, and agricultural products that contain nanoparticles must be monitored (Card et al., 2011). There is an urgent need for regulatory systems worldwide to develop methods to take science-based decisions on safety of nanotechnology-based food applications. In India, as of now, there is no specific regulation for nanomaterials. All packaged foods including novel foods are regulated by the Food Safety and Standard Act of 2006 by the Food Safety and Standard Authority of India.

4.34 CONCLUSIONS

Consumption of nutritious food is important for human survival and well being. Contaminated food has the opposite effect. Food safety is a worldwide issue affecting hundreds of millions of people who suffer from foodborne diseases. According to WHO, it is one of the most widespread health problems and an important cause of reduced economic productivity. In developed nations, consumers are now well aware of food safety issues and in developing nations there is a need to create more awareness.

Innovation in food-processing technology can prove advantageous to the consumers and contribute to food safety. Innovations in production of convenience foods packaged in a manner satisfactory to the consumer are beginning to occupy a center place in food business. Products will have greater likeliness of success when food producers address consumer needs, respond to consumer concerns, and offer tangible benefits.

Communication to consumer plays a pivotal role in determining the acceptance of a given product by consumer. Food labels give all the information that is essential. Factual information, statements (Bruhn, 2008) about safety, and benefits will increase consumer acceptance. Regulation will have major impact on food innovation. It involves exhaustive and complex process and countries all over the world have their national regulatory bodies who are actively engaged in ensuring the safety of foods and face the challenges due to innovations in food safety.

REFERENCES

Alfadul, M. 2010. Use of nanotechnology in food processing, packaging and safety—Review. *African Journal of Food Agriculture Nutrition and Development* 10: 2719–2739.

Annual Report. 2003–04. *Ministry of Food Processing Industries*. Government of India. http://mofpi.nic.in.

Arthur, M.H. 2002. Emerging microbiological food safety issues: Implications for control in the 21st century. *Food Technology* 56(2): 48–51.

Bruhn, C.M. 2008. Consumer and regulatory impacts on food related innovation (Section 3). In editorial. Consumer acceptance of food innovations. *Innovation: Management, Policy and Practice* 10: 91–95.

Card, J.W., Jonaitis, J.W., Tafazoli S., and Magnuson, B.A. 2011. An appraisal of the published literature on the safety and toxicity of food related nanomaterials. *Critical Reviews in Toxicology* 41: 20–49.

Codex. 1985. Codex Stan. 146–1985. General standard for the labeling and claims for prepackaged foods for special dietary uses.

Codex. 1997. CAC/GL 23–1997. Guidelines for use of nutrition and health claims. http://www.codexalimentarus.net.

Codex. 1999. GL32–1999. Guidelines for the production, processing, labeling and marketing of organically produced foods. www.codexalimentarius.net.

Codex. 2003. CAC/AC 45–2003. Guideline for the conduct of food safety assessment of foods derived from recombinant DNA plants. www.codexalimentarius.net.

Codex. 2003. CAC/RCP-1, 1969. Rev.4–2003. Recommended international code of practice general principles of food hygiene. http://codexalimentarius.net.

Codex. 2006. CAC/GL 60–2006. Principles for traceability/product training as a tool within a food inspection and certification system. http://www.codexalimentarius.net.

Diez-Gonzalez Z.F. and Karaibrahimoglu. 2005. Rapid analysis techniques in food microbiology. In *Methods of Analysis of Food Components and Additives*. (Ed.) Otles, S. Chemical and functional properties of food components series. CRC Taylor & Francis, FL, USA.

Dingman, J. 2008. Nanotechnology: Its impact on food safety. *Journal of Environmental Health* 70: 48–50.

Environment Protection Act, India. 1986. www:http://envfor.nic.in/legis/env/env1. html

Ernst and Young/FICCI. 2009. Nutraceuticals critical supplement for building a healthy India. http://www.fubuews.com/article/print.asp?articleid=26111 (accessed on January 12, 2010).

FAO/WHO. 1991. *Strategies for Assessing the Safety of Foods Produced by Biotechnology*. Report of a Joint FAO/WHO Consultation. Geneva, Switzerland, World Health Organization.

FAO. 2003. FAO/WHO Consultation on the Safety assessment of foods derived from genetically modified animals, including fish.

FDA. 2009. Appendix C: Health claims. http://ww.fda.gov/ffodd/guidance Compliance Regulatory Information/ Guidance Documents/ Food Labeling Guide/ucmob4919 htm.

FDA. 2011. Recalls, market withdrawals and safety alerts. http://www.fda.gov/safety/ recalls/default.htm.

Food Safety and Standards Act. 2006. Government of India. www.fssai.gov.in.

Food Safety and Standards Authority of India. 2010. Operationalizing the regulation of genetically modified foods in India. www.fssai.gov.in.

Gibson, G.R. and Williams, C.M. (Eds.) 2003. *Functional Foods, Concept to Product CRC Press*. Woodhead Publishing Ltd., UK.

Hasler, C.M. (Ed) 2005. *Regulation of Functional Foods and Nutraceuticals. A Global Prespective*. IFT Press and Blackwell Publishing, Ames, Iowa, USA.

Hayward, D.C. 2005. Determination of pollutants in foods. In *Methods of Analysis of Food Components and Additives*. (Ed.) Otles, S. Chemical and functional properties of food components series. CRC Taylor & Francis, FL, USA.

Kuiper, H.A., Kleter, G.A., Noteborn, H.P.J.M., and Kok, E.J. 2002. Substantial equivalence—An appropriate paradigm for the safety assessment of genetically modified foods. *Toxicology* 181/182: 427–431.

Lehotay, S.J. and Mastovska, K. 2005. Determination of pesticide residues. In *Methods of Analysis of Food Components and Additives*. (Ed.) Otles, S. Chemical and functional properties of food components series. CRC Taylor & Francis, FL, USA.

Lichtenberg. 2003. Impact of food safety on world trade issues. In *Food Safety Handbook* (Eds.) Schmidt, R.H. and Rodrick, G.E., pp. 725–740. Wiley Interscience, NJ, USA.

Lund, BM., Baird Parker, T.C., and Gould, G.W. (Eds.) 2000. *The Microbiological Safety and Quality of Food*. Volume I. An Aspen Publishers, Inc.

Moraru, C.I., Panchapakesan, C.P., Huang, Q., Takshistov, P., Liu, S., and Kokini, J.L. 2003. Nanotechnology: A new frontier in food science. *Food Technology* 57: 24–29.

NLEA. 1990. http//www.fda.gov/ICECI/Inspectionguides/ucmo74948.htm. Accessed on 20 March 2011.

Polasa, K. and Sudershan Rao, V. 2009. Functional Foods. In *Text Book of Human Nutrition*. (Eds.) Bamji, M.S., Krishnaswamy, K., and Brahmam, G.N.V. Oxford & IBH Publishing Co Pvt. Ltd., New Delhi, India.

Robert (Skip), A. and Steward. I.I. 2003a. Definition of food safety. In *Food Safety Hand Book*. (Eds.) Schmidt R.H. and Rodrick, G.E., pp. 3–9. Wiley Interscience, NJ, USA.

Robert (Skip) A. and Steward. I.I. 2003b. Characterization of food hazards. In *Food Safety Hand Book* (Eds.) Schmidt R.H. and Rodrick, G.E., pp. 3–9. Wiley Interscience, NJ, USA.

Rooney, M.L. 2003. Food safety and innovation food packaging. In *Food Safety Hand Book*. (Eds.) Schmidt R.H. and Rodrick, G.E., pp. 3–9. Wiley Interscience, NJ, USA.

Rupp, H. 2003. Chemical and physical hazards produced during food processing, storage and preparation. In *Food Safety Handbook.* (Eds.) Schmidt R.H. and Rodrick, G.E., pp. 3–9. Wiley Interscience, NJ, USA.

The British Standards Institution. 2011. ISO 22000 Food Safety. http://www.bisgroup.co.in/en-in/Assessment-and certification-services/management-systems/standards-and-schemes/ISO 22000.

Tunick, M.H. 2005. Selection of techniques used in food analysis. In *Methods of Analysis of Food Components and Additives.* (Ed.) Otles, S. Chemical and functional properties of food components series. CRC Taylor & Francis, FL, USA.

World Health Organization. 1984. *The Role of Food Safety in Health and Development.* Technical Report Series 705. Expert Committee on Food Safety, Geneva; WHO; pp. 1–79.

5 Creating and Establishing Networks for the Commercialization of Innovations

Leena Aarikka-Stenroos and Birgitta Sandberg

CONTENTS

5.1 INTRODUCTION

The development and marketing of innovations are known to be highly demanding tasks (Chiesa and Frattini 2011). Overcoming the technological challenges in the research and development phase does not in itself deliver an innovation. For an invention to become an innovation, it has to be commercially successful (Schumpeter 1934), which presumes both a successful launch and diffusion into the market. Commercialization typically brings critical new challenges to innovator firms (Easingwood and Koustelos 2000), and existing research shows that many companies and products tend to fail in this phase (Di Benedetto 1999, Chiesa and Frattini 2011). Investment in the innovation may be considerable by that time, and the risk of rejection is still very high. Commercialization challenges originate from the novelty of innovations that makes customers and other actors in the business environment resist them (Chiesa and Frattini 2011). Nevertheless, successful diffusion requires adoption among users, complementors, and intermediaries; the new product easily fails if it does not attract support from the adoption networks (Chiesa and Frattini 2011). This makes the manner in which the commercialization is handled as important and emphasizes the critical role of creating and establishing the networks for commercialization.

The basic premise of this study is that a single company is rarely capable of generating success-ful diffusion in the commercialization phase of a new product, and therefore networking is crucial to commercialization. However, networking has in this respect focused largely on R&D activities (e.g., Ritter and Gemünden 2003). Our study suggests that networks can also facilitate marketing, commercialization, and the launch of innovations by providing manifold complementary resources and establishing a supportive context in which a new product might survive. The role of network-ing and extensive arrangements between industries and authorities are important in many indus-tries, and particularly in the functional food industry (Mark-Herbert 2004, Matthyssens et al. 2008). We see that knowledge of how to utilize networks in the commercialization and market creation for innovations becomes increasingly important for companies facing tightening financial conditions and increasing competition. Small innovator firms in particular may lack financial and personnel resources, and the legitimacy that enables them to reach potential customers and rele-vant market actors.

Commercialization comprises the development of the product/concept, its successful launch, and interaction activities with potential buyers that demonstrate its potential benefits (see Jolly 1997, Di Benedetto 1999). Product development and marketing/commercialization activities may overlap during the innovation process. The linear innovation model suggests that the whole innovation process begins with an idea, proceeds with product development, and ends when the product creates wealth. However, firms are increasingly employing a nonlinear approach, according to which the interaction with users and partners occurs throughout the whole process (Sandberg 2008). In either case, the innovation process includes both development and marketing activities. In moving toward commer-cialization, the innovator firm needs to shift its focus from technical development to marketing. So, the key tasks are the creation of demand, acquisition of marketing resources, effective communication with end users to facilitate adoption, building national and international distribution channels, and accessing market and customer information (Di Benedetto 1999, Easingwood et al. 2006).

Even though network relations may facilitate bringing innovations to market, commercialization as a function of a network has been mentioned only very briefly (Bullinger et al. 2004, Millson and Wilemon 2008, Möller and Svahn 2009). Moreover, user involvement is a topic of growing interest, but this research tends to focus on customers' contribution to product development (von Hippel 1989), not on commercialization. The focus is on getting the technology to the stage at which it is ready for the market, even though innovator firms also need commercialization competence to ensure that the market accepts the product (Story et al. 2009, Aarikka-Stenroos and Sandberg 2012).

When the firm moves toward commercialization, it needs to gain and mobilize diverse support-ers for commercialization. The commencement of commercialization activities will presumably transform the set of the innovator firm's relations because it needs different resources for commer-cialization compared to R&D. However, knowledge about transformations of innovation networks is still sparse, and empirical studies are few in number (e.g., Heikkinen et al. 2007). Network com-petence is a crucial aspect of innovation success in R&D (Ritter and Gemünden 2003), and particu-larly in commercialization as the innovator firms need to be able to access and mobilize the required resources through their network relations (Aarikka-Stenroos and Sandberg 2012). In the innovation context, this is often challenging due to problems of trust (e.g., Story et al. 2009). Furthermore, Heikkinen et al.'s (2007) findings on how a new product development network broke up during the commercialization phase because of diverging goals indicate that innovation networks face particu-lar management challenges in the commercialization phase.

This study presumes that networking may help to overcome the challenges inherent in commer-cialization and therefore it analyzes *how a network may help a firm in its commercialization efforts.* In contribution, the study (1) identifies relevant commercialization tasks and network actors who can contribute to those tasks and (2) analyzes how an R&D network can be transformed into a com-mercialization network. The theoretical background of the study is based mainly on the network and innovation management literature. The key concept commercialization network refers to a group of actors involved formally or informally in the commercialization of an innovation. This study concentrates on product innovations, and adopts the word innovation to mean a successfully developed and launched, new or improved product (Trott 2002). The study can be characterized as exploratory. The empirical part provides three cases from the wellness and functional food industries describing how innovator firms are utilizing networks in commercialization and market creation to ensure the success of their inventions. On the basis of research results and conclusions, we suggest implications for managers within innovator firms and industries in the development of their innovation networks.

5.2 MOVING TOWARD COMMERCIALIZATION

5.2.1 COMMERCIALIZATION ACTIVITIES AND NEW TASKS

The commencement of commercialization changes the focus of relevant activities: the innovator firm cannot concentrate only on product development issues in order to create a new product that satisfies end-user needs, it must focus on overcoming the resistance of end users, intermediaries, and complementors (cf. Woodside and Biemans 2005, Chiesa and Frattini 2011). Commercialization involves diverse strategic and tactical marketing tasks such as demonstrations, advertising, brand development, promotional events, organizing distribution, and gathering customer feedback (Guiltinan 1999, Easingwood et al. 2006).

Relevant commercialization tasks depend first and foremost on the features of the innovation (Rogers 1983), namely, its complexity, trialability, relative advantage, observability, and compatibility. If the invention appears to be easy to understand and use, adoption tends to be faster. The ability to test the innovation enhances its adoption (Robertson, 1971). Customers will evaluate the relative advantage and therefore need convincing of the potential benefits (Rogers 1983). The more observable the benefits, the faster the innovation tends to be adopted (Rogers 1983). Moreover, the more compatible the innovation is with previously introduced ideas and the needs of potential adopters, the faster the adoption tends to be (Rogers 1983). The role of communication becomes inevitable as synergetic marketing communication and supporting brands, together with word-of-mouth communication, facilitate adoption (Chiesa and Frattini 2011). Hence, awareness building, customer education, and the provision of trial opportunities are critical factors of innovation success (Easingwood and Koustelos 2000, Easingwood et al. 2006). All of these tasks are fairly demanding and usually require a significant sacrifice of scarce resources.

Customers are not the only objects of commercialization tasks; commercialization activities need to be directed also toward other market actors who impact how the innovation diffuses to the markets. For example, because resistance among distributors can hinder commercial success, they will need convincing of the innovation's value to their customers (see Parthasarathy et al. 1994, Woodside and Biemans 2005).

5.2.2 NETWORK ACTORS WITH CONTRIBUTION POTENTIAL TO COMMERCIALIZATION

Various actors could contribute to commercialization. Support and resources can be provided in R&D activities by competitors, distributors, buyers, consultants, suppliers, research institutes and universities, government agencies, and industry associations (Ritter and Gemünden 2003, Möller et al. 2005). Similarly, in commercialization activities, network actors such as these could be of value and are discussed next.

Users can contribute to the commercialization in terms of identifying other potential users, in demonstrating and teaching how the new product works, assessing its market potential, evaluating the extent to which it meets a significant user need, and acting as references (Biemans 1991, Harrison and Waluszewski 2008). With regard to consumer products, vertically linked *intermediaries* are crucial actors because they provide distribution resources and make the product available to users (Parthasarathy et al. 1994, Easingwood et al. 2006). Also, actors beyond the traditional supply chain can play an important role in bringing innovations successfully to market (Story et al. 2009, Aarikka-Stenroos and Sandberg 2012, Chiesa and Frattini 2011). *Competitors* or *partners* are potential sources of strategic collaboration: for example, *innovative firms with complementary resources, products, and channel relationships* may together create future demand and markets and thus push/pull the innovation through (Möller and Svahn 2009). *Companies that supply products or services complementary* to the innovation also tend to fortify demand for a new product (Chiesa and Frattini 2011). *Public organizations and educational institutions* may contribute to commercialization if they articulate encouraging visions for the use of the innovation in society (Troshani and Doolin 2007). *Local municipalities and universities can establish trust and expertise, and foster relations with political authorities* that could provide information within their own areas of expertise and facilitate the development of new business fields (Partanen et al. 2008, Möller and Svahn 2009). *Established firms* as partners and supporters may also play an important role throughout the commercialization as their stability, credibility, and good reputation often spread to their partners (Anderson et al. 1994).

Particular *key persons* are an important group of potential contributors in commercialization as the literature on adoption and diffusion emphasizes that certain individuals determine the success of innovations. *Lead users, mavens, expert opinion leaders*, and *hub persons* (with large numbers of contacts) are people who have a substantial influence on opinion formation/change and who therefore can accelerate or block the adoption of the product (Woodside and Biemans 2005, Harrison and Waluszewski 2008, Goldenberg et al. 2009). These persons can provide publicity, demonstrate the product, and explain its unique benefits over what is currently available (Harrison and Waluszewski 2008).

In sum, the commencement of commercialization pushes the innovator firm to collaborate with diverse actors for the following activities: trust creation, credibility establishment, awareness building, customer education, trial opportunities, distribution, and the provision of complementary offerings. Diverse actors could provide new resources related to experience of the industry, customer and market knowledge, the ability to identify the optimal functionality of the product and brand, communication, distribution, and strategic alignment. Such actors could also provide established relations that facilitate the building of new relations (Anderson et al. 1994). However, the challenge lies in how to get these potential network actors interested and mobilized within the commercialization network. The move from R&D to commercialization requires transformations and renewal of network relations which must be managed. These aspects are discussed in the following section.

5.2.3 TRANSFORMATION FROM R&D TO COMMERCIALIZATION NETWORK

When the firm moves from R&D to commercialization, it needs to manage its relations with diverse actors effectively. Network competence is a company-specific ability to build and use inter-organizational relationships so that the different relationships complement and fit well with each other (Ritter and Gemünden 2003). An innovator firm with commercialization-related network competence is able to build new relations, identify new areas of collaboration in existing relationships, and mobilize key actors; it may thus realize first mover advantages, ensure innovation success, and cope with considerable challenges related to the newness of innovations (Aarikka-Stenroos and Sandberg 2012).

The commencement of commercialization often changes earlier network relations (Heikkinen et al. 2007, Aarikka-Stenroos and Sandberg 2012). These changes and transformations may originate from internal and endogenous factors, such as when the firm gains an insight that could enable it to collaborate in a novel way, or exogenous factors, when economic or political changes in the business environment concern several network actors simultaneously (Halinen et al. 1999). The changes may be incremental, when the existing relationship is used in a new way, or radical, when a relationship between two actors breaks down or a new actor appears (Halinen et al. 1999). Sometimes an incremental dyadic change may lead to a larger radical change in networks if other actors consider it important, and consequently react by building or untying their relationships (Halinen et al. 1999).

Changes and transformations are, however, often effected by earlier conventions. For example, path dependence restricts and facilitates changes in networks since technical solutions, for example, are developed and adapted in relation to each other (Håkansson and Waluszewski 2002). At some junctures, it becomes evident that there could be new ways to collaborate; existing collaboration can assume new dimensions, or it may be possible to collaborate with new actors in completely new ways. However, creating reformative collaboration with novel partners requires the deformation of earlier conventions (Håkansson and Waluszewski 2002). Moreover, existing relations often facilitate the creation of new relations, but they can also constrain further networking by locking actors into collaboration with certain actors and locking them out of collaboration with others (Anderson et al. 1994, Ritter and Gemünden 2003). Diverse risks and incredulity, embedded in innovations, may also restrain any potentially new collaboration. Due to uncertainties, users and intermediaries more easily adopt imitation tactics as they do not dare to be innovative adopters (Parthasarathy et al. 1994, Harrison and Waluszewski 2008), and thus do not rush into collaboration. These aspects all provide challenges when the firm aims to build up its commercialization network.

Despite the challenges, several reasons may motivate network actors to be involved in commercialization networks: Actors may share mutual goals and common involvement in the particular issue; networking provides potential growth and profit; relations offer access to new business relationships, new markets and information; collaboration generates learning and the opportunity to adopt new ideas; collaboration enhances reputation and image; actors need collaboration on account of the complexity of the product; collaboration facilitates the alignment of strategies and roadmaps; and collaboration enables the acquisition of negotiation power (see Ritter and Gemünden 2003, Bullinger et al. 2004).

Even though there are good reasons to collaborate for commercialization, diverse fears and distrust may also emerge. It is particularly challenging for innovative firms to engage in collaboration if there is no common history, with a resulting lack of trust (Story et al. 2009). Consequently, accessing and mobilizing prospective network actors for commercialization may be difficult (Aarikka-Stenroos and Sandberg 2012). Moreover, collaboration among innovator industries may also result in coordination difficulties and the creation of future competitors (Millson and Wilemon 2008). Trust is therefore a critical component when parties seek to collaborate on new offerings and concepts, but wish to avoid opportunism and competition. Initial trust can be grounded in preexisting social relations among managers and employees, and in the firm's or key person's reputation (see Larson 1992, Partanen et al. 2008). Organizational achievements such as awards and good stakeholder relationships (Zott and Huy 2007) could also facilitate building new collaboration for commercialization and market creation. Trust emerges more easily through choosing the same kinds of partner with similar strategic goals or technology, products, markets or cultures, and similar administrative systems, often found to enhance success in collaboration (Biemans 1991, Dhanaraj and Parkhe 2006). However, dissimilarity may also be a predictor of success: weak ties between dissimilar actors convey more new information and therefore innovator firms should not only utilize strong ties providing similar ideas, but also weak ties with actors whose different ideas introduce more new information (originally Granovetter 1973, Möller and Rajala 2007).

A firm pursuing new relationships needs to identify and convince potential partners by profiling their own resources and the potential benefits of collaboration. In order to mobilize actors, they need to see sufficient benefit and synergy potential in collaboration. However, if innovation concerns a very new concept it may be difficult to determine the details of necessary collaboration clearly in advance (Möller and Svahn 2009). There is also the matter of how and by whom collaboration is managed. This makes power issues important: the dependence between networked actors often leads to a situation in which the more powerful firm is freer to choose its options with the dependent firm being a follower, adapting to its wishes (Ritter et al. 2004). Highly centralized innovation networks often have a hub firm orchestrating the interaction. In the absence of a dominant

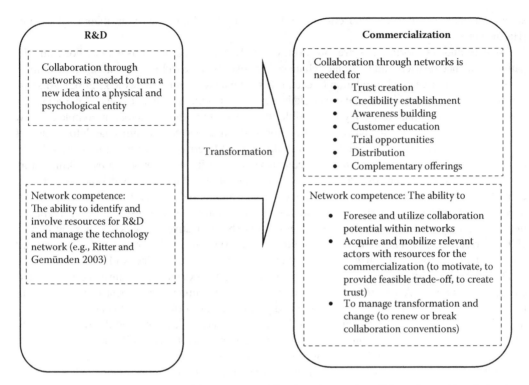

FIGURE 5.1   Transformation from R&D to commercialization: changes in collaboration and in relations.

hub player, the actors must agree on the way to organize collaboration with reciprocity, coherence in goals, and trust apparently being more important than formal agreements (Larson 1992, Dhanaraj and Parkhe 2006).

Figure 5.1 shows the main aspects of commercialization networks. When new commercialization activities emerge, new collaboration is needed and therefore the R&D network needs to transform into the commercialization network. This transformation requires new abilities from the innovator firm as it needs to cope with commercialization tasks and be able to identify, access, and mobilize diverse network actors to get their support for the new product/service in the commercialization.

5.3   METHODS

The empirical part of the study is a multiple case study, where three commercialization networks are described and analyzed. The reason for choosing a case study strategy is that it facilitates holistic understanding of complex phenomena that are not easily separable from their context (cf. Yin 1989). Case study research maximizes the realism of the context at the expense of precision and generalizability (McGrath 1982). The three cases enable both valuable description and comparison and concern the commercialization of "Nordic Walkers" (poles for fitness walking), "Benecol" (a functional food ingredient), and the "Bone Health Exercise Monitor" (a device for monitoring bone exercise). In all cases, Finnish firms developed the innovations that differed substantially from the firm's existing products and targeted them at international consumer markets.

The study is longitudinal and relies mainly on retrospective data. The case data included both semistructured interviews of key actors and extensive archival and media-originated data. The data collection took place between 2002 and 2011 with the researchers conducting 11 face-to-face interviews among key actors representing the innovator firms and other organizations involved in the R&D and commercialization activities. All the interviews covered the following: (1) the characteristics of the innovation; (2) the actors and tasks in the R&D; (3) the actors and tasks in the commercialization; and (4) the nature of and reasons for the actors' collaboration at different stages. The case data also included numerous telephone discussions, email correspondence, company reports and hundreds of newspaper articles and web pages concerning the product, the company, and the focal markets.

During the analysis phase, the researchers cross-checked the data in order to eliminate possible errors. Data triangulation helped enhance the trustworthiness of the results. Initially within-case analysis was employed for each case, followed by cross-case analysis. The first step in the within-case analysis was to classify the data in the form of a chronological listing of events, and to identify the critical incidents in both R&D and commercialization. Then the data were organized in themes such as the key actors and activities involved in the R&D and the commercialization. Cross-case analysis was done by comparing different R&D and commercialization networks, relevant commercialization tasks and actors and thus allowed comparison of similarities and differences between the cases. The analysis resulted in three case descriptions and delineation of commercialization networks, which are presented next.

5.4   CASES

The following three cases illustrate how companies apply a network approach in the commercialization of new products. The emphasis is on the relevant actors and tasks, the shift from R&D to commercialization and managing network relations for commercialization.

5.4.1   EXEL AND NORDIC WALKING

The Finnish firm Exel successfully commercialized Nordic Walkers poles. In the 1990s, the market for cross-country skiing equipment began to decline slowly which encouraged the firm to generate ideas for new products related to walking. Collaboration by three actors between 1995 and 1997 generated the idea of special poles that everyone could use throughout the year for exercise purposes and thus they comprised the R&D network. The innovator firm Exel plc specializes in designing, manufacturing, and marketing the composite sports equipment; The Sports Institute of Finland (hereafter The Sports Institute) is a science- and training-based center of education for leisure and sports activities, which also develops and markets exercise and educational services for top level sports actors and coaches; The Central Association for Recreational Sports and Outdoor Activities (hereafter The Central Association) is a nonprofit organization whose aim is to encourage ordinary people's interest in outdoor activities. The resources of these actors were complementary: Exel, a widely known sports brand, had pole manufacturing expertise, and could provide equipment for the new sport; The Sports Institute had sports-related scientific knowledge about different training methods, and contacts with experts and opinion leaders (e.g., trainers and doctors), and the Central Association had knowledge of outdoor sports. The actors all shared the common goal of changing attitudes toward sport.

Following the development of the product and the concept Exel started its commercialization activities, but then problems started to arise. The first production run was only a couple of thousand pairs of poles, and it was initially difficult to sell even that amount. There was resistance from the distribution actors, and because the trade did not believe in the product the retailers were reluctant to display it on their shelves. The actors realized that it was also necessary to collaborate in the commercialization of the new product and concept, to make the sport attractive to customers and other relevant actors in the network. The atmosphere was favorable for further collaboration in commercialization, due to strong social links and trust between the main actors involved in the R&D collaboration. The commercialization through the network began in autumn 1997. The Central Association started to organize mass events in which trial opportunities and education were offered enabling people to try the sport and to learn to use the poles. Actually, the biggest problem was not a lack of awareness, as the media provided a massive amount of publicity by keenly profiling "the new strange sport." The major problem was getting people to walk with poles.

Little by little, the actors started to expand the commercialization network by actively forging new relations with diverse actors such as national sports and health associations, experts and instructors, associations, community fitness centers, and sports clubs. A range of actors took care of various commercialization tasks: awareness building involved all the core actors and also those involved in the media, health associations, and the medical profession. Nonprofit expert actors in particular generated trust and credibility: health associations (e.g., The Rheumatism Association, The Allergy and Asthma Federation) conveyed the message that walking with poles was good for the health, and doctors publicly highlighted the benefits of the sport. The Cooper Institute in the United States provided test results on the positive health effects of the Nordic Walking concept. Complementary offerings started to emerge from sports apparel manufacturers and fitness clubs. The actors also built a sports instructor network: through sports and health associations they found instructors, educated them about the new sport, and provided them with training material and poles. The Sports Institute introduced the sport to its visitors. Word-of-mouth communication among users and experts further accelerated innovation diffusion: lead users in particular built awareness, gave instruction on the use of poles, and communicated the benefits further. Through this multidimensional expanding commercialization network, the innovator firm was able to achieve a breakthrough:

> They had people coming into their store asking "Have you got any Nordic walking poles?" and at first, many offered them hiking poles ... but people started insisting that "They have to be Exel Nordic Walkers." Then store managers started calling us to say that "We"ve got some people here who want to buy those Nordic walking poles of yours. Would you mind sending some, please?
>
> *Senior Vice President, Exel*

Demand started to grow in the winter of 1997. Nordic Walkers achieved commercial success extremely quickly and Exel started to export them to almost 30 countries in which it has basically utilized the same commercialization tactics.

5.4.2 Raisio and Benecol

Raisio specializes in plant-based foods such as groceries and functional food ingredients. The company invented an ingredient, used in Benecol products, that lowers the LDL cholesterol level in the human body. The development of Benecol products started at the end of the 1980s when the R&D department unintentionally uncovered the benefits of sitosterol, a form of plant sterol, while seeking solutions to Raisio's problem of having a continuous supply of rapeseed oil as a by-product being sold at a low price, while at the same time needing the healthier but more expensive sunflower oil for its margarine production. In 1989, one of Raisio's chemists finally discovered how sitosterol could be transformed into a form suitable for addition not only to vegetable spreads but also to all kinds of food. The R&D activities were supported by several industrial partners, such as Kaukas who provided the original idea of using sitosterol ester, and research parties such as that of Dr. Miettinen, which provided medical information and the North Karelia Project (a national health organization) which enabled medical testing of the population.

The invention was radically new and among the first products in a new product category, functional foods. The company was able to patent the ingredient's manufacturing method. The Finnish Food Safety Authority did not initially accept the addition of the plant sterol to food, but changed its position after hearing from Finnish medical experts. The medical effects of sitostanol ester-based products were clinically tested over several years before launching it in Finland in 1995. The *New England Journal of Medicine* published research on sitostanol ester's benefits on the same day the product was launched.

From the beginning of commercialization, it was evident that the product offered worldwide promise, since there is a global need to develop health-maintaining nutrition for the aging population and to prevent major cardiovascular diseases. Since Raisio had no experience of global markets, it started to collaborate with McNeil under Johnson & Johnson in 1998; they agreed on a licensing contract to use sitostanol ester in food industries worldwide, with the international launch to commence in the United States, the United Kingdom, Ireland, and Benelux countries. Benecol was launched in 1999, but consumers in the United States did not "buy" the product and legislation in the United States raised critical challenges:

> This was a classic example of how in the beginning there are massive sales expectations, but cash flow does not come easily after all. It takes time to learn how a really new product needs to be commercialized and brought to market.

Commercial Director, Benecol

Benecol decided to buy back its licenses and take the concept to international markets itself. Further expansion beyond Europe started in 2000 through licensing agreements whereby partners got the ingredient produced in both Finland and the United States, rights to the Benecol brand, and support from the Benecol network which continuously develops marketing practices. Since the ingredient, used in Benecol products, could be added to anything eatable, diverse partners were gradually attained. By 2003, 13 new Benecol products were launched around the world and by 2007 Benecol was the market leader in the United Kingdom. Plant stanol ester was chosen as one of the 10 greatest health-enhancing nutritional innovations worldwide in the *European Journal of Clinical Nutrition*.

Distribution is the partners' responsibility since they know their home markets while, at the same time, marketing practices are developed by all licensing partners and Raisio Benecol. Best practices and accumulated knowledge are openly shared with the inner actors, who add the ingredient to a variety of foods from margarine to yoghurt in their local markets, and thus are not competitors. Since the credibility of the benefits is important for partners, customers and statutory regulators, scientific clinical testing played a crucial role during commercialization. Almost 60 clinical tests of the ingredient's effects have been conducted up to 2011, backed up by 15 years of safe usage.

In Finland, where cardiovascular disease is common, the motivation to use cholesterol-lowering products is strong, but other markets have required much education on cholesterol problems and cholesterol-lowering products. Benecol has built a Health Care Promotion group, comprising expert parties that share credible knowledge on cholesterol-lowering issues, which educates markets around the world and works particularly closely with doctors and nurses who are normally in the front line when it comes to identifying the need for the product. Furthermore, Benecol has attracted exceptional attention in medical publications as a result of several clinical studies that proved the health claims to be true, boosted by public media; this all built awareness and credibility for the product. Regulators have also been important actors during commercialization, as they determine how and with what kinds of argument the product can be sold. As legal definitions for functional foods are often lacking or inconsistent, authorities are in effect involved in market creation (see Mark-Herbert 2004). For example, regulation in Europe permits the addition of the Benecol ingredient to yoghurt but not to juice, and this also impacts who can be Benecol-licensing partners.

The current situation is that even in a challenging economic climate sales have grown, and Benecol has become Raisio's flagship product selling in 30 countries on five continents.

5.4.3 NEWTEST AND BONE HEALTH

Newtest is a small wellness high-tech company specializing in the development, manufacture and sales of human performance testing, and assessment products. Its R&D activities with Oulu University and the VTT Technical Research Centre of Finland resulted in the Newtest Bone Exercise Monitor. This patented innovation (an accelerometer combined with a microprocessor) estimates whether the amount and quality of daily exercise are sufficient to develop bone density and prevent osteoporosis, which is becoming a serious health threat, especially in industrialized countries. The monitor's contribution to bone health was proven through award-winning scientific research conducted by the University of Oulu Faculty of Medicine and the Oulu Deaconess Institute.

When Newtest launched the monitor, all the media were present. However, in order to launch successfully it also had to raise interest in bone issues among customers and partners. For this purpose, Newtest started to create a commercialization network from scratch. The idea came from two sources: A potential customer in Japan suggested testing the idea in Finland with a view to later replication in Japan and, second, Newtest knew of the successful Nordic Walkers case and wanted to reproduce this networking pattern. The basis for such networking seemed solid because consumers, the media, international organizations, and governments are increasingly interested in wellbeing, and the diversity of wellness industries provided versatile potential collaborators from health care services to health supplements and vitamins.

In 2006, Newtest started a project to build a network of diverse bone health-related industry actors from electronics to the food industry with synergistic offerings. In fact, it was originally about bone exercise, but the theme soon extended to bone health in order to include food companies because, for example, milk products containing calcium contribute to bone health. Together the firms involved could create markets for bone health offerings by building a clear concept and raising awareness, gathering research information on bone health for participating organizations, producing common promotional material, and creating new synergistic concepts. Newtest's idea was that the actors could also promote its new monitor and thus built awareness, trust, and credibility. Some actors such as pharmacies, sports equipment retailers, and providers of fitness club and health care services would organize trial opportunities, and handle education and distribution matters.

The CEO of Newtest and the project manager contacted the market leaders in each bone health-related industry: providers of osteoporosis diagnostic equipment, private health clinics, various sports and health associations, sports clubs, aerobic associations, food manufacturers, functional foods manufacturers, pharmacy chains, pharmaceutical industry actors such as calcium and D vitamin manufacturers, insurance companies, and also some nonprofit organizations (e.g., national osteoporosis foundations, innovation promotion organizations). Given Newtest's focus on international markets, global firms were also targeted. Food group D, the global leader in fresh dairy products, showed interest but later withdrew from the negotiations because its marketing strategy emphasized product lightness, not bone health.

Networking for bone health proved to be rather difficult. Most of the contacted actors expressed their interest and support but were not willing to enter into formal collaboration for multiple reasons: Their target groups varied from teenagers to elderly people, which would have complicated potential common activities; the novelty of the collaboration, and the small size and unfamiliarity of Newtest itself made firms suspicious; some firms were looking for short-term returns and clear private trade-offs, and were not willing to commit to the common long-term goal of creating bone health markets. The vague line between competition and collaboration also complicated the situation:

> The main principle has been not to involve competitors in the net. But, actually, what and where is a competitor? It's difficult to define.
>
> *CEO of one of the recruited firms*

Nevertheless, some actors did understand the potential. For example, a device rental company realized that it and Newtest had similar strategic goals and agreed to utilize the market potential of the monitor in their business by selling or renting it to their customers. An orthopedic hospital was also willing to rent out equipment and provide instruction on its use.

Following the negotiations, there was a meeting in 2007 to formalize collaboration as The Bone Health Association. Along with Newtest, the seven committed actors included, for example, an insurance company and a nutrient wholesaler. However, fatal problems emerged: not one of the actors wanted to take an active role, and the blurred nature of the goals and roles further complicated the situation. As a consequence, formal interaction promoting bone health ceased. Newtest brought its product to the market in 2005, and in spite of its recognized potential it has still not broken through.

5.5 DISCUSSION AND CONCLUSIONS

5.5.1 SUMMING UP AND COMPARING CASES

In all cases, a variety of complementary actors were able to contribute to commercialization by supporting awareness creation, benefit confirmation, and distribution. Awareness creation was not, in fact, a problem in any of the cases described above as the media tend to be interested in innovations. The innovations gained more credibility when the support came from two different actor groups: medical-related actors (e.g., doctors) and wellness-related actors (e.g., health associations) in the Nordic Walkers case, and medical-related actors (e.g., research institutes) and food industry actors (partners) in the Benecol case. In Nordic Walkers, such actors also made their divergent relations available to reach new relevant actors. Expert opinion leaders and nonprofit organizations would have made an important contribution in all cases, but only Exel collaborated with both profit and nonprofit organizations to convince customers of its innovation's benefits. Distribution and the availability of supporting complementary offerings were also key issues. Nordic Walkers represent an extreme case (see Parthasarathy et al. 1994) in that the innovator firm had to circumvent intermediaries, because they did not adopt the product, and to activate actors beyond them in order to enable distribution of the innovation. It is worth noting that despite the increased emphasis on user involvement, users were not included in the Bone Health and Benecol cases, whereas in the Nordic Walkers case they played a major role as lead teachers.

The shift from R&D to commercialization through networks occurred in a different fashion in all cases. In the Nordic Walkers case, the network was an extension of the R&D innovation network. With "developers" turning into "promoters" the network gradually extended as the actors involved forged new relations and, as a result, the network grew easily and quickly. In the Benecol case, the innovator firm started to develop new relations with diverse actors, progressing step by step and offering clear trade-offs and benefits for involved actors. In the Bone Health case, the commercialization network was more in the nature of innovative marketing collaboration for new value (to enhance bone health), but because collaboration started from scratch without established relations and clearly defined benefits, no radical collaboration occurred. These cases illustrate how a gradual shift in innovation networks is easier to realize than revolutionary, radical change. In hindsight, involving one or two commercialization actors at the development stage might have helped Newtest in the commercialization process. Table 5.1 summarizes the key actors and tasks in the three commercialization networks, and the main features of the network transformation.

5.5.2 CONCLUSIONS

This study generated new knowledge for managers and researchers on how innovator firms can collaborate through networks to ensure the successful commercialization of new products. The contribution of the study lies in analyzing their manifold actors and their contribution to commercialization activities, as previous research on innovation networks has mainly focused on R&D networks (Heikkinen et al. 2007, Möller and Svahn 2009). The results show that collaboration for commercialization in health-related industries can vary from pursuing strategic long-term goals, such as market creation, to synergetic co-marketing.

TABLE 5.1

Main Findings on Commercialization Networks

Case	Key Actors and Key Tasks in Commercialization	Features of Transformation
Nordic Walking—Exel	Key actors: Sports and health-related (both business and nonprofit) actors and lead users Key tasks: To promote awareness, teaching and learning, benefit illustrations, events, demonstrations	Driver of transformation: Rejection of poles → need for new launch tactics Transformation: First collaboration within the R&D network continued but shifted toward commercialization, and then the network was gradually expanded as new relations were forged through existing relations Grounds for collaboration: Common goal (to get ordinary people to exercise outdoors) and clear trade-offs existed; collaboration was strategic for all actors Management of transformation and commercialization: Informal interactive management, evolutionary task planning, task development Main challenge: To overcome rejection by distributors and users
Benecol—Raisio	Key actors: Research organizations, partners, regulators, medical and public media, expert promoters Key tasks: To build credibility and validate benefits, educate markets, share best practices on how to market the product	Driver of transformation: Failure in the major licensing partnership → need for diverse licensing partners around the world Transformation: Totally new relationships with diverse partners and actors were forged; R&D and commercialization relations were partly isolated. Grounds for collaboration: Reaching the goal "to get people to lower cholesterol" offered diverse benefits (such as profit, sales, and increased health in the community) for all involved actors; collaboration is strategic for many actors Management of transformation and commercialization: Licensing agreements and informal management of Benecol network, reciprocal information sharing Main challenges: To educate partners, experts and users in order to evoke needs and create markets
Bone Health—Newtest	Key actors: Diverse actors providing bone health-related products and services from various industries (emphasis on business actors) Key tasks: To provide marketing communications, branding, information and knowledge, to distribute the monitor	Driver of transformation: Need to launch the product, and identification of "bone health" markets Transformation: Radical changes were pursued: the key actor aimed to forge totally new collaborations on the basis of new value arguments without common histories; R&D and commercialization relations were totally isolated

TABLE 5.1   (continued)
Main Findings on Commercialization Networks

Case	Key Actors and Key Tasks in Commercialization	Features of Transformation
		Grounds for collaboration: Common goal (to get people to take care of their bone health) existed but individual rewards were blurred due to a new "value innovation"; collaboration held strategic relevance for only some actors
		Management of transformation and commercialization: Informal discussion and formal management through association. Disagreement occurred on relevant actors.
		Main challenges: To create trusting multi-industry collaboration for a new value concept and to break conventions: potential actors were easy to identify but hard to gain and mobilize despite the potential

Commercialization of a product appears to be more complicated than the literature depicts. The results of this study show how various actors can facilitate awareness and credibility building, customer education, distribution, marketing communication, brand development, reputation, and forging new relationships, which all need to be mastered in order to overcome resistance to newness (see Figure 5.2). Network relations are crucial, particularly in communicating multifaceted benefits that prospective users may not otherwise understand or trust—an aspect that is common in functional foods industries (see Mark-Herbert 2004).

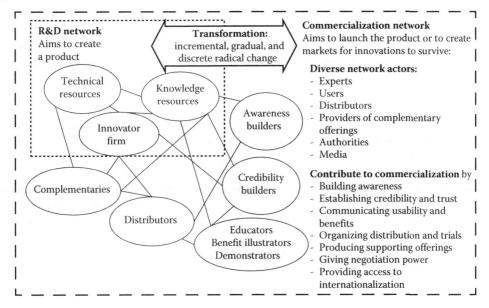

FIGURE 5.2   The transformation toward commercialization networks. (Modified from Aarikka-Stenroos, L. and B. Sandberg. 2012. *Journal of Business Research* 65(2):198–206.)

In the optimal situation, a commercialization network combines the complementary resources of service and product providers in different kinds of related industries and profit and nonprofit organizations. In any case, the innovator firm needs to interact not only with customers and users but also with leading partners such as distributors, complementors and opinion leaders, whose contribution to diffusion, adaptation, and market creation is crucial.

Our results indicate that the potential actors and resources were easy to identify, but often difficult to mobilize on account of diversity in strategic orientation, size, industry, and markets. It seems that the more heterogeneous the actors and the more path-dependence breaking the new collaboration, the more difficult it is to evidence the potential goals and benefits of collaboration, and to recognize the actors' roles in commercialization. The diversity of actors may not only boost commercialization, but also create challenges. The results show that the challenges in networking for commercialization originate from the different goals of relevant actors, uncertainty regarding rewards, a lack of trust and the fear that collaboration will turn into competition, differences concerning the relevance of focal collaboration, and disagreement about the organizing systems. It is challenging to overcome path dependence and create relations between actors who have not previously collaborated. Common goals, values, and offering complementarity facilitate collaboration for commercialization as actors are only committed if it aligns with their own activities, strategies, and business models, and if clear and often rapid trade-offs motivate them to collaborate. In addition, the results indicate that the move toward commercialization demands a new kind of network competence, in other words the ability to identify and access the required resources, mobilize and organize collaboration, and manage the transformation.

5.5.3 IMPLICATIONS FOR MANAGERS

The findings will help innovator firms and new product developers optimize collaboration throughout the whole process from R&D to commercialization. The study may help managers better realize the full potential of the actors in their existing networks and purposefully create networks of value in commercialization. Managers should especially employ network resources to create awareness, build trust, and provide trialability, education and complementary offerings. There are various paths to creating a network for commercialization: the firm can find new collaboration aspects concerning commercialization from its existing R&D relations; use existing relations to access and mobilize new collaboration with novel actors; or build completely new relations with novel collaborators, but that is the most challenging path. In any case, managers should be aware of the value of their R&D network actors so, when forming the R&D network, it would be beneficial to involve those who would be important in the different tasks required or who already have relations to other actors that are required for commercialization.

Two strategies for the application of the network approach to the commercialization of new products emerge from this research. The first is that the innovator firm could use a portfolio of interorganizational relationships to commercialize their innovations and thus provide clear benefits and resource trade-offs for actors who are able to make a contribution. Alternatively, innovator firms could collaborate proactively and use network relations to create markets and new fields of business, but this kind of network should focus on issues, values and new business models rather than particular innovations.

Networking and collaboration with external marketing contributors does not necessarily reduce the marketing costs, but may increase the success of marketing efforts as they enable the communication of the benefits and use of the new product in a credible and understandable fashion, offer complete solutions instead of only product-related solutions, and ease internationalization—all of which are crucial in the wellbeing and health industries.

REFERENCES

Aarikka-Stenroos, L. and B. Sandberg. 2012. From new-product development to commercialization through networks. *Journal of Business Research* 65(2):198–206.

Anderson, J.C., H. Håkansson, and J. Johanson. 1994. Dyadic business relationships within a business network context. *Journal of Marketing* 58:1–15.

Biemans, W.G. 1991. User and third-party involvement in developing medical equipment innovations. *Technovation* 11:163–182.

Bullinger, H.-J., K. Auernhammer, and A. Gomeringer. 2004. Managing networks in the knowledge-driven economy. *International Journal of Production Research* 42:3337–3353.

Chiesa, V. and F. Frattini. 2011. Commercializing technological innovation: Learning from failures in high-tech markets. *Journal of Product Innovation Management* 28:437–454.

Dhanaraj, C. and A. Parkhe. 2006. Orchestrating innovation networks. *Academy of Management Review* 31:659–669.

Di Benedetto, C.A. 1999. Identifying the key success factors in new product launch. *Journal of Product Innovation Management* 16:530–544.

Easingwood, C. and A. Koustelos. 2000. Marketing high technology: Preparation, targeting, positioning, execution. *Business Horizons* 43:27–34.

Easingwood, C., S. Moxey, and H. Capleton. 2006. Bringing high technology to market: Successful strategies employed in the worldwide software industry. *Journal of Product Innovation Management* 23:498–511.

Goldenberg J., S. Han, D.R. Lehmann, and J.W. Hong. 2009. The role of hubs in the adoption process. *Journal of Marketing* 73:1–13.

Granovetter, M. 1973. The strength of weak ties. *American Journal of Sociology* 78:1360–1380.

Guiltinan, J.P. 1999. Launch strategy, launch tactics, and demand outcomes. *Journal of Product Innovation Management* 16:509–529.

Halinen, A., A. Salmi, and V. Havila. 1999. From dyadic change to changing business networks: An analytical framework. *Journal of Management Studies* 36:779–794.

Heikkinen, M., T. Mainela, J. Still, and J. Tähtinen. 2007. Roles for managing in mobile service development nets. *Industrial Marketing Management* 36:909–925.

Harrison, D. and A. Waluszewski. 2008. The development of a user network as a way to re-launch an unwanted product. *Research Policy* 37:115–130.

Heikkinen, M.T., T. Mainela, J. Still, and J. Tähtinen. 2007. Roles for managing in mobile service development nets. *Industrial Marketing Management* 36:909–925.

Håkansson, H. and A. Waluszewski. 2002. Path dependence: Restricting or facilitating technical development? *Journal of Business Research* 55:561–570.

Jolly, V.K. 1997. *Commercializing New Technologies. Getting form Mind to Market*. Boston, MA: Harvard Business School Press.

Larson, A. 1992. Network dyads in entrepreneurial settings: A case study of the governance of exchange relationships. *Administrative Science Quarterly* 37:76–104.

Mark-Herbert, C. 2004. Innovation of a new product category—Functional foods. *Technovation* 24:713–719.

Matthyssens, P., K. Vandendempt, and L. Berghman. 2008. Value innovation in the functional foods industry. Deviations from the industry recipe. *British Food Journal* 110:144–155.

McGrath, J.E. 1982. Dilemmatics. The study of research choices and dilemmas. In *Judgement Calls in Research*, eds. McGrath J.E., Martin J., and Kulka R.A. Beverly Hills: Sage Publications.

Millson, M. and D. Wilemon. 2008. Designing strategic innovation networks to facilitate global NPD performance. *Journal of General Management* 34:39–56.

Möller, K. and A. Rajala. 2007. Rise of strategic nets—New modes of value creation. *Industrial Marketing Management* 36:895–908.

Möller, K. and S. Svahn. 2009. How to influence the birth of new success fields—Network perspective. *Industrial Marketing Management* 38:450–458.

Möller, K., A. Rajala, and S. Svahn. 2005. Strategic business nets—Their type and management. *Journal of Business Research* 58:1274–1284.

Partanen, J., K. Möller, M. Westerlund, R. Rajala, and A. Rajala. 2008. Social capital in the growth of science-and-technology-based SMEs. *Industrial Marketing Management* 37:513–522.

Parthasarathy, M., R. Sohi, and R.D. Hampton. 1994. Dual diffusion: Analysis and implication for sales force management. *Journal of Marketing Theory and Practice* 2:1–14.

Ritter, T. and H.G. Gemünden. 2003. Network competence: Its impact on innovation success and its antecedents. *Journal of Business Research* 6:745–755.

Ritter, T., I. Wilkinson, and W. Johnston. 2004. Managing in complex business networks. *Industrial Marketing Management* 33:175–183.

Robertson, T.S. 1971. *Innovative Behavior and Communication*. New York: Holt, Rinehart and Winston.

Rogers, E.M. 1983. *Diffusion of Innovations*. 3rd ed. New York: The Free Press.

Sandberg, B. 2008. *Managing and Marketing Radical Innovations. Marketing New Technology.* London: Routledge.

Schumpeter, J.A. 1934. *The Theory of Economic Development. An Inquiry into Profits, Capital, Credit, Interest, and the Business Cycle.* Cambridge, MA: Harvard University Press.

Story, V., S. Hart, and L. O'Malley. 2009. Relational resource and competences for radical product innovation. *Journal of Marketing Management* 25:461–481.

Troshani, I. and B. Doolin. 2007. Innovation diffusion: A stakeholder and social network view. *European Journal of Innovation Management* 10:176–200.

Trott, P. 2002. *Innovation Management and New Product Development.* 2nd ed. Harlow: Pearson Education.

von Hippel, E. 1989. move this reference after "Trott, P. 2002. *Innovation Management and*" & *Technology Management* 32:24–27.

Woodside, A.G. and W.G. Biemans. 2005. Modeling innovation, manufacturing, diffusion and adoption/rejection processes. *Journal of Business & Industrial Marketing* 20:380–393.

Yin, R.K. 1989. *Case Study Research. Design and Methods.* Newbury Park: Sage Publications.

Zott, C. and Q.N. Huy. 2007. How entrepreneurs use symbolic management to acquire resources. *Administrative Science Quarterly* 52:70–105.

Section II

Market and Trends

6 Regulation and Marketing of Nutraceuticals and Functional Foods in Europe
The Broader Impact of Nutrition and Health Claims Regulation

Patrick Coppens

CONTENTS

6.1 LEGAL FRAMEWORK FOR NUTRACEUTICALS AND FUNCTIONAL FOODS IN THE EUROPEAN UNION

In the European Union (EU), nutraceuticals and functional foods do not exist as legal concepts. Together with food supplements and dietetic foods, such products are considered and regulated under general food law. The food safety provisions of the General Food Law Regulation (Regulation 178/2002) and the Novel Foods Regulation (Regulation 258/97) apply to cover their safety. The Nutrition and Health Claims Regulation (NHCR) (Corrigendum to Regulation 1924/2006) covers rules on claims. Compositional requirements, including rules for the addition of nutrients to foods and food supplements, are subject to specific Regulations: the Addition of vitamins and minerals and other substances to foods Regulation (AVMF) (Regulation 1925/2006) and the Food Supplements Directive (FSD) (Directive 2002/46/EC). The EU is lacking harmonized rules on the use of other food components—the so-called other substances with a nutritional or physiological effect—including botanicals. These are covered by diverging national legislation. The Mutual Recognition Regulation (MRR) (Regulation 764/2008) specifies that such products that are lawfully marketed in one Member State can be sold in all other Member States even if they would not respect existing national requirements in those other Member States.

In principle, therefore, the legal framework appears clear, consistent, and complete. However, in reality, many problems exist. National rules create frequent trade barriers for products containing substances other than vitamins and minerals and the principle of mutual recognition is often ignored by the Member States that have widely divergent views on safety. The existing notification procedures are often used as authorization procedures resulting in prohibitions or restrictions to the marketing of certain products. In addition, the legal classification of many substances, in particular botanicals, also represents a major obstacle to entering the European Market. A number of Member States consistently continue to consider certain ingredients as only acceptable in medicinal products, despite extensive case-law by the Court of Justice of the European Union (CJEU) to the effect that judgements on the status must be carried out on a case-by-case basis and that an ingredient as such cannot be considered as either food or medicine (Silano et al. 2011).

Although the call for further harmonized EU rules increases, the European Commission continues to support its 2008 report in which it concludes that further harmonization is not only feasible given the wide variety of different rules applicable in the Member States but also not necessary because of a number of new legislative texts that would help facilitate acceptance of products between the Member States, in particular the AVMF, NHCR, and MRR (EC 2008).

These legislative texts date from 2007 to 2009 and their effect on the market to date is fairly limited. It remains to be seen in how far they will be able to create a more harmonized EU market. It is clear that at least the implementation of the NHCR has been hampered by many implementation problems and has led to many unanticipated consequences, many of which seem contrary to the intended objectives of the Regulation.

This chapter describes some of the major issues that have arisen and will give an insight on how the implementation is impacting the various objectives of the legislation. It shows that the developing Regulations in this area are extremely difficult and complex and that principles of proper law-making are hard to apply. It confirms the findings of a recent report by the European Responsible Nutrition Alliance that the EU claims regulation is hardly meeting any of its initial objectives (ERNA 2011a).

6.2 NUTRITION AND HEALTH CLAIMS REGULATION: THE DIFFICULT ROAD TO IMPLEMENTATION

The NHCR is undisputably one of the most complex and difficult pieces of legislation the EU has ever adopted in the field of food law. It starts from the basic principle that all nutrition and health claims used on product labels and in the publicity of foodstuffs need to be pre-approved.

The objectives of the NHCR have been described in the proposal and include (EC 2003):

- To achieve a high level of consumer protection by providing further voluntary information, beyond the mandatory information foreseen by EU legislation.
- To improve the free movement of goods within the internal market.
- To increase legal security for economic operators.
- To ensure fair competition in the area of foods.
- To promote and protect innovation in the area of foods.

During the discussions with the European Parliament, concern was also raised on its implications for small and medium-sized enterprises (SMEs).

The development of the NHCR took nearly 6 years since it was first announced and consultations started. The actual legislative process itself took nearly 3 years before the text finally came into application on July 1, 2007. It was the result of years of discussions and negotiations and it can be observed that many aspects are unclear or incoherent because they are largely the result of compromises between the EU Member States and the European Parliament. This has resulted in a final text the implementation of which has been hampered by numerous and significant interpretation issues. The law has already been complemented by an important number of implementing and guidance texts.

One of the main aspects at the origin of many of the implementation problems is the fact that the NHCR is very prescriptive and only permits the use of claims after they have been approved and put on specific positive lists. It contains three different authorization procedures depending on the type of claim, but the application of these in practice has turned out to be virtually identical. The assessment of the scientific data underlying a claim is entrusted to the European Food Safety Authority (EFSA) but the criteria for the scientific substantiation of a claim have not been included in the law. The approach taken by EFSA has led to the rejection of most claims for food components other than essential nutrients and has been the focus of controversy.

At this point in time, 5 years after the law entered into force little of the NHCR is being applied and enforced, with many transition periods still in place and the full impact of this legislation is yet to be seen. A number of fundamental aspects of the law that should have been fully in effect are not operational. These include the so-called "*Article 13 list of claims*" and the concept of nutrient profiles. In addition, the Member States are still discussing many interpretation issues and several guidance documents are still under development to clarify the main issues to both companies and enforcement authorities. The way in which the Regulation is interpreted, applied, and enforced has therefore been appropriately referred to by many as a "*learning process.*"

6.2.1 Need for Extensive Post Hoc Clarification

Despite the Interinstitutional Agreement on the quality of drafting EU legislation specifying that Community legislative acts shall be drafted clearly, simply, and precisely, the NHCR is nothing like that and has required more than 10 documents of clarifications and guidance on the implementation of its various provisions (EC 1999).

It started with the publication of the wrong version of the NHCR on December 30, 2006 in the *Official Journal of the European Union* (Regulation 1924/2006). A corrigendum with the right text was soon published on January 19, 2007 (Corrigendum to Regulation 1924/2006).

Since then, this text has seen several amendments (Regulation 107/2008, Regulation 109/2008, Regulation 116/2010).

Furthermore, the legislation has also required clarification and implementing rules:

- A first set of guidelines clarifying certain aspects of the NHCR was adopted and published on the EC website and at least two additional sets were under discussion in the first half of

2012 (EC 2007, EC 2009, EC 2010). Also some Member States have developed guidelines on national level (Swedish Food Administration 2009, UK FSA 2011).

- Implementing rules for the application of the applicant-linked authorization process have been published as Regulation 353/2008 in 2008 (Regulation 353/2008). These were largely based on guidance that has been developed by EFSA on the content of applications under the Article 14 procedure.
- Further guidance was needed on the aspects relating to the applications for authorization. EFSA issued several guidance documents, briefing notes, submission templates to be used as background for the compilation of applications for authorization. Some examples:
  - Pre-submission guidance for applicants intending to submit applications for authorization of health claims made on foods (March 2007) (EFSA 2007a).
  - Scientific and technical guidance for the preparation and presentation of the application for authorization of a health claim (July 2007, updated in June 2011) (EFSA 2007b).
  - Templates for claims submissions (July 2007) (EFSA 2007c).
- A number of guidance documents relating to the scientific criteria applied for Articles 13, 13.5, and 14 applications and for specific fields of health (EFSA 2011a–g).

In summary, despite the Regulation being in application for almost five years, implementation is slow and many aspects still need clarification, making the application of the Regulation by companies cumbersome and uncertain. It can be argued that legislation that needs this amount of guidance and clarification is not an example of clear, simple, and precise legislation. It is hardly surprising that it therefore is leading to numerous interpretation and implementation issues.

6.2.2 LOGIC FOR CREATING CLAIMS CATEGORIES AND RESULTING BORDERLINES

A major problem with the EU NHCR is undoubtedly its unclear definitions of the claims that are actually covered. Although one would at first glance estimate that the NHCR covers three types of claims ("*nutrition claims*," "*health claims*," and "*reduction of disease risk claims*") as these are the ones that have been explicitly defined, it actually covers no less than 16 different categories of claims. Each of these categories not only presents interpretation issues, but also creates borderlines with each other that again need further clarification (see Table 6.1).

As the type of claim determines the rules and procedures to be followed, it is of the utmost importance to be able to classify claims correctly. This multitude of definitions however leads to a number of classification issues between the various claims, some of which have been addressed in a general way by the EC and the Member States but others remain to be resolved on a case-by-case basis.

6.2.3 DISCUSSIONS ON WHAT IS COVERED AND WHAT IS NOT?

When following the implementation of the NHCR, one cannot avoid wondering if it is clear what will be covered and what not. The NHCR covers claims in all "*commercial communications*," but this concept is not defined. This oversight already gave rise to debates and unresolved discussions relating to specific communications (e.g., the description or referral to health claims in scientific publication, communication to medical professionals).

This leads of course to the crucial question of what is to be regarded as commercial and what as noncommercial information. Given that the restrictive outcome of the claims approval process is likely to result in the rejection of many claims for many food components currently in use, this may lead to companies exploring ways of communication that may or not fall out of the scope of commercial communication. Enforcement is left to the discretion of the Member States, potentially resulting in diverging application of the law, a major source of legal uncertainty.

TABLE 6.1

Overview of the Different Types of Claims Covered by the NHCR and Associated Interpretation Issues

Claim	Status	Associated Issues	Status
Nutrition claim	Defined in Article 2.2.4	Borderline with "function claims"	Interpretation guidelines
Health claim	Defined in Article 2.2.5	Broad definition. Covers also general nonspecific health benefits	Lack of clarification
Reduction of disease risk claim	Defined in Article 2.2.6	Risk factor	Interpretation guidelines
Claims relating to children's development and health	Not defined. Referred to in relation to Article 14	Scope	Interpretation guidelines
Health claims describing or referring to the role of a nutrient or other substance in growth, development and the functions of the body	Not defined. Referred to under Article 13	Borderline with reduction of disease risk claims	Interpretation guidelines
Health claims describing or referring to psychological and behavioral functions	Not defined. Referred to under Article 13	Borderline with reduction of disease risk claims	Interpretation guidelines
Health claims describing or referring to slimming or weight-control or a reduction in the sense of hunger or an increase in the sense of satiety or to the reduction of the available energy from the diet	Not defined. Referred to under Article 13	Borderline with foods for particular nutritional uses	Interpretation guidelines
Claims based on newly developed scientific evidence and/or which include a request for the protection of proprietary data	Not defined. Referred to under Article 13.5.	What is newly developed scientific evidence?	Lack of clarification
Comparative claims	Not defined. Referred to under Article 9	Scope	Interpretation guidelines
General, nonspecific benefits of the nutrient or food for overall good health or health-related well-being	Not defined. Referred to under Article 10.3	Scope	Lack of clarification
Recommendations of or endorsements by national associations of medical, nutrition or dietetic professionals and health-related charities	Not defined. Referred to under Article 11	Scope	Lack of clarification
Claims which suggest that health could be affected by not consuming the food	Not defined. Referred to under Article 12	Scope	—
Claims which make reference to the rate or amount of weight loss	Not defined. Referred to under Article 12	Scope	—
Claims which make reference to recommendations of individual doctors or health professionals and other associations not referred to in Article 11	Not defined. Referred to under Article 12	Scope	—
Generic descriptors (denominations)	Referred to under Article 1.4	Scope	—
Trade mark, brand name or fancy name which may be construed as a nutrition or health claim	Referred to under Article 1.3	Scope	—

6.2.4   THREE AUTHORIZATION PROCEDURES APPLIED AS ONE

The NHCR provides for three distinct authorization procedures, each with their specific rules and process for authorization:

- The so-called *"Article 13 list"* or *"Article 13.1 list"* was intended as an approval procedure for generally accepted *"function claims."* These are claims based on generally accepted scientific evidence that are well understood by the average consumer. The intention was simple: The Member States must submit their list of accepted claims to the EC; the EC asks EFSA for advice; and the final adopted list is used by all companies wanting to make the allowed claims in conformity with the conditions of use. It was argued by the EC that this list specifically accommodates the needs of SMEs who do not have the resources to invest in innovative research to develop applications for authorization.
- The so-called applicant-linked *"accelerated"* procedure of Article 18 covering *"function claims"* that are based on new data and/or those including a request for the protection of proprietary data, to enable a quick assessment of the evidence underlying new claims to promote innovation based on investments in research.
- And the *"full"* authorization procedure of Article 14 for RDRC that hitherto had not been allowed because they were considered of a medicinal nature and therefore needed a thorough assessment. (It should be noted that claims referring to children's development and health were added to the art 14 procedure as part of the final compromise between the EP and Council without much consideration of the practical consequences of this decision.)

This choice for three procedures of different length and burden was intentional and represented a proportionate approach relative to the various strengths of the claims. However, following the approach for assessment of the scientific evidence adopted by EFSA, the differences intended by the law only exist on paper. EFSA's initial guidance for applications, referred only to Article 14 claims. The same way of working had by 2010 been explicitly extended to both article 13.5 and article 13.1 claims (EFSA 2009a).

The fact that the implementation of these procedures is now almost identical can make one wonder about the consistency of the various procedures included in the NHCR. There seems to be little logic or need left for such complex classification: The data required are the same, the process for scientific assessment is the same and the process of authorization is in reality also virtually the same.

6.2.5   MAJOR ADJUSTMENTS OF THE PROCESS NEEDED

Because of the lack of clarity and the fact that no impact assessment has been performed to address the consequences of the provisions adopted, the implementation of the NHCR has already required a number of major adjustments. This shows how open to interpretation the implementation of the NHCR is and adds significantly to the sense of legal insecurity. Some examples:

A fundamental change in the application of the Article 13.5 procedure from February 28, 2008: Article 13.5 and the procedure of Article 18 foresee a quicker procedure for *"function claims"* that are based on newly developed scientific evidence and/or contain a request for the protection of proprietary data. It came as a complete surprise when EFSA indicated in its presubmission guidance in March 2007 that this procedure would only take effect after the establishment of the Article 13 list, that is, after January 31, 2010 at the earliest.

This was apparently based on an unclear and disputed legal interpretation of the specific provisions. It led to changed expectations and consequences for companies that had counted on submitting an application under this procedure instead of under the article 13.1 list. Faced with these criticisms and inconsistencies, the EC was forced to change its interpretation in October 2007 and to accept that applications for authorisation could be introduced from February 1, 2008.

A fundamental change in the decision-making process: Commitology procedure with scrutiny: The original NHCR foresaw that decisions on claims approval or refusal are taken by "*comitology*." This means that a decision is taken in the Standing Committee for the Food Chain and Animal Health (SCFCAH), a regulatory committee composed of Member State experts to assist the EC in taking decisions. This process would enable a decision to be taken within 8–10 months for an Article 13.5 and 10–12 months for an Article 14 submission.

However, in July 2006, the EU institutions reached an agreement for a new procedure relating to the delegation of powers to the EC. This new process, the "comitology procedure with scrutiny," foresees that certain decisions by the SCFCAH are submitted to Council (Member States) and the European Parliament (EP), both of which have the power to veto such decisions (Decision 2006/512/EC). This extra step in the procedure was known at the moment that the NHCR was adopted, but no adjustments were made at that time. The effect is a delay to adoption of a decision by potentially 4–6 months and the introduction of an additional possibility for stopping any decision to allow or reject a claim, resulting in additional legal uncertainty.

Batchwise decision taking: One of the outcomes of the NHCR is the establishment of the list of claims under Article 13. The vast number of claims submitted in this process (over 44,000) led EFSA to decide it would publish its opinions on these claims in batches. This came as a surprise to everyone, including the EC who asked EFSA not to do so because of the distortive effect this would have on the market. EFSA refused because its statutes oblige EFSA to publish opinions once adopted. After an exciting exchange of letters on this topic, the EC decided to accept and follow this with the batchwise taking of decisions to allow or refuse claims.

This caused a high level of concern because of the arbitrary nature of the selection of the claims covered and the potential economic damage to the operators concerned. Consequently, the EC announced on September 27, 2010 that it had decided to adapt this approach once again and take one decision on the Article 13 list of claims for all substances except botanicals. It is now clear that, not only botanicals but also other claims, the assessment of which is not yet finalized will be exempted, leading again to unequal treatment of a substantial number of claims.

Removing botanicals from the process to address their specific issues: Botanicals present a specific group of food ingredients, mainly used in food supplements but also in medicinal products. Under European medicinal law, traditional herbal medicinal products benefit from a simplified registration procedure under which no proof of efficacy needs to be provided on the basis that sufficient bibliographic or expert evidence is available on the traditional use of the medicinal product (Directive 2004/24/EC). This is obviously in sharp contrast to the reliance on randomized controlled trials (RCTs) under the provisions of the NHCR to demonstrate health effects. It creates an unfair competitive situation between two important economic sectors. The EC has realized this and has decided to remove botanicals from the assessment process pending clarification and possible correction of this situation.

"Second chance" for specific claims (probiotics, insufficient claims): Claims have failed to receive positive opinions by EFSA for various reasons. One is lack of sufficient characterisation of the substance. This was the case for probiotics, for which EFSA only published guidance on the requirements for characterization after all submissions had been made. The EC has therefore accepted that these claims may benefit from an opportunity to submit the missing information, thereby giving them a fair chance to be reassessed.

For several other claims, EFSA has concluded that there was "insufficient" evidence to establish a cause–effect relationship. Since the submission of these claims had been compiled in 2006 and 2007 and opinions only became available starting from 2009, it could be possible that in the meantime further evidence has become available and therefore also for these claims, the EC has provided an opportunity to complement further data.

This process ran from June 1, 2011 to September 31, 2011 and 91 claims are now being reassessed. However, there are many more claims for which the evidence has not been considered by EFSA for other reasons and these claims have not been given this possibility.

Transition periods for implementation: The various transition periods specified in Article 28 of the NHCR are perhaps one of the most difficult aspects to understand. One can wonder about the need for these differences (e.g., between Articles 13.1a and 13.1b and c). The reason is that the transition periods have not been properly adjusted to the last minute changes of the compromise between the institutions. Fortunately the EC and most Member States have adopted pragmatic solutions and applied in practice the same transition period to all claims.

But one oversight needed a legal correction: the lack of a transition period for claims referring to children's development and health. The inclusion of this category of claims under the Article 14 procedure was also part of the last minute compromise but the transition period had been overlooked. It took quite a long time for the necessary adjustment to be drafted and approved (Regulation 109/2008) and it was actually published after this end date for the transition period it actually established. Fortunately here also, the Member States took a pragmatic approach and continued to allow such claims on the market.

Lack of clarity of the roles of the Member States and the EC, especially in relation to the Article 13 list and the validity check of applications: Another adjustment, still in the process of discussion is clarification on the role of the Member States for the verification of the validity of an application. This obligation was introduced officially by Regulation 1169/2009, but only in general terms. Five years after the entry into force of the NHCR, there still is no clarity on what this validity verification actually would need to be and guidelines are still under discussion.

Adjustment of the scientific principles: Perhaps the major field where adjustment is needed but which is not yet addressed is relating to the scientific principles underlying the scientific assessment of the claims. This is obviously the cornerstone of the NHCR, determining in great part its effectiveness. The approach adopted has been criticized by some as being too pharmaceutically based and not appropriate to address nutritional sciences. Others have argued that this approach does not respect the proportionality and original intention of the NHCR and that alternative ways of assessing the strength, consistency, and plausibility of the scientific evidence are more appropriate and still in line with the ECs Terms of Reference (Richardson 2005, Ames et al. 2007, Heaney 2008, Jones et al. 2008, Blumberg et al. 2010, Gallagher et al. 2011, Biesalski et al. 2011). At the end of 2011, a complaint has been submitted before the European Ombudsman and judged admissible. The judgement of the ombudsman may give significant indications as to whether the NHCR has been properly implemented in this respect (EHPM 2011).

6.2.6 FLEXIBILITY OF THE DEADLINES

The speed of decision making in the EU has always been a weak point, hampering innovation in many fields. This is illustrated by the usual reluctance for the EC to propose clear deadlines for the various steps in a given process leading to decisions. Clear deadlines have been requested and proposed by the EP during the legislative procedure on the NHCR. It was therefore one of the first legislations in the food area where the institutions involved are bound by deadlines. However, there are so many gaps and the existing deadlines are interpreted with so much flexibility that predictability as to the completion of the process is virtually impossible (see Table 6.2). A decision that initially was intended to be taken within a reasonable timeline of 8–10 months will in reality easily take double that time.

6.2.7 NUTRIENT PROFILES

The development of nutrient profiles, that is, criteria allowing or disallowing foods to make nutrition and health claims, depending on the quantities of certain nutrients and other food components, is a fundamental component of the NHCR. However, given its political nature, the setting of these profiles is blocked at the highest political level after fundamental objections were raised by certain Member States on the basis of the proposals developed by the EC.

TABLE 6.2

Overview of the Time Limits of the Procedures and the Actual Application of These Limits, Starting from the Submission to the National Competent Authority of a Member State

Step in the Procedure	Time Limit Set Article 18	Time Limit Set Article 14–17	Application of the Time Limit
Acknowledgment of receipt of the application in writing within 14 days of its receipt	14 days	14 days	
Validity check by the Member State before sending to EFSA	Not specified	Not specified	Can take days/weeks
MS to notify EFSA	n.a.	Without delay	?
EFSA to notify EC and MS	n.a.	Without delay	?
EFSA administration (completeness check)	Not specified	Not specified	Can take days/weeks
EFSA opinion	5 months	5 months	EFSA does only consider to fall within this time period the assessment work by the scientific panel from receipt of the application until adoption of its opinion, although it should start from the date of receipt of the request
Company to submit information upon a request for further information by EFSA	15 days	Not specified	
EFSA opinion time limit can be extended	1 month	2 months	
Stop the clock	Not specified	Not specified	Both on the initiative of EFSA or on request of an applicant, EFSA can stop the clock during which time the official time limit of 5 months is temporarily suspended
EFSA publication of the opinion and sending it to the EC and MS	Not specified	Not specified	Can take days/weeks
Submitting of a draft decision to the SCFCAH	The SCFCAH is actually lot necessary, but is used anyway to consult the Member States	2 months	
Discussion and adoption of the decision	Not specified In principle the chair of the SCFCAH should determine a deadline for the delivering of each decision to be taken	Not specified In principle the chair of the SCFCAH should determine a deadline for the delivering of each decision to be taken	Can take weeks/months

continued

TABLE 6.2 (continued)

Overview of the Time Limits of the Procedures and the Actual Application of These Limits, Starting from the Submission to the National Competent Authority of a Member State

Step in the Procedure	Time Limit Set Article 18	Time Limit Set Article 14–17	Application of the Time Limit
Sending decision to EP for scrutiny	Not specified	Not specified	Can take weeks
Administration for the scrutiny procedure	Not specified	Not specified	Can take weeks
Scrutiny procedure	3 months	3 months	
Translation and publication of the decision	Not specified	Not specified	Can take weeks

Note: n.a. = not applicable.

6.2.8 UNSATISFACTORY AUTHORIZATION PROCESS

Finally, it should be noted that also the procedure for claims assessment is not optimal and several aspects are often criticized, including:

- *Lack of transparency.* Companies have no insight into their application once it is submitted and into what happens with complementary data they are asked to submit during the assessment process.
- *Lack of predictability in the process.* Not only is there little clarity on the expectations, despite the guidance and templates published by EFSA, it is also unclear how the criteria will be applied and the outcome often comes as an unpleasant surprise.
- *Lack of pre-submission meetings.* The fact that there is no opportunity to discuss the requirements and criteria that EFSA would consider acceptable prior to an application has been considered by many as an important weakness. EFSA has recently taken steps to improve the possibilities for interaction with applicants by the creation of an application help desk.
- *Lack of exchange during the process.* One of the frequently heard criticisms by applicants is the lack of possibility for exchange during the process. In response EFSA has gradually introduced the principle of the "*stop the clock*" to allow more time for clarification. Still applicants have indicated that requests for further information are selective and often do not consider the fundamental elements that lead to a negative opinion.
- *Lack of opportunity for the applicant to be informed of the outcome.* A further legitimate critique is that the applicant learns about the outcome of its opinion only a few hours before everyone else and has little time to prepare its reaction.
- *Lack of possibility to have scientific discussions.* There is no possibility for the scientists that have conducted the scientific studies to discuss relevant issues directly with the scientists that carry out the assessments.
- *Lack of involvement of experts in the field.* It is noted by the scientific experts in the field that their area of expertise is often not represented in background of the experts involved in the assessment of claims application in EFSA.
- *Lack of opportunity for the applicant to be heard.* The only possibility that exists for commenting on an opinion as an applicant is by using the 30-day period following publication that is granted to everybody. This has proven quite unsatisfactory not only because it remains a written procedure and not all comments are sent to EFSA for a response, but also because the information in the opinion is often concise and not sufficient to appreciate all nuances of the reasoning.

6.3 PRINCIPLES FOR THE SCIENTIFIC ASSESSMENT OF HEALTH CLAIMS

One of the most visible outcomes of the EU NHCR is the high number of claims for which EFSA has rejected the scientific justification. The NHCR specifies that health claims should only be authorized after a scientific assessment of the highest possible standard and that the totality of the available scientific data should be taken into account and the evidence weighed. The criteria for assessment are not specified by the NHCR itself, but have been established by EFSA without much consultation with stakeholders or academic peers.

It is therefore not surprising that the whole Article 13 list process started without any indication or guidance on the scientific requirements and that many of the earlier applications for authorization failed to succeed.

6.3.1 FAILURE OF THE ARTICLE 13 LIST PROCESS

The deadline for submission of Article 13 claims was very ambitious: January 31, 2008, leaving only 7 months after the date of application. No guidance on requirements was available and no common process determined by the Member States.

For this reason, the main representative European food/food supplements federations (CIAA (www.fooddrinkeurope.eu), EHPM (www.ehpm.org), ERNA (www.erna.org), and EBF (www. botanicalforum.eu) took the initiative to try and coordinate this massive exercise from the industry side. Already in 2006, these federations commissioned scientific experts to develop a template and guidelines for companies to submit entries (Richardson et al. 2007). These entries were vetted by a group of independent experts and compiled into a final list of 776 claims entries, the outcome of the EU-wide coordination exercise (ERNA 2007). The guidance and template were presented to the Members States and used by most to coordinate their collection of claims entries on national level.

But then the process went astray. The Member States accepted submissions from all parties without doing a proper quality check and this resulted in over 40,000 submissions landing on the desk of the EC, many of these duplicates and of very poor quality. The concerted industry effort was completely wasted in this multitude of claims. The EC took almost 1 year to sort out the list, remove and compile the duplicates and put them in a proper format. During this process, claims were modified, changed, combined, went missing and mysteriously reappeared and the end result was a list of 4185 and about 10,000 similar claims that were sent to EFSA for assessment in July 2008. The final list was later, in March 2010, extended with a further 452 claims that had gone missing bringing the final total to 4637 claims entries.

The first sign of the major discrepancy between the criteria used by the submitters and the expectations by EFSA came almost as soon as EFSA received the list, when it sent more than half of this list back for further clarification. This was based on a quick screening and, despite the criteria for the screening being published by EFSA, many incoherencies were observed in the selection of claims that were included for clarification or not (EFSA 2008, ERNA 2009a). In view of the missing guidance, this clarification round was rather unsatisfactory and not capable of correcting most of the entries concerned.

A further sign of the unpreparedness of the EC and Member States to cope with the massive amount of information was that EFSA was not able to get access to the 250,000 references that accompanied the submissions. A process was therefore initiated to ask companies to provide EFSA with physical or electronic copies of all these references.

The real amplitude of this discrepancy came with the publication of the first batch of EFSA opinions on October 1, 2009 with many claims for vitamins and minerals receiving positive opinions, but very few of the other substances.

The trend of mainly negative opinions was confirmed in further batches, published during 2010–2011. Extensive comments have been raised as to the appropriateness of the approach (ERNA

2009b, 2010, 2011a). Of particular relevance is that a high number of submissions have been rejected mainly because of formalistic reasons (insufficient characterization of the food component or the claimed effect, or the claims being out of the scope of the article 13 list).

6.3.2 DIFFICULT WAY TOWARD CLARITY

It may sound strange that EFSA never clearly published in advance the methodology it was planning to use for the assessment of claims nor submitted this to public consultation (in contrast with most if not all other new methodologies). EFSA just started applying a methodology that was not known to the submitters of entries and applications. That this methodology had considerable weaknesses only became clear with the gradual publication of opinions.

The first and only initiative EFSA organized in relation to the scientific substantiation, before it adopted its approach, was a conference on nutrition and health claims in Bologna in November 2006 (EFSA 2006). Subsequently, after having adopted the approach, EFSA has tried to explain this methodology in various guidelines and explanatory documents and through a number of specific meetings:

- The publication and subsequent consultation on a 42-page template providing guidance on the information to be submitted for the assessment of an application for authorization under Article 14 of the NHCR (so aimed primarily to reduction of disease risk claims), submitted to consultation and finally published on July 26, 2007 (EFSA 2007d). These guidelines are very detailed and complex.
- EFSA provided further clarification and explanation on its approach in a technical report to address a number of frequently asked questions and in several technical meetings with stakeholders (EFSA 2009b). But a fundamental discussion on the appropriateness of the chosen approach has never taken place. It could have prevented many of the problems that are creating major challenges in the implementation of the NHCR.
- On the Article 13 list of claims, the first time that EFSA presented and discussed its approach in an official way was at a meeting organized on October 6, 2009 for the EC and the Member States. This was after the first batch of opinions had already been published. To accompany this meeting, a briefing document was published for comments only few days before the actual meeting (EFSA 2009c).
- Given the need for still further information, EFSA finally published its *modus operandi* explaining its approach on May 7, 2010, after three batches of opinions covering almost half of the Article 13 claims had already been published (EFSA 2010a).
- An updated briefing document was submitted to a consultation on May 17, 2010 and finally published on the website on April 26, 2011 (EFSA 2011a).

In addition to this meeting for EC and Member States, EFSA organized a number of technical meetings to explain and discuss its approach with the stakeholders. However, these meetings all had in common that they hardly offered a possibility for discussion.

Nevertheless, EFSA is committed to provide more information and has published a number of specific guidance documents, open to consultation and technical meetings on a number of specific scientific topics:

- Gut and immune health. An accompanying technical meeting was organized in Amsterdam on December 2, 2010 (EFSA 2011b).
- Antioxidants, oxidative damage, and cardiovascular health (EFSA 2011c).
- Bone, joints, and oral health (EFSA 2011d).
- Appetite ratings, weight management, and blood glucose concentrations (EFSA 2011e).

- Neurological and psychological functions (EFSA 2011f).
- Physical performance (EFSA 2011g).

The guidance documents and the meeting have made it painfully clear that while the approach may be high level scientific, it has considerable limitations.

6.3.3 LIMITATIONS OF THE PHARMACEUTICAL STYLE ADOPTED WHEN APPLIED TO FOOD RESEARCH

Except for the well-established roles of vitamins and minerals in the body, the EFSA approach for virtually all other food components relies mainly on the availability of RCTs, demonstrating statistically significant and biologically relevant changes in validated biomarkers of functions that are considered beneficial for health in a healthy population.

There is no doubt that this is the highest attainable standard for demonstrating health effects, as it is also the gold standard for pharmaceutical efficacy demonstration. However, in particular, academics have stated it may not be appropriate for many areas of food research because of its inherent limitations.

- It is clear that except for vitamins and minerals, the roles of which are considered generally accepted, very few other food components are capable of obtaining positive opinions.
- Many submissions are rejected for formalistic reasons. The evidence is not even considered. Examples of formalistic reasons include:
  - *Lack of precise characterization.* Opinions have illustrated that EFSA addresses characterization in an absolute way. This means that generally accepted claims, for example, for whole grain and dietary fiber, are not considered eligible. This is in contrast to the approach of other organizations (e.g., World Health Organization/Food and Agriculture Organization (WHO/FAO) report of 2003 on Diet, Nutrition and the Prevention of Chronic Diseases) (WHO/FAO 2002).
  - *Lack of precise definition of the claimed effect.* Health effects can be worded in various ways that reflect consumer understanding. However, the EFSA opinions appear to require very precise health effects that are measurable. Health benefits relating to immune function, gastrointestinal functioning, liver or kidney function, and so on are not considered, as no precise mechanistic measurement is possible.

    In addition, it is observed that the vast majority of claims that have received positive opinions (apart from vitamins and minerals) do relate to markers that are linked to chronic diseases (e.g., cholesterol, blood pressure and platelet aggregation to cardiovascular disease, calcium and vitamin D to osteoporosis, oral acid neutralization, and tooth mineralization to dental caries).
  - *Nonacceptance that the claimed effect is beneficial.* To date, most claimed effects have been judged to be beneficial or potentially beneficial by EFSA. Nevertheless, some effects are not considered as beneficial. A notable example is the *increase of potentially beneficial microorganisms in the gastrointestinal tract.* EFSA indicates that this is a scientific judgment, but there are no or limited criteria available which demonstrate that this is not a beneficial physiological effect *per se.*
- The EFSA approach makes it nearly impossible to have claims approved relating to the maintenance of a certain physiological function in the absence of data demonstrating an improvement of such function (or a reduction of the risk factor).
- With the exception of vitamins and minerals, EFSA does not accept the weight of authoritative statements, recognized textbooks and monographs, when assessing a claim. It relies on the individual papers and study reports and often highlights flaws in design and data treatment to consider the studies of limited value.

In justifying their approach, EFSA claims that the scientific criteria used for the assessment of claims are similar to those of other systems (e.g., US FDA and Codex Alimentarius) (EFSA 2010b). This clearly is a matter of interpretation as the systems are fundamentally different:

- In the United States, no pre-marketing assessment takes place on health claims other than reduction of disease risk claims (which are called *"Health Claims"* under US legislation). The FDA guidelines on an Evidence-Based Review System for the Scientific Evaluation of Health Claims therefore only apply to the equivalent of the EU Article 14 reduction of disease risk claims and not to the function claims covered by Article 13. Such claims are at least in part covered by other guidelines, which relate to manufacturers obligations, not to FDA assessment criteria (FDA 2008, 2009).

  Furthermore, the US system specifically accepts qualified health claims, which the EFSA assessment does not (FDA 2006). Finally, one can only observe that the US system is capable of accepting general claims for dietary fiber-containing foods, which is not the case with the EFSA assessment methodology.

- Also the similarity with the *Codex Alimentarius* guidelines should be nuanced (Codex Alimentarius 1997). These guidelines explicitly foresee that claims should be possible for categories of foods with a common property. Furthermore, the guidelines specifically consider that some health claims, such as those involving a relationship between a food category and a health effect, may be substantiated based on observational evidence such as epidemiological studies. Such studies should provide a consistent body of evidence from a number of well-designed studies. Evidence-based dietary guidelines and authoritative statements prepared or endorsed by a competent authoritative body and meeting the same high-scientific standards may also be used. This is clearly not the case with EFSA's approach.

This led the European Responsible Nutrition Alliance (ERNA) to propose and suggest an alternative methodology that they consider would be more appropriate to address the quality and consistency of the scientific evidence to assess the plausibility of the claimed effect (ERNA 2009c).

Table 6.3 gives an overview of the EU approach for the assessment of claims as adopted by EFSA and the consequences it has for certain areas of health effects.

6.4 IMPACT AND UNANTICIPATED CONSEQUENCES

It may seem strange that the NHCR has never been subject to a proper quantitative impact assessment. It assumed that since it concerns voluntary information, there would not be any impact on the market while it would allow companies to make accepted claims in the whole EU.

The European Health Claims Alliance, a group created by concerned companies in 2009 to address the implementation of the claims Regulation, commissioned an independent impact assessment to assess the economic impact of the NHCR. It shows serious consequences both in terms of effectiveness of the NHCR and on economic level (see Table 6.4) (Brookes 2010).

In addition numerous further consequences have arisen, many unexpected and even contrary to the objectives of the NHCR in terms of consumer protection, fair competition, legal certainty, research and innovation, free movement of goods and small- and medium-sized enterprises.

6.4.1 IMPACT ON CONSUMER PROTECTION

Protection of the consumer against misleading claims is undoubtedly the main element that has driven the NHCR. It was felt that many claims used by companies were not sufficiently substantiated and that this was undermining the credibility of genuine health effects and induced consumers to spending money on products that did not deliver the purported benefits. However, the way in which the NHCR is being implemented is likely not to achieve this objective. It is likely to lead to

TABLE 6.3

Overview of the EU Approach for the Assessment of Claims as Adopted by EFSA and the Consequences It Has for Certain Areas of Health Effects

General Principles Applied by EFSA	Consequences
1. The food/constituent must be defined and characterized. Studies to substantiate the claimed effect must be on the food/constituent.	EFSA considers characterization of a food or food component in an absolute way and only accepts studies performed with individual substances or foods with well-defined amounts of those substances as pertinent.
• If the claim is for a constituent, studies to substantiate the claim need to be presented on that constituent.	This leads to a situation where claims accepted by other organizations are not acceptable in the EU:
• If the claim is on a specific product formulation/combination of constituents, studies need to be presented on this formulation.	• The process is not able to reach positive conclusions on complex foods or mixtures of food components in the diet.
• A rationale for the role of each constituent relevant to the claimed effect should be provided.	• E.g., Claims for dietary fiber[a] are not accepted, despite links between the intake of dietary fiber and body weight regulation and reduction of obesity having been judged as convincing and between the reduction of type 2 diabetes and cardiovascular disease as probable by WHO/FAO.[b]
Studies on the food/constituents must include the conditions of use.	• E.g., Claims relating to various health benefits of whole grain[c] are not acceptable.
Evidence must show how variability would influence the effect, how differences between members from a category would influence the effect.	• The strong focus on well-defined substance characterization leads EFSA to consider much of the observational studies that have been performed with the foods as such as not pertinent for the assessment of the claims.
Consistency of the final product for those characteristics pertinent to the claimed effect, batch-to-batch stability must be shown.	• E.g., For soy protein[d] EFSA could not draw conclusions for the scientific substantiation of the claimed effect because the scientific evidence does not allow one to distinguish between the effects of the protein component of soy and those of soy isoflavones on lipid peroxidation.
	• E.g., *Camellia sinensis* (L.) Kuntze (tea)[e] is not sufficiently characterized for health benefits to be accepted, but catechins from green tea (including Epigallocatechin-galate) would.
	• The strong focus on pure food components makes it difficult to accept natural variability associated with the composition of foodstuffs.
	• E.g., EFSA considered that pomegranate, its juice, and even the polyphenols it contains[f] are not sufficiently characterized for a health benefit to be accepted. Only punicalagin and ellagic acid would.
	• E.g., Propolis[g] could not be sufficiently characterized because differences are observed in the qualitative and quantitative values of constituents in the propolis from various geographical origins.
	• The strong focus on well characterized food components favors effects that can be demonstrated by interventions with substances on top of the normal diet but largely fails to assess beneficial effects of modifications of the diet itself.
	• E.g., For hydroxypropylmethylcellulose[h] and pectin, EFSA accepts that the addition of 4 g of HPMC and at least 10 g of pectin respectively have been shown to reduce post-prandial glycemic responses. In contrast carbohydrates that induce a low/reduced glycemic response and carbohydrates with a low glycemic index (e.g., <55) are not sufficiently characterized.

continued

TABLE 6.3 (continued)

Overview of the EU Approach for the Assessment of Claims as Adopted by EFSA and the Consequences It Has for Certain Areas of Health Effects

General Principles Applied by EFSA	Consequences
2. The claimed effect must be a beneficial physiological effect.	EFSA considers characterization of a claimed effect in terms of the potential for the effect to be measured or tested.
The claimed effect must be clearly defined.	Although EFSA considers effects relating to the maintenance of many physiological functions as beneficial, the evidence therefore needs to rely on improvements of the function under consideration (e.g., vision) or the reduction of a related risk factor (e.g., cholesterol).
The chosen outcome measure(s) must be appropriate to allow an assessment if (and to what extent) the effect has occurred. Not every demonstrated statistically significant effect is beneficial.	This leads to a number of consequences for specific fields of health:
The claimed effect needs to be specific enough to be testable and measurable by generally accepted methods. EFSA does the assessment on a case-by-case basis using scientific judgement based on the evidence provided and generally accepted scientific knowledge.	• Many health relationships are judged to be insufficiently characterized to be assessed, which eliminates whole areas of health benefits from the scope of the NHCR. The essential problem is that it is difficult to describe psychological health effects in terms that can be addressed on the basis of RCTs.
The better an effect is defined and measured by choosing appropriate endpoints and methodology, the better can the relevance of the effect to health be assessed.	Examples of not sufficiently characterized health effects (considered to be general and nonspecific and not referring to any specific health claim):
Beneficial effect is defined as the probability of a positive health effect and/or the probability of a reduction of an adverse health effect in an organism, system, or (sub) population in reaction to exposure to an agent.	• Cell membrane permeability.[j]
	• Immune system, immunity, immune health, immune system function, natural defences, support immune defences.[k]
	• Maintenance of, or contribution to, a healthy and balanced digestive system.[l]
	• Energy, vitality, vitalizing, invigoration of the body, rejuvenation, tonic, stimulant.[m]
	• Purification, purifying/detoxifying, urinary elimination, depurative, detoxificant, detoxification, supports the natural mechanism for body's purification, toxin elimination.[n]
	• Antioxidative effects relating to cell aging.[o]
	• Health effects are often selected on the basis of their measurability and not accepted because the evidence only supports a general health relationship. The choice of claims taken for assessment is biased towards claims indicating improvements of physiological functions rather than maintenance.
	• E.g., For EPA/DHA,[p] skin health is translated not to maintenance of normal skin but to protection of the skin from photo-oxidative (UV-induced) damage.
	• E.g., Also for EPA/DHA[p] immune function and normal immune system function are translated not into maintenance of the normal function of the immune system but to supporting a normal/healthy immune function in the context of decreasing the level or production of eicosanoids, arachidonic acid-derived mediators and pro-inflammatory cytokines.
	• E.g., for zeaxanthin[q] (and other substances such as lutein), EFSA is looking for evidence of an improvement of vision upon supplementation, not for the role in the maintenance for normal vision and protection of the retina.

- Certain health effects are considered not to be beneficial based on unclear criteria and the evidence is not considered in these cases. Examples include:
  - Effects related to diuretic function (water elimination from the body).[r]
  - Changes in parameters of the immune system (e.g., stimulating macrophages and increasing circulating lymphocytes).[s]
  - Antioxidant properties.[o]
  - Increase of potentially beneficial microorganisms in the gastrointestinal tracts.[s]

Only for essential nutrients (vitamins, minerals, and essential fatty acids), their role in the body is accepted based on "well-established consensus among scientific experts." This is not accepted for health benefits of other substances. For such health effects, the reliance on intervention studies, demonstrating statistically and biologically significant improvements of a biological function or validated biomarker in the general population (or specific target group), leads to a situation where only effects that relate to the reduction of a disease risk factor are considered acceptable. Most health claims (other than for essential nutrients) receiving a positive EFSA opinion to date relate to reduction of disease risk.

- Lowering or maintenance of cholesterol levels
  - Maintenance of normal cholesterol is only acceptable if the substance also has a lowering effect. Cholesterol is an accepted risk factor for cardiovascular disease.
- Maintenance of blood pressure
  - Maintenance of blood pressure is only accepted because the substances (EPA and DHA) were shown to be able to decrease blood pressure.
- Decreasing platelet aggregation
  - The claim relates to the maintenance of normal platelet aggregation, contributing to healthy blood flow. Decreasing platelet aggregation was explicitly considered a risk factor for the development of cardiovascular disease, relevant in the context of delaying atherosclerosis progression and cardiovascular complications.
- Decreasing bone mineral density
  - Increasing bone mineral density is a risk factor for osteoporosis.
- Plaque acid neutralization, tooth mineralization, reduction of oral dryness and reduction of dental plaque
  - These are all factors, clearly involved as (risk) factors in the development of caries.

Reduction of disease risk claims are only acceptable when the data are able to identify a risk factor and a reduction of this risk factor is demonstrated.

continued

3. A cause and effect relationship must be established between the consumption of the food/constituent and the claimed effect (for the target group under the proposed conditions of use).

Elements that are considered include:
- The extent to which a cause and effect relationship is established between consumption of the food/constituent and claimed effect for the target group under the proposed conditions of use.

Weighing of all of the evidence from pertinent studies addressing their overall strength, consistency, and biological plausibility
- Quality of individual studies.
- Applicability of studies to the target group.
- Conditions of use proposed by the applicant.

Human data are central for substantiation (EFSA has established a hierarchy of evidence).
- Studies must be carried out with the food/constituent.
- Appropriate outcome measure(s) of the claimed effect must be assessed.
- The conditions for human studies vs conditions of use (e.g., food/constituent quantity) must be addressed.

TABLE 6.3 (continued)

Overview of the EU Approach for the Assessment of Claims as Adopted by EFSA and the Consequences It Has for Certain Areas of Health Effects

General Principles Applied by EFSA	Consequences
• Study group must be representative of the target group. Extrapolation of studies in patients on a case-by-case basis. Studies in animals or *in vitro* may provide supportive evidence. No pre-established formula (number/type of studies needed). For reduction of disease risk claims, wording should refer to the specific risk factor for disease. Opinions indicate nature and quality of evidence but do not provide grades of evidence.	For reduction of disease risk claims, only claimed effects that relate to the reduction (or beneficial alteration) of a risk factor for the development of a human disease (not reduction of the risk of disease) are acceptable. • This leads to a situation that such claims would not be accepted if only a direct effect on the reductions of the disease would be demonstrated, something of much more value for public health than the reduction of a risk factor. 　• E.g., For a reduction of disease risk claim related to gastrointestinal infections, a relevant reduction of specific pathogenic microorganisms or their toxins in the gastrointestinal tract, as measured in suitable samples (e.g., stools), is required. The reduction of signs and symptoms of the infection in itself is not sufficient. In addressing the quality of the studies, many flaws of study design and methodology are identified which lead to rejection of the studies as evidence in support of the claimed effect. Such weaknesses and flaws include: 　• Small number of subjects 　• Lack of control groups 　• Short duration of the studies 　• High drop-out rate 　• Lack of statistical power 　• Lack of adequate randomization 　• Intervention matrices (e.g., capsules) differing from the foods specified in the application 　• Lack of proper validation of questionnaires 　• Inappropriate markers for the chosen end point 　• Insufficient blinding 　• … The reliance on pharmaceutical style study protocols ignores many of the practical problems of designing intervention trials with foods in the general (healthy) population to show statistically and biologically significant changes in physiological parameters. A systematic assessment and weighing of the totality of the evidence would be a more appropriate way to address the strength, consistency, and plausibility of nutritional effects.

a *EFSA Journal* 2010; 8(10):1735.
b WHO/FAO 2002 Technical Report Series 916.
c *EFSA Journal* 2010; 8(10):1766.
d *EFSA Journal* 2010; 8(10):1812.
e *EFSA Journal* 2010; 8(10):1791.
f *EFSA Journal* 2010; 8(10):1750.
g *EFSA Journal* 2010; 8(10):1810.
h *EFSA Journal* 2010; 8(10):1739.
i *EFSA Journal* 2010; 8(10):1747.
j *EFSA Journal* 2010; 8(10):1725.
k *EFSA Journal* 2010; 8(10):1799.
l *EFSA Journal* 2010; 8(10):1767.
m *EFSA Journal* 2010; 8(10):1738.
n *EFSA Journal* 2010; 8(10):1733.
o *EFSA Journal* 2010; 8(10):1752.
p *EFSA Journal* 2010; 8(10):1796.
q *EFSA Journal* 2010; 8(10):1724.
r *EFSA Journal* 2010; 8(10):1742.
s *EFSA Journal* 2010; 8(10):1809.

TABLE 6.4

Main Conclusions of the Impact Assessment in Relation to the NHCR's Main Objectives

Objective	Delivery of Objective Rating	Reasons for Rating
Achieve high level of consumer protection and ensure consumers not misled, claims made are clear and accurate, consumers can make informed and meaningful choices	Poor	Fewer product choices Increased advertising spend may result in more vague messages to consumers (less informed) Increased share of 3rd country suppliers who can avoid EU legislation requirements in country of origin
To increase legal security for economic operators	Poor	Lack of clarity/transparency in approval process = increased legal uncertainty
To improve free movement of foods/products and ensure fair competition	Weak	Batch handling of decisions hinders competition Extra costs of supporting products/bringing to market = raising barriers to entry and reduces competition
To promote, encourage, and protect innovation	Poor	Uncertainty and expected increased costs of bringing products to market = discourages innovation
Recognition of the importance of SMEs in maintaining quality and preservation of different dietary habits across the EU	Poor	SMEs likely to be most affected by expected negative economic impacts

claims on the market, the context of which is difficult to understand. It will deny informed consumers' essential information to judge upon the relevance of emerging scientific findings and it will shift communication on health benefits to less controllable information sources.

6.4.1.1   Will There Be Less Unsubstantiated Claims on the Market?

Because all health claims made on food should be subject to a pre-marketing authorization, this would logically need to lead to only scientifically substantiated claims on the market. However, it is considered by many that the vast number of rejected claims is likely to lead companies to look for alternative ways of communication (other than commercial communications, e.g., via media and press, Internet, social networks, etc.) that will either fall out of the scope or be more difficult to control. The result may very well be even less controlled and scientifically justified information than is the case today.

6.4.1.2   Will Claims Be More Understandable to the Consumer?

It was anticipated that control over the wording would make claims better understandable to the consumer. However, enforcement of accepted claims will require officials to judge on the flexibility of the wording of claims and consumer understanding, without any criteria in place. This is likely to focus on details of the claims wording, based on subjective impressions.

In addition, consumer understanding is dependent on the level of knowledge of the consumer, not on the claim. Despite the intention of the EC to allow flexibility of the wording, Member States continue to raise doubts on the comprehensibility of certain words (e.g., "neurotransmitter," "homocysteine metabolism," "energy-yielding metabolism," "macronutrient metabolism," "connective tissues," "protection of cell constituents against oxidative damage," "maternal tissue growth during pregnancy," etc.). Whether legitimate or not, there are no criteria on the basis of which consumer understanding of these terms and potential alternatives can be assessed.

The disparate approach taken by EFSA on claims for essential nutrients as opposed to other food components has led to the acceptance of rather strong claims for vitamins and minerals, such as

"Vitamin B6 contributes to the normal function of the immune system," which can be made on a product containing 15% of the RDA (EFSA 2009d). However, it is not clear if such a claim will be understood to have the same relevance as a similar claim for a probiotic product (should such a claim be approved). Another example is the fundamentally different nature of a cholesterol-lowering effect of phytosterols/stanols as compared to that of essential fatty acids (linoleic acid).

The term "Qualified Health Claims" comes from the claims system that is applicable in the United States. Such claims describe health effects that are supported by scientific evidence, but do not meet the "significant scientific agreement" standard. As a result, to ensure that they are not false or misleading to consumers, they must be accompanied by a disclaimer or other qualifying language to accurately communicate the level of scientific evidence supporting the claim. This approach has not been applied in the EU, leaving only claims for which conclusive evidence exists.

Grading of the evidence has been advocated as an alternative approach, essential for product innovation. It is not an inferior standard but a different methodology. The scientific assessment of the totality of the available data and weighing of the evidence using grading of evidence requires an equally rigorous, if not higher standard of scientific judgement and this would be consistent with a legislation advocating the use of the highest standard. Grading of evidence has been applied by the World Health Organisation and World Cancer Research Fund, has been addressed by the European Medicines Agency in the context of the assessment of the efficacy of medicinal products, and was even at a certain moment proposed by the authorities of The Netherlands in the context of the Article 13 list (WCRF 1997, EMEA 1999, WHO/FAO 2002, EMEA 2004, Netherlands 2004).

Furthermore, grading of the evidence is a system that enables systematic reporting on the strength, consistency, and plausibility of the evidence for a health effect and does not necessarily need to lead to qualified health claims. The EU claims system is apparently not able to confirm the health effects for dietary fiber or whole grain that are part of many if not all national food recommendations (EFSA 2010c, EFSA 2010d). These claims received negative opinions because EFSA was not able to characterize these food components and match them with intervention trials. It can legitimately be questioned if a system that is not able to confirm the health benefits of dietary fiber is suitable to be applied to foods and many limitations of this approach have been published.

Furthermore if health effects are only considered valid when they are convincingly demonstrated, this also raises the question whether consumers do not have the right to be informed about health effects for which there are indications but no consensus yet. The public health dimension may even be more important. Some have raised the question if it would not be appropriate to apply the "inverse precautionary" principle to such claims, which means that in cases where there are indications of a beneficial effect, it would be legitimate to give the benefit of the doubt to the effect because, if further research would show the effect cannot be confirmed, no harm would have been done and the claim could be disallowed (Biesalski et al. 2011). If the claimed effect would be confirmed by further research, at least consumers would have had the information and have benefited from the effect.

6.4.2 IMPACT ON INNOVATION

Innovation obviously is an important aspect of economic strength. It was promoted as the motor for economic change in the EU Lisbon Strategy (http://ec.europa.eu/information_society/eeurope/i2010/ict_and_lisbon/index_en.htm) and is at the heart of the Europe 2020 blueprint for re-establishing the competitiveness of the EU economy (http://ec.europa.eu/europe2020/index_en.htm).

It is inescapable that the NHCR and in particular its implementation will have a considerable impact on research efforts in this field. The very fact that the legislation includes a system for generic approvals (i.e., a claim is submitted by a company, but the approval is valid for the whole industry) is in itself an anti-innovative principle.

The NHCR has aimed at compensating this by a system of proprietary data protection to grant a form of exclusivity for a claim for a 5-year period of time. However, at the current state of implementation, there are clear signs that this is not sufficient to foster innovation. Several other issues actively hinder innovation and make companies hesitate to initiate research investments into new health products. Some examples include

- The fact that the type of scientific evidence needed is so narrow and specific means that chances of success, and thus innovation, are restricted only to those food components that have the chance of meeting the pharmaceutical style requirements adopted by EFSA. Such research may not be possible or feasible for complex food components because of the costs of the large intervention trials required. The lack of validated biomarkers in various fields of health further limits the possibilities.
- The uncertainty relating to the expectations of EFSA on what will be acceptable and what not is another important factor that greatly hinders decisions to engage in new research. In view of such uncertainties and the unpredictability of the outcome of the authorization process companies are not able to ascertain the return on investment and may be looking to abandon research projects and shift budgets toward marketing activities.
- The fact that mainly claims relating to vitamins and minerals have received positive EFSA opinions, often relating to very important fields of health including immune function, cognitive function and tiredness, in combination with the very low chances for approval of claims for other substances, may create a situation where companies chose to use claims for vitamins and minerals in their products rather than to engage in research into new components with essentially the same health benefits as those already allowed.
- The establishment of the Article 13 list in itself will in effect establish a health effect for a food component that will last as long as it remains included in the list and, taken together with the failure of the approach to acknowledge emerging science, may lead to a standstill on most, if not all new research for that food component, because there would not be a need any longer for further diversification of the health effect.
- The approval process in itself is long and a positive EFSA opinion is not a guarantee for a final approval, as the Member States need to take a decision and the decision may still be rejected through EP scrutiny. During this process, competition may already prepare to capture parts of the market by other means (e.g., by using already approved claims for other food components or brand marketing in combination with generic advertising for the food component).
- Finally, the system of proprietary data protection itself is turning out to be far weaker than initially anticipated, in particular by the curious and unanticipated interpretation that published data are not eligible for protection.

6.4.3   IMPACT ON FAIR COMPETITION

The aim of the NHCR to promote fair competition was obviously inspired by the fact that unscrupulous manufacturers making misleading claims can gain illegitimate profit and compete with and undermine the credibility of genuine health effects of foods. One important element to ensure fair competition is to create a level playing field not only in relation to the rules applying to claims, but also in relation to the claims itself.

At this stage in the implementation process, it is doubtful if this aim will be achieved:

- Harmonized legislation in the EU is often flawed by diverging national interpretations and issues are rarely clarified on EU level or before the relevant court. It is practically unavoidable that the sensitivity of various Member States for some specific wordings, perceived differences in consumer understanding, the national interpretations of the borderline with medicinal products and in particular the lack of harmonization of food composition, will be elements leading to restrictions in the free circulation of foods bearing claims.

- The Food Supplements Directive harmonizes the composition of food supplements but only provides for specific rules for vitamins and minerals. The use of other substances is subject to national rules. As long as diverging national rules exist and mutual recognition is not applied (despite the existence of the mutual recognition legislation), this will greatly hinder the free movement of foods with approved nutrition and health claims.
- Another element is that various claims have not been treated equally during the process. The possibility to provide further information for some and not for other claims, the batch-wise publications of opinion on claims, the removal of botanicals from the assessment process, the putting on hold of certain claims are all examples of discrepancies that create competitive advantages and disadvantages for companies depending on the composition of their products.
- The approach for assessment adopted by EFSA creates an even more fundamental discrepancy between claims. By relying mainly on RCTs demonstrating statistically and biologically significant improvements of bodily functions based on measurements of validated biomarkers in a healthy population, the approach in itself limits the potential for many health effects to be recognized. Certain fields of health (e.g., cholesterol lowering) are favored by multiple positive opinions, while other fields, where markers are not accepted (e.g., probiotics, antioxidants, immune effects, etc.), have not seen many positive opinions to date. This is clearly to the advantage of companies active in the favored sectors and disadvantageous for those that have built their product portfolio in the not favored sectors.
- Finally and for completeness sake, the intended adoption of nutrient profiles may also have a considerable distortive potential on the food sector.

6.4.4   IMPACT ON LEGAL CERTAINTY

Uncertainty undoubtedly ranks at the very top of the difficulties companies experience with the NHCR. Uncertainty about the interpretation of the definition and many of the general provisions of the law, uncertainty about the expectations of EFSA and the chances of success of an application, uncertainty whether proprietary data protection will be accepted, uncertainty about whether the application will survive the discussions of the EC and Member States and the scrutiny of the EP, uncertainty on how national authorities will enforce a claim, uncertainty on transition periods and actions to be taken at the current time. It can therefore be safely said at this point that legal certainty is far from achieved.

6.4.5   IMPACT ON RESEARCH

The approach as adopted by EFSA has set a trend toward medicalization of food and its appropriateness for nutritional research has been questioned and the limitations demonstrated. The resulting probable reduction of research efforts and investments will undoubtedly lead to less research commissioned in academic centers and certain fields of research may be abandoned altogether. This will almost inevitably lead to losses in jobs, a brain drain to regions where emerging science still has a chance and weakening of EU's functional food research capacity.

Another criticism heard from academics is that by its ruling on the quality and usefulness of scientific research done by others, EFSA is fundamentally undermining the peer review without giving the possibility of the researchers involved to directly discuss and defend their work.

Finally the application of the NHCR provisions is a strong stimulus for keeping data unpublished. In order not to lose the possibility for data protection, companies commissioning research will refrain the researchers from publishing their results. EFSA will be the first to see and judge them and after the opinion there will not be much incentive to publish the data either.

6.4.6 IMPACT ON SMALL- AND MEDIUM-SIZED ENTERPRISES

Fundamentally, the claims Regulation is strongly biased toward applications for authorization, a complex and resource intensive process, hardly accessible to most SMEs. This will lead to claims for other substances moving away from SMEs into the hands of companies with research capacities, thereby creating new challenges to their competitive position.

6.5 CONCLUSION

Although on paper the EU has a fairly consistent and complete legal system to regulate products such as nutraceuticals, functional foods and food supplements, in reality the market is hampered by the divergent application of these rules and further national legislation and enforcement practices. More recent EU legislation has not been able to affect this much at this time. The Mutual Recognition Regulation is not being applied to its full extent and companies remain affected by subjective considerations in the various Member States. The fortification Regulation contains a process to address safety concerns relating to the use of particular ingredients in foods when exposure would increase substantially, but implementing rules have just been agreed upon and the process has not been used.

The main instrument seen by the EC to regulate these products is the Nutrition and Health Claims Regulation. It is a legislation that requires pre-marketing approval for all claims. It has been fraught with implementation problems and it is gradually becoming clear it will fail to achieve many of its objectives. The development of the article 13 list has suffered more than 2 years delay already and a first, only partial list is scheduled to come into application in the second half of 2012. Work on nutrient profiles has shown a delay of over 3 years already and is still blocked at political level. The application has seen so many adjustments and the lack of clarity of many provisions create much legal uncertainty and is likely to lead to enforcement problems. The scientific standard adopted by EFSA has been criticized as being not realistic for food research and has led to many claims for other substances being rejected and botanicals taken out of the process. As a consequence, the NHCR is expected to lead to substantial economic consequences for the food sector in the EU and potentially internationally. The uncertainty of the criteria, the length of the authorization procedure, the lack of transparency and interaction on applications, the cost of the research needed, the limited value of data protection and the unpredictability of the decision-making process are all factors that will lead to reduced investments in research and innovation. It is likely that in the end no single one of the NHCR's objectives will be met and that the EU claims experiment will have led to little added value at a considerable economic cost.

REFERENCES

Ames, B.N., McCann, J.C., Stampfer, M.J., and Willett, W.C. 2007. Evidence-based decision making on micronutrients and chronic disease: Longterm randomized controlled trials are not enough. Letter to the editor. *The American Journal of Clinical Nutrition* 86, 522–523.

Biesalski, H.K., Aggett, P., and Anton, R. et al. 2011. *26th Hohenheim Consensus Conference*, September 11th 2010. Scientific substantiation of health claims: Evidence-based nutrition. *Nutrition* 27, S1–S20.

Blumberg, J., Heaney, R.P., Huncharek, M. et al. 2010. Evidence-based criteria in the nutritional context. *Nutrition Reviews* 68, 478–484.

Brookes, G. Economic Impact Assessment of the European Union (EU)'s Nutrition & Health Claims Regulation on the EU food supplement sector and market. September 2010. GBC Ltd, UK. http://www.ehpm.org/userfiles/file/Impact%20Assessment/Impact%20Assessment%20FINAL.pdf

Codex Alimentarius. 1997. Guidelines for use of nutrition and health claims; Annex: Recommendations on the scientific substantiation of health claims. CAC/GL 23-1997. http://www.codexalimentarius.net/download/standards/351/CXG_023e.pdf

Corrigendum to Regulation (EC) No. 1924/2006 of the European Parliament and of the Council of 20 December 2006 on nutrition and health claims made on foods. *Official Journal of the European Union* L12/3, 18 January 2007.

Decision 2006/512/EC of 17 July 2006 amending Decision 1999/468/EC laying down the procedures for the exercise of implementing powers conferred on the Commission. *Official Journal of the European Community* L200/11, 22 July 2006.

Directive 2002/46/EC of the European Parliament and of the Council of 10 June 2002 on the approximation of the laws of the Member States relating to food supplements. *Official Journal of the European Union* L136/85, 12 July 2002.

Directive 2004/24/EC of the European Parliament and of the Council of 31 March 2004 amending, as regards traditional herbal medicinal products, Directive 2001/83/EC on the Community code relating to medicinal products for human use. *Official Journal of the European Union* L136/85, 30 April 2004.

EC. 1999. European Parliament, Council, Commission Interinstitutional Agreement of 22 December 1998 on common guidelines for the quality of drafting of Community legislation. *Official Journal of The European Union* C73/1, 17 March 1999.

EC. 2003. Proposal for a regulation of the European Parliament and of the council on nutrition and health claims made on foods Brussels, 16.7.2003. COM (2003) 424 final 2003/0165 (COD).

EC. 2007. Guidance on the implementation of Regulation (EC) No. 1924/2006 on nutrition and health claims made on foods. Conclusions of the Standing Committee on the food chain and animal health. 14 December 2007.

EC. 2008. Commission of the European Communities. Report from the commission to the Council and the European Parliament on the use of substances other than vitamins and minerals in food supplements. COM (2008) 824 final. Brussels, 5 December 2008. Available online: http://ec.europa.eu/food/food/labellingnutrition/supplements/documents/COMM_PDF_COM_2008_0824_F_EN_RAPPORT.pdf

EC. 2009. Working paper [on the admissibility check] tabled as agenda item 5 at the meeting of the claims working group on 20 April 2009.

EC. 2010. Guidance on using authorised nutrition and health claims in accordance with Regulation (EC) 1924/2006 on nutrition and health claims made on foods, tabled as agenda item 4 at the meeting of the claims working group on 18 October 2010.

EFSA. 2006. Summary report: EFSA Conference on Nutrition and Health Claims, 8–10 November 2006, Bologna, Italy. http://www.efsa.europa.eu/en/supporting/doc/nutritionhealthclaims.pdf

EFSA. 2007a. Pre-submission Guidance for applicants intending to submit applications for authorisation of health claims made on foods. 14 March 2007. Last updated (Rev.): 21 December 2007 http://www.efsa.europa.eu/EFSA/efsa_locale-1178620753812_1211902594478.htm

EFSA. 2007b. Scientific and technical guidance for the preparation and presentation of the application for authorisation of a health claim. Opinion of the scientific panel on dietetic products, nutrition and allergies. adopted on 6 July 2007. *The EFSA Journal* 530, 1–44.

EFSA. 2007c. Templates for claims submissions. http://www.efsa.europa.eu/EFSA/efsa_locale-1178620753812_1211902594460.htm

EFSA. 2007d. Scientific and technical guidance for the preparation and presentation of the application for authorisation of a health claim. *The EFSA Journal* 530, 1–44.

EFSA. 2008. Criteria for the initial screening of Article 13 (3) health claims of Regulation (EC) No. 1924/2006 agreed by the NDA panel on 7 October 2008. 2 October 2008. http://www.efsa.europa.eu/en/ndaclaims13/docs/ndaart13torax01.pdf

EFSA. 2009a. Briefing document for Member States and European Commission on the evaluation of Article 13.1 health claims. Technical report. *EFSA Journal* 7(11), 1386.

EFSA. 2009b. Frequently Asked Questions (FAQ) related to the assessment of Article 14 and 13.5 health claims applications on request of EFSA. *EFSA Journal* 7(9), 1339.

EFSA. 2009c. Briefing document for Member States and European Commission on the evaluation of Article 13.1 health claims on request of EFSA. *EFSA Journal* 7(11), 1386.

EFSA. 2009d. Scientific Opinion on the substantiation of health claims related to vitamin B6 [...]. *EFSA Journal* 7(9),1225.

EFSA. 2010a. EFSA's Modus Operandi for Article 13 (3) Health Claims of Regulation (EC) No. 1924/2006. 07 May 2010. http://www.efsa.europa.eu/en/ndaclaims13/docs/art13modusoperandi.pdf

EFSA. 2010b. Flynn A. Presentation on EFSA's evaluation of health claims: Scientific substantiation at the 1 June Stakeholder meeting in Parma. http://www.efsa.europa.eu/en/events/event/nda100601.htm

EFSA. 2010c. Scientific Opinion on the substantiation of health claims related to dietary fibre [...]. *EFSA Journal* 8(10), 1735.

EFSA. 2010d. Scientific Opinion on the substantiation of health claims related to whole grain [...]. *EFSA Journal* 8(10),1766.

EFSA. 2011a. General guidance for stakeholders on the evaluation of Article 13.1, 13.5 and 14 health claims. *EFSA Journal* 9(4), 2135. Available online: www.efsa.europa.eu/efsajournal

EFSA. 2011b. Guidance on the scientific requirements for health claims related to gut and immune function. *EFSA Journal* 9(4), 1984. Available online: www.efsa.europa.eu/efsajournal

EFSA. 2011c. Guidance on the scientific requirements for health claims related to antioxidants, oxidative damage and cardiovascular health. *EFSA Journal* 9(12), 2474. Available online: www.efsa.europa.eu/efsajournal

EFSA. 2011d. Draft guidance on the scientific requirements for health claims related to bone, joints, and oral health. 26 April 2011. Final version to be published in the course of 2012.

EFSA. 2011e. Draft guidance on the scientific requirements for health claims related to appetite ratings, weight management, and blood glucose concentrations. 26 April 2011. Final version to be published in the course of 2012.

EFSA. 2011f. Draft guidance on the scientific requirements for health claims related to neurological and psychological functions. 17 October 2011. Final version to be published in the course of 2012.

EFSA. 2011g. Guidance on the scientific requirements for health claims related to physical performance. 19 December 2011. Final version to be published in the course of 2012.

EHPM. 2011. Press release (23/11/2011) Ombudsman judges EHPM claims complaint valid. http://www.ehpm.org/News.aspx?NewsID=114

EMEA. 1999. Working party on Herbal Medicinal Products. Updated draft points to consider on the evidence of safety and efficacy required for well-established herbal medicinal products in bibliographic applications EMEA/HMPWP/23/99. London, 25 October 1999.

EMEA. 2004. Working party on Herbal Medicinal Products. Final concept paper on the implementation of different levels of scientific evidence in core-data for herbal drugs. EMEA/CPMP/HMPWP/1156/03. London, 3 March 2004.

ERNA. 2007. Joint CIAA-ERNA-EHPM-EBF list of article 13 entries. http://www.erna.org/Industry-article-13-list.aspx

ERNA. 2009a. Joint ERNA-EHPM-EBF Response and comments in relation to the request for clarification from EFSA on certain article 13 entries. Letter to the EC sent on 18 May 2009. http://www.erna.org/Industry-article-13-list.aspx

ERNA. 2009b. Joint ERNA-EHPM-EBF comments in relation to the first batch of article 13.1 claims opinions. Letter sent to the EC on 15 October 2009. Available on-line at www.erna.org

ERNA. 2009c. Model for the assessment of article 13.1 health claims in the framework of the EU Nutrition and Health Claims Regulation in relation to the terms of reference. June 2009. http://www.erna.org/UserFiles/Claims%20Model%20Final.pdf

ERNA. 2010. Joint ERNA-EHPM-EBF comments in relation to the second batch of article 13.1 claims opinions. Letter sent to the EC on 15 May 2010. Available on-line at www.erna.org

ERNA. 2011a. Nutrition and Health Claims in the EU. A review of the consequences of implementation. 2011. http://www.erna.org/ERNA-Report-on-Claims.aspx

ERNA. 2011b. Joint ERNA-EHPM-EBF comments in relation to the third batch of article 13.1 claims opinions. Letter sent to the EC on 20 March 2011. Available on-line at www.erna.org

FDA. 2006. Guidance for Industry: FDA's Implementation of "Qualified Health Claims": Questions and Answers; Final Guidance. 12 May 2006. www.fda.gov/Food/GuidanceComplianceRegulatoryInformation/GuidanceDocuments/FoodLabelingNutrition/ucm053843.htm

FDA. 2008. FDA. Guidance for Industry: Substantiation for Dietary Supplement Claims Made Under Section 403(r) (6) of the Federal Food, Drug, and Cosmetic Act. December 2008. www.fda.gov/Food/GuidanceComplianceRegulatoryInformation/GuidanceDocuments/DietarySupplements/ucm073200.htm

FDA. 2009. Guidance for Industry: Evidence-Based Review System for the Scientific Evaluation of Health Claims—Final. January 2009. www.fda.gov/Food/GuidanceComplianceRegulatoryInformation/GuidanceDocuments/FoodLabelingNutrition/ucm073332.htm

Gallagher, A.M., Meijer G.W., and Richardson, D.P. et al. 2011. A standardised approach towards PROving the efficacy of foods and food constituents for health CLAIMs (PROCLAIM): Providing guidance. 2011. *British Journal of Nutrition* 106, S16–S28.

Heaney, R.P. 2008. Nutrients, endpoints, and the problem of proof. *Journal of Nutrition* 138, 1591–1595.

Jones, P.J.H., Asp, N-G., and Silva, P. 2008. Evidence for health claims on foods: How much is enough? (Editorial) *Journal of Nutrition* 138, 1189S–1191S.

Netherlands 2004. Proposal for a systematic approach for a generic list of Health Claims. Draft December 2004.

Regulation 107/2008 of the European Parliament and of the Council of 15 January 2008 amending Regulation (EC) No. 1924/2006 on nutrition and health claims made on foods as regards the implementing powers conferred on the Commission. *Official Journal of the European Union* L39/8, 13 February 2008.

Regulation 109/2008 of the European Parliament and of the Council of 15 January 2008 amending Regulation (EC) No. 1924/2006 on nutrition and health claims made on foods. *Official Journal of the European Union* L39/14, 13 February 2008.

Regulation 116/2010 of 9 February 2010 amending Regulation (EC) No. 1924/2006 of the European Parliament and of the Council with regard to the list of nutrition claims. *Official Journal of the European Union* L37/16, 10 February 2010.

Regulation 178/2002 of the European Parliament and of the Council of 28 January 2002 laying down the general principles and requirements of food law, establishing the European Food Safety Authority and laying down procedures in matters of food safety. *Official Journal of the European Union* L31/1, 1 February 2002.

Regulation 258/97 of the European Parliament and of the Council of 27 January 1997 concerning novel foods and novel food ingredients. *Official Journal of the European Union* L043/1, 14 February 1997.

Regulation 353/2008 of 18 April 2008 establishing implementing rules for applications for authorisation of health claims as provided for in Article 15 of Regulation 1924/2006 of the European Parliament and of the Council. *Official Journal of the European Union* L109/11, 19 April 2008.

Regulation 764/2008 of the European Parliament and of the Council of 9 July 2008 laying down procedures relating to the application of certain national technical rules to products lawfully marketed in another Member State and repealing Decision No. 3052/95/EC. *Official Journal of the European Union* L218/21. 13.08, 2008.

Regulation (EC) No. 1169/2009 of 30 November 2009 amending Regulation (EC) No. 353/2008 establishing implementing rules for applications for authorisation of health claims as provided for in Article 15 of Regulation (EC) No. 1924/2006 of the European Parliament and of the Council. *Official Journal of the European Union* L314/34. 1 December 2009.

Regulation 1924/2006 of the European Parliament and of the Council of 20 December 2006 on nutrition and health claims made on foods. *Official Journal of the European Union* L404/9, 30 December 2006.

Regulation 1925/2006 of the European Parliament and of the Council of 20 December 2006 on the addition of vitamins and minerals and of certain other substances to foods. *Official Journal of the European Union* L404/26, 30 December 2006.

Richardson, D.P., Binns, N.M., and Viner, P. 2007. Guidelines for an evidence-based review system for the scientific justification of diet and health relationships under Article 13 of the new European legislation on nutrition and health claims. *Food Science and Technology Bulletin: Functional Foods* 3(8), 81–95.

Richardson, D.P. 2005. The scientific substantiation of health claims with particular reference to the grading of evidence. *European Journal of Nutrition* 44, 319–324.

Silano, V., Coppens, P., Larrañaga-Guetaria, A. et al. 2011. Regulations applicable to plant food supplements and related products in the European Union. *Food and Function* 2, 710_719.

Swedish Food Administration. 2009. Näringspåståenden och hälsopåståenden om livsmedel Förordning (EG) nr 1924/2006 5 November 2009. http://www.slv.se/upload/dokument/livsmedelskontroll/vagledningar/vagledning_narings-_och_halsopastaenden.pdf

UK FSA. 2011. European Regulation (EC) No. 1924/2006 on nutrition and health claims made on foods. Food Standards Agency guidance to compliance version 2 (November 2011). http://www.dh.gov.uk/en/Publicationsandstatistics/Publications/PublicationsPolicyAndGuidance/DH_130972

WCRF 1997. World Cancer Research Fund/American Institute for Cancer Research (1997). *Food, Nutrition and the Prevention of Cancer: A Global Perspective*. Washington D.C.

WHO/FAO 2002. World Health Organization/Food and Agriculture Organization (WHO/FAO) 2002. *Diet, Nutrition and the Prevention of Chronic Diseases*. WHO Technical Report Series 916.

7 Market and Marketing of Functional Foods and Dietary Supplements in America

Philip E. Apong

CONTENTS

7.1 INTRODUCTION

We live in an era where technology is rapidly advancing in many aspects of our daily lives, running the gamut from the latest feats of architectural engineering to cutting-edge smart phones and electronics, from the astronomical achievement of sending automated probes into deep space, to medical breakthroughs right here on terra firma. So it comes as no surprise that over the decades of scientific achievements in biology and nutrition, scientists today have seemingly developed a fundamental grasp of the most rudimentary nutritional requirements for the maintenance of basic human health and survival. However, as our understanding of human physiology faces constant evolution, there continues to be a commensurate development of nutritional sciences involving strategies designed to manipulate human physiology beyond that of merely providing basic daily nourishment. Nutritionists and health professionals are unraveling the beneficial role of proper nutrition, including the incorporation of nutraceuticals and health foods in disease prevention and health promotion, and this is facilitating an increase in the number of nutrition and functional food companies in the United States and globally (Bagchi, 2006).

Today, nutrition-savvy personnel at various companies are diligently pushing the ideas behind conventional nutrition to a whole new level, by designing advanced dietary interventions to promote health and well-being, and even support maximum human performance and physical potential. Many companies are fervently bringing these latest innovations to the American marketplace in the form of technologically advanced food items dubbed "functional foods" or in other formats in the form of "dietary supplements." Often in designing these functional foods and dietary supplements, companies will collaborate with the scholarly minds of academia at various university or research facilities. Companies will then promote their goods in a barrage of advertising, hitting Americans with persuasive claims, with their marketing efforts facilitated by media such as the Internet (now accessible almost everywhere on convenient smart phones and tablet computers), television, radio, and print. All of this publicity has served to create a generally positive public perception, resulting in a demand for these items across America and perhaps even globally.

Although over the last three decades the functional food market has been deeply rooted in Japan and Asia, it is continuously growing in Europe and America (Tomomatsu, 1994; Hasler, 1996, 2000; Farr, 1997; Milner, 2000; Arai, 2002; Roberfroid, 2002; Goffin et al., 2011). Functional foods and dietary supplements are available to Americans across a variety of sales channels, including natural/ specialty retail, mass market retail, mail order, multilevel marketing, and health practitioners (NBJ, 2010, 2011). This wide array of availability has likely contributed to the persistent growth of the nutrition industry in the United States in recent years (NBJ, 2010, 2011). In fact, the United States currently boasts the largest most rapidly expanding functional food and nutraceuticals market in the world (Evani, 2009; Vergari et al., 2010). Likewise, the use of dietary supplements among Americans has shown continuous growth over the years (Bailey et al., 2011). The increase in demand for dietary supplements and functional foods is almost certainly being propelled by various factors, including the increasing cost of healthcare, the increase in life expectancy, and desire for improved quality of life with aging, and the increasing awareness involving the link between diet and health (Evani, 2009; Vergari et al., 2010).

In order to continue to bring successful functional foods and dietary supplements to the high-stakes American marketplace, it would be advantageous for industry staff, including marketers, researchers, and product development specialists, among other personnel, to have an appreciation of the many ramifications of marketing their products in the United States. This chapter will delve more into the definition of a functional food and dietary supplement. Furthermore, we will discuss some of the pertinent points of consideration to keep in mind when bringing these nutrition-based products to the American market. Some of the current trends in the U.S. functional food and dietary supplement industry are also presented.

7.2 DEFINITION OF FUNCTIONAL FOOD

Everyone knows that food is necessary for basic sustenance. However, functional foods differ from regular foods in that these items may be envisioned as the luxurious next-generation nutrition of sorts, since they contain ingredients with intended efficacy superseding basic nutrition (Dwyer, 2007). That is to say, functional foods are intended not only to satisfy hunger and provide necessary nutrients, but also to target and improve upon physiological function (Diplock et al., 1999). In addition, functional foods may even prevent or reduce the risk of chronic disease while increasing physical and mental well-being (Huggett and Schliter, 1996; Vergari et al., 2010). Functional foods are recognized by the International Food Council as foods with components that provide health benefits beyond basic nutrition (Dwyer, 2007). Diplock et al. (1999) published a nice definition of functional food that is widely accepted as consensus, which is well articulated as follows:

A food can be regarded as functional if it is satisfactorily demonstrated to affect beneficially one or more target functions in the body, beyond adequate nutritional effects, in a way that is relevant to either improved stage of health and well-being and/or reduction of risk of disease.

A functional food must remain food and it must demonstrate its effects in amounts that can normally be expected to be consumed in the diet: it is not a pill or a capsule, but part of the normal food pattern.

The *Nutrition Business Journal* defines functional food as food fortified with added or concentrated ingredients to a functional level, which improves health and/or performance of products marketed for their "inherent" functional qualities (NBJ, 2010). Unlike pharmaceutical drugs which are often designed to be potent acute remedies to specific health concerns, functional foods are meant to promote and support health and wellness by providing functional nutrients often over a more prolonged duration (NBJ, 2010).

7.3 EXAMPLES OF FUNCTIONAL FOODS

There are numerous categories of functional foods designed to emulate traditional foods. Some of the prominent categories include the following.

7.3.1 PROBIOTICS

Probiotics are foods which contain a single or mixed culture of microorganisms that beneficially contribute to health by improving the body's microbial balance (Fuller, 1989). Various health benefits have been ascribed to the inclusion of probiotic functional food in the diet, including metabolism of lactose, control of gastrointestinal infections, suppression of cancer, reduction of serum cholesterol, and immune stimulation (Gilliland, 1990; Shortt, 1999; Saarela et al., 2000). Dairy products are the key products in this sector (Vergari et al., 2010) and often these dairy products contain human-derived *Lactobacillus* and *Bifidobacterium* species (Charalampopoulos et al., 2002). Recently, probiotics have been appearing in foods other than dairy and yogurts and these include probiotic bars, juices, and muffins, among others (Evani, 2009).

7.3.2 PREBIOTICS AND FIBERS

Prebiotic foods contain ingredients that are not hydrolyzed by the digestive enzymes in the upper gastrointestinal tract and these foods beneficially affect the host by selectively stimulating the growth and/or activity of one or a limited number of bacteria in the colon that can improve host health (Gibson and Roberfroid, 1995). Prebiotics usually comprise fiber derived from plant cell walls and these are the components which are resistant to human digestion. Research suggests that dietary fiber can promote a range of benefits, including laxative effects, blood cholesterol reduction (Spiller, 1994), blood glucose attenuation (Bijlani, 1985), cancer prevention (Wang et al., 2001), and reduce the risk of heart disease (Fernandez, 2001) and obesity (Charalampopoulous et al., 2002). Fiber may even promote satiety and reduce digestive complaints.

7.3.3 FUNCTIONAL FATS

With the media as well as food labeling constantly berating and demonizing the untoward effects of trans and saturated fats, the American public is becoming more aware of the potential deleterious consequences of consuming excessive amounts these unhealthy components in their diets. Consumers with this basic understanding seem to be avoiding these types of food (Evani, 2009). Manufacturers of functional foods are addressing the trans and saturated fat dilemma by introducing healthier fats such as omega-3 and omega-6 to their functional foods. Omega-3 fatty acids might help to maintain normal blood pressure and influence the fats in the blood in a way that is healthier for the heart (Hilliam, 1998).

7.3.4 ANTIOXIDANTS

The prevalence of antioxidants is becoming more visible in functional foods. Carotenoid compounds are among the highly demanded ingredients in this category with ingredients such as astaxanthin becoming popular (Vergari et al., 2010). Other popular ingredients making their debut in functional food products include "super fruits" with high antioxidant capacity such as açai, pomegranate, blueberry, and even spices such as turmeric (Evani, 2009).

7.3.5 OTHER FUNCTIONAL FOOD CATEGORIES

Various other categories ranging from functional spreads containing phytostanol esters to lower cholesterol (Vergari et al., 2010) to functional drinks fortified with vitamins and ingredients have emerged on the market. Blood pressure maintenance, beautifying, and eye health drinks with lutein, and other antioxidants, are currently being advertised (NBJ, 2010; Vergari et al., 2010). Even concepts such as functional bakery products, meats, and eggs have been introduced, all with fortified ingredients to make them healthier options to conventional products of the same nature (Vergari et al., 2010).

7.4 DEFINITION OF DIETARY SUPPLEMENT

The distinction between functional foods and dietary supplements is that the former must emulate conventional food products and be consumed as typical traditional food items, whereas dietary supplements are designed to bolster nutrition and take on forms not related to foods. In fact, the Food and Drug Administration has laid out the definition of a dietary supplement in the Dietary Supplement Health Education Act (DSHEA), which states that dietary supplements are defined as vitamins, minerals, herbs, or other botanicals, amino acids, and other dietary substances intended to supplement the diet by increasing the total dietary intake, or as any concentrate, metabolite, constituent, extract, or combination of these ingredients (Ross, 2000). Dietary supplements are meant for oral ingestion and can be in the form of a tablet, capsule, powder, softgel, gelcap, and liquid. Therefore, unlike functional foods, dietary supplements are not represented as a conventional food or as the sole item of a meal or of the diet and they are labeled as dietary supplements (Ross, 2000).

7.4.1 POPULAR DIETARY SUPPLEMENT CATEGORIES IN THE UNITED STATES

Recent market analysis indicates that vitamins and mineral sit among the top-selling supplements within the U.S. market, along with various dietary supplement ingredients such as fish oils, green tea, echinacea, açai, saw palmetto, mangosteen, melatonin to name a few (NBJ, 2010). Moreover, current trends show emerging public interest in the sports nutrition dietary supplement arena (NBJ, 2010). Estimates of sports nutrition sales in America in 2009 and for 2010, for example, range from $2.9 to US$3.2 billion (NBJ, 2010, 2011; Heller, 2010). The trend in sports nutrition growth may be due to a continued interest from bodybuilders, athletes, and recreational athletes to a newly categorized demographic who are being coined "lifestyle users" (Heller, 2010). This demographic comprises people who consume sports nutrition products in order to provide a refreshing beverage or fast meal replacement, or support or for a quick energy boost (Heller, 2010).

7.5 SOME CONSIDERATIONS IN THE DEVELOPMENT AND MARKETING OF FUNCTIONAL FOODS AND DIETARY SUPPLEMENTS IN AMERICA

Since functional foods and dietary supplements offer consumers' targeted nutrition with the promise of safety and efficacy, there are various points to consider in the development of these innovations in order to ensure compliance and successful long-term viability within the U.S. market. Below are some of the main points of concern.

7.5.1 RESEARCH AND DEVELOPMENT

With the pledge of bolstering health, well-being, and/or unlocking the human physical potential, specific resources need to be allocated in the development of functional foods and dietary supplements in order to ensure that they work and do so in a safe manner. In-depth efforts in nutritional research and product development are required to facilitate product longevity in the market (Menrad, 2003). These efforts can be financially costly and can lead to increased cost to the consumer. Due to the economic burden in the development and marketing of functional foods, the challenge of introducing them to the American market may be better suited to larger companies (Farr, 1997) such as pharmaceutical companies wishing to venture into and capture shares of the functional food market, or large food companies looking to introduce biotechnology as a means to stay innovative (Belem, 1999). Because of the extra resources required for functional food development, it is easy to see why they are generally more expensive than conventional food items. For example, the total cost from the product idea to market introduction of a new conventional food product is estimated to be up to US$1 million or US$2 million, whereas the development and marketing costs of functional food products may greatly exceed this level (Menrad, 2003; Vergari et al., 2010). This cost may present a challenge since consumers may only be willing to pay up to a certain premium to purchase functional foods (Menrad, 2003; Verbeke, 2005; Vergari et al., 2010). Moreover, there is mounting expenses in dietary supplement manufacturing associated with newly instituted Goods Manufacturing Practices (NBJ, 2010, 2011).

Companies who wish to be successful in developing a diverse product portfolio will need to foster strong interdepartmental teamwork and employ visionary research and development staff as well as imaginative marketing personnel. These individuals will need to work cooperatively to design successful business strategies with innovative products intended to fit particular niches with robust and convincing health claims. Proper marketing research prior to market entry is absolutely necessary since the functional foods market is extremely competitive and surprisingly pockmarked with a high degree of failures (Menrad, 2003; Stewart-Knox and Mitchell, 2003; NBJ, 2010). Moreover, the dietary supplement market is also very competitive and seems to be saturated with many products claiming to support various outcomes, ranging from enhancing mental focus and memory, to supporting weight loss, to enhancing beauty from within, to facilitating enhanced muscle growth and sports performance, just to name a few indications. With so many competitors in the American functional nutrition marketplace, innovation seems to be one critical factor in capturing market share. As an adjunct corollary to this incessant need for continual innovation, the introduction of knock-off products may not always be viable for companies, since the originator usually will have garnered brand equity and consumer loyalty. In fact, Stewart-Knox and Mitchell (2003) reported that, at least for food products, there is a growing body of evidence to indicate that original concepts are more successful than "copy-cat" or "me-too" products. Thus, companies with brand new concepts who can be the first to sway customer attitudes in favor of their products will be candidates for longevity and growth of their brands in the U.S. market and perhaps even globally.

The key to establishing brand equity will be persuasive marketable claims designed to capture the attention of the American public. Additionally, since these claims are subject to regulatory scrutiny, they must be scientifically sound, especially in the stringent eyes of the American regulators. To support safety and efficacy, companies will need to continue to fund research in the form of gold-standard randomized clinical trials. Company-sponsored, publically available peer-reviewed studies published in high-impact journals will definitely help companies distinguish themselves as credible in the eyes of both the American public, who use the products, and federal regulators, who consistently review marketing claims for veracity and authenticity. Furthermore, to corroborate safety and efficacy, it would be advantageous to have extensive safety data on ingredients within the products.

7.5.2 MARKETING CLAIMS AND REGULATIONS FOR FUNCTIONAL FOODS/DIETARY SUPPLEMENTS

In the United States, functional foods are regulated as a category of food and need to satisfy the provisions for conventional foods as specified in the Federal Food Drug and Cosmetic Act (Eussen et al., 2011). Health claims on the efficacy of functional foods are contingent upon successful regulatory review of peer-reviewed data with the benchmark of success resting in the provision of sound peer-reviewed data, which are compared to a set of criteria necessary for permissible claims (Jones and Jew, 2007). In order to meet the strict requirements of scientific verification of the efficacy and safety of functional food and dietary supplement ingredients, statistically validated data from various model systems, from retrospective and prospective epidemiological studies, as well as from clinical intervention studies on humans need to exist (Menrad, 2003).

With regard to permissible ingredients, dietary supplement ingredients sold in the United States before the implementation of the Dietary Supplement Health and Education Act (DSHEA) on October 15, 1994 are considered as "grandfathered" and generally accepted as safe, whereas dietary ingredients marketed after October 15, 1994 are considered new dietary ingredients requiring premarket review of safety by the Food and Drug Administration (Taylor, 2004; US FDA, 2011). DSHEA amended the Federal Food Drug and Cosmetic Act by adding various provisions with two notable provisions defining the terms "dietary supplement" and "new dietary ingredient" or NDI. It has been instated that the manufacturer or distributor of an NDI or supplement containing an NDI submit premarket notification to the FDA at least 75 days before introducing the supplement into interstate commerce or delivering it for introduction into interstate commerce unless the NDI and any other dietary ingredients in the dietary supplement have been present in the food supply as an article used for food in a form in which the food has not been chemically altered (US FDA, 2011).

In the United States, there are essentially three types of labeling claims that can be made on functional foods and dietary supplements (Agarwal et al., 2008; Hoadley and Rowlands, 2008). First, there are the nutrient content claims, which essentially characterize the level of a specific nutrient(s). An example of this would be "good source of calcium" (Agarwal et al., 2008). Second, there are the structure/function claims, which describe the nutrient's role in health maintenance. An example of this would be "calcium helps build strong bones" (Agarwal et al., 2008). Third, there are health claims, which describe the nutrient's role in disease risk reduction. An example of this would be "calcium may reduce the risk of osteoporosis" (Agarwal et al., 2008). The FDA has regulations to govern each of these types of claims. Moreover, all food labeling statements must be truthful and not misleading (Agarwal et al., 2008; Hoadley and Rowlands, 2008). In addition to the FDA, the U.S. Federal Trade Commission (FTC) regulates claims about all products, including those with functional ingredients (Dwyer, 2007).

With such rigid guidelines governing marketing claims, companies who wish to launch successfully products with sound claims in the United States need to do their due diligence in accumulating data on the efficacy and safety of their functional food or dietary supplement product. This is where collaborative efforts between the nutritional experts in academia and a company's research and product development teams will definitely prove to be a boon. It is likely that only the top-tier companies with sizeable budgets will be able to fund clinical research at leading universities or contract research organizations and submit their findings for peer review and publication. Publically available, published, peer-reviewed gold-standard studies can unquestionably help support brands as many scientifically minded consumers can access the literature and form their own positive opinion regarding the usage of the functional food or dietary supplement. Moreover, marketing departments can leverage their company's publically available clinical studies as real robust science, since the studies will have been reviewed by competent members of the scientific community. This type of approach seems indispensable in facilitating the formation and solidification of positive consumer attitudes toward new functional foods and dietary supplements.

7.5.3   American Consumer Attitudes toward Functional Food/Dietary Supplements

The image of health promotion of a functional food product or dietary ingredient is certainly a prerequisite for success but it is by no means enough to ensure a commercial triumph (Vergari et al., 2010). Several criteria need to be met in order to ensure a marketing victory and product viability. It is indeed necessary to educate the American consumer of the benefits of the product. Public education is of critical importance since one of the best predictors of functional food use is the perceived reward from using the functional food, as consumers may feel as if they are taking care of themselves and making the correct acceptable choices for their own health (Urala and Lahteenmaki, 2003). Belief in the health benefits conferred by functional foods is the main determinant in the product's acceptance (Verbeke, 2005). In fact, various studies have found correlations between peoples' opinions or beliefs about health benefits and acceptance of functional foods (Hilliam, 1996; Childs, 1997; Verbeke, 2005). Functional food-related attitudes and the willingness to use them are contingent upon the type of functional food as it has been noted in the literature that consumers do not view functional foods as one specific homogeneous group but rather as separate products within various food categories (Urala and Lahteenmaki, 2004). For example, consumers may be amenable to adopting dairy-based functional foods for skeletal health promotion because of the natural association of dairy and calcium content, whereas a calcium-enriched orange juice may not resonate well with consumers.

Since functional foods are modeled after conventional foods, choosing the correct format or carrier for the actives can play a role in securing positive attitudes regarding the item in question. As functional foods are classified in different categories, partly determined by the matrix or carrier within which they deliver their efficacious ingredients, it is necessary for product developers to choose the correct carriers to ensure successful product acceptance by Americans. Some research suggests that carriers with a good health image are more attractive than carriers deficient in healthy connotations (Ares and Gámbaro, 2007). For example, Van Kleef et al. (2005) found that margarine, yogurt, and brown bread were rated as attractive functional food carriers rather than chewing gum, ice cream, and chocolate. Moreover, consumer surveys seem to show that for many people, the "functional" component of functional food is mainly viewed as value added, but may not determine the choice of the food product per se (Vergari et al., 2010). Marketing analysis studies in the United States and Europe show that general success factors for function foods appear to coincide with the success factors of regular food and these include taste, convenience product variety, and packaging (Menrad, 2003; Urala and Lahteenmaki, 2003; Vergari et al., 2010). It should be emphasized that in general, contrary to the whole notion of changing lifestyle habits to improve health, many consumers are somewhat obstinate and do not seem willing to change their daily lifestyles or eating patterns for the consumption of a specific functional food product (Menrad, 2003). Therefore, besides cost, convenience, and overall health connotations, functional food taste and sensory appeal will be primary success factors for market penetration.

There are various demographic and social issues to functional food and dietary supplement use which become apparent from sociodemographic studies conducted within the United States. Data from the United States suggest that the functional food consumers tend to be predominantly female, well educated, on a higher income, and over the age of 35 (Childs, 1997; Gilbert, 1997; Verbeke, 2005). Females seem to be more attune with health concerns and amenable to the use of functional foods to promote health (Verbeke, 2005). Therefore, more efforts to design functional foods catering to male health issues, with a marketing campaign addressing more virile consumer messages, may be beneficial to capturing the U.S. male audience. It has also been noted that the presence of children and aging family members in the household may positively affect attitudes toward functional food acceptance, as people may be looking to actively promote longevity and family health and disease prevention (Verbeke, 2005).

With regard to dietary supplement usage, in a recent analysis of NHANES 2003–2006 data, Bailey et al. (2011) observed that dietary supplement use was reported by one-half of all Americans.

The NHANES is a nationally representative, cross-sectional survey that samples noninstitutional-ized, civilian U.S. residents using a complex, stratified, multistage probability cluster sampling design (Bailey et al., 2011). The data as presented by Bailey et al. (2011) suggest a high prevalence of dietary supplement use in the U.S. population which has increased over the years. However, it seems that dietary supplement use is not homogeneously dispersed among the American popula-tion, with some disparity existing from a sociodemographic standpoint. In fact, Bailey et al. (2011) indicated that dietary supplement use was lowest in obese adults and highest among non-Hispanic whites, older adults, and those with more than a high-school education. Since it is evident that dietary supplements and functional foods' usage is heterogeneous among the American population, companies marketing in the United States may need to continually spend money to persuade vari-ous demographics or create demographic-specific market offerings.

The growth of the functional food and dietary supplement industry in the United States is not without its challenges. Besides the economic hardships recently befalling the United States, various other consumer attitudinal factors may be adding a few checks and balances to the growth of the functional foods, dietary supplements, and overall nutrition industry (NBJ, 2010). These include stricter regulators, determined critics, and litigious consumer advocacy groups who may legiti-mately be targeting some unscrupulous companies marketing less than rigorous products (NBJ, 2010). With this type of volatility inherent within the American system, it is best for companies to comply with FDA and FTC regulations and market their products honestly.

7.6   FUTURE OF THE FUNCTIONAL FOOD AND DIETARY SUPPLEMENT INDUSTRY AND KEYS TO SUCCESS IN AMERICA

The increase in demand for functional foods and dietary supplements across America is multifac-eted and is a likely contingent upon many factors, including the increasing cost of healthcare, the aging baby boomer demographic, along with the increase in life expectancy, the desire for improved quality of life, the desire for targeted nutrition to increase physical performance, and the increasing awareness involving the link between diet and health (Evani, 2009; Vergari et al., 2010). Despite recent economic hardships plaguing the United States, the American nutrition industry continues to grow in most product categories and sales channels (NBJ, 2010, 2011). In fact, functional foods continue to hold the largest share of the nutrition market with U.S. consumer sales of functional foods and beverages having increased 4.6% to $39.1 billion in 2010 (NBJ, 2011). This was up from 2.7% growth in 2009 (NBJ, 2011). Forecasted sales are expected to reach up to nearly $45 billion for functional foods and nearly $32 billion for dietary supplements in 2013 (NBJ, 2011). Recently, popular categories in the functional food business consist of a variety of mainstays, including func-tional sweeteners such as stevia, digestive health products such as probiotics, prebiotics, and fiber-based products, immune system support, and functional spices (Evani, 2009; NBJ, 2010). The dietary supplement market also seems to be surviving the tough economic times in America. Items among the general trends driving the maintenance and growth in the American dietary supplement market include vitamins, minerals, fish oil, and essential fatty acids, and antiaging dietary supple-ment products (NBJ, 2010, 2011). Moreover, there seems to be a steady growth rate in the sports nutrition supplement arena and condition-specific supplements (NBJ, 2010, 2011).

Since Americans are becoming more cognizant of the link between functional nutrition and health and performance, the functional food and dietary supplement market within the United States seems to be an indelible bastion of steadily growing high-stakes business opportunities. In order to ensure its continued success, key stakeholders within the competitive American nutrition industry will have to put forth concerted efforts to meet the demands of a growing body of educated consumers. Researchers and product development specialists working within the functional food and dietary supplement industry will have to work closely with marketing personnel to find new ways to design and promote their products. Successful marketing of the products will continue to entail educating potential consumers with persuasive, yet truthful, claims regarding health promotion or other structure/function claims associated with key ingredients or formulas. Successful functional foods will be designed to fit the American dietary lifestyle with cost, convenience, and food attributes that render them desirable from a financial, flavor, and overall sensory perspective. This is especially important since, as mentioned earlier, many consumers are not willing to change their daily lifestyles or eating patterns for the consumption of a specific functional food product.

7.7 CONCLUSION

In conclusion, it will be new innovations in functional food and dietary supplement products that will continue to propel the U.S. functional nutrition industry forward. All products will continue to require rigorous science behind the safety and efficacy of their formulations or key ingredients in order to be able to withstand the scrutiny of the adapting regulatory framework of the FDA and FTC, and serve to build an image of company credibility as well as reinforce positive consumer attitudes. Companies within the functional nutrition industry should continue to foster an environment of collaboration where bright-minded creative staff members constantly expand upon and leverage their knowledge of nutrition to serve as competitive ammunition in the next big-budget marketing campaigns. Moreover, it will take an in-depth understanding and appreciation of various aspects of marketing within the United States, as well as an understanding of the American regulatory framework, to facilitate successful product launches and build indelible brands which can be embraced by potentially millions of people across the vast American landscape.

REFERENCES

Agarwal, S., Hordvik, S., and Morar, S. 2008. Health and wellness related labeling claims for functional foods and dietary supplements in the USA. In *Nutraceutical and Functional Food Regulations in the United States and around the World*, ed. D. Bagchi, pp. 133–141. New York: Elsevier Inc.

Arai, S. 2002. Global view on functional foods: Asian perspectives. *Br J Nutr* 88(S2): S139–S143.

Ares, G. and Gámbaro, A. 2007. Influence of gender, age and motives underlying food choice on perceived healthiness and willingness to try functional foods. *Appetite* 49: 148–158.

Bagchi, D. 2006. Nutraceuticals and functional foods regulations in the United States and around the world. *Toxicology* 221(1): 1–3.

Bailey, R., Gahche, J., Lentino, C., Dwyer, J., Engel, J., Thomas, P., Betz, J., Sempos, C., and Picciano, M. 2011. Dietary supplement use in the United States, 2003–2006. *J Nutr* 141(2): 261–266.

Belem, M. 1999. Application of biotechnology in the product development of nutraceuticals in Canada. *Trends Food Sci Technol* 10: 101–106.

Bijlani, R. 1985. Dietary fiber: Consensus and controversy. *Prog Food Nutr Sci* 9(3–4): 343–393.

Charalampopoulos, D., Wang, R., Pandiella, S., and Webb, C. 2002. Application of cereals and cereal components in functional foods review. *Int J Food Microbiol* 79(1–2): 131–141.

Childs, N. 1997. Functional foods and the food industry: Consumer, economic and product development issues. *J Nutraceuticals Functional Med Foods* 1: 25–43.

Diplock, A., Aggett, P., Ashwell, M., Bornet, F., Fern, E., and Roberfroid, M. 1999. Scientific concepts of functional foods in Europe: Consensus document. *Br J Nutr* 81(suppl. 1): S1–S27.

Dwyer, J. 2007. Do functional components in food have a role in helping to solve current health issues? *J Nutr* 137: 2489S–2492S.

Eussen, S.R., Verhagen, H., Klungel, O.H., Garssen, J., van Loveren, H., van Kranen, H.J., and Rompelberg, C.J. 2011. Functional foods and dietary supplements: Products at the interface between pharma and nutrition. *Eur J Pharmacol* 668(suppl. 1): S2–S9.

Evani, S. 2009. Trends in the US Functional Foods, Beverages and Ingredients Market: Institute of Food Technologists—Show report. Agriculture and Agri-Food Canada. http://www.ats.agr.gc.ca/eve/5289-eng.htm. (accessed September 29, 2011).

Farr, D. 1997. Functional foods. *Cancer Lett* 114: 59–63.

Fernandez, M. 2001. Soluble fiber and non-digestible carbohydrate effects on plasma lipid and cardiovascular risk. *Curr Opin Lipidol* 12: 35–40.

Fuller, R. 1989. Probiotics in man and animals. *J Appl Bacteriol* 66(5): 365–378.

Gibson, G. and Roberfroid, M. 1995. Dietary modulation of human colonic microbiota: Introducing the concept of probiotics. *J Nutr* 125(6): 1401–1412.

Gilbert, L. 1997. The consumer market for functional foods. *J Nutraceuticals Functional Med Foods* 1(3): 5–21.

Gilliland, S. 1990. Health and nutritional benefits from lactic acid bacteria. *FEMS Microbiol Rev* 87: 175–188.

Goffin, D., Delzenne, N., Blecker, C., Hanon, E., Deroanne, C., and Paquot, M. 2011. Will isomalto-oligosaccharides, a well-established functional food in Asia, break through the European and American market? The status of knowledge on these prebiotics. *Crit Rev Food Sci Nutr* 51(5): 394–409.

Hasler, C. 1996. Functional foods: The Western perspective. *Nutr Rev* 54(11 Pt 2): S6–S10.

Hasler, C. 2000. The changing face of functional foods. *J Am Coll Nutr* 19(5 suppl): 499S–506S.

Heller, L. 2010. Sports nutrition market driven by non-sporty consumers. Nutraingredients.com. http://www.nutraingredients.com/content/view/print/306382 (accessed September 1, 2011).

Hilliam, M. 1996. Functional foods: The Western consumer viewpoint. *Nutr Rev* 54 (11), S189–S194.

Hilliam, M. 1998. The market for functional foods. *Int Dairy J* 8: 349–353.

Hoadley, J. and Rowlands, J. 2008. FDA perspectives on food label claims in the USA. In *Nutraceutical and Functional Food Regulations in the United States and around the World*, ed. D. Bagchi, pp. 115–132. New York: Elsevier Inc.

Huggett, A. and Schliter, B. 1996. Research needs for establishing the safety of functional foods. *Nutr Rev* 54: S143–S148.

Jones, P. and Jew, S. 2007. Functional food development: Concept to reality. *Trends Food Sci Technol* 18: 387–390.

Menrad, K. 2003. Market and marketing of functional food in Europe. *J Food Process Eng* 56: 181–188.

Milner, J. 2000. Functional foods: The US perspective. *Am J Clin Nutr* 71: 1654–1659.

NBJ, *Nutrition Business Journal*. (2010) Supplemental Business Report. http://www.nutritionbusiness.com.

NBJ, *Nutrition Business Journal*. (2011) Supplemental Business Report. http://www.nutritionbusiness.com.

Roberfroid, M. 2002. Global view on functional foods: European perspectives. *Br J Nutr* 88: 133–138.

Ross, S. 2000. Functional foods: The food and drug administration perspective. *Am J Clin Nutr* 71(suppl): 1735S–1738S.

Saarela, M., Mogensen, G., Fonden, R., Matto, J., and Mattila-Sandholm, T. 2000. Probiotic bacteria: Safety functional and technological properties. *J Biotechnol* 84: 197–215.

Shortt, C. 1999. The probiotic century: Historical and current perspectives. *Trends Food Sci Technol* 10: 411–417.

Spiller, R. 1994. Pharmacology of dietary fiber. *Pharmacol Ther Field* 62: 407–427.

Stewart-Knox, B. and Mitchell, P. 2003. What separates the winners from the losers in new food product development? *Trends Food Sci Technol* 14: 58–64.

Taylor, C. 2004. Regulatory frameworks for functional foods and dietary supplements. *Nutr Rev* 62: 55–59.

Tomomatsu, H. 1994. Health effects of oligosaccharides. *Food Technol* 48: 61–65.

Urala, N. and Lahteenmaki, L. 2003. Reasons behind consumers' functional food choices. *Nutr Food Sci* 33(4): 148–158.

Urala, N. and Lahteenmaki, L. 2004. Attitudes behind consumers' willingness to use functional foods. *Food Quality Preference* 15: 793–803.

US FDA. 2011. Draft Guidance for Industry: Dietary Supplements: New Dietary Ingredient Notifications and Related Issues, http://www.fda.gov/food/guidancecomplianceregulatoryinformation/guidancedocuments/dietarysupplements/ucm257563.htm (accessed August 25, 2011).

Van Kleef, E., Van Trijp, H., and Luning, P. 2005. Functional foods: Health claim—Food product compatibility and the impact of health claim framing on consumer evaluation. *Appetite* 44: 299–308.

Verbeke, W. 2005. Consumer acceptance of functional foods: Socio-demographic, cognitive and attitudinal determinants. *Food Quality Preference* 16: 45–57.

Vergari, F., Tibuzzi, A., and Basile, G. 2010. An overview of the functional food market: From marketing issues and commercial players to future demand from life in space. *Adv Exp Med Biol* 698: 308–321.

Wang, Y., Wang, Y., and Li, C. 2001. Effect of dietary fibre on diabetes patient. *Shipin Gongye Keji* 22: 25–27.

8 Dairy Innovations and Market Growth in India

Raka Saxena, A.K. Srivastava, and A.K. Singh

CONTENTS

In the present era, processing and new distribution options provide increasing opportunities available to food marketers to provide the consumer with convenient and nutritious products. The rapid economic and income growth, urbanization, and globalization are leading to a dramatic shift of diets away from staples and increasingly toward livestock and dairy products, vegetables and fruit, and fats and oils (Pingali 2004). The current food consumption patterns are showing signs of convergence toward a nutritious diet. The main determinants of the changes in the demand for food are: income growth, which leads to major shifts in demand across different types of food; the process of urbanization, which brings about new dietary needs; and more generally lifestyle changes (Pingali 2004).

All these factors, which are responsible for change or shift in consumer demand, have led to change in the product mix of the dairy products over a period of time. A number of innovations have taken place in the past and many health-oriented dairy products have appeared in the market. The recent examples of these are probiotic curds and drinks launched by major dairy players. The research is undergoing to integrate the millets with the dairy products so that a wholesome food can be provided to the consumer. This paper broadly discusses the changes in consumption pattern of dairy products along with major innovations in dairy sector.

8.1 GLOBAL DIRECTIONS IN MILK PRODUCTION AND CONSUMPTION

The world milk production more than doubled during the span of 50 years and increased from 344 million tonnes in 1961 to 703 million tonnes in 2009 (Figure 8.1). If the public and private stock

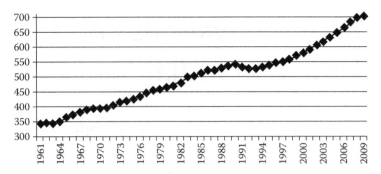

FIGURE 8.1   World milk production (million tonnes). (Compiled from www.faostat.org/prodstat.)

changes are not taken into account, the world milk consumption can be equated to the world milk production. The world milk production/consumption registered a consistent increase, leaving aside some fluctuations because of the global and or regional shocks.

The global increase in milk production and consumption is appreciable; the regional patterns in consumption would throw more light on the situation of various regions. Globally, there has been increasing pressure on the livestock sector to meet the growing demand for high-value livestock products and animal protein. The growth in livestock sector is driven by the population growth, rising incomes and urbanization. It has been observed that there is a strong positive relationship between the level of income and the consumption of livestock products and the consumption of livestock products is increasing at the expense of staple foods. The high-value protein from the livestock sector improves the nutrition of the vast majority of the world. Livestock products are also important sources of a wide range of essential micronutrients, in particular minerals such as iron and zinc, and vitamins such as vitamin A.

Table 8.1 provides a clear stock of regional situation in terms of production and consumption shares of milk. Some regions are self-sufficient in terms of milk production, which is clearly evident through higher share of a particular region in world production as compared to the share in world consumption. Asia is the biggest consumer as well as producer of milk. Asia, Africa, and Central America rely on imports for meeting out some of their domestic consumption requirements, whereas Europe, North America, South America, and Oceania are self-sufficient. Oceania is the only region in the world, where consumption is lower than net exports volume. About 60% of the production is exported outside Oceania (IDF 2010).

TABLE 8.1
Regionwise Global Milk Consumption: 2009

	Consumption (Million Tonnes)	Share in World Consumption (%)	Share in World Production (%)
Asia	268.3	38.4	36.0
Europe	206.8	**29.6**	30.8
North America	93.0	**13.3**	13.4
South America	58.3	**8.3**	8.5
Africa	42.6	6.1	5.2
Central America	19.7	2.8	2.3
Oceania	10.6	**1.5**	3.7
World	699.5	100.0	100.0

Source: Adapted from IDF 2010. *Bulletin of International Dairy Federation*, No. 446.
Note: The bold values indicate the self sufficiency of regions in terms of milk production.

8.2 INDIAN DAIRY SITUATION

Livestock sector is an integral part of farming system of Indian economy, adding value to the tune of more than Rs. 170 thousand crore (4.4%) to the country's gross domestic product (GDP) (CSO 2009). The share of livestock sector in value of output from agricultural and allied activities has increased from 25.8% in TE2001/02 to 27.4% in TE2008/09. India is the number one milk producer in the world and has made rapid strides in milk production. The milk production has increased from 17 million tons in 1950–1951 to 112.5 million tons in 2009–2010, registering a steady growth rate of 3.5–4.5% during this period as against the world average growth rate of about 1%. Figure 8.2 presents the information regarding trends in milk production and availability. The per capita milk availability has also increased from 130 g/day in 1950–1951 to 263 g/day in 2009–2010 despite considerable increase in the human population.

With increase in availability of milk and milk products, the consumption basket of the Indian consumer has also witnessed lot of changes over the period of time. Promoting healthy diets and lifestyles to reduce the burden of diseases requires a multifaceted and multisectoral approach involving the various relevant sectors in societies. The strategies must not merely be ensuring food security for all, but must also achieve the consumption of adequate quantities of safe and good quality foods that together make up a healthy diet. It would be therefore useful to examine trends in consumption patterns.

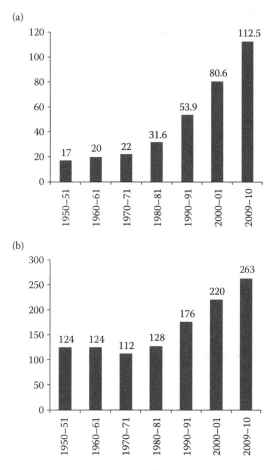

FIGURE 8.2 Trend in production and availability of milk: (a) milk production (million tonnes) and (b) per capita availability (g/day).

In India, the surveys carried out by the National Sample Survey Organization (NSSO) set up in the Department of Statistics of the Government of India in 1950 provide data on food consumption patterns. NSSO collects data on various aspects of Indian economy through nationwide large-scale sample surveys with an objective to assist in socioeconomic planning and policy making. NSSO carried out Consumer Expenditure Surveys quinquennially since 1972–1973 (27th, 32nd, 38th, 43rd, 50th, 55th, and 61st rounds of NSS, at roughly 5-year intervals). Lately, NSSO has also started publishing the annual consumption expenditure data on food and nonfood items. The information extracted from various National Sample Survey rounds on consumption expenditure is presented in Table 8.2.

During last three decades, there has been a decline in the proportion of expenditure on food items in both urban and rural areas. The proportion of expenditure on nonfood items has increased from 35.65% (1977–1978) to 47.7% (2007–2008) in rural areas and from 40.02% (1977–1978) to 60.4% (2007–2008) in urban areas. However, the consumption expenditure on food remained higher in rural areas as compared to urban areas. During 1977–1978 and 2007–2008, the share of food in total consumer expenditure has fallen from 64.35% to 52.3% in rural areas and from 59.98% to 39.6% in urban areas.

Despite significant decline in consumption expenditure on food category, the proportion of consumption expenditure on milk and milk products exhibited marginal changes. Though, the share of

TABLE 8.2
Household Consumption Expenditure on Milk and Milk Products

		Rural		Urban	
NSS Round	**Year**	**Milk and Milk Products**	**Total Food**	**Milk and Milk Products**	**Total Food**
32nd	1977–1978	7.68	64.35	9.53	59.98
38th	1982	7.51	65.57	9.24	58.57
42nd	1986–1987	9.57	65.67	10.48	57.93
43rd	1987–1988	8.62	63.77	9.53	55.92
44th	1988–1989	8.94	63.85	10.02	57.14
45th	1989–1990	9.69	64.28	9.91	55.52
46th	1990–1991	9.42	65.97	9.9	56.85
47th	1991	8.99	63.07	10.04	56.1
48th	1992	9.4	65	10.4	56
49th	1993	9.4	65.2	10.7	57.6
50th	1993–1994	9.5	63.2	9.8	54.7
51st	1994–1995	8.9	61	9.7	53.4
52nd	1995–1996	9.4	60.34	9.42	50.06
53rd	1997	9.95	58.73	9.72	49.62
54th	1998	9.56	60.83	9.45	49.64
55th	1999–2000	8.8	59.4	8.7	48.1
56th	2000–2001	8.7	56.3	8.3	43.8
57th	2001–2002	8.4	55.5	8.1	43.1
58th	2002	8.5	55	7.7	42.5
59th	2003	8	54	7.8	42
60th	2004	8.4	53.9	7.8	41.6
61st	2004–2005	8.47	55.05	7.92	42.51
62nd	2005–2006	8.2	53.3	7.3	40.0
63rd	2006–2007	8.1	52.3	7.4	39.4
64th	2007–2008	7.8	52.3	7.2	39.6

Source: Information compiled from GOI. 2010. Basic Animal Husbandry Statistics, 2010. Govt. of India.

food expenditure was higher in rural areas, the share of consumption expenditure on milk and milk products category was relatively higher in urban areas due to greater consumer awareness toward healthy foods and availability of variety products. The studies indicate that dietary diversification has taken over time and the diets have shifted in favor of high-value products. However, wide variations exist across states and income groups in terms of consumption expenditure.

8.3   MILK UTILIZATION PATTERN IN INDIA

The household sector and unorganized sector in India account for >80% of milk produced in India and remaining is handled by the organized sector. About 45% of India's milk production is utilized for making indigenous milk products such as ghee, butter, khoa, paneer, chhana, and curd (Sharad, 2007). The productwise milk utilization pattern is given in Table 8.3. The household sector makes the products of shorter shelf life, whereas the organized sector manufactures the Western dairy products such as cheese, butter, milk powders, ice cream, ghee which have longer shelf life.

The traditional milk products are the largest-selling products and account for 95% of all products consumed in India. There are a large number of unorganized dairy manufacturing enterprises handling production of traditional dairy products with a low capital base and little concern for food standards and good manufacturing practices. The demand for traditional milk products increases during the winter season and coincides with major festivals and ceremonies. Now, most of the dairy companies in organized sector have started production of sweets on a commercial scale. The major push has come from big brands such as Amul, Mother Dairy, Nestle, Britannia, Haldiram, Bikanerwala, and so on.

The Indian milk-based sweets are finding their place overseas also. In North America alone, this market is estimated at US$500 million (Sharad, 2007). Indian sweets have a good market in developed countries, where the share of food is small in the overall household expenditure.

8.4   INNOVATIONS IN FOOD CATEGORY

Owing to changes in consumers' lifestyles, the expectations are fast changing and the demand for innovative products is increasing rapidly. Now the attention of scientific investigations has moved toward exploring the role of biologically active components on human health. Basic temptation in human beings toward nature and the products that are natural, for every little disturbances related to health, resulted in flourishing of market with products containing various therapeutic ingredients. Functional foods, pharma foods, designer foods, and nutraceuticals are synonymous for foods that

TABLE 8.3
Milk Utilization Pattern in India: 1943–2005 (in %)

	1943	1956	2001	2005
Milk production (million tones)	23.5	17.8	84.6	94.5
Milk utilization (%)	100	100	100	100
Liquid milk	**28.0**	**39.2**	**46.0**	**50.0**
Traditional products	**72**	**60.8**	**50.0**	**45.0**
Ghee/Makkhan	58.7	46.0	33.0	
Dahi	5.2	8.8	7.0	
Khoa	5.0	4.4	7.0	
Chhana and paneer	3.1	1.6	3.0	
Western products: Milk powder, etc.	Negligible	Negligible	4.0	5.0

Source: Dairy India 2007.

Note: The bold values indicate the categories of milk products.

can prevent and treat diseases. Epidemiological studies and randomized clinical trials carried out in different parts of the world have been demonstrated or at least suggested numerous health effects related to functional food consumption, such as reduction of cancer risk, improvement of heart health, enhancement of immune functions, lowering of menopause symptoms, improvement of gastrointestinal health, anti-inflammatory effects, reduction of blood pressure, antibacterial and antiviral activities, reduction of osteoporosis, and so on.

Nutritional significance of milk molecules is well documented and increasing cases of cancers, coronary heart diseases, osteoporosis, and many other chronic diseases, have been attributed to our diet. Known nutrients, that is, vitamins, proteins, milk and milk constituents, clearly have more to offer and scientists are scurrying to discover exactly which milk components might fend off specific diseases.

8.4.1 Functional Foods

In recent years, there has been a vast and rapidly growing body of scientific data showing that diet plays an important part in diseases. Thus, the functional foods have entered the global market in the past decade. The functional foods present new economic opportunities in addition to the health benefits. The functional foods are generally offered at a premium price. The global market size of functional foods has been estimated between US$30 and US$60 billion with Japan, the United States, and Europe as the biggest markets (Williams et al. 2006). Since the market for global functional foods is growing at a rapid pace, the developing countries are also emerging to cater to the increasing demand.

There is an increasing demand by consumers for quality of life, which is fueling the nutraceutical revolution. Functional foods are viewed as one option available for seeking cost-effective health care and improved health status. Moreover, the large segment of the population is aging and considerable health care budget in most country is focused on treatment rather than prevention. Thus, the use of nutraceuticals in daily diets can be seen as means to reduce escalating health care costs that will contribute not only to a longer lifespan, but also more importantly, to a longer health span.

CONDITIONS FOR FUNCTIONAL FOOD

- It is a food (not capsule, tablet, or powder) derived from naturally occurring ingredients.
- It should be consumed as part of daily diet.
- It has particular when ingested, serving to regulate a particular body process. Such as
  - Improvement of biological defense mechanisms
  - Prevention and recovery of specific disease
  - Control of mental and physical conditions
  - Retarding the aging process

Functional foods may improve the general conditions of the body or decrease the risk of some diseases and could even be used for curing some illnesses. Functional foods have been defined as "foods that, by virtue of the presence of physiologically active components, provide a health benefit beyond basic nutrition." However, The Institute of Medicine's Food and Nutrition Board (IOM/FNB 1994) defined functional foods as "any food or food ingredient that may provide a health benefit beyond the traditional nutrients it contains (IOM/NAS, 1994)."

Since time immemorial, dairy products have been an integral part of human diet. Milk is the only food, which has got the power to sustain life in all the stages of development, and is considered an important part of a balanced diet. Besides being a source of quality proteins and energy-rich fat, it contains important micronutrients like calcium, potassium, sodium, magnesium, and vitamins, which are vital for overall development of the human body. Also, several health attributes are associated with milk or its constituents, such as the role of calcium in controlling hypertension and

TABLE 8.4

Examples of Functional Components in Milk and Milk Products

Class/Components	Source	Potential Benefit
	Probiotics	
Lactobacilli, Bifidobacteria	Yogurt, other dairy and nondairy applications	May improve gastrointestinal health and systemic immunity
	Fatty Acids	
CLA	Fat-rich dairy products, fermented milk products	Anticancer, antiatherosclerosis
	Whey Proteins	
β-Lactoglobulin	Whey	Enhance glutathione synthesis
Lactoferrin	Whey, colostrums	Antibacterial, increase bioavailability of iron
	Prebiotics	
Lactulose	Heated milks, synthesized from lactose	Bifodgenic factor, improve GIT conditions in infants, laxative, prevent allergy
GOS	Fermented foods, galactosyltransferase activity of microbes	Promote growth of probiotic bacteria, anticancer, increase mineral bioavailability
	Bioactive Peptides	
Caseino-phosphopeptides	Fermented milks, proteolysis of casein	Mineral binding specially calcium
Casomorphins	Proteolysis of α- and β-casein	Increase intestinal water and electrolyte absorption, increase GI transit time

colonic anticarcinogenicity, protective roles of carotenenoids and conjugated linoleic acid (CLA) against cancers (Table 8.4). Butyric acid, the short-chain fatty acid of milk fat has been shown to regulate cell growth and enhance the antitumor activities. Certain minor milk components either naturally occur or formed during processing have also been endowed with many unique health benefits. Examples include lactoferrin, lactulose, galacto-oligosaccharides (GOS), β-lactoglobulin, and bioactive peptides. Some of the important segments of functional dairy foods and nutraceuticals have been discussed hereunder.

8.4.2 PROBIOTIC DAIRY FOODS

The human gastrointestinal tract (GIT) harbors >100 trillion microorganisms belonging to 400 different bacterial species. The number of cells are almost 10 times than the rest of the body cells. A delicate balance exists between beneficial and harmful bacteria present in GIT and any disturbance may lead to abnormalities. About 70% of the body's immune system is localized in GIT. Incorporation of beneficial bacteria into foods to counteract harmful organisms in the GIT has been the most visible component of this new area. Such microorganisms are termed as "Probiotics." There is growing scientific evidence to support the concept that beneficial gut microflora may provide protection against gastrointestinal disorders, including gastrointestinal infections, inflammatory bowel diseases, and even cancer.

The basis for selection of probiotic microorganisms include safety, functional aspects (survival, adherence, colonization, antimicrobial production, immune stimulation, antigenotoxic activity, and prevention of pathogens), and technological details such as growth in milk and other food base, sensory properties, stability, phage resistance, and viability. Newer avenues as carriers of probiotic organisms are being sought. Fermented milk products being a "live" food is potentially an excellent vehicle for these beneficial microbial cultures. Considering the beneficial properties of probiotic organisms these organisms may produce end products that may be different from those produced by the normal starters in these products; several attempts have been made to manufacture probiotic milk products such as probiotic dahi, probiotic cheese, probiotic yoghurt, and yoghurt drinks. Probiotic dahi developed at our Institute containing *Lactobacillus acidophilus* and *Lactobacillus casei* was found to delay the onset of glucose intolerance, hyperglycemia, dyslipidemia, and oxidative stress in high fructose-induced diabetic rats. It indicates reduced risk of diabetes and its complications.

8.4.3 FORTIFIED MILK PRODUCTS

Milk in its natural form is almost unique as a balanced source of man's dietary need. The various steps in processing and storage have a measurable impact on some specific nutrients. Liquid milk fortification with vitamins A and D is mandatory in several countries. β-Carotene is added as a color-enhancing agent to some milk products such as butter. Dried milk is often fortified with vitamins A and D, calcium, and iron. Milk-based infant formula and weaning foods are fortified with a range of vitamins, minerals, and other nutrients such as polyunsaturated fatty acids. Powdered milk used for complementary feeding in Chile is fortified with vitamin C, iron, copper, and zinc. However, the milk fortification usually impaired its sensory and processing quality characteristics. Moreover, bioavailability of fortified nutrients is another major concern. Investigations carried out at the National Dairy Research Institute (NDRI) suggest possibilities of fortification of liquid milk with calcium and iron.

8.4.4 WHEY PROTEINS AND PEPTIDES

Whey proteins are termed as "wonder proteins" and may find applications in nutritional, functional, dietetic, sports, and infant foods. They possess excellent amino acids profile, high PER and biological value, easier digestibility and assimilability, bland taste, and excellent functional properties. Dietary whey proteins have a number of putative, biological effects when ingested. The ability of whey proteins to increase the level of natural antioxidants within the body and possibly in stabilizing DNA during cell division is emerging as premier contribution to population health. The anticarcinogenic properties of whey proteins are related to compounds rich in sulfur containing amino acids, methionine, and cysteine. Methionine is utilized for glutathion synthesis in times of cysteine deficiency and it also acts as methyl donor. Hypomethylation of a DNA is an important risk factor for cancer at number of sites. Glutathion is, believed to act as an antioxidant, anticarcinogenic and in stabilization and repair of DNA.

8.5 UNDERSTANDING THE INDIAN CONSUMER MARKET

The study of demographics involves understanding statistical characteristics of a population, which will help firms to understand the current market for novel foods especially dairy foods and predict the future trends. The food marketers must consider several issues affecting the structure of population. The social classes can also be used in the positioning of food products.

The Indian consumer market, primarily dominated by young generation, is becoming increasingly sophisticated and brand conscious. India has the largest population of the young in the world—over 890 million people are below 45 years of age. India has more English-speaking people than in the whole of Europe. With rising incomes, aggregate consumption in India is expected to grow fourfold in real terms—from $420.7 billion in 2006 to $1.73 trillion in 2025 (India brand equity foundation (IBEF)). India has entered a long-term virtuous cycle in which rising income leads to rising consumption, which in turn creates more business opportunities and employment. Different social classes satisfy different needs from different categories of processed foods (Table 8.5).

This holds tremendous importance for the novel food marketers. Designing the marketing mix will depend upon the distribution of households across various strata, their basic needs, and

TABLE 8.5

Needs of Indian Consumer from Processed Food

Annual Household Income	Number of Households (Million)	Need from Processed Food
>INR 10.0 lakhs	1.2	Lifestyle and aspiration (cheese, wine, gourmet food, etc.)
INR 5.0–10.0 lakhs	2.4	Convenience & time saving (RTE, RTC, purees, etc.)
INR 2.0–5.0 lakhs	10.9	Food inflation protection (frozen fruits and vegetables, fruit juices, etc.)
INR 0.5–2.0 lakhs	91.3	Wholesome nutrition (milk, juices, meat, etc.)
<INR 0.5 lakhs	101.0	Basic nutrition (fortified atta, iodized salt, etc.)

Source: Information compiled from Gupta, R. 2009. Indian Palate: Changing Food Habits & Consumer Behavior, Presentation browsed from World Wide Web.

purchasing power. Slight product innovations may increase the market share and can increase the profitability.

8.6 MAJOR STRATEGIES IN DEVELOPMENT OF INNOVATIVE/NOVEL DAIRY FOODS

8.6.1 TECHNOLOGICAL CHALLENGES

Four different technological hurdles have to be overcome before launch of a product containing bioactive substances:

- Isolation of the desired components
- Preestablishment of the biological activity
- Incorporation of the bioactive components into a formulated product
- Verification of efficacy and safety of final product

Such a sequence of experimental events is also required for the introduction of new food additives; additional is a thorough proof of the claimed benefit of the bioactive components. This applies especially when the bioactive component is a completely new substance never consumed before in significant amounts. Separation, purification, and production at industrial level of such nutraceuticals must be thought in terms of integrated and high-added value. Membrane technologies (MF, UF, NF) provide key opportunities to manufacture milk nutraceuticals in native state. The incorporation of bioactive components into processed foods, its delivery, and bioavailability are other important issues that need reprisal.

The scientific evidence for functional foods and their physiologically active components can be categorized into four distinct areas: (a) clinical trials, (b) animal studies, (c) experimental *in vitro* laboratory studies, and (d) epidemiologic studies. Much of the current evidence for functional foods lacks well-designed clinical trials; however, the foundational evidence provided through the other types of scientific investigation is substantial for several of the functional foods and their health-promoting components.

8.6.2 SAFETY ISSUES

Although increasing the availability of healthful foods including functional foods in the diet is critical to ensuring a healthier population, safety is a critical issue. The optimal levels of majority of the biologically active components currently under investigation have yet to be determined. The benefits and risks to individuals and populations as a whole must be weighed carefully when considering the widespread use of physiologically active functional foods. Knowledge of toxicity of functional food components is crucial to decrease the risk:benefit ratio. The safety issues related to probiotic microorganisms that have to be considered include

- Intrinsic properties of the probiotic strains
- Pharmacokinetics of probiotic strains
- Interaction between probiotic strains and the host
- Knowledge of toxicity of functional food components is crucial to decrease the risk: benefit ratio

8.6.3   REGULATORY FRAMEWORK

A suitable regulatory framework is needed for proper market development of innovative products. The clear-cut regulation at each critical point related to production, certification, promotion, and marketing is required for ensuring consumers' trust in the novel products. This will also provide a level-playing field fostering competition and encouraging competition.

8.6.4   CREATING INSTITUTIONAL CAPACITY

The National Agricultural Research System in India consists of number of institutions conducting basic and applied research in the fields of food science and dairy science. The institutional capacity building becomes very important for sustained innovation framework. Creation of research capacity will be helpful in screening the local resources and uncover potential new sources for innovative food and dairy products.

8.6.5   UNDERSTANDING DEMAND AND BUILDING EFFICIENT MARKETING NETWORK

Consumer interest in the relationship between diet and health has increased the demand for information on functional foods. Rapid advances in science and technology, increasing healthcare costs, changes in food laws affecting label and product claims, an aging population, and rising interest in attaining wellness through diet are among the factors fueling interest in functional foods. Credible scientific research indicates many potential health benefits from milk components. It should be stressed, however, that functional foods are not a magic bullet or universal panacea for poor health habits.

Launch of any new food product in the market requires extensive market research. The market requirements will be helpful in strategic decision making for the market players. The marketing of novel products also requires significant research efforts because most markets scientific evidence and proof of health and wellness. There is need to establish an efficient supply chain. The major factors will be consumer awareness toward health, their dietary pattern, responsiveness toward innovative food and health solutions, the disposable incomes, existence of specialized markets, and the retail network.

Regulations will have to evolve to promote R&D, ensure validation, and prevent exploitation of consumers. Companies will also have to be sincere and honest in their claims while marketing and communicating with consumers till appropriate regulations for scientific validation are evolved. Processors will need to provide an optimal merger between taste, convenience, and health attributes. Companies will require expert knowledge in flavor-masking fortification know-how and delivery systems.

REFERENCES

CSO. 2009. National Accounts Statistics, 2008–09. Central Statistical Organization, Govt. of India.
GOI. 2010. Basic Animal Husbandry Statistics, 2010. Govt. of India.

Gupta, P. R. 2007. *Dairy India Yearbook*, Priyadarshini Vihar, New Delhi.

Gupta, R. 2009. Indian Palate: Changing Food Habits & Consumer Behavior, Presentation browsed from World Wide Web.

IDF. 2010. World Dairy Situation 2010. *Bulletin of International Dairy Federation*, No. 446, pp. 24–25.

IOM/NAS. 1994. In: Thomas, P. R. and Earl, R. (eds.), *Opportunities in the Nutrition and Food Sciences,* Institute of Medicine/National Academy of Sciences, National Academy Press, Washington, D.C., p. 109.

Pingali, P. 2004. Westernization of Asian Diets and the transformation of food systems: Implications for research and policy, ESA Working Paper No. 04–17, Agricultural and Development Economics Division, The Food and Agriculture Organization of the United Nations.

Sharad, J. 2007. Making food processing viable, In: Gupta, P. R. (ed.), *Dairy India Yearbook*, Dairy India, New Delhi.

Williams, M., Pehu, E., and Ragasa, C. 2006. *Functional Foods: Opportunities and Challenges for Developing Countries*, ARD, The World Bank, Washington.

www.faostat.org/prodstat

9 Changing Global Food Consumption Patterns
An Economic Perspective

Srikanta Chatterjee*

CONTENTS

9.1 INTRODUCTION AND OUTLINE OF CHAPTER

As a basic necessity of life, the availability, quality, and affordability of food are of great concern to both individuals and nations alike. The world enjoyed several decades of relative stability in the price of basic items of food, including food grains, following the introduction of some new, high-yielding seed varieties, better irrigation, and use of fertilizers in the 1960s. This helped raise the production of wheat and other grain cereals quite dramatically, and the world came to enjoy a much improved food environment with reliable and affordable supply of several basic items of food. The period from the early 1970s to 1990 saw world food grains and oilseeds output rise steadily, by an

* The research toward this chapter started when the author was a Visiting Senior Fellow at the Center for International Studies of the London School of Economics (LSE) in May and June 2011. He wishes to acknowledge the hospitality of the Center, especially for the access he enjoyed to the British Library of Social Sciences, which is located at the School. He also wishes to record his appreciation to The Riddet Institute and to Massey University for granting him the leave to take up the Fellowship at the LSE.

average of 2.2% a year, with periodic fluctuations. With the exception of parts of the African continent, the rate of growth of food crops exceeded that of the world population, leading to an increase in their per capita availability, and to their relatively stable prices. Indeed, world food prices in real terms were at their lowest in 100 years in 2000 [1]. For much of the world's population, cereals are the main source of nutrition; so any adverse change particularly in the production and the prices of cereals is cause for worry.

Since the early 1990s, the rate of growth of grains and oilseeds has declined, globally, to 1.3% a year, and is projected to decline further to around 1.2% over the next decade. This and a few other adverse factors have contributed to the rapid rise in the world market prices for major food products since early 2006, recording an increase of around 60% in just 2 years to early 2008. More recently, the FAO food price index (FFPI) has averaged 221 points in August 2011, 26 points higher than a year earlier [2]. The climate of rising retail prices of food items globally has raised the specter of another global food crisis, especially in the poorer countries, where the drive for food security has suffered a major jolt.

Side by side with these changes in the patterns of food production and supply, there have been significant changes to the patterns of food consumption around the globe. Many of these changes are continuing, and are spreading to populations which had not previously experienced them. Some of these changes are related to changing patterns of human habitation and life style or global demographic changes. These influences on food demand are usually referred to as "structural" in nature. Significant changes to dietary preferences are also observed to result from growing affluence, especially in the developing world. These changes are induced by income changes and changes in the relative prices of food items. Such changes indicate improvements in the quality and quantity of food consumption, which, generally, is a positive and desirable outcome. However, not all of the newly evolving dietary preferences and patterns have been beneficial from human health or nutrition perspectives. Indeed, some of these such as the increasing incidences of obesity and other harmful afflictions in many countries, both developed and developing, are causing concern amongst policymakers [2]. The issue of nutrition is an important one, and is almost always of relevance in the context of food, but it is not within the scope of this chapter.

In the light of these changes, this chapter aims to examine several interrelated developments and issues relating to the fast-changing global food situation. Its main focus is food consumption and the observed and projected changes thereto. It starts, however, by examining briefly the factors and forces that have influenced the production of food crops and how they have changed over the recent decades. A quick look at the pattern of expected changes in food production in the future rounds off this section. The chapter goes on, then, to look at the influences behind the changes in the consumption of food in different countries and regions of the world. The last couple of decades have seen some significant improvements in the living standards of large numbers of people in the developing world—first in some of the Southeast Asian economies, and then in China, India, and a few other countries. Rising living standards naturally lead to changes in the pattern of food consumption which, in turn, has implications for food quality, prices, availabilities, and trade. Some of these issues, in their relationships with food consumption, will be examined to understand the changes that have already occurred and to look into their possible evolution in the future. Some issues of policy, at the national, regional, and global levels, will be addressed to conclude the chapter.

9.2 GLOBAL FOOD SUPPLY IN CONTEXT

There are different methods of measuring agricultural production because it comprises a heterogeneous bundle of commodities including crops and other food items. The index of total agricultural production from 1990 to 2006 recorded a rising trend for the world as a whole, although there were considerable regional variations. For example, there had not been much of an increase in the agricultural output of the developed countries [3]. Perhaps a more meaningful measure than the total output is the per capita agricultural output, that is, the total output divided by the relevant population. The per capita output of three major cereals—rice, wheat, and maize—increased steadily from the early 1960s to the early 1990s, flattened off after that, and then went on a slowly declining trend over the period 2000–2006, but recovered over the next 3 years. Its performance in the future would of course depend on the growth in both the total output and the population.

Growth in the total agricultural output is a function of the land area harvested and the growth in productivity, measured as the change in the aggregate average yield, per acre. The land area suitable for agriculture, including animal grazing, is around 3 billion hectares, which is less than one-half of the world's land area [4]. Much of the land suited for agriculture is already being used in agriculture and farming activities. Any increase in world cropland would therefore need to come from other land-based activities, such as forestry and range-based uses, for example. Since the 1970s, the average annual growth rate of the area harvested was around 0.15%, achieved mostly through deforestation and by land-switching from pastoral and other uses. More intensive cultivation, such as multiple cropping, and the use of previously unused fallow or marginal land have also made a contribution to the observed increase in agricultural production.

There is also always some loss of cultivated land occurring through such natural processes as soil erosion, salinization, and nutrient depletion, and also through conscious decisions to transfer land to nonagricultural uses. These losses of course adversely affect agricultural output, at least potentially.

The steady rise in the total agricultural output over the last few decades has therefore been the result mainly of improved productivity, as mentioned earlier. The declining trend in the growth rate of agricultural output, also alluded to earlier, is a matter of particular concern when viewed in conjunction with the increasing scarcity of cultivable land.

World population grew at an annual average rate of 1.7% over the period 1970–1990, falling to 1.4% over the period 1990–2007. The declining trend is expected to continue into the future, falling to 1.1% by 2017 [2]. But, despite this decline in the growth rate of population, the total world population has of course been increasing. The growth rate of average per capita production of food grains and oilseeds has therefore been declining, and is expected to continue doing so into the future as the decline in yields and the increase in population impact together.

9.3 GLOBAL FOOD CONSUMPTION TRENDS

9.3.1 QUICK NOTE ON THE MEASUREMENT ISSUE

The consumption of food needs to be examined at a number of levels and on different criteria. At a crude macro level, with the growth in world population, the demand for food must rise over time. In addition, since much of the increase in world population in recent decades has been occurring in the developing countries where food availability has generally been scarce, the impact on the demand for food has been stronger with rising populations and levels of affluence. To make better sense, information on food consumption or availability is often expressed in terms of its energy content at the per capita level. This enables food from different major sources such as cereals; meat and other animal products; milk and dairy products; vegetables and fruits, and oils and fat, for example, to be converted to a uniform unit, namely calories, for purposes of comparison within and across countries and/or over periods of time. As an example of the usefulness of the calorie-based measurement of food available for consumption worldwide, let us note that, over three decades to the end of the 1990s, despite a 70% increase in world population, enough agricultural products were produced globally to make available 17% more calories per person. This, if evenly distributed, would have been enough to provide around 2700 kcal per person daily. There were considerable regional variations in the rate of growth of food calorie production, but all regions except sub-Saharan Africa registered noticeable gains over this period [5].

Statistical data on the availability of the broad groups of food items in different countries are collected by the Food and Agricultural Organisation (FAO) of the United Nations from a large number of countries on a regular basis (FAOSTAT). These are then processed to produce annual food balance sheets (FBS) for these countries. The FBS are based on information on the supply of food items, which includes production, net exports, and inventory changes. It also provides information on the utilization of food items using figures on final consumption demand, intermediate use, such as animal feed; nonfood industrial use and waste for each commodity. It is possible to calculate from this database the per capita average supplies of calories from the food items. However, the actual per capita availabilities of the food items, as opposed to their supplies, would depend on several other factors such as the price levels at which the commodities are available in a country and the income levels of the consumers which would determine the ease of access, or "entitlement" to food, as Sen [6] has termed it. The FAO database, being sourced from data at the national level, cannot provide information on the distribution of the nationally available food within the country or at the household level. For these reasons, the FAO uses the description "national average apparent food consumption" to capture food consumption in kilocalories per capita per day.

At the national level, many countries conduct frequent cross-sectional surveys to monitor the nature of dietary intake and changes thereto over time. Most countries also conduct smaller surveys in single locations and/or with smaller sample sizes with questions that help elicit specific information that the large nationwide surveys may not cover.

While the calorie measure helps to capture food intake from different food sources in terms of a single quantifiable unit, it is still necessary to understand the importance of a "balanced diet" for human health and nutrition. This, in turn, necessitates quantifying not just the total calorie intake, but also intake from specified food items categorized as such broad types as cereals, meat products, milk and dairy products, vegetables and fruits, oils and fats, etc. Many national governments around the world have developed dietary guidelines for people to use in choosing their diets for required nutrition. Internationally too, organizations such as the FAO and the World Health Organisation (WHO) issue dietary guidelines and recommendations for balanced eating for health and nutrition. These organizations also monitor the changes taking place in global food production and consumption to identify the potential problems and shortfalls and alert policymakers to the needs for the adoption of appropriate policies to deal with them [7].

Another convenient way to measure the consumption of food, of course, is to use the expenditure of a spending unit, such as a household, on food over a given period of time. Countries that conduct regular surveys of household behavior usually seek information on the respondent's budget, and how the budget is split over different items of expenditure, food, and nonfood. The budget share of food tends to decline as the level of affluence improves, in line with Engel's law [8], which predicts a proportionate decline in the food share of the household budget with rising income. The insight of this observation is useful in numerous contexts. For example, if the budget shares of equivalent rural households on food are observed to change differently from those of the urban households within a country over time, it would indicate uneven changes in the real living standards in the two sectors.

The advantage of the money measure is that it is easy to use, and it lends itself to useful interpretations of observed expenditure patterns at different locations within a country at a given point of time, or over a period of time. But comparing expenditures incurred over time and/or across dispersed geographic locations involves the need to correct them for prices and changes in prices which may be different. Nevertheless, its wide use around the world testifies to its attraction as a measuring device.

9.3.2 STRUCTURAL CHANGES TO GLOBAL CONSUMPTION PATTERNS

World population, which has just crossed the 7 billion mark, is projected to reach 7.5 billion by 2020 [8]. Almost all of the net increase in world population over the coming decades will be in the developing countries where some 6 billion people currently live, about a half of them in the rural areas. Demographers have been observing an accelerating process of urbanization of the populations of developing countries. This process is projected to continue and result in the doubling of the urban population from 1.7 billion in 1995 to 3.4 billion by 2020 [8]. Together with the impact of the generally increasing populations, the projected increase in urbanization would affect the demand for food in significant ways.

There are many reasons why the food habits and dietary practices of people change when they move from a rural to an urban environment. For example, urban consumers typically encounter a wider choice of available food in the market place; they experience a greater variety of culinary choices reflecting a more cosmopolitan urban social environment; being usually more time conscious and time constrained in their urban habitats, they tend to develop a preference for food that requires less preparation time; with a generally more sedentary lifestyle that urban living entails, the dietary choices may change to reflect a lower calorie intake, and with little or no opportunity to grow any food in their urban settings, urban dwellers' consumption is less restricted by the necessity to make use of home-grown food which they would have had when living in the rural areas. This greater dependence on the market tends to affect the quantity, quality, and variety of the urban dwellers' consumption basket, subject to the constraints of their food budgets. However, the dominance of supermarket-type shopping facilities offering more processed, ready-to-eat food may induce increased calorie intake, despite the possible reduction in the aforementioned urban dwellers' calorie needs.

All these and other influences on the consumption of food operate slowly over time to make an observable difference in the dietary practices. This is sometimes referred to as "nutrition transition" which reflects both quantitative and qualitative aspects of changing patterns of food consumption [9].

Over the last three decades of the twentieth century, per capita food consumption had improved steadily at the global level and also across most regions. In calorie terms, average intake increased by some 400 kcal between 1969/1971 and 1999/2001, although many developing countries, especially in sub-Saharan Africa, experienced a decline from an already low per capita energy consumption over the period [10].

A major aspect of the nutrition transition concerns the changes that occur in the sourcing of the total calorie intake from different major categories of food. In the developing world as a whole, this transition is observed mainly in terms of a move away from a cereal-based diet to a more varied one in the direction of animal products and oils and sugar, for example. Thus, over the four decades from 1963 to 2003, calorie intake from meat increased by 199%, from sugar by 127%, and from vegetable oil by 199% in the developing countries [2]. In the developed countries by contrast, significant increase in the calorie source was observed only from vegetable oils, indicating perhaps that these countries had already gone through their nutrition transition. In global terms, dietary patterns have become more energy- and sugar-rich over the years as substitution in favor of processed food, and away from food rich in fiber, has been gathering pace.

A related aspect of the observed dietary shift in favor of animal products (meat, milk, and egg in the main) is the effect this has on total cereal use, which includes the use of cereals as animal feed. This is demonstrated rather dramatically by the fact that the per capita annual consumption of cereals in the United States was 953 kg over the period 2004–2006, which was over three times the world average, while China's cereal consumption, at 288 kg, is only slightly above the world average, and India's 175 kg, significantly lower than it. These figures reflect the patterns of animal product consumption of the three countries. The conversion rates of feed to edible animal product vary depending on the type of product. For example, to produce 1 lb of chicken meat requires 2.6 lb, beef requires 7 lb, and pork 6.5 lb of corn [11].

9.3.3 EVOLVING FUTURE SCENARIO

Given the changing global demographic transition scenario detailed earlier, increased food demand will come mostly from the developing countries, according to the FAO [12]. This increase will cover all major food items as diets become more varied and calorie intakes continue improving across countries. The International Food Policy Research Institute (IFPRI) projects that, between

1995 and 2020, about 85% of the global demand for cereals is expected to come from the developing countries. Their demand for meat will also account for an equally large proportion of the global increase [13].

In the development literature of recent times, China and India have loomed large mainly because of their sustained and high growth performance in recent times. Not surprisingly, therefore, the changes in these two countries' food habits will continue to have a major impact on the global food situation. China alone, according to the IFPRI, will account for a quarter of the increase in the demand for cereals, and as much as two-fifths of that in meat demand over the 25 years to 2020. The impact of India's faster economic growth on the global food demand has so far been less spectacular than China's, as noted before. India's lower average consumption of meat—a mere fifth of the average meat consumption of 127 kg a year in the United States, for example—is probably related to its food preferences which are, partly at least, culturally determined; proportionately more Indian households than Chinese may be vegetarian.

Given the projected changes in the levels of per capita incomes, changing food preferences, and demographic transitions discussed earlier, world meat demand is projected to grow much faster than the demand for cereal, and meat consumption is expected to double in the developing world between 1995 and 2020. These changes referred to as a "Livestock Revolution"—analogous with the "Green Revolution" of the 1960s—have some significant implications for global land-use patterns, agriculture, agri-food industries, and the environment, among others. A sustained increase in the production of cereals to be used as animal feed would be needed to allow this transition to succeed. Using data from FAOSTAT and other sources, IFPRI's International Model for Policy Analysis of Commodities and Trade (IMPACT) suggests

> ... under most likely scenario global demand for cereals will increase by 39 percent between 1995 and 2020 to reach 2,466 million tons; demand for meat will increase by 58 percent to reach 313 percent; and demand for roots and tubers will increase by 37 percent to reach 864 million tons [13, p. 8].

While food demand is predicted to keep growing in volume and in the variety of its composition, the required increase in the supply of food would be a more difficult problem to resolve. The IFPRI projections suggest that 40% more grain would need to be produced by 2020, and much of it would need to result from increased productivity of the farmed land. Improved availability of fertilizers and irrigation facilities, additional investment in infrastructure, and agricultural research—especially in the agricultural sectors of the poorly performing economies—would be needed to achieve a noticeable improvement in agricultural output. Additional farmland available for raising cereals would be very limited, according to the projections of IMPACT. Only about 7.4% increase, or 51 million hectares, of extra land, can be expected by 2020.

The combination of increased demand for cereals and limited scope for increased supply in the developing world would necessitate increased net import of cereals by them from the developed countries, South Asia being the leading developing area needs to import more cereals. About 60% of the increased demand for cereals would be supplied by the United States. According to the IMPACT projections, although Russia, some of the Eastern European countries and Australia are likely to increase their market share too.

These changes will have significant impact on the availability of dietary energy supply (DES) in different countries. Projections of future DES prepared prior to the recent, rapidly rising, food price inflation scenario starting around 2006 were decidedly more optimistic than they are now. A study prepared by two FAO economists in 2005 [14], for example, suggested:

> ... Some developing countries will have even reached the very high calorie supply brackets of developed countries today. Overall, 43 countries, home of 3.5 billion people, will have reached average calorie availabilities of 3200 kcal per day at their disposal [10].

The continuing upward trend in the real price of major food products globally, alluded to earlier, introduces serious doubts about the prospects of continuing improvements in food supply and its consequential impact on DES in the near future. The demand and supply factors referred to earlier will interact together to determine how the net supply positions are going to change, and how the changes will be distributed across different countries and regions of the world. The future of global and regional food security is threatened by several relatively new factors too. A brief review of these factors is warranted here and will be addressed a little later in the chapter; but attention is focused first on the nature and extent of consumption involving food items which may be termed "speciality foods," which are of interest mainly to a somewhat "select and distinct" group of affluent consumers. These involve the consumption of functional and organic foods, and also genetically modified foods, the appeal of which is less clear, both at the individual consumer level and also at the national level.

9.4 TRENDS IN THE CONSUMPTION OF SPECIALITY FOODS

The role of food as a source of life-sustaining energy is well understood. Food also provides the nutrition necessary for general health and resistance to diseases—indeed, it helps survival itself. As food and nutrition sciences have progressed beyond dealing with food for mere survival and basic nutrition, newer uses of food for promoting what may be termed "optimal health" have come to evolve over time. There are consumers who, for example, wish to minimize or avoid eating foods which they perceive to be not as "close to nature" as they would like. They may be motivated by their desire to avoid certain ingredients inherent in ordinary, conventional, or mass-produced foods for reasons of health and/or other considerations which they value. Such food products are of course in the nature of "niche items," and of interest to relatively small sections of consumers. But the evidence suggests that their impact is growing, and that their implications extend beyond just those who directly patronize them. Three loosely interrelated categories of such foods are discussed briefly here.

9.4.1 FUNCTIONAL FOODS

9.4.1.1 Concept

As the term implies, functional foods are meant to confer certain health and/or lifestyle benefits beyond providing energy and basic nutrition [15]. Such benefits may derive from dietary supplements consumed as such, or from the consumption of conventional foods—fortified, enriched, or enhanced—to achieve some specific health objectives. Increasing urbanization, rising longevity, higher incidences of noncommunicable diseases, and high and growing costs of healthcare around the world have made people more conscious of the importance of "good diet" as an ongoing factor in healthcare and prevention of diseases. In most cultures, health and medicinal qualities of many traditional food products remain well-entrenched, and are usually passed down by word of mouth or regular practice from generation to generation.

With increasing commercialization of the food industries globally, research and development have gone into encouraging and promoting innovations around food products to cater for specific health and lifestyle needs. In these developments, science and technologies have combined to (i) identify the contributions that specific ingredients in given items of food make to human health and nutrition; (ii) reproduce these ingredients artificially in laboratories; (iii) trial them to test for their efficacies, and, if successful; and (iv) mass produce and market them.

It is of course necessary for independent regulatory oversight and control of these activities to ensure their safety and to ascertain the accuracy of the claims the agents responsible for their development might make. Many countries have governmental agencies that exercise such control. The Food and Drug Administration (FDA) of the United States, for example, has wide-ranging authority and regulatory power to ensure product safety and accuracy in the areas of food and pharmaceutical products. Similar functions are performed by the European Food Safety Authority (EFSA) for the European Union (EU) countries.

There are also specialist, nonprofit organizations in different countries lending their professional expertise to evaluate the products and processes in the food and related areas. The US based Institute of Food Technologists (IFT), for example, plays an important role in providing a scientific perspective on food-related issues. In 2005, the IFT released a Report, *The Promise of Functional Foods: Opportunities and Challenges (www.ift.org/reports/expert-reports/science)* containing insights from the extensive deliberations of a multidisciplinary panel on a variety of issues concerning the functional food. The report made several recommendations to promote the development of functional foods. The details of this elaborate report, which is readily available, are not gone into here. Instead, some aspects of the evolving market for functional foods are summarized here.

9.4.1.2   Some Broad Facts and Figures

Because functional foods are, by definition, distinct from the mainstream food products, detailed statistical information relating to them is not easily available from standard official sources. Nevertheless, there exist research bodies or commercial groups with interest and involvement in the functional food areas. These organizations monitor relevant developments, often for their own use; but the information is also often available in the public domain. Use is made here of such information.

The UK based research organization, Leatherhead Food Research, has recently released a report, *Future Directions for the Global Functional Foods Market (www.leatherheadfood.com/functional-foods)*, containing some useful information, which we make use of here.

The Report defines functional foods as "food and drink products making a specific health claim." It values the market for such foods at US$24.2 billion in 2010; estimates that it has grown 1.5 times since 2003, and observes that the growth rate of this market has been much faster than the market for food and drinks generally.

In proportionate terms, dairy products, with its share of 38.1%, lead the functional foods market, followed by bakery and cereals (22.7%); beverages (12.5%); fats and oils (8.1%); meat, fish, and eggs (7.4%); and soya products (5.8%). The countrywise distribution of the market for functional foods shows the Japanese consuming 38.4%, the United States 31.1%, Europe 28.9%, and Australia a very modest 1.6% of the global consumption. The growth rates of demand have also varied from country to country, Japan registering the strongest growth at over 46% and Australia 39% over the period 2006–2010.

There is evidence of a slowdown in the growth in the market for functional foods in recent years. This must partly be due to the decline in global economic activity over the last few years. It is also a fact, however, that authorities in many countries have tended to get stricter in their monitoring of the health benefits claimed by functional foods, leading to reduction in the proliferation of new products and a reduction in the sales of some of the existing ones. Nevertheless, the attraction of food products offering distinct health benefits is unlikely to fade away. If anything, stricter control by specialized authorities could well help enhance their marketability by improving their reliability.

9.4.2   ORGANIC FOODS

As agricultural practices have got technologically more complex, its dependence on chemical fertilizers, pesticides, and other inputs of industrial origin has increased. In the ever-growing demand for food and the natural desire for increased variety in human dietary preferences, the need to achieve increased food supply has been the main driving force behind the farming activities. However, there are individual consumers as well as activist groups in many countries who champion the cause of environmental protection and animal welfare which, they feel, are neglected by conventional methods of agricultural and pastoral farming. This is where organic farming on the production side and organic food on the consumption side of the agri-food system fit in.

Organic food of agricultural origin must avoid using pesticides that are known to be harmful to human health, and organic animal foods must come from animals that are not treated with antibiotics or growth hormones. The advocates of organic food place a strong emphasis on maintaining and improving the natural environment, and promoting biodiversity. These, they claim, are achieved better by using organic farming methods. There is also the belief that organic food is "better for the health," although, to our knowledge, no conclusive scientific evidence exists to prove the nutritional superiority of organic food items from conventionally produced ones [16].

Organic foods tend to be more expensive than their conventional substitutes because of the lower crop yields, higher feed prices, and higher labor intensities associated with the required production methods. Nevertheless, sales of organic food and drinks are rising rapidly and at a much faster rate than foodstuffs in general. One estimate puts the global sales figure for organic food at $54.9 billion in 2009, rising from $50.9 billion in 2008. Not surprisingly, much of the demand for organic foods is in the more affluent countries of the world, with the Group of 7 (G7) countries accounting for 80% of the total global sales. The largest markets are in the United States, Germany, and France, and the highest per capita consumption is in Denmark, Switzerland, and Austria. Fresh produce, such as fruits and vegetables, lead the organic food consumption category, followed by dairy products and drinks, according to the *Organic Monitor 2006* (http://www.organicmonitor.com/700240.htm).

The total organically managed land area was around 37.2 million hectares in 2009, largest being in Australia (12 million hectares), followed by Argentina (9.4 million hectares) and the United States (1.9 million hectares). The growth rates of agricultural land used for organic farming have been the fastest in some of the developing countries—in Asia, Africa, and Latin America—which experienced triple-digit growth since 2000, while other regions saw double-digit growth rates [17]. Given the dominance of the affluent countries in the consumption of organic foods, their production in the developing countries is highly export-oriented. While this may seem to make sense, given the higher prices organic foods command, lower yields and potential volatilities in the export markets are among the risk factors such farming must take into consideration.

9.4.3 GENETICALLY MODIFIED FOODS

The need to raise the global output of food products, of both plant and animal origin, is urgent in the face of the growing population, increasing urbanization, and rising affluence around the world, as this chapter has elaborated. Conventional methods to achieve this have been, and are being, tried, with varying success. Applying new scientific knowledge and/or technological innovations to solve or avert difficult problems has always been part of the story of human evolution and progress. In recent times, biological sciences have achieved major breakthroughs in understanding the functioning and interactions of genes of both plants and animals. These insights have come to be used in agri-food activities in a variety of ways—the aims being to improve yields and enhance certain desired qualities or avoid certain harmful traits in crops and/or animals [18].

The label GM foods or GMOs, meaning genetically modified organisms, has come to be used to refer to cereal or other crop plants developed with the help of newly developed molecular biological techniques. The purpose of such biotechnological intervention in plant growth is usually to enable these plants to avoid high doses of chemical herbicides and/or to produce one or more pesticidal proteins themselves. If successful, these developments have the potential to increase crop yields by reducing pest damage and also, in some cases, damage from other impediments such as frosts, salinity, and droughts, for example. Other benefits of GM foods, claimed by their protagonists, include improving general or specific nutritional qualities of crops, fruits, and vegetables. Those who counsel a more cautious approach to venturing into this new and relatively unknown territory tend to argue that they may unleash harmful environmental and health consequences. In poorer countries, many farmers grow crops mainly for their own consumption, with very little surplus for commercial marketing. If patented GM technology develops plants that are incapable of producing seeds for replanting, farmers would be forced to purchase them every sowing season from the companies that hold the patent. This would, obviously, interfere with their traditional livelihood by making them dependent on the suppliers of seeds, a crucial item of their economic functioning.

The international community has paid heed to such concerns, especially those concerning environmental protection, from the early days of the application of GM technologies to agriculture, especially in the agri-food areas. A long process of intergovernmental and/or expert group consultations preceded the adoption of The Cartagena Protocol on Biodiversity (Secretariat of the Convention on Biological Diversity 2000, http://bch.cbd.int/protocol), which came into force in September 2003. Although the Protocol does not cover food safety issues—there are other, national, regulatory frameworks to address them—it does provide an international forum for discussions on the handling of living modified organisms (LMOs) resulting from the application of biotechnology that may affect biodiversity adversely. The primary focus of this chapter being food consumption from a global perspective, the issue of GM foods in its multiple perspectives is not of direct relevance to it, and is not therefore gone into any further.

Detailed information on the production and, especially, consumption and also international trade involving GM foods as such are not plentiful. The vast bulk of such food crops grown around the world can be sourced to the United States (53%) and Argentina (17%); with smaller proportions found in other countries such as Brazil (11%), Canada (6%), China and India (4% each), as of 2006. The main crops involved are herbicide and pest-resistant soya beans, sweet corn, cotton, canola, and alfalfa.

It would probably be fair to observe that the applications of molecular biology and its related biotechnology are still in their early stages, and a lot more will need to be learnt before more extensive uses of them become acceptable. Concerns about their implications for the natural environment and human and animal health are also very real, and would need to be addressed if they are to make a lasting contribution to human welfare.

9.5 SOME EMERGING INFLUENCES AND THE FUTURE OF THE GLOBAL FOOD ECONOMY

The continuing concern about the upward trend in global food prices has been alluded to earlier in this chapter. This has spawned numerous studies exploring the factors and forces behind the steady price rise. These studies have helped to identify some distinctive influences confronting the global food economy as it struggles to find a new steady state in its disturbed equilibrium. Among these influences are (a) the increased demand for biofuels, with its consequential diversion of food crops and cultivable land away from food to nonfood uses, (b) climate change and its impacts on food production, and (c) globalization of the food economy characterized by the dominance of large multinational companies with enormous market powers to control entire food supply chains. These influences will continue to affect the food economy from both demand and supply sides. The following discussion explores how these forces have been affecting the consumption aspects of food and how they are likely to do so into the future. However, where appropriate, the discussion goes beyond just food prices, and covers other issues pertinent to the global food economy.

9.5.1 Rising Price of Fossil Fuels and the Search for Alternatives

9.5.1.1 Use of Fossil versus Bioenergy: A Brief Background

Until well into the twentieth century, the use of fossil fuels as a source of energy was not large; much of the energy necessary in farming activities for example used to be derived from draught animals, biomass such as tree and plant products, organic wastes, and residues. Industrial processes were reliant mainly on steam power fuelled usually by coal. With the increasing use of the internal combustion engine, industrial activities and road transport came to depend more on fossil fuels—petroleum, natural gas, and diesel. Farming activities too switched to using fossil fuels for their farm machinery and fertilizers. With the discovery of new oil and gas reserves in different locations around the world, dependence on petroleum and its related products steadily increased in the second half of the twentieth century. The process was hugely helped by the "low" real price of fossil fuels in the decades immediately following the World War II when the demand for energy was rising rapidly as the affluent world was recovering from the ravages of the war. Many of the poorer countries too, having emerged from colonial rule in this period, started on their development paths over this period.

Following the brief Arab-Israeli war in late 1973, the world faced its first oil shock, which saw crude oil prices quadrupling over a short few years as a result of the imposition of oil embargo by the large Arab oil exporters. This led to a global economic downturn; prompting renewed search for fresh oilfields and also for alternatives to fossil fuels.

Since the first oil shock, there have been several other episodes of oil price rise, but new oil fields came to be developed in different locations around the world leading to steady increase in the supply of oil too. The global supply of oil seems now to have reached a plateau around 2005, and significant increases are probably not likely to occur in the way they did in the past. In any case, the rising costs of extraction and processing of hydrocarbon have also been a factor in the observed price rise of recent times. The oil shocks of the period up to the 1980s were mostly supply-induced. More recent price rises have stemmed increasingly from the sharply increased demand for energy in the high-growth economies, such as those of China and India in recent decades.

The steady increase in the price of oil has been a factor in the observed rise in the price of food since 2006. Agricultural activities are energy-intensive as oil, diesel, natural gas, and fertilizers are amongst its inputs, and transporting its inputs from, and produce to, markets or processors also use fossil fuels as energy.

9.5.1.2 Impact of Biofuels on Food and Nonfood Crops

The search for alternative fuels has involved developing renewable energy sources ranging from solar, wind and tidal, to biofuels, such as ethanol and biodiesel, or biogas and hydrogen. The incentive to use plant-based inputs to produce liquid or gaseous energy derives mainly from cost considerations; "high" hydrocarbon prices have therefore been a factor in the move toward biofuels in recent years. Also, the environmental concerns—the emission of greenhouse gases, associated with fossil fuels—are mitigated at least to some extent when they are replaced by biofuels [19].

The impact on the supplies and prices of some food items derive from the diversion of a few crops to producing biofuels. The efforts to produce biofuels started in the 1970s, when, following the first oil shock, Brazil got into using sugarcane to produce ethanol as a response to the sudden rise in the price of fuel oils. It is only in recent years that concerns have come to be expressed by policy makers both at national and global levels about the observed surge in some countries in the direction of producing more and more biofuels. Currently, biofuel production is dominated by the United States, followed by the EU and Brazil. Between them, the United States and Brazil produce over 70% of the world's ethanol; while the EU and the United States are the main producers of biodiesel. The EU alone consumes some two-thirds of the available global supply of biodiesel [19]. Diverting corn for ethanol or soya bean for biodiesel obviously raises their price and reduces their availability as food. The potential seriousness of such diversion can be guessed from the fact that in 2007, the United States used over 20% of its entire corn crop to produce ethanol.

The main crops used in these activities are maize, soya beans, and sugarcane; wheat, barley, rapeseed, and a few other food crops are also used in a limited way. The United States is the major producer of both corn and soya bean in the world. Any major diversion of these crops to biofuel production in the United States has a significant effect on the global availability and price of corn. To take just two examples of how sharply such diversion has occurred in recent years, in the United

States, between 2004 and 2007, the share of soya beans used in biodiesel production increased from 1% to 12% of production, and that of corn used in the production of ethanol increased from 11% to 25%. The diversion of food crops to the production of biofuels is assisted by production and consumption subsidies in many countries—the rationale being to promote energy security and to mitigate the climate change-related effects. There are also governmental mandates in many countries to include a proportion of biofuels in fuels for use in road transport. The current mandate in the EU is to continue till 2020, and that in the United States to 2022. These factors combine to cause competition between alternative uses of food crops to get more and more unfavorable for food. Land use patterns change over time to reflect the attraction of (privately) more profitable activities such as production of inputs for biofuels. Consumers facing rising prices of several food items, some of which are amongst the daily necessities such as cooking oil, cereals, and sugar, for example, have few cost-effective substitutes to turn to.

9.5.2 CLIMATE CHANGE AND THE GLOBAL FOOD ECONOMY

Of all the emerging influences affecting the food sector, the implications of climate change are probably the most complex to understand, to mitigate or to use for purposes of predicting how it might affect the global food economy. It is now generally accepted that the global climate has been warming, and that its impact is likely to increase in the medium-to-long term into the future. What is within the realms of possibility, according to experts working with global economic models incorporating different scenarios of average temperature change, is to anticipate that the steadily warming climate will seriously alter crop yields, particularly in the tropics and subtropics by the end on the twenty-first century. This implies that nearly half the world's population will face serious food shortages. Results from the testing of various models simulating the impact of temperature changes for a range of locations show that, in low-latitude regions, even moderate increases in temperature (1–2°C) are likely to reduce the yields of major cereals. In the mid-to-high latitudes, however, similar increases in temperature are likely to improve crop yields. Taken as a whole, such results project potential improvements in food production as long as the local average temperature increases are in the 1–3°C range. Above that range, food production will decrease. Several studies have foreshadowed worsening conditions in respect of food availabilities, stability in the supply and the price of food, food utilization, and access to food because of both the long-term gradual changes in climate and also the episodes of climatic extremes such as heat-waves, floods, and other natural hazards which are predicted to occur with increasing frequency [20].

There will also be significant changes to the distribution of global hunger and malnutrition, with sub-Saharan Africa and South Asia possibly faring the worst. All developing countries, because of their location in the tropical and subtropical regions of the planet (35°C north to 35° south latitudes), are likely to experience reduced crop yields, while more affluent countries at higher, temperate, latitudes may experience improved crop yields. There will therefore be the need to increase trade flows involving the exports of food and forestry products from richer countries to poorer ones, indicating increased dependence of the latter.

Climate scientists and modellers studying the phenomenon of gradual global warming point out that some of the adverse changes can be mitigated by consciously seeking to adapt to the changes. In large countries such as Brazil and India, for example, there are regional variations in temperature and precipitation. Some crops may actually benefit from mild warming if they are grown in areas which are less vulnerable. Policy makers will need to consider the potential for measures such as changing the plant varieties and planting times, utilizing lands according to their most productive use—if necessary, in nonfarm activities, and developing strategies that integrate development and poverty alleviation aims with policies specifically for mitigating the effects of climate change. Precisely because the problem involves the whole planet, international collaboration in policymaking and in the sharing of expertise would be a vital ingredient in the mitigation of the adverse effects of climate change.

9.5.3 GLOBALIZATION OF THE FOOD ECONOMY: EVOLUTION AND IMPLICATIONS

Assisted by a few favorable technological and economic developments in recent decades, the process of integration of the global economy has gathered pace. These developments include increasing containerization of bulky cargo for long-distance cross-border transportation, improved and faster airfreight facilities, and the availability of new and more efficient methods for gathering and transmitting information and communication, made possible by the information and communication technology (ICT) revolution. All this has resulted in a decline in the real cost of conducting business internationally, which has helped increase the global trade, including trade in usually bulky agricultural and farm products. This phenomenon of increased global connectedness is often referred to as globalization. Amongst other effects, it has helped boost the global concentration of agribusiness, involving both the output and input sectors of the food economy [21].

Transnational involvement in the food industry is not new. A limited number of processed food items such as instant coffee, chocolates, and biscuits, for example, have been produced over many years by well-known multinational companies in selected countries around the world. Such products were usually meant for a small group of affluent and sophisticated consumers in those countries or in their neighborhoods. But, as the average consumption of basic staple food items started reaching their limits in richer countries, their growth prospects dimmed, with slowing population growth and stable or reducing average and incremental spending on food in these countries. This encouraged a process of concentration in the processed food industry which, in turn, saw an oligopolistic market structure, characterized by a few large transnational conglomerates, evolved from the mid-1970s.

A parallel, but complementary, development in the poorer countries has been characterized by faster population growth and urbanization, improving prosperity, and its resulting nutrition transition, alluded to earlier. A very rapid increase in the number and variety of processed food products is observed since the decade of the 1970s as a response to these complementary changes in the economies and societies of the rich and the poor countries. The developing countries have often been utilized as major suppliers of raw materials, which they grow or possess, for food to be processed into specialized brands ready for consumption in both developed and developing economies. A process of acquisition, merger, and take overs has resulted in these transnational companies, both in upstream and downstream activities in the agri-food economy, consolidating their positions in the global market place.

For example, 30 companies account for one-third of the world's processed food; five companies control 75% of international grain trade, and six companies manage 75% of the world's pesticides market [22].

The industries processing food, of course, need to acquire the necessary raw materials. They often seek a vertically integrated production system that connects them to the local farmers and the suppliers of other inputs, directly in competition (often unequal), with other purchasers of these goods and services. Taking the recent Indian experience as a case study, one observes how the food grains market, long dominated by the public sector, has seen a steady increase in the participation of the private sector. This process has involved several foreign-owned MNCs, such as Glencore, Toepfer, and Cargill, as well as Indian-owned companies such as the Reliance group, buying wheat directly from the farmers. This activity has come to coincide with the government having to import, in 2008, wheat for the first time in several years to replenish its buffer stocks. The objective of this measure was to ensure adequate supplies to the food-based welfare programs. India's (reducing) food security has come to be seen as an issue of concern in consequence of these developments.

While different developing countries offer different advantages to the global agri-food industries, the larger and faster growing economies have become these industries' major targets as they offer potentially large domestic markets as well as useful inputs and other resources. Thus, Brazil has emerged as a leading global supply source for a number of important agri-food commodities such as red meat, poultry, and coffee, and China as a leading exporter of seafood, fruits, and vegetables, and a leading importer of soy. India has been somewhat slow in its uptake of transnational-dominated food-processing activities. Thus, while China processes around 40% of its agricultural produce, Brazil 70%, Malaysia 80%, and Thailand around 30%, value addition to agricultural produce in India is only around 20%.

In the developing economies, the penetration of the agri-food multinationals has gone beyond the production and processing stages to the retail sector as well. For example, just as in the Indian domestic food sector such well-known names as Unilever, Cadbury, Nestle, and Pepsi have been involved in the processing side. The retail giant Wal-Mart has been seeking to get involved in the retailing side, "to partner with India's Reliance Industry Ltd (RIL) to build super market stores in 784 Indian towns, 1600 farm supply hubs, and move the produce with a 40-plane air cargo fleet" [23]. If these efforts were to succeed and proliferate, there will be even more intense competition at the starting points of India's food supply chain, namely, the farmers and growers of farm products. Given the unequal nature of the competition, the farmers and growers, especially the smaller ones, are likely to suffer the most.

China too has, until recently, encouraged foreign investment in its agri-food sector in partnership with its domestic firms. The global transnational companies, understandably, have been active in this large and fast-growing economy in the processing, trade, and retail areas. More recently, however, China has become less welcoming to foreign direct investment, as evidenced by its removal, in 2008, of fiscal incentives to such investments. This will enable China's domestic firms to compete better in the domestic market, and become more competitive internationally too.

A further development in the international dimension of the global food economy has been the effort many countries have started to make in leasing or acquiring land outright in other countries with the aim of improving the security of their future food supplies. Countries as different as the populous China and India, on the one hand, and the sparsely populated, but arid, Saudi Arabia, the Emirates, and Libya, on the other, have been acquiring farmlands in Africa and elsewhere. There is no accurate estimate of the amount of land acquired so far by one country in another in this "scramble." One report notes "20 million hectares of land—twice the size of Germany's croplands—have been sold since 2006 in more than four dozen land deals, mainly in Africa. So far, most of the buyers are a mix of private investors, US private equity houses such as Sanlam Private Equity, the Saudi Kingdom Zephyr fund, the UK's CDC, and sovereign wealth funds" [24]. While the rationale for such actions in a world of increasing food insecurity is understandable, their ramifications are almost certain to extend well beyond just the food sector.

9.6   CONCLUDING OBSERVATIONS

This chapter has examined a number of interrelated aspects of the global food economy as it has evolved over the last few decades and also how it might change over the next few decades in response to the factors and forces affecting it in the contemporary national, regional, and global contexts. Several useful conclusions emerge from the detailed discourse. First, the world food situation has worsened in recent times in the sense that the growth in demand for food that has already occurred has not been met with an equivalent increase in its supply. There has also emerged a regional mismatch between where food is scarce and where it is in surplus. More importantly perhaps, while it is certain that the demand for food will continue to grow, it is by no means certain that the supply response will prove adequate. If the supply response continues to be inadequate, the rising trend in the prices of food will not be reversed; indeed it may deteriorate. This will be cause for serious worry as increasing hunger is the single most potent factor challenging the political and social stability, both locally and globally.

The much acclaimed Green Revolution of the 1960s, as this chapter has explained, helped ease the global food situation in a way that enabled many countries enjoy a period of improved security and stable prices of food. While it would be the most welcome to have a similar technological breakthrough in the global food economy, it would need to have a somewhat different outcome. It must enable the observed "nutrition transition" to continue—and, possibly, to accelerate—extending its benefits to larger proportions of the world population over the next few decades.

The keys to the required productivity growth involving the agricultural and farming sectors include additional investment in agricultural R&D; removal of policy-induced distortions affecting agricultural production and trade; globally coordinated approach to issues like climate change and the diversion of food crops to biofuels, and the use of new knowledge gained from bioscience and biotechnology in a manner that does not compromise food safety or the quality of the natural environment.

A global commitment to improve food security for the vast majority of the world's population, living mainly in the developing countries, is an ideal whose time has come. Whether human ingenuity and human compassion can be directed at solving the problem of global hunger and nutrition remains to be seen.

REFERENCES

1. Trostle, R. 2008. Global agricultural supply and demand: Factors contributing to the recent increase in food commodity prices. *A Report from the Economic Research Service*, United States Department of Agriculture.
2. Food and Agricultural Organisation. 2011. *World Food Situation: FAO Food Price Index*. http://www.fao.org/worldfoodsituation/wfs-home/foodpricesindex/en.
3. Food and Agricultural Organisation 2006. World agriculture towards 2030/2050. Interim Report.
4. Kendall, H. W. and D. Pimentel 1994. Constraints on the expansion of the global food supply, *Ambio*, 23(3), Reprinted in *The Royal Swedish Academy of Sciences*. http://dieoff.org/page36.htm
5. Food and Agricultural Organisation 2003. Diet, nutrition and the prevention of chronic diseases. Report of a Joint FAO/WHO Expert Group. WHO Technical Report Series 916.
6. Sen, A. K. 1981. *Poverty and Famines: An Essay on Entitlement and Deprivation*. Oxford: Oxford University Press.
7. World Health Organisation 2003. *WHO Global Database on National Nutritional Policies and Programmes*. Geneva: Department of Nutrition, World Health Organisation.
8. Perthel, D. 1975. Engel's law revisited. *The International Statistical Review*, 43(2), 211–218.
9. *The Economist* 22nd October 2011. Now we are seven billion.
10. Food and Agricultural Organisation 2002. World Agriculture toward 2015/2030, Summary Report.
11. Chand, R. 2008. The global food crisis: Causes, Severity and outlook, *The Economic and Political Weekly*, June 28, 2008.
12. Food and Agricultural Organisation 2006. *The State of Food Insecurity in the World 2006*.
13. Pinstrup-Andersen, P., R. Pandya-Lorch, and M. W. Rosegrant 1999. World food prospects: Critical issues for the twenty-first century. Food Policy Report, International Food Policy Research Institute, Washington D.C.
14. Schidhuber, J. and P. Shetty 2007. The nutrition transition to 2030: Why developing countries are likely to bear the major burden. *Food Economics—Acta Agriculturae Scandinavia Section C*, 2(34), 150–166.
15. Heasman. M. and J. Melentin 2001. *The Functional Food Revolution*. London: Earthscan Publishers, 2001.
16. Kearney, J. 2010. Food consumption trends and drivers. *Philosophical Transactions Royal Society London B*, 365(1554), 2793–2807.
17. Organic Trade Association June 8, 2011. Industry statistics and projected growth. (http://www.ota.com/organic/mt/business.htm). Accessed July 20, 2011.
18. Whitman, D. B. 2000. Genetically modified foods: Harmful or helpful? (http://www.csa.com/discoveryguides/gmfood/overview.php). Accessed 20 July 2011.
19. Sharma, A. 2008. Is higher demand for biofuels fuelling food prices? *Economic and Political Weekly*, August 9, 37–40.
20. Battisti, D. S., and R. L. Naylor 2009. Historical warnings of future food insecurity with unprecedented seasonal heat. *Science*, 323, 240–244.
21. Anderson, K. 2010. Globalisation effects on world agricultural trade, 1960–2050. *Philosophical Transactions of the Royal Society B*, 365, 3007–3021.

22. Chatterjee, S. 2011. Globalisation, India's evolving food economy and trade prospects for Australia and New Zealand. In M. Tonts and M.A.B. Siddique (eds.), *Globalisation, Agriculture and Development: Perspectives from the Asia-Pacific*. Cheltenham: Edward-Elgar, pp. 102–130.

23. Shiva, V. 2006. *WTO Is Dead, Long Live Free Trade: Globalisation and Its New Avatars*. Findland, MA: Organic Consumers Association, accessed at http://www.organicconsumers.org/articles/article_1254.cfm. Accessed on 20 October 2008.

24. Wilkinson, J. 2009. Globalisation of agribusiness and developing world food systems. *Monthly Review*, 61(04), http: monthlyreview.org/archives/2009/page 2 (accessed on 30 April 2012).

10 Influence of Regulations on the Commercialization and Marketing of Functional Foods and Nutraceuticals in Canada and the United States

Lina Paulionis, Alex Kocenas, Manki Ho, Karen Ly, Larry McGirr, and Ilana Platt

CONTENTS

10.1 INTRODUCTION

Science and technology are modernizing the face of consumable products, such as conventional foods and dietary supplements, and constantly changing our perceptions of "healthy." Two main scientific areas—safety and efficacy—that fall under the purview of regulatory authorities, such as Health Canada and the United States Food and Drug Administration (the U.S. FDA), are key determinants of how quickly and effectively marketing and commercialization initiatives can be pursued in Canada and the United States, respectively.

Health Canada and the U.S. FDA have established regulations, policies, and guidance documents that describe the breadth and depth of scientific evidence required to support the safety and/or efficacy of consumable products. These pertinent scientific and regulatory requirements will be discussed in this chapter, since they are fundamental to safe and lawful product innovation and commercialization. Further, since these requirements vary depending on the product category (e.g., foods vs. dietary supplements), and since a key consideration in developing a regulatory strategy for product commercialization is the regulatory classification of a product, the defining features of each category of consumable products (foods vs. dietary supplements vs. drugs) will additionally be discussed.

10.2   CANADA

10.2.1   CLASSIFICATION OF FOODS, NATURAL HEALTH PRODUCTS (NHPs), AND DRUGS AND RELATED LEGISLATION AND REGULATORY AUTHORITIES

Canada's *Food and Drugs Act** categorizes consumed products as foods or drugs, with drugs including the subcategory of NHPs. A food is defined as "any article manufactured, sold, or represented for use as a food or drink for human beings, including chewing gum, and any ingredient that may be mixed with food for any purpose whatever" (*Food and Drugs Act*, s. 2).

The definition of drugs and NHPs clearly communicates their intended purpose and the intended effects of drugs and NHPs are indeed identical. A product is classified as a drug if it includes any substance or mixture of substances manufactured, sold, or represented for use in: (a) "the diagnosis, treatment, mitigation, or prevention of a disease, disorder, or abnormal physical state, or its symptoms, in human beings or animals; (b) restoring, correcting or modifying organic functions in human beings or animals; or (c) disinfection in premises in which food is manufactured, prepared, or kept" (*Food and Drugs Act*, s. 2).

NHPs are similarly defined as drugs and are "manufactured, sold, or represented for use in (a) the diagnosis, treatment, mitigation, or prevention of a disease, disorder, or abnormal physical state or its symptoms in humans; (b) restoring or correcting organic functions in humans; or (c) modifying organic functions in humans, such as modifying those functions in a manner that maintains or promotes health" (*Natural Health Products Regulations*).

NHPs are differentiated from drugs in that they must be substances listed in Schedule 1 of the NHP Regulations [*Natural Health Products Regulations*; *Regulations Amending the Food and Drug Regulations (1385—Vitamin K)*] and thus must be

1. A plant or a plant material, an alga, a bacterium, a fungus, or a nonhuman animal material
2. An extract or isolate of a substance described in item 1, the primary molecular structure of which is identical to that which it had prior to its extraction or isolation
3. Any of the following vitamins: biotin, folate, niacin, pantothenic acid, riboflavin, thiamine, vitamins A, B_6, B_{12}, C, D, E, K_1, K_2
4. An amino acid
5. An essential fatty acid
6. A synthetic duplicate of a substance described in any of items 2–5
7. A mineral
8. A probiotic

---

* Canada's Food and Drugs Act is the primary documentation governing the safety and quality of foods sold in Canada. The Act includes legislation pertaining to food labeling, advertising, and claims; food standards and compositional requirements; fortification; foods for special dietary uses; food additives; chemical and microbial safety; veterinary drugs; packaging material; and pesticides. The primary objective of the Food and Drugs Act is to protect the public against health hazards and fraud from the sale of foods, beverages, drugs, NHPs, medical devices, and cosmetics.

Since the definition of an NHP does not place limitations on its required format or matrix, there has been a plethora of products sold and advertised as NHPs in food formats—energy drinks are an example. As such, in 2009, Health Canada's Natural Health Products Directorate and Food Directorate published a guidance document: *Classification of Products at the Food-Natural Health Product Interface: Products in Food Formats* (Health Canada, 2010a) to help industry determine whether a product is a food or an NHP. The following criteria are used to determine whether a product is a food or an NHP: (i) product composition, (ii) product representation, (iii) product format, (iv) public perception, and (v) history of use. The application of these criteria to the classification of a product as a food or an NHP is shown in Table 10.1. Agriculture and Agri-Food Canada has also developed a question/answer document (Agriculture and Agri-Foods Canada, 2011a) to facilitate the differentiation of these two product categories.

Foods, drugs, and NHPs are regulated under the *Food and Drugs Act* and its associated regulations: the *Food and Drug Regulations* and the *Natural Health Products Regulations*. Products that meet the definition of an NHP, as defined in the *Natural Health Products Regulations*, are subject to the *Food and Drugs Act* as it applies to a drug and to the *Natural Health Products Regulations*. Products that are foods as defined in the *Food and Drugs Act* are subject to the *Food and Drugs Act*

TABLE 10.1

Criteria Applied by Health Canada to Differentiate Foods from NHPs

Criteria	Food	NHP
Product composition	• Product has known food purposes—it is solely intended to provide nourishment, nutrition, hydration, or to satisfy hunger, thirst or a desire for taste, texture, or flavor	• Products (or its ingredient) have no known food purpose[a] but only therapeutic uses[b] • Products (or its ingredient) have known food purpose but are present at a level incompatible with uses as a food and compatible only with a therapeutic use
Product representation[c]	• Claims made on product are based only on the use of the product as a food	• Product is represented as having therapeutic use (e.g., claims refer to therapeutic uses)
Product format	• Product is sold in a format and serving size consistent with food use (e.g., chewing gum, hard candy, candy bar, or beverage) • Lack of dosing information (implies that product can be consumed freely and without regard to quantity)	• Product format allows for it to be consumed in measured or controlled doses (e.g., capsules, pills, or tablets) • Product sold in single dose units or with a measure that indicates that it is to be consumed in controlled amounts (even if the product is in a food format)
Public perception	• Product is perceived by the public as a food	• Product is perceived by the public as having therapeutic purposes
History of use	• Product has historical pattern of use as a food	• Product has historical pattern of use consistent with therapeutic purposes

Source: Data from Health Canada. 2010a. *Classification of Products at the Food–Natural Health Product Interface: Products in Food Formats*. Health Canada, Natural Health Products Directorate, Food Directorate. http://www.hc-sc.gc.ca/dhp-mps/alt_formats/hpfb-dgpsa/pdf/prodnatur/food-nhp-aliments-psn-guide-eng.pdf (Version 2.0, June 2010).

[a] A product solely intended to provide nourishment, nutrition, hydration, or to satisfy hunger, thirst or a desire for taste, texture or flavor has a known "food purpose."

[b] Therapeutic use means a product is intended to be used for the diagnosis, treatment, mitigation, or prevention of a disease, disorder, or abnormal physical state or its symptoms in humans, or restoring or correcting organic function in humans, or modifying organic functions in humans (Health Canada, 2010a).

[c] Representation includes indications of use; claims expressed or implied in words, sentences, pictures, symbols, paragraphs, product labels, package inserts or advertisement; and the product's placement and location of sale.

as it applies to food and to Parts A, B, and D of the *Food and Drug Regulations* (Health Canada, 2010a). A product that is both an NHP and a food (some products may be classified as both) is subject to the *Natural Health Products Regulations* but is exempted from the *Food and Drug Regulations* as they apply to a food (Health Canada, 2010a).

The Food Directorate (FD), Therapeutic Products Directorate (TPD), and the Natural Health Products Directorate (NHPD), all part of the Health Products and Food Branch of Health Canada, are the federal health authorities responsible for regulating foods, drugs, and NHPs, respectively (Health Canada, 2011a). Any amendments or regulatory proposals made by the Directorates in the Health Products and Food Branch are posted online in *Canada Gazette* Part I and open for public comment. Newly approved regulations are then published online in *Canada Gazette* Part II.

Three main government bodies are involved in the development, interpretation, or enforcement of the *Food and Drugs Act and its Regulations*: Health Canada, the Canadian Food Inspection Agency (CFIA), and Agriculture and Agri-Food Canada (AAFC).*

10.2.2 SAFETY CONSIDERATIONS FOR FOODS AND NHPS

Following the development of a new substance, be it a bioactive or another substance with a technical or functional effect, which is intended for incorporation in either a food or natural health product (NHP), decisions regarding its route of approval must be made. These decisions are dependent on substance's classification as a food ingredient, novel food/novel food ingredient, food additive, processing aid, flavoring agent, or medicinal ingredient (for use in a natural health product); these classifications will be discussed in greater detail below.

10.2.2.1 Food Ingredients and Novel Foods

In Canada, food ingredients are defined as "an individual unit of food that is combined as an individual unit of food with one or more other individual units of food to form an integral unit of food that is sold as a prepackaged product" (CFIA, 2010a). The use of a food ingredient does not require premarket approval unless it does not have a history of use, in which case the food ingredient is referred to as a novel food ingredient.

Novel foods, which include whole foods and food ingredients, are defined in section B.28.001 in the *Food and Drug Regulations* as: "(a) a substance, including a microorganism, that does not have a history of safe use as a food; or (b) a food that has been manufactured, prepared, preserved, or packaged by a process that (i) has not been previously applied to that food and (ii) causes the food to undergo a major change; or (c) a food that is derived from a plant, animal, or microorganism that has been genetically modified such that (i) the plant, animal, or microorganism exhibits characteristics that were not previously observed in that plant, animal, or microorganism, (ii) the plant, animal, or microorganism no longer exhibits characteristics that were previously observed in that plant, animal, or microorganism, or (iii) one or more characteristics of the plant, animal, or microorganism no longer fall within the anticipated range for that plant, animal, or microorganism." To ensure their safety, novel foods are subject to premarket notification, as described in B.28.002 of the *Food and Drug Regulations*. That is,

---

* Health Canada is responsible for the development of policies, regulations, and standards regarding health, nutritional, and safety aspects of foods, and also the development of guidance documents to assist the industry in compliance with the regulations (Agriculture and Agri-Foods Canada, 2010; Canadian Food Inspection Agency, 2010). The CFIA is responsible for the enforcement of the *Food and Drugs Act*, as well as other food-related policies, standards, and regulations established by Health Canada (e.g., those regarding agriculture, consumer goods, licensing and arbitration, packaging, and labeling). The CFIA maintains the *Guide to Food Labeling and Advertising* to aid industry, consumers, and CFIA inspectors with the interpretation of food policies and regulations (Agriculture and Agri-Foods Canada, 2010; Canadian Food Inspection Agency, 2011). AAFC is not involved in the development or enforcement of regulations pertaining to agriculture, foods, or related consumer goods, but provides information and guidance to industry to assist in their compliance with relevant policy and regulations, particularly those pertaining to innovative foods with potential health benefits (e.g., health claims and novel foods/ingredients) (Agriculture and Agri-Foods Canada, 2010, 2011b; Canadian Food Inspection Agency, 2010, 2011).

a novel food application is required for submission to Health Canada that characterizes the novel food and its manufacturing process, and that includes data on dietary exposure, history of use, and safety. A guidance document prepared by Health Canada: *Guidelines for the Safety Assessment of Novel Foods Derived from Plants and Microorganisms* (Health Canada, 2006a) outlines the data requirements for a novel food application. However, even with the availability of published resources, consultation with Health Canada's Food Directorate is encouraged during the development phase of a product to determine the specific safety data requirements. Once a novel food is approved, petitioners receive a "no objection letter." The sale of the novel food in Canada is then permitted and the approval of the novel food is published online on the Health Canada website (Health Canada, 2011b).

10.2.2.2   Food Additives and Food-Processing Aids

According to B.01.001 in the *Food and Drug Regulations*, "a food additive means any substance the use of which results, or may reasonably be expected to result, in it or its by-products becoming a part of or affecting the characteristics of a food, but does *not* include (a) any nutritive material that is used, recognized, or commonly sold as an article or ingredient of food; (b) vitamins, mineral nutrients, and amino acids other than those listed in the tables in Division 16 in the *Food and Drug Regulations*; (c) spices, seasonings, flavoring preparations, essential oils, oleoresins, and natural extractives; (d) agricultural chemicals other than those listed in the tables in Division 16 in the *Food and Drug Regulations*; (e) food-packaging materials and components thereof; and (f) drugs recommended for administration to animals that may be consumed as food."

According to the Food Directorate, a food-processing aid is "a substance that is used for a technical effect in food processing or manufacture, the use of which does not affect the intrinsic characteristics of the food and results in no or negligible residues of the substance or its by-products in or on the finished food" (Health Canada, 2008). Processing aids are permitted for use without premarket approval provided they meet the specific criteria for the definition of a processing aid (i.e., results in no or negligible residues in the food). Although the use of a processing aid does not require a submission, petitioners may seek a "Letter of Opinion" from the Bureau of Chemical Safety of Health Canada's Food Directorate, confirming that under its conditions of use, the substance in question is indeed considered to be a processing aid and is acceptable for use. If the definition of a processing aid is not met, the processing aid is considered to be a food additive and the approval process for food additives would be applicable.

A substance not present in the final food but which has affected the characteristics of that food would be regulated as a food additive. If the use of the substance does not affect the characteristics of the food, and further it does not remain in the final food, the substance is considered a processing aid. A submission for a food additive is required if a petitioner is seeking approval for use in Canada of a new food additive not currently regulated in the *Food and Drug Regulations*. A petitioner is also required to prepare a submission for an extension of the use of an existing food additive such as, for example, to extend the use of an existing food additive to a different food, or to extend the use of a food additive to a higher maximum level, or to add a new organism to the list of permitted sources of enzymes used as food additives. The submission requires detailed data and scientific information meeting the requirements of *B.16.002* of the *Food and Drug Regulations*. Health Canada's Bureau of Chemical Safety has prepared a guidance document: *Policy for Differentiating Food Additives and Processing Aids* (Health Canada, 2008) to help differentiate food additives from processing aids.

10.2.2.3   Flavoring Agents in Foods

Standards are available in Division *B.10* of the *Food and Drug Regulations* pertaining to specific flavoring preparations, such as essences or extracts obtained from aromatic plants. Flavors or flavoring preparations that are not mentioned in *Division B.10* are considered unstandardized food ingredients. Upon request by the petitioner, the Bureau of Chemical Safety of Health Canada's Food Directorate can evaluate the safe use of these unstandardized ingredients and can issue a

"Letter of Opinion." The intent of a "Letter of Opinion" is to confirm that under its conditions of use, the substance in question is indeed considered to be a flavoring agent and is acceptable for use. Unlike food additives, flavoring agents do not require a premarket submission to Health Canada.

10.2.2.4 NHPs

The *Natural Health Products Regulations* were developed with the principle of self-care, such that products controlled by these regulations could be selected by consumers without the need to consult a health care practitioner and obtain a prescription. To ensure their safe use by the general population, standards for their efficacy, safety, and quality have thus been established. To assist industry in meeting these standards, the NHPD has published several guidance documents: *Evidence for Safety and Efficacy of Finished Natural Products* (Health Canada, 2006b) and *Evidence for Quality of Finished Natural Health Products* (Health Canada, 2007a).

The safety of the NHP as a whole, or for each ingredient, must be demonstrated for the product's recommended conditions of use: dose, dosage form, route of administration, targeted health effect (i.e., health claim). Moreover, the type of evidence required to support the safety of an NHP will depend on the health claim of interest.

All NHPs sold in Canada require a product license before being marketed, which is an eight-digit product license number preceded by the letters NPN (Natural Product Number) or, in the case of a homeopathic medicine, by the letters DIN-HM (Drug Identification Number for Homeopathic Medicines) (Health Canada, 2009a). A produce license is granted following a favorable review of a Product License Application (PLA) by the NHPD (Health Canada, 2010b).

A PLA includes scientific information pertaining to efficacy, safety, and quality. Several guidance documents are available on NHPD's website to facilitate the completion of PLAs (Health Canada, 2010c). An important consideration in preparing a PLA is that the NHPD allows applicants to reference monographs in support of the safety and efficacy of their ingredient/product (Health Canada, 2007b, 2009b). Monographs, available for both single ingredients (e.g., garlic) and products (e.g., multivitamin/mineral supplements), characterize an ingredient/product (e.g., its source and specifications), and its conditions of use (e.g., dose, dosage form, route of administration), and provide known safety and efficacy information (Health Canada, 2007c). Thus, rather than requiring applicants to provide evidence on safety and efficacy for ingredients/products that are already known to be safe and efficacious, when used under the conditions specified in the monographs, the NHPD allows monographs to be cited in a PLA in support of their safety and efficacy (Health Canada, 2009a).

10.2.3 Health Claim Categories Applicable to Foods and NHPs

A consideration in developing a regulatory strategy for a new product and/or ingredient is its eligibility for claims. The applicable health claim categories on both foods and NHPs and the scientific requirements for their substantiation are thus briefly discussed below and in Section 10.2.4.

In Canada, health claims made on foods and NHPs are not specifically defined in regulations; rather, guidance documents (Health Canada, 2006a, 2009b) and CFIA's *Guide to Food Labeling and Advertising* (CFIA, 2003) describe the different claim categories that apply to foods or NHPs. See Table 10.2 for an outline of these claim categories.

Both foods and NHPs similarly permit therapeutic, disease-risk reduction, and function (or structure/function) claims. Whereas all claims made on NHPs require approval by the NHPD following the submission of a PLA, only therapeutic and disease-risk reduction claims made on foods require approval by the Food Directorate. For these food health claims, an application that meets the requirements set forth in Health Canada's *Guidance Document for Preparing a Submission for Food Health Claims* (Health Canada, 2009c) requires submission to Health Canada's FD. Function claims (nutrient function or other function claims) do not require Health Canada's approval albeit voluntary submissions on their substantiation can be submitted to the FD. Should voluntary

TABLE 10.2

Categories of Permissible Claims in Canada on Foods and NHPs and Their Definitions

Product Category	Claim Category	Definition	Regulatory Approval Required
Food[a]	Therapeutic	Claims regarding the diagnosis, treatment, or prevention of a disease, disorder, abnormal physical state or its symptoms; or, claims about restoring or correcting abnormal functions of the body or modifying body functions beyond the normal physiological effects of food.	Yes
	Disease-risk reduction	Claims regarding the reduction of the risk of developing a diet-related disease or condition.	Yes
	Nutrient function	Claims regarding known nutrients or energy essential for the maintenance of good health or normal growth and development.	No
	Other function	Claims regarding the specific beneficial effects that the consumption of a food or a constituent of a food (nutrient or other component) has on the normal functions or biological activities of the body or on performance (physical or mental).	No
	General health	Claims regarding healthy eating or dietary patterns that do not refer to a health effect.	No
NHP[b]	Therapeutic	Claims regarding the diagnosis, treatment, mitigation, or prevention of a disease, disorder, abnormal physical state, or its symptoms.	Yes
	Disease-risk reduction	Claims regarding the relationship between the NHP and the reduction of the risk of developing a specific disease or abnormal physiological state.	Yes
	Structure–function	Claims regarding the effect of the NHP on a structure or physiological function, or the NHP's support of an anatomical, physiological, or mental function.	Yes
	Nonspecific structure–function[c]	Claims regarding broad statements indicating that the NHP promotes overall health.	Yes

Note: NHP = Natural Health Product.

[a] Data from CFIA (2003).

[b] Data from Health Canada, 2006a. In addition to the categories of NHP claims listed, claims on NHPs may be further divided into traditional and nontraditional use claims. If the NHP has a history of use of at least 50 consecutive years within a cultural belief system or healing paradigm, it may be considered "traditional," a designation which must be indicated as a part of the product's health claim (e.g., "Traditionally used for ..."). The types of claims permitted for NHPs and their definitions listed in this table apply regardless of whether an NHP has been traditionally used for medicinal purposes (Health Canada, 2006a).

[c] The NHPD prefers the use of specific claims that provide consumers with more information regarding the NHP. Nonspecific claims are only accepted when there is adequate evidence to demonstrate safety.

submissions not be made to Health Canada, "in house" substantiation dossiers must be made available to enforcement agencies (i.e., CFIA) upon their request.

An important difference between foods and NHPs relates to Section 3 (1) of the *Food and Drugs Act* which states that "No person shall advertise any food, drug, cosmetic, or device to the general public as a treatment, preventative, or cure for any of the diseases, disorders, or abnormal physical states referred to in Section 3, Schedule A." As of June 2008, NHPs are permitted to make preventative claims (but not treatment or curative claims) for Schedule A diseases (included in Schedule A are diseases such as depression, hypertension, cancer, obesity). Foods, however, have not been granted a similar exemption from Section 3 (1) of the *Food and Drugs Act* and thus cannot make any claims related to Schedule A diseases, unless a regulatory amendment is sought. [Provisions have been included in the *Food and Drugs Act* (s. 30 (j)) and *Food and Drug Regulations* to exempt foods from Section 3 of the *Food and Drugs Act* (Schedule A) (Health Canada, 2009c).]

Although not related to "health claims" per se, it is of interest to note that nutrient content claims (e.g., "source of calcium") that are permitted on foods (CFIA, 2003, Chapter 7) are not permitted on NHPs, as all NHPs must be associated with representations indicating a relationship between the NHP and a health effect.

10.2.4 HEALTH CLAIM SUBSTANTIATION STANDARDS APPLICABLE TO FOODS AND NHPS

Health claims made on foods and NHPs must be scientifically substantiated. Two documents exist to guide the process of substantiating health claims on foods: *Guidance Document for Preparing a Submission for Food Health Claims* (Health Canada, 2009c) and Chapter 8 in CFIA's *Guide to Food Labeling and Advertising* (CFIA, 2003, Chapter 8). The former guidance document (Health Canada, 2009c) articulates the overarching scientific standard for claim substantiation that applies to therapeutic, disease-risk reduction, and other function claims,[*] which is a "high level of certainty," defined as "the majority of high-quality human studies supports a statistically significant (i.e., significance achieved at $p \leq 0.05$) favorable effect." This scientific standard expresses Health Canada's requirement for: (i) high-quality evidence from human studies (Health Canada provides guidance in the form of a standardized tool, for rating the quality of human studies[†]); (ii) the achievement of statistical significance at $p \leq 0.05$; and (iii) the demonstration of a favorable effect (i.e., a biologically/physiologically relevant effect expected to benefit the health of the target population). Other required criteria for claim substantiation on foods are outlined in Table 10.3 and compared with requirements set forth by the NHPD for health claims made on NHPs.

To guide the substantiation of health claims on NHPs, the data of which are included in a Product License Application, the NHPD has prepared a guidance document: *Evidence for Safety and Efficacy of Finished Natural Health Products* (Health Canada, 2006b). Unlike the defined scientific standard for food health claim substantiation, the NHPD states that evidence for claim substantiation on NHPs must be "adequate"—a term which is open to interpretation but nevertheless defined by the NHPD as: (i) specifically supports the claim and all recommended conditions of use; (ii) is from relevant levels of evidence (NHPD states five different levels of evidence[‡]); (iii) reflects the concept of self-care; (iv) reflects the totality of evidence; (v) is from reputable and well-recognized

---

[*] General health claims do not require substantiation and nutrient function claims have unique requirements for substantiation that are described in CFIA's Guide to Food Labelling and Advertising (Canadian Food Inspection Agency, 2003, Chapt. 8, Section 8.6.5).

[†] For health claims on foods, study quality is evaluated using an explicitly defined qualitative and quantitative checklist tool, the implementation of which results in each study being assigned a score based on the percentage of quality criteria fulfilled. Intervention studies with quality scores ≥8/15 (≥53.3%), and prospective observational studies with quality scores ≥7/12 (≥58.3%), are considered to be "high quality."

[‡] For health claims on NHPs, five types of evidence (listed in decreasing order of strength) are accepted for claim substantiation: (a) well-designed systematic reviews and meta-analyses of randomized controlled clinical trials or other clinical trials, or at least one well-designed randomized controlled clinical trial (preferably multicentered); (b) well-designed clinical trials without randomization and/or control groups; (c) well-designed descriptive and observational studies, such as correlational studies, cohort studies, and case-control studies; (d) peer-reviewed published articles, conclusions of other reputable regulatory agencies, or previous marketing experience, expert opinion reports, referenced textbooks, or web site (if the information is peer-reviewed and there is a hardcover version of the site, for example, Natural Medicines Comprehensive Database); and (e) references to a traditional use or pharmacopoeias.

TABLE 10.3

Criteria Required for the Substantiation of Health Claims on Foods and NHPs in Canada

Factor	Definition	Food	NHP
Systematic approach	A methodical, consistent approach is applied to substantiate a health claim.	Required	Not required
Systematic, well-constructed literature search	A methodical, consistent approach is applied to identify literature pertinent to the health claim.	Required	Encouraged
Transparency	Search strategies, literature selection criteria, and literature evaluation procedures are fully disclosed, to increase the credibility of the submission and to permit reproducibility	Required	Not required
Comprehensiveness	All original and relevant research in humans is captured, including evidence in favor and not in favor of the health claim (i.e., the totality of evidence).	Required	Required
Human evidence	The focus of claim substantiation is on original research in humans that investigates the product and health effect of interest.	Required[a]	Required[b]
Appraisal of study quality	The application of a systematic, consistent approach to evaluate the scientific quality of studies pertinent to the health claim.[c]	Required	Recommended
Demonstration of causality	Scientific evidence that component X independently causes health outcome Y, in human studies.	Required	Not required[d]
Generalizability	Evidence exists to support the claimed effect, the dose, and conditions of use of the product in the target population of interest.	Required	Required
Physiological relevance of the claimed effect	The claimed effect of the product is physiologically relevant and beneficial to the health of the target population. To ensure physiological relevance of the claimed effect, surrogate biomarkers of the claimed effect must have methodological and physiological validity, and must be favorably affected by the consumption of the product.	Required	Not required
Feasibility of consumption of effective dose	The amount of food to be consumed to achieve a beneficial effect can be incorporated into a healthy, balanced diet by the target population.	Required	N/A
Demonstration of safety	Under the recommended conditions of use, the product poses minimal risk to human health and well-being.	Required[e]	Required[f]

Note: N/A = not applicable; NHP = Natural Health Product.

[a] For health claims on foods, only certain types of human studies are permitted as the basis for claim substantiation: controlled human intervention and prospective observational studies (Health Canada, 2009c).

[b] For health claims on NHPs, five types of evidence (listed in decreasing order of strength) are accepted for claim substantiation: (a) well-designed systematic reviews and meta-analyses of randomized controlled clinical trials or other clinical trials, or at least one well-designed randomized controlled clinical trial (preferably multicentered); (b) well-designed clinical trials without randomization and/or control groups; (c) well-designed descriptive and observational studies, such as correlational studies, cohort studies, and case-control studies; (d) peer-reviewed published articles, conclusions of other reputable regulatory agencies, or previous marketing experience, expert opinion reports, referenced textbooks, or web site (if the information is peer-reviewed and there is a hardcover version of the site, for example, Natural Medicines Comprehensive Database); and (e) references to a traditional use or pharmacopoeias.

[c] For health claims on foods, study quality is evaluated using an explicitly defined qualitative and quantitative checklist tool, the implementation of which results in each study being assigned a score based on the percentage of quality criteria fulfilled. Intervention studies with quality scores $\geq 8/15$ ($\geq 53.3\%$), and prospective observational studies with quality scores $\geq 7/12$ ($\geq 58.3\%$), are considered to be "high quality." No formal checklist exists for the quality appraisal of studies used to substantiate a health claim on an NHP; however, the NHPD states 13 questions that can be used to determine and compare the quality of evidence from various studies within a particular level of evidence (Health Canada, 2006b).

continued

TABLE 10.3   (continued)
Criteria Required for the Substantiation of Health Claims on Foods and NHPs in Canada

ᵈ   As stated in Footnote "b" to this table, substantiation of a health claim on an NHP may be based on studies from which it is not possible to deduce causality (e.g., retrospective observational studies), authoritative body statements (including textbooks, pharmacopeias, websites, and marketing experience), or traditional use. Since these resources are ranked by the NHPD as being weaker types of evidence, it is implied that they are permissible, but not preferred, sources of claim substantiation.

ᵉ   For food health claim submissions, dietary intake estimates are required so that changes in usual dietary patterns with potential approval of the health claim can be assessed. Further, quality assurance information is required to demonstrate the food is produced according to quality standards and consistently meets predefined specifications. However, detailed safety information is not provided in a health claim application since the subject of a health claim application must be for a food approved for safe use; or, if a novel food is the subject of the health claim, a novel food application must be completed and submitted to Health Canada preceding or concurrent with the health claim application (Health Canada, 2009c).

ᶠ   Standards for safety are provided in NHPD's guidance document *Evidence for Safety and Efficacy of Finished Natural Products* (Health Canada, 2006b). The safety information is to be presented together with the efficacy information in a Product License Application. Further, documentation regarding chemical composition and contamination of NHPs (i.e., quality) is required, and guidance is provided in *Evidence for Quality of Finished Natural Health Products* (Health Canada, 2007a).

sources; (vi) is mostly of high quality;* and (vii) supports the safety of the product when used according to the recommended conditions of use (Health Canada, 2006b).

For NHPs, it is explicitly stated by the NHPD that the quality and quantity of evidence required to substantiate a claim and its conditions of use can vary depending on the type of claim (i.e., claim category) (Health Canada, 2006b). A similar principle is not articulated for food health claims and thus it can be assumed that the substantiation criteria outlined in Health Canada's guidance document for food health claim submissions (Health Canada, 2009c) are similarly applied to all health claim categories (i.e., therapeutic, disease-risk reduction, or other function claims). An important similarity between foods and NHPs with respect to claim substantiation is that the "totality of evidence"—that is, evidence in favor and not in favor of the health claim of interest—should be reviewed and discussed.

10.3   THE UNITED STATES

10.3.1   CLASSIFICATION OF FOODS, DIETARY SUPPLEMENTS AND DRUGS, AND RELATED LEGISLATION AND REGULATORY AUTHORITIES

In the United States (U.S.), the *Federal Food, Drug, and Cosmetic Act* (sect. 201) categorizes consumed products as foods, dietary supplements, and drugs. Interestingly, the classification of products in U.S. is slightly different than Canada's. In U.S., dietary supplements are a subcategory of foods while in Canada, NHPs are a subcategory of drugs.

In the *Federal Food, Drug, and Cosmetic Act* (sect. 201), foods are defined as: "(a) articles used for food or drink for man or other animals, (b) chewing gum, and (c) articles used for components of any such article." Dietary supplements are defined as products (other than tobacco) intended to supplement the diet that are labeled as dietary supplements, and that contain one or more of the following "dietary ingredients:" "(a) a vitamin; (b) a mineral; (c) an herb or other botanical; (d) an

* No formal checklist exists for the quality appraisal of studies used to substantiate a health claim on an NHP; however, the NHPD states 13 questions that can be used to determine and compare the quality of evidence from various studies within a particular level of evidence (Health Canada, 2006b).

amino acid; (e) a dietary substance for use by humans to supplement the diet by increasing the total dietary intake; (f) or a concentrate, metabolite, constituent, extract, or combination of any ingredient described in (a) to (e) above." Dietary supplements must not be represented for use as a conventional food or as a sole component of a meal or diet. This is an important point that is elaborated below. Moreover, although they are "intended for ingestion" in tablet, capsule, powder, softgel, gelcap, or liquid form (*Federal Food, Drug, and Cosmetic Act*, sects. 201 & 411), they can be ingested in other forms as long as the dietary supplement is not represented for use as a conventional food and is not represented for use as a sole item of a meal or the diet (*Federal Food, Drug, and Cosmetic Act*, s. 411).

A guidance document published by the U.S. Food and Drug Administration (FDA): *Draft Guidance for Industry: Factors that Distinguish Liquid Dietary Supplements from Beverages, Considerations Regarding Novel Ingredients, and Labeling for Beverages and Other Conventional Foods* (FDA, 2009a) summarizes key factors to consider in deciding whether a dietary supplement would have "representation for use as a conventional food," which are (i) a product's name, (ii) packaging, (iii) serving size, (iv) recommended conditions of use, and (v) other representations about the product. Using "liquids" (that are stated by the U.S. FDA to be an acceptable form for dietary supplements) and "beverages" (a conventional food) as examples, the FDA states that liquid products can be "represented as conventional foods" as a result of factors such as their packaging,* the volume in which they are intended to be consumed,† their product or brand name,‡ and statements in labeling or advertising. Moreover, even with a label on a liquid product that characterizes the liquid product as a dietary supplement, the product may be misbranded as a dietary supplement (FDA, 2009a).

In U.S., drugs are defined as: "(a) articles recognized in the U.S. Pharmacopoeia, Homeopathic Pharmacopoeia of the United States, or National Formulary, or any supplement to them; and (b) articles intended for use in the diagnosis, cure, mitigation, treatment, or prevention of disease in humans or other animals; and (c) articles (other than food) intended to affect the structure or any function of the body of humans or other animals; and (d) articles intended for use as components of any article specified in clauses (a), (b), or (c)" (*Federal Food, Drug, and Cosmetic Act*, s. 201). It is noteworthy that, although affecting the structure/function of humans is a drug effect as per the third point (c) in the drug definition, structure/function statements on foods and dietary supplements do not cause these products to be regulated as drugs. This exemption is stated in the *Federal Food, Drug, and Cosmetic Act* (sect. 201).

The *Federal Food, Drug, and Cosmetic Act* provides the U.S. FDA with the authority to regulate foods, drugs, devices, and cosmetics. A number of major amendments have been made to the *Federal Food, Drug, and Cosmetic Act* since its enactment in 1938, due to deficiencies in existing provisions, changes brought upon by technological advances, and evolving public policies. For example, the *Food Additive Amendment (FAA) of 1958* introduced important provisions regarding the regulation of food additives; the *Dietary Supplement Health and Education Act (DSHEA)* enacted in 1994, introduced provisions for dietary supplements (e.g., the permissibility of structure/function claims) and the concept of "new dietary ingredients"; and, the *U.S. Food and Drug Administration Modernization Act (FDAMA)*, enacted in 1997, which affected regulations pertaining to food (e.g., regarding health and nutrient content claims), drugs, devices, and biological products.

---

* The packaging of liquid products in bottles or cans similar to those in which single or multiple servings of beverages like soda, bottled water, fruit juices, and iced tea are sold, suggests that the liquid product is intended for use as a conventional food (FDA, 2009a).

† Liquid products that suggest through their recommended daily intake that they are intended to be consumed in amounts that provide all or a significant part of the entire daily drinking fluid intake of an average person in the United States are represented as conventional foods (i.e., beverages) (FDA, 2009a).

‡ Product or brand names that use conventional food terms such as "beverage," "drink," "water," "juice," or similar terms represent the product as a conventional food (FDA, 2009a).

Eight product/service-oriented centers carry out the mission of the U.S. FDA,* one of which is the Center for Food Safety and Applied Nutrition (CFSAN). Within CFSAN is the Office of Nutritional Products, Labeling, and Dietary Supplements (ONPLDS), which is responsible for developing policy and regulations for dietary supplements and nutrition labeling, the development of food standards, and the scientific evaluation of health claim petitions (FDA, 2011a).

An additional organization of importance in U.S. is U.S. Federal Trade Commission (FTC), which is a federal agency that actively enforces laws, specifically laws outlawing "unfair or deceptive acts or practices" (Federal Trade Commission, 2001, 2010). The FTC's authority is embodied in the *Federal Trade Commission Act* (Federal Trade Commission, 1994). Under this Act, the Commission is empowered to: prevent unfair methods of competition and unfair or deceptive acts or practices; seek monetary redress for conduct injurious to consumers; and, prescribe trade regulation rules that establish requirements to prevent unfair or deceptive acts or practices (Federal Trade Commission, 2011a). All of FTC's enforcement actions are publicly listed (Federal Trade Commission, 2011b). The FTC and U.S. FDA work together under a long-standing liaison agreement governing the division of responsibilities between the two agencies under which the FTC has assumed primary responsibility for regulating food and dietary supplement *advertising*, while U.S. FDA has taken primary responsibility for regulating food and dietary supplement *labeling* (Federal Trade Commission, 1994, 2001).

10.3.2   SAFETY CONSIDERATIONS FOR FOODS AND DIETARY SUPPLEMENTS

10.3.2.1   Food Additives and Generally Recognized as Safe (GRAS) Substances

The *Food Additive Amendment (FAA) of 1958* divides food additives into four major categories: color additives, prior-sanctioned substances, GRAS substances, and other food additives. The regulatory framework pertaining to color additives is beyond the scope of this chapter, and more information can be found on U.S. FDA's website (FDA, 2011b–http://www.fda.gov/ForIndustry/ColorAdditives/default.htm). The majority of the discussion below will focus on GRAS substances and food additives.

In U.S., a food additive is broadly defined as any substance added to food, including substances used in the production, processing, treatment, packaging, transportation, and storage of foods. The legal definition of a food additive, outlined in Sect. 201(s) of the *Federal Food, Drug and Cosmetic Act*, is "any substance the intended use of which results or may reasonably be expected to result, directly or indirectly, in its becoming a component or otherwise affecting the characteristics of any food (including any substance intended for use in producing, manufacturing, packing, processing, preparing, treating, packaging, transporting, or holding food; and including any source of radiation intended for any such use)." Substances excluded from the definition of a food additive include pesticides, color additives, new animal drugs, ingredients intended for use in dietary supplements, and "prior sanctioned substances"—that is, substances granted approval prior to the enactment of the Food Additive Amendment (*FAA) of 1958*.

By legal definition, a food additive is subject to premarket approval by the U.S. FDA, following the submission of a food additive petition in accordance with the *Code of Federal Regulations*, title 21, sect. 171.1. If approved by the U.S. FDA, a Federal Register final rule is drafted, issuing a regulation that prescribes the conditions under which the additive may be safely used (FDA, 2003). Details of the food additive petition process are discussed in Rulis and Levitt (2009).

As a result of the *Food Additive Amendment (FAA) of 1958*, a new category of substances that are considered GRAS was created. Any substance that is intentionally added to food is a food

---

* The eight centers are: The Office of Regulatory Affairs, Center for Food Safety and Applied Nutrition, Center for Veterinary Medicine, National Center for Toxicological Research, Center for Drug Evaluation and Research, Center for Devices and Radiological Health, Center for Biologics Evaluation and Research, and the Center for Tobacco Products (FDA, 2011a).

additive that is subject to premarket review and approval by the U.S. FDA in accordance with the *Code of Federal Regulations*, title 21, sect. 170.30, *unless* the substance is GRAS among "qualified experts" through "scientific procedures"* for its "intended conditions of use." Whether a substance has been used in foods prior to January 1, 1958 determines the quality and quantity of data required to demonstrate safety in the GRAS assessment process. However, the recognition of safety in the GRAS process, based upon "scientific procedures," requires the same quantity and quality of scientific evidence as is required to obtain approval as a food additive (*Code of Federal Regulations*, title 21, sect. 170.30).

On April 17, 1997, the FDA published a *Federal Register* Proposal to reform the GRAS assessment process (FDA, 1997–62 FR 18938). In this document, the FDA proposed to replace the resource-intensive GRAS Affirmation Petition Process that was put into place in the 1970s, with a more streamlined voluntary GRAS Notification Process; the GRAS Notification Process currently exists.

As part of the current GRAS Notification Process, documentation supporting the safe use of a food ingredient under intended conditions of use is submitted to a group of qualified experts (often called the Expert Panel).† Once a conclusion is reached among the qualified experts on the ingredient's safety, a consensus statement is drafted summarizing their findings. A GRAS may be "self-affirmed" without notification to the U.S. FDA or, alternatively, the U.S. FDA may be voluntarily "notified" of the GRAS assessment. Should a notification be made, the U.S. FDA has the opportunity to object to the GRAS status. The notification itself and the information to support the safety of a GRAS substance is publicly available on FDA's website and thus subject to public scrutiny (FDA, 2011c). The GRAS determination and notification processes have been reviewed extensively in Rulis and Levitt (2009).

Although the safety determination of food additives and GRAS ingredients follows different procedures (see Figure 10.1), the basis on which safety is concluded is the same. Both food additive petitions and GRAS determinations require scientific evidence on the characterization of the substance and its manufacturing process, specifications, the intended conditions of use, stability data, dietary exposure data (i.e., estimated daily intakes), and safety data.

10.3.2.2   Dietary Ingredients

Regarding dietary supplements, whether notification to the U.S. FDA is required for the use of a dietary ingredient in a dietary supplement depends on whether the dietary ingredient was marketed prior to or after October 15, 1994—the date *Dietary Supplement Health and Education Act (DSHEA)* was enacted (FDA, 2011d). Dietary ingredients marketed prior to October 15, 1994 as a dietary supplement, or for use in dietary supplements, are excluded from premarket notification, unless there have been changes made to the manufacturing process that may have altered the identity of the ingredient. In contrast, dietary ingredients marketed after October 15, 1994 are considered to be new dietary ingredients (NDIs) and are subject to premarket notification in accordance with the *Code of Federal Regulations*, title 21, sect. 190.6, unless they have been present in the food supply as an article used for food (FDA, 2011d).

There is no authoritative list of dietary ingredients that were marketed in dietary supplements before October 15, 1994; therefore, manufacturers and distributors are responsible for determining if an ingredient is an NDI (FDA, 2011d). Details on what constitutes an NDI, when an NDI notification is required, and the types of data and information recommended by the U.S. FDA as evidence to support the safety of an NDI are available in U.S. FDA's draft guidance document: *Draft Guidance for Industry—Dietary Supplements—New Dietary Ingredient Notifications and Related Issues* (FDA, 2011e). In general, an NDI notification should include characterization of the dietary

---

* "Scientific procedures" refer to the evaluation of safety data by qualified experts (i.e., qualified by scientific training and experience). The data are ordinarily published studies but corroborating data may also come from unpublished studies.
† It is stated in regulations (*Code of Federal Regulations*, title 21, sect. 170.3) that experts are "qualified by scientific training and experience to evaluate the safety of food and food ingredients."

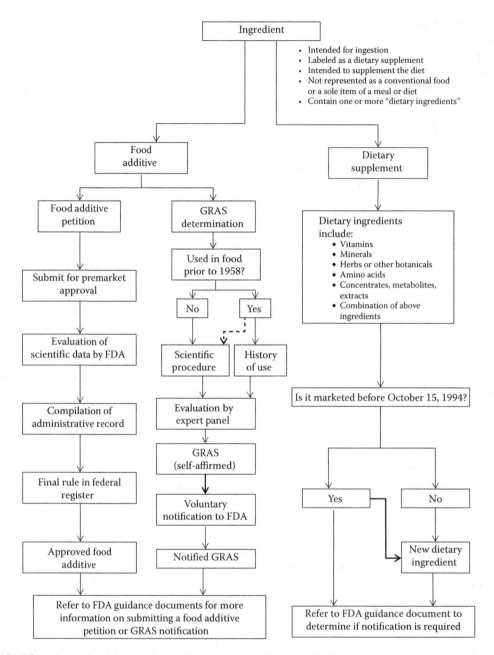

FIGURE 10.1 A visual representation of important considerations for food and dietary supplement ingredients. (Adapted from FDA. 2011f. *Food Additives.* Food and Drug Administration, U.S. http://www.fda.gov/Food/FoodIngredients. Packaging/FoodAdditives/default.htm [Last updated: 05/04/2011]; FDA. 2011g. Generally Recognized as Safe (GRAS). Food and Drug Administration, U.S. http://www.fda.gov/Food/FoodIngredientsPackaging/GenerallyRecognizedasSafeGRAS/default.htm [Last Updated: 06/10/2011].)

supplement, the level of NDI in the dietary supplement, intended conditions of use of the dietary supplement, and safety data to support the use of the NDI under intended conditions of use. Information on history of use can also be included.

Once the U.S. FDA receives the NDI notification, for 75 days following that date, the notifier cannot market the dietary supplement that contains the NDI (FDA, 2011d). Although U.S. FDA may not comment on an NDI notification, U.S. FDA states that its failure to respond to a notification does not constitute a finding by the agency that the use of the NDI under the intended conditions of use is safe or unadulterated. NDI notifications received by the U.S. FDA are publicly listed (FDA, 2011d).

Figure 10.1 provides a visual depiction of important considerations for food (i.e., food additives and GRAS substances) and dietary supplement ingredients.

10.3.3 Health Claim Categories Applicable to Foods and Dietary Supplements

Unlike in Canada, in U.S., a health claim is defined in regulations (*Code of Federal Regulations*, title 21, sect. 101.14) as "any claim made on the label or in labeling of a food, including a dietary supplement, that expressly or by implication,* including third-party references, written statements (e.g., a brand name including a term such as "heart"), symbols (e.g., a heart symbol), or vignettes, characterizes the relationship of any substance to a disease or health-related condition."† It is noteworthy that this definition applies to both foods and dietary supplements and thus "substance" can be a specific food, a component of food, a dietary supplement or an ingredient in a dietary supplement. Requirements for health claim petitions to the U.S. FDA are specified in the Code of Federal Regulations, title 21, sect. 101.70, and the general requirements for health claims are in the Code of Federal Regulations, title 21, sect. 101.14.

There are three main categories of health claims in the United States, as outlined in Table 10.4 below: *Nutrition Labeling and Education Act* (NLEA)-authorized health claims,‡ FDAMA-authorized Health Claims,§ and Qualified Health Claims. One additional category of claims—structure/function claims—is not considered a "health claim" category in U.S.; as such, these claims cannot state or imply effects on disease/disease risk.

NLEA-authorized claims and qualified health claims, which apply to both foods and dietary supplements, are reviewed and approved by the U.S. FDA while the U.S. FDA must only be "notified" of FDAMA-authorized claims (which only apply to foods and not dietary supplements), at least 120 days before the first market introduction of the food with the claim.

Structure–function claims can be made on both foods and dietary supplements and do not require review and approval by the U.S. FDA; however, the U.S. FDA must be notified of these claims if they are made on dietary supplements, and the notification must be no later than 30 days following market introduction of the dietary supplement (FDA, 2009b). No such notification is required when structure/function claims are made on conventional foods. Further, when structure–function claims are made on dietary supplements, a disclaimer must be included on the product label that states: *This statement has not been evaluated by the Food and Drug Administration. This product is not intended to diagnose, treat, cure, or prevent any disease.* This disclaimer is not required when conventional foods include structure/function claims.

For NLEA-authorized claims, U.S. FDA publishes a regulation authorizing the use of a specific claim. For qualified claims, a "letter of enforcement discretion," in which U.S. FDA indicates that it

---

* Implied health claims include those statements, symbols, vignettes, or other forms of communication that suggest, within the context in which they are presented, that a relationship exists between the presence or level of a substance in the food and a disease or health-related condition (*Code of Federal Regulations*, title 21, sect. 101.14).

† *Disease or health-related condition* means damage to an organ, part, structure, or system of the body such that it does not function properly (e.g., cardiovascular disease), or a state of health leading to such dysfunctioning (e.g., hypertension); except that diseases resulting from essential nutrient deficiencies (e.g., scurvy, pellagra) are not included in this definition (Code of Federal Regulations, title 21, sect. 101.14).

‡ The NLEA of 1990 was designed to give consumers more scientifically valid information about foods they eat. Among other provisions, the NLEA directed U.S. FDA to issue regulations providing for the use of statements (i.e., health claims) that describe the relationship between a substance and a disease in the labeling of foods, including dietary supplements, after such statements have been reviewed and authorized by U.S. FDA (FDA, 2009a).

§ Prior to the FDAMA of 1997, companies could not use a health claim or nutrient content claim in food labeling unless the U.S. FDA published a regulation authorizing such a claim. Provisions of FDAMA, which amended the *Federal Food, Drug, and Cosmetic Act*, permit distributors and manufacturers to use claims if such claims are based on current, published, authoritative statements from certain federal scientific bodies, as well as from the National Academy of Sciences. These provisions are intended to expedite the process by which the scientific basis for such claims is established (FDA, 1998).

TABLE 10.4
Categories of Permissible Claims in the United States on Foods and Dietary Supplements and Their Definitions

Product Category	Claim Category	Definition	Regulatory Approval Required
Foods and dietary supplements	Structure–function claims[a]	Correspond to claims that describe the role of a nutrient or dietary ingredient intended to affect the structure or function in humans (e.g., "calcium builds strong bones"), or that characterize the documented mechanism by which a nutrient or dietary ingredient acts to maintain such structure or function (e.g., "fiber maintains bowel regularity," or "antioxidants maintain cell integrity") or describe general well-being from consumption of a nutrient or dietary ingredient. Structure/function claims may also describe a benefit related to a nutrient deficiency disease (like vitamin C and scurvy), as long as the statement also tells how widespread such a disease is in the United States.	No[b]
	NLEA-authorized Health Claims	Describe or imply a relationship between a food, food component, dietary supplement or dietary supplement ingredient, and a disease or health-related condition.	Yes
Foods[e]	Qualified Health Claims		Yes[c]
	FDAMA-authorized Health Claims	Describe or imply a relationship between a food, food component, dietary supplement or dietary supplement ingredient, and a disease or health-related condition.	No[d]

Note: FDAMA = Food and Drug Administration Modernization Act of 1997; NLEA = Nutrition Labeling and Education Act.

[a] These claims are not considered health claims and thus cannot state effects that are permissible for health claims (e.g., effects on disease risk).

[b] In accordance with the Code of Federal Regulations, title 21, 101.93 (c), a disclaimer must be used on dietary supplements that states: "This statement has not been evaluated by the Food and Drug Administration. This product is not intended to diagnose, treat, cure, or prevent any disease." This disclaimer is not required on conventional foods that make structure/function claims. Further, in accordance with the Code of Federal Regulations, title 21, 101.93(a)(2), the U.S. FDA must be notified of structure/function claims on dietary supplements no later than 30 days following market introduction of the dietary supplement. The notification must include: the name and address of the manufacturer; the exact claim to be used; the name of the dietary ingredient or supplement that is the subject of the claim; the name of the dietary supplement; a signed certification that the notice is complete and accurate, and that the notifying firm has substantiation that the claim is truthful and not misleading. No such notification to the U.S. FDA is required for structure/function claims made on conventional foods.

[c] Unlike NLEA-authorized and FDAMA-authorized health claims, qualified health claims do not need to meet the significant scientific agreement standard for claim substantiation.

[d] These claims are based on a published "authoritative statement" (i.e., formal declaration) from a federal scientific body. The U.S. FDA must be notified at least 120 days before the first market introduction of the food with the claim. The content of the notification can be found in U.S. FDA's guidance document: *Guidance for Industry: Notification of a Health Claim or Nutrient Content Claim Based on an Authoritative Statement of a Scientific Body* (FDA, 1998).

[e] FDAMA does not provide for health claims based on authoritative statements for dietary supplements (FDA, 1998).

does not object to use of the claim so long as it follows U.S. FDA's specifications for claim wording, is issued. For FDAMA-authorized claims, the claim may be made 120 days following the date of submission of the notification of the claim to the U.S. FDA without the requirement of a published regulation. However, the U.S. FDA can issue a regulation prohibiting or modifying the FDAMA claim (FDA, 1998).

10.3.4 HEALTH CLAIM SUBSTANTIATION STANDARDS APPLICABLE TO FOODS AND DIETARY SUPPLEMENTS

In U.S., the substantiation standard (i.e., the quality, quantity, and type of evidence required for substantiation) differs depending on the claim category; however, as will be discussed below, there are similar principles/considerations made in the claim substantiation process regardless of the claim of interest.

FDAMA-authorized claims can be substantiated based on a published "authoritative statement" from a U.S. federal scientific body. Acceptable scientific bodies and appropriate "authoritative statements" are described in FDA's *Guidance for Industry: Notification of a Health Claim or Nutrient Content Claim Based on an Authoritative Statement of a Scientific Body* (FDA, 1998). The key point regarding this claim category is that the U.S. FDA applies the standard of "significant scientific agreement" (SSA) in determining whether a FDAMA-claim is indeed substantiated. Similarly, the U.S. FDA applies the SSA standard to NLEA-authorized health claims in contrast to qualified health claims that need not meet the SSA standard (Table 10.5).

The SSA standard and the process the U.S. FDA uses in determining whether it is met by a body of evidence are outlined in its guidance document: *Guidance for Industry: Evidence-Based Review System for the Scientific Evaluation of Health Claims–Final* (FDA, 2009c). As indicated in this document, the process* used to decide whether a claim meets the SSA standard or does not meet the SSA standard (thus making it potentially eligible for a qualified health claim) is the same, the difference lies in the level of uncertainty in the final stages of evaluation of the relevant evidence.

The SSA standard indicates a "high level of confidence," among qualified experts, in the validity of a health claim, as a result of a demonstrated consistency in the effect of a substance (food or dietary supplement) across different human studies and different investigators (FDA, 2009b). A health claim that meets the SSA standard is unlikely to be reversed by subsequent/new studies. In contrast, for a body of evidence that is credible but does not meet the SSA standard (e.g., qualified health claims), as a result of inconsistencies in the effect of a substance across studies, a limited

---

TABLE 10.5
Comparison of Claim Substantiation Standards in the United States

Claim Category	Product Category	Substantiation Standard
Structure–function claims	Dietary supplements	"Competent and reliable scientific evidence"
Structure–function claims	Foods	Not defined
NLEA-authorized health claims	Foods and dietary supplements	SSA
Qualified health claims	Foods and dietary supplements	Less than SSA
FDAMA-authorized health claims	Foods	SSA

---

* The evaluation "process" involves a series of steps to: assess scientific studies and eliminate those from which no accurate scientific conclusions can be drawn; rate the remaining studies for methodological quality; and evaluate the strength of the totality of scientific evidence by considering: study types, methodological quality, quantity of evidence for and against the claim (taking into account the numbers of various types of studies and study sample sizes), relevance to the U.S. population or target subgroup, replication of study results supporting the proposed claim, and overall consistency of the evidence (FDA, 2009a).

number of studies, or uncertainties as to whether the claimed effect would be physiologically relevant, the U.S. FDA would specify "qualifying language" that identifies the limitations in the scientific evidence. For example, for the qualified health claim on selenium and thyroid cancer, U.S. FDA is exercising "enforcement discretion" for the following claim wording: "One weak, small study suggests that selenium intake may reduce the risk of thyroid cancer. Based on this study, U.S. FDA concludes that it is highly uncertain that selenium supplements reduce the risk of thyroid cancer" (FDA, 2009d). All NLEA- and FDAMA-authorized health claims (Appendix C) and qualified health claims are available on U.S. FDA's website (FDA, 2009e).

For structure–function claims, since they were originally intended for dietary supplements, the U.S. FDA does not discuss, nor provides guidance on their substantiation on conventional foods but rather only discusses substantiation standards for dietary supplements.

The substantiation of structure–function claims on dietary supplements is guided by two documents written by the U.S. FDA and FTC respectively: *Substantiation for Dietary Supplement Claims Made Under Section 403(r)(6) of the Federal Food, Drug, and Cosmetic Act* (FDA, 2008); and, *Dietary Supplements: An Advertising Guide for Industry* (Federal Trade Commission, 2001). The substantiation standard of "competent and reliable scientific evidence," described in these documents, is applied by both the U.S. FDA and FTC (FDA, 2008). "Competent and reliable scientific evidence" has been defined in FTC case law as "tests, analyses, research, studies, or other evidence based on the expertise of professionals in the relevant area, that has been conducted and evaluated in an objective manner by persons qualified to do so, using procedures generally accepted in the profession to yield accurate and reliable results (FDA, 2008)."

The key considerations made by both the U.S. FDA and FTC in determining whether evidence is sufficient to support a structure–function claim on dietary supplements are the same considerations made by the U.S. FDA in determining whether health claims are substantiated, which are

- The proposed claim wording (e.g., the health effect being claimed and its degree of specificity) and its multiple interpretations
- What experts in a relevant area (i.e., related to the claimed health effect) would generally consider to be "adequate evidence"
- The totality and consistency of the evidence and whether inconsistencies can be explained*
- The quality of the evidence [All 3 guidance documents for health claims or structure/function claims on dietary supplements provide factors that the U.S. FDA or U.S. FTC consider in appraising the quality of studies (Federal Trade Commission, 2001; FDA, 2008, 2009c).]
- The quantity of the evidence
- The relevance of the evidence (i.e., whether the product/ingredient of interest has been investigated in humans; the relevance of the study population and the study's setting to the target population and the U.S.; and the relevance of the investigated product to the product intended for marketing)

A noteworthy point made by the FTC in their guidance document on structure–function claim substantiation on dietary supplements (Federal Trade Commission, 2001), is that "there is no fixed formula for the number or type of studies required" and that "although there is no requirement that a dietary supplement claim be supported by any specific number of studies, the replication of research results in an independently conducted study adds to the weight of the evidence" (Federal Trade Commission, 2001). These statements do not preclude the possibility of substantiating a structure–function claim on a dietary supplement with only one human study.

Since no specific guidance document has been issued for structure–function claims on conventional foods, it is logical to defer to the guidance documents written for the same claim category of

---

* Where there are inconsistencies in the evidence, it is important to examine whether there is a plausible explanation for them—e.g., inconsistencies may be due to differences in dosage, the form of administration (e.g., oral or intravenous), the population tested, or other aspects of study methodology (Federal Trade Commission, 2001).

interest (structure–function claims) albeit for a different product category (dietary supplements) (Federal Trade Commission, 2001; FDA, 2008). However, that said, since foods, unlike dietary supplements, are consumed ad libitum, it is recommended that documents prepared by the U.S. FDA to guide health claim substantiation for foods also be referred to (FDA, 2009c).

10.4 CONCLUSIONS

The existing legislation and regulatory frameworks in Canada and the U.S. support the innovation and marketing of foods and dietary supplements (or NHPs). Differences between the two countries' interest in civil rights (i.e., freedom of speech) are, however, apparent. Unlike in Canada, the U.S. has the "First Amendment"* which is the basis for the permissibility of a larger range of claims, specifically claims not supported by strong science—that is, qualified health claims. Another major jurisdictional difference relates to the permissible mechanisms for approving ingredient safety. Unlike in Canada, the U.S. does not solely rely on regulatory authorities to conduct safety approvals; rather, it additionally has a self-affirmation method of approval (i.e., GRAS).

Similarities do indeed exist between the two jurisdictions with respect to data requirements to demonstrate safety and efficacy. These similarities can be capitalized upon in the marketing and commercialization of new products and/or ingredients.

REFERENCES

Agriculture and Agri-Foods Canada. 2010. *Food Regulations*. http://www4.agr.gc.ca/AAFC-AAC/display-afficher.do?id=1277744358829&lang=eng [Last modified: 2010–07–28].

Agriculture and Agro-Foods Canada. 2011a. *Classification of Products at the Food-Natural Health Product Interface: Questions and Answers.* http://www4.agr.gc.ca/AAFC-AAC/display-afficher.do?id=1288285991143&lang=eng [Last modified: 2010–11–22].

Agriculture and Agri-Foods Canada. 2011b. *Agriculture and Agri-Foods Canada.* Online. http://www4.agr.gc.ca/AAFC-AAC/display-afficher.do?id=1175599418927&lang=eng [Last modified: 2011–06–10].

Canada Gazette, Part I. 1998–2011. http://www.gazette.gc.ca/rp-pr/p1/index-eng.html.

Canada Gazette, Part II. 1998–2011. http://www.gazette.gc.ca/rp-pr/p2/index-eng.html.

Canadian Food Inspection Agency. 2003. *Guide to Food Labelling and Advertising.* http://www.inspection.gc.ca/english/fssa/labeti/guide/toce.shtml [Last modified: 2010–07–28].

Canadian Food Inspection Agency. 2010. *Science and Regulation... Working Together for Canadians.* http://www.inspection.gc.ca/english/agen/broch/broche.shtml [Last modified: 2010–11–25].

Canadian Food Inspection Agency. 2010a. List of Ingredients. http://www.inspection.gc.ca/english/fssa/labeti/ingrede.shtml [Last modified: 2010-04-09].

Code of Federal Regulations, title 21. 2011. http://ecfr.gpoaccess.gov/cgi/t/text/text-idx?sid=440ad1542ceb04f96cb46d175274ae77&c=ecfr&tpl=/ecfrbrowse/Title21/21tab_02.tpl.

Dietary Supplement Health and Education Act (DSHEA). 1994. Public Law 103–417, 103rd Congress. http://ww.fda.gov/RegulatoryInformation/Legislation/FederalFoodDrugandCosmeticActFDCAct/SignificantAmendmentstotheFDCAct/ucm148003.htm.

FDA. 1997. Substances Generally Recognized as Safe [Docket No. 97N–0103] (Food and Drug Administration, U.S.). 62 Fed. Reg. 18938 (Apr. 17, 1997). http://www.gpo.gov/fdsys/pkg/FR-1997–04–17/html/97–9706.htm.

FDA. 1998. *Guidance for Industry: Notification of a Health Claim or Nutrient Content Claim Based on an Authoritative Statement of a Scientific Body.* Food and Drug Administration, U.S. (FDA), Center for Food Safety and Applied Nutrition (CFSAN), Office of Nutrition, Labeling, and Dietary Supplements. http://www.fda.gov/Food/GuidanceComplianceRegulatoryInformation/GuidanceDocuments/FoodLabelingNutrition/ucm056975.htm [June 11, 1998].

FDA. 2003. *Guidance for Industry: Questions and Answers about the Petition Process.* Food and Drug Administration, U.S. (FDA), Center for Food Safety and Applied Nutrition (CFSAN), Office of Food Additive Safety. http://www.fda.gov/Food/GuidanceComplianceRegulatoryInformation/GuidanceDocuments/FoodIngredientsandPackaging/ucm253328.htm [Sep. 2003; Revised: Apr. 2006 & Apr. 2011].

---

* The First Amendment does not permit the U.S. FDA to reject health claims that they determine to be potentially misleading unless they also determine that a disclaimer would not eliminate the potential deception.

FDA. 2008. *Guidance for Industry: Substantiation for Dietary Supplement Claims Made Under Section 403(r) (6) of the Federal Food, Drug, and Cosmetic Act.* Food and Drug Administration, U.S. (FDA), Center for Food Safety and Applied Nutrition (CFSAN), Office of Nutrition, Labeling, and Dietary Supplements. http://www.fda.gov/Food/GuidanceComplianceRegulatoryInformation/GuidanceDocuments/DietarySupplements/ucm073200.htm [Dec. 2008].

FDA. 2009a. *Draft Guidance for Industry: Factors that Distinguish Liquid Dietary Supplements from Beverages, Considerations Regarding Novel Ingredients, and Labeling for Beverages and Other Conventional Foods.* Food and Drug Administration, U.S. (FDA), Center for Food Safety and Applied Nutrition (CFSAN). http://www.fda.gov/Food/GuidanceComplianceRegulatoryInformation/GuidanceDocuments/DietarySupplements/ucm196903.htm [Page Last Updated: 05/25/2011].

FDA. 2009b. *Health Claim Notification for the Substitution of Saturated Fat in the Diet with Unsaturated Fatty Acids and Reduced Risk of Heart Disease.* Food and Drug Administration (FDA). http://www.fda.gov/Food/LabelingNutrition/LabelClaims/FDAModernizationActFDAMAClaims/ucm073631.htm [Last updated: 06/18/2009].

FDA. 2009c. *Guidance for Industry: Evidence-Based Review System for the Scientific Evaluation of Health Claims–Final.* Food and Drug Administration, U.S. (FDA), Center for Food Safety and Applied Nutrition (CFSAN), Office of Nutrition, Labeling and Dietary Supplements. http://www.fda.gov/Food/GuidanceComplianceRegulatoryInformation/GuidanceDocuments/FoodLabelingNutrition/ucm073332.htm [Jan. 2009].

FDA. 2009d. *Selenium and a Reduced Risk of Site-specific Cancers, FDA-2008-Q-0323.* Food and Drug Administration, U.S. (FDA), Center for Food Safety and Applied Nutrition (CFSAN), Office of Nutrition, Labeling and Dietary Supplements. http://www.fda.gov/Food/LabelingNutrition/LabelClaims/QualifiedHealthClaims/ucm168527.htm [Jun. 19, 2009].

FDA. 2009e. *Label Claims.* Food and Drug Administration, U.S. http://www.fda.gov/Food/LabelingNutrition/LabelClaims/default.htm [Last updated: 04/30/2009].

FDA. 2011a. [Organization Chart]. Food and Drug Administration, U.S. http://www.fda.gov/downloads/AboutFDA/CentersOffices/OrganizationCharts/UCM254312.pdf [Approved: 5/9/11].

FDA. 2011b. *For Industry: Color Additives.* Food and Drug Administration, U.S. FDA. http://www.fda.gov/ForIndustry/ColorAdditives/default.htm [Last updated: 06/03/2011].

FDA. 2011c. GRAS Notice Inventory. Food and Drug Administration, U.S. http://www.accessdata.fda.gov/scripts/fcn/fcnNavigation.cfm?rpt=grasListing [Last updated: 05/31/2011].

FDA. 2011d. *New Dietary Ingredients in Dietary Supplements–Background for Industry.* Food and Drug Administration, U.S. (FDA), Center for Food Safety and Applied Nutrition (CFSAN). http://www.fda.gov/Food/DietarySupplements/ucm109764.htm [Last updated: 06/14/2011].

FDA. 2011e. *Draft Guidance for Industry: Dietary Supplements: New Dietary Ingredient Notifications and Related Issues.* Food and Drug Administration, U.S. (FDA). http://www.fda.gov/Food/GuidanceComplianceRegulatoryInformation/GuidanceDocuments/DietarySupplements/ucm257563.htm [Last updated: 07/01/2011].

FDA. 2011f. *Food Additives.* Food and Drug Administration, U.S. http://www.fda.gov/Food/FoodIngredientsPackaging/FoodAdditives/default.htm [Last updated: 05/04/2011].

FDA. 2011g. Generally Recognized as Safe (GRAS). Food and Drug Administration, U.S. http://www.fda.gov/Food/FoodIngredientsPackaging/GenerallyRecognizedasSafeGRAS/default.htm [Last Updated: 06/10/2011].

Federal Food, Drug, and Cosmetic Act (FD&C Act). U.S. *Code*, 21 U.S.C. (2010). http://www.fda.gov/regulatoryinformation/legislation/federalfooddrugandcosmeticactfdcact/default.htm

Federal Trade Commission. 1994. *Enforcement Policy Statement on Food Advertising.* Federal Trade Commission, U.S. http://www.ftc.gov/bcp/policystmt/ad-food.shtm [May 1994].

Federal Trade Commission. 2001. *Dietary Supplements: An Advertising Guide for Industry.* Federal Trade Commission, U.S., Bureau of Consumer Protection. http://business.ftc.gov/documents/bus09-dietary-supplements-advertising-guide-industry [Apr. 2001].

Federal Trade Commission. 2010. *About the Federal Trade Commission.* http://www.ftc.gov/ftc/about.shtm [Last modified: June 17, 2010].

Federal Trade Commission. 2011a. *Legal Resources–Statutes Relating to Both Missions.* Federal Trade Commission, U.S. http://www.ftc.gov/ogc/stat1.shtm [Last modified: Feb. 3, 2011].

Federal Trade Commission. 2011b. *Commission Actions . . .* Federal Trade Commission, U.S. http://www.ftc.gov/os/actions.shtm [Last modified: July 15, 2011].

Food Additive Amendment (FAA) of 1958. Public Law 85–929; *U.S. Statutes at Large* 72(1958), Stat. 1784. http://www.cq.com/graphics/sal/85/sal85–929.pdf.

Food and Drug Administration Modernization Act (FDAMA) of 1997. Public Law 105–115; U.S. Statutes at Large 105(1997):111, Stat. 2296. http://www.fda.gov/RegulatoryInformation/Legislation/FederalFood DrugandCosmeticActFDCAct/SignificantAmendmentstotheFDCAct/FDAMA/default.htm.

Food and Drug Regulations, Consolidated Regulations of Canada, c. 870 (2011). http://laws.justice.gc.ca/eng/ regulations/C.R.C.,_c._870/index.html [last amended on 2011–04–01].

Food and Drugs Act, Statutes of Canada, c. F-27 (1985). http://laws.justice.gc.ca/eng/acts/F-27/ [last amended on 2008–06–16].

Health Canada. 2006a. *Guidelines for the Safety Assessment of Novel Foods Derived from Plants and Microorganisms.* Ottawa, ON: Health Canada, Health Products and Food Branch, Food Directorate. http://www.hc-sc.gc.ca/fn-an/legislation/guide-ld/nf-an/index-eng.php [June 2006].

Health Canada. 2006b. *Evidence for Safety and Efficacy of Finished Natural Health Products.* Ottawa, ON: Health Canada, Natural Health Products Directorate. http://www.hc-sc.gc.ca/dhp-mps/prodnatur/legisla-tion/docs/efe-paie-eng.php [Dec. 2006].

Health Canada. 2007a. *Evidence for Quality of Finished Natural Health Products.* (Guidance document, ver-sion 2). Ottawa, ON: Health Canada, Natural Health Products Directorate. http://www.hc-sc.gc.ca/dhp-mps/prodnatur/legislation/docs/eq-paq-eng.php [June 2006].

Health Canada. 2007b. *Compendium of Monographs.* (Version 2.1). Ottawa, ON: Health Canada, Natural Health Products Directorate. http://www.hc-sc.gc.ca/dhp-mps/alt_formats/hpfb-dgpsa/pdf/prodnatur/ compendium_mono_v2–1-eng.pdf [Nov. 2007].

Health Canada. 2007c. *Natural Health Products Ingredients Database.* Ottawa, ON: Health Canada, Natural Health Products Directorate. http://webprod.hc-sc.gc.ca/nhpid-bdipsn/monosReq.do?lang=eng [Modified: 2007–04–18].

Health Canada. 2008. *Policy for Differentiating Food Additives and Processing Aids.* Ottawa, ON: Health Canada, Health Products and Food Branch, Food Directorate, Bureau of Chemical Safety. http://www. hc-sc.gc.ca/fn-an/pubs/policy_fa-pa-eng.php.

Health Canada. 2009a. *Product Licensing.* Ottawa, ON: Health Canada. http://www.hc-sc.gc.ca/dhp-mps/prod-natur/applications/licen-prod/index-eng.php [Modified: 2009–08–11].

Health Canada. 2009b. *Compendium of Monographs.* Ottawa, ON: Health Canada, Natural Health Products Directorate. http://www.hc-sc.gc.ca/dhp-mps/prodnatur/applications/licen-prod/monograph/index-eng. php/ [Modified: 2009–03–12].

Health Canada. 2009c. *Guidance Document for Preparing a Submission for Food Health Claims.* Health Canada, Food Directorate, Health Products and Food Branch, Bureau of Nutritional Sciences. http:// www.hc-sc.gc.ca/fn-an/alt_formats/hpfb-dgpsa/pdf/legislation/health-claims_guidance-orientation_alle-gations-sante-eng.pdf.

Health Canada. 2010a. *Classification of Products at the Food–Natural Health Product Interface: Products in Food Formats.* Health Canada, Natural Health Products Directorate, Food Directorate. http://www. hc-sc.gc.ca/dhp-mps/alt_formats/hpfb-dgpsa/pdf/prodnatur/food-nhp-aliments-psn-guide-eng.pdf (Version 2.0, June 2010).

Health Canada. 2010b. *Product Licence Application Form.* (Version 2). Ottawa, ON: Health Canada. http://www. hc-sc.gc.ca/dhp-mps/prodnatur/applications/licen-prod/form/index-eng.php [Modified: 2010–06–30].

Health Canada. 2010c. *Drug and Health Products Guidance Documents.* Ottawa, ON: Health Canada. http:// www.hc-sc.gc.ca/dhp-mps/prodnatur/legislation/docs/index-eng.php [Modified: 2010–10–26].

Health Canada. 2011a. *Health Products and Food Branch* Online. http://www.hc-sc.gc.ca/ahc-asc/branch-dirgen/hpfb-dgpsa/index-eng.php [Last modified: 2011–06–24].

Health Canada. 2011b. *Approved Products.* Ottawa, ON: Health Canada. http://www.hc-sc.gc.ca/fn-an/gmf-agm/appro/index-eng.php [Modified: 2011–03–07].

Natural Health Products Regulations, SOR/2003–196. http://laws-lois.justice.gc.ca/eng/regulations/SOR-2003–196/index.html [last amended on 2008–06–01].

Nutrition Labeling and Education Act of 1990 (NLEA). Public Law 101–535, U.S. House of Representatives Bill 3562.

Regulations Amending the Food and Drug Regulations (1385—Vitamin K), Canada Gazette 2005, II, SOR/2005–307 (Food and Drugs Act). http://gazette.gc.ca/archives/p2/2005/2005–10–19/html/sor-dors307-eng.html.

Rulis, A.M. and Levitt, J.A. 2009. FDA'S food ingredient approval process: safety assurance based on scientific assessment. *Regul. Toxicol. Pharmacol.* 53(1):20–31.

Section III

Consumer Perspective on
Innovation versus Need

11 Functional Food Trends in India

Rekha R. Mallia

CONTENTS

11.1 INTRODUCTION

Food goes beyond nourishment, as it encompasses a multitude of human experiences and emotions, and these vary between cultures and religions. As we gain knowledge about the health aspects of food, we discover new ways of preparing and using biomaterial for food, and also rediscover the value of some of the old practices. Despite the low level of public awareness in India when compared to the Western markets, functional foods and ingredients are finding growth across India, as consumers switch on to the promise of healthier foods, beverages, and supplements. This has led to the coining of a new term—Nutraceuticals, which means "functional food."[1-4] Functional Foods/ Nutraceuticals in recent years have witnessed a tremendous increase in interest among the consumers due to their potential of providing health benefits. The likes of probiotics-fortified dairy products and omega-3-fortified health drinks and baby foods are winning over swathes of Indian consumers according to the new reports.

11.2 REGULATIONS IN INDIA

India is the second largest producer of food, with surfeit of nutritive and therapeutic compounds whose value is yet to be realized in modern market places. Though there had been multiple laws and regulations covering the foods market in India, there has been no single law that significantly regulated the functional food market. As a result of the lapse and disordered health policies, the morbidity and mortality levels in the country are still high. Low investments in health are indicated as being the primary reason for poor quality and an uneven healthcare delivery system across the country. The poor people seek private health services at the cost of essential expenditure, such as nutrition, the report continued.

The Indian government passed the Food Safety and Standard Act in 2006 to integrate and streamline the many regulations covering nutraceuticals, foods, and dietary supplements. The act calls for the creation of the Food Safety and Standards Authority (FSSA). Once established, the FSSA will be in charge of drafting and governing rules and regulations for the food industry and assign local authorities, and a system of regular audit, including product-recall procedures, enforcements, and penalties. A significant augmentation is necessary for the act to have a magnitude of impact on the Indian functional food and nutraceutical industry like the Dietary Supplements Health Education Act (DSHEA) 1994 had on dietary supplement industry in the United States.[5]

The Food Safety and Standard Act 2006 aims to establish a single reference point for all matters relating to Food Safety and Standards, by moving from multilevel, multidepartmental control to a single line of command. It incorporates the salient provisions of the Prevention of Food Adulteration Act 1954 and is based on international legislations, Instrumentalities, and Codex Alimentarius Commission.[6]

Regulation broadly defines the intervention of Government in industry and primarily controls the product quality in case of food products. Unlike the United States, where the DSHEA is in place to regulate these products, in India, the Government is in the process of drafting a law to regulate manufacturing, importing, and marketing of health foods, dietary supplements, and other nutraceuticals.[7,8]

The United States and Europe are going to be the emerging markets for nutraceutical exports from India because an existing large market base is already in place and consumers are looking for better and healthier options to prevent lifestyle-related diseases.[9,10] The market potential for the U.S. and European markets alone for nutraceutical exports from India by 2013 are expected to raise over $75 billion.

There is currently no official harmonized definition or harmonization of the technical requirements and guidelines for functional food products in Asia. Academics and food companies generally understand functional foods to contain or to be fortified with nutrients or other bioactive compounds that help to maintain and promote health. Functional foods in Asia tend to be regulated under the conventional food category. However, health claims regulatory environment is evolving and significant changes in the next 5 years are expected.[11,12]

Big companies are utilizing direct multilevel marketing, to reach new consumers with their products delivered by someone known and trusted. However, most of the large companies have not ventured into nutraceuticals or dietary supplements due to regulatory confusion, lack of adequate awareness and understanding, and poor vision of the market.[9,13] Several companies are reportedly waiting in the wings until these guidelines are defined.

The Indian nutraceutical supplement and functional food industry is set to open up new opportunities for international companies, with the new regulatory guidelines for these product lines coming under the discrete food category. This would boost the level of science behind products by defining the scope of acceptable health and nutritional claims which have to be on the basis of clinical trials, protocols, and systematic scientific studies carried out as a part of R&D and new product development. There would be greater opportunities for marketing tie-ups with Indian companies and a greater array of products available for Indian consumers.

11.3   AYURVEDIC SUPPORT

The basic objective of Ayurveda is "to maintain the health of the healthy and to mitigate the disease in the diseased ones." Ayurveda's strength lies in the fact that it states clearly "anna—anna aushadhi—aushadhi" continuum, which means diet—diet as medicine—medicine continuum. Such wisdom has helped in tapping traditional knowledge for developing new actives for health maintenance, which is the most common aim of food supplements.[14] The Drugs and Cosmetics Acts of India recognizes 57 such books, which collectively contain about 35,000 ayurvedic recipes and processes to make them. These recipes are said to have been documented only after conducting numerous trials on humans from different corners of the Indian subcontinent since the inception of Ayurveda and 70% of the population in this region still relies on Ayurveda for its primary healthcare. Large numbers of recipes are used today and their safety is ensured. These recipes have helped in identifying new leads for specific health benefits much quicker than the conventional drug discovery route.

The use of Ayurveda, however, is not restricted to India alone. In the United States, over 751,000 people have received ayurvedic treatment according to the National Center for Health Statictics, 2004. Besides the United States, ayurvedic products are also exported from India to Canada, Germany, Japan, Malaysia, Australia, New Zealand, the Middle East, France, Switzerland, South Africa, and Russia in the form of ingredients and functional foods.

Several drug companies have rolled out a series of ayurvedic and health treatment centers across the country and abroad in the past 5 years. Various specialized centers have sprung up in providing complete packages including health treatments by the use of ayurvedic methods and dietary food packages made under brands of ayurvedic preparations. Kits containing such preparations are available at various outlets in major cities of the country and abroad. As a part of the tourism promotion in the country, the development authority has sanctioned such centers to be set up in clubs, premier hotels, and resorts with strict intervention by the authority. This has in turn increased the preferential demand of food which supports the therapeutic and health benefits in the country.

11.4   HEALTH AWARENESS AND MARKET ATTITUDE

With the increasing understanding of the nutritive value of various food items, and the basic biochemical roles that they play, consumers appreciate the values of the menu that various societies have adopted around the world. Personalized medicine appears to be the way of the future.

The importance of prevention has to be treated equally for diagnosing and treating acute and chronic medical conditions. It already has been demonstrated that alteration in lifestyle (e.g., diet and exercise) can influence the onset and severity of disease for a significant percentage of individuals. Therefore, a new wave of consumers is challenging the industry by demanding foods based upon their disease-preventive functions. With consumers becoming more health conscious and recognizing the need to take more responsibility to protect their own health, the functional food and drink markets have grown exponentially across the globe.

Analysts say the growth of India's nutritional supplement market is being driven by the changing lifestyle of the country's consumers and increased knowledge about nutritional supplements. Today's consumer demand for functional foods is influenced by several factors, not the least of which are the scientific and clinical findings supporting the claims. In this age when the dissemination of scientific findings is made easy by the electronic interface and its information superhighways, the consumers are more informed on the subjects of health, chronic illness, prevention, and nutrition. Scientific advances in these areas, as well as in food technology, allow the food industry to satisfy the increased demand for functional foods by consumers. The traditional free size concept has evolved into even-more-challenging product development that currently targets specific demographics, including age, race, and sex.

Even though developing countries are a rich source of raw materials for functional food products because of their vast biodiversity and cost advantages in crop production, developing a functional foods industry in these countries faces significant barriers. The cost of bringing a new product to the market can be significant, especially the upfront costs associated with high-value food processing and exporting including search for markets, product research and certification, meeting regulatory demands, consumer research, and public relations.

Demographics are a useful start in defining the consumer target but are inadequate alone.

Consumers can be categorized into the kind of diet they are on, as healthy or very healthy. When it comes to contemplating dietary improvement, consumers aged between 30 and 39 years are more likely than those in any other age group to want to eat healthy foods more often (over 85%).[15] The functional food industry trends largely depend on this segment of the consumer population. Younger shoppers are less likely to eat health food than older ones. Knowing the attitudinal designators of each age group will help functional food manufacturers find the right market for their products.

As a result of the increased media attention to the relationship between food and health, there is an increased sense of nutritional confusion. Majority of the consumers are often confused about what they should eat to stay healthy. Nutritional confusion increases somewhat with age. Most consumers still prefer naturally nutritious foods to supplements or fortified foods. In addition, a defined part of these consumer groups who face an acute health condition would be more concerned on the diet. As shoppers get older, they are much more likely to be concerned about heart disease, cancer, high cholesterol levels, osteoporosis, and diabetes. Other health concerns, such as stress and menopause, can also be charted across generations.

Though the key challenge for the functional food industry lies in increasing the awareness among the public, a lot of work is already being done in the manufacturing industry, catering to the local and international world market through new product development in this line opening wider opportunities for the future.

REFERENCES

1. *International Food Information Council Functional Foods Now*. Washington, DC: International Food and Information Council; 1999.
2. Kalra, E.K. Nutraceutical: Definition & introduction, *AAPS Pharmsci.*, 2003, 5(2) Article 25 (DOI.10.1208/PS/0500225).
3. Hardy, G. Nutraceutical and functional food: Introduction and meaning, *Nutrition*, 2000, 16, 688–689.
4. Brower, V. Nutraceuticals: Poised for healthy slice of healthcare market? *Nat. Biotechnol.*, 1998, 16, 728–731.
5. Regulation of functional food in Indian Subcontinent, food and beverages news. http://www.efenbeon-line.com/view_story.asp?type=story&id=880).
6. LII of India, http://www.commonlii.org/in/.
7. India together: Legislative brief. http://www.indiatogether.org/.
8. FICCI Study on Implementation of Food Safety and Standard Act 2006: An industry perspective. http://www.indiaenvironmentportal.org.in.
9. Jacobs, K. India: Nutraceutical market sees 40% growth, *Just-Food*, 17 June 2008.
10. Mehta, A.G. Untapped wealth of nutraceutical exports. *The Hindu Business Line*, August 15, 2008.
11. Lim, W.W. and Tsi, D. Defining functional food claims, regulatory environment for functional food claims in Asia. *Asia Food Journal*, September 2008. http://www.asiafoodjournal.com/article-5565-definingfiunctionalfoodclaims-Asia.html.
12. Williams, M., Pehu, E., and Ragasa, C. Functional foods- opportunities and challenges for developing countries. *Agricultural and Rural Development Notes*, September 2006, 19, 1–4.
13. Kaushik, D. and Kaushik N. *Functional food/Nutraceuticals Regulation in India, Review on Pharmainfo*, 2009, 7(5).
14. Narayana, A.D.B., Smith, J., and Charter, E. Reverse Pharmacology for Developing Functional Foods/Herbalc Supplements: Approaches, Framework and Case Studies. In *Functional Food Product Development*, Smith, J. and Charter, E. (Eds). John Wiley and Sons, 2009, Chapter 12, p. 244.
15. Gilbert, L. Marketing functional foods: How to reach your target audience. *AgBioForum*, 2000, 3(1), 20–38.
16. Ayurvedic Medicine: An Introduction. *National center for complementary and alternate medicine*, NCCAM Pub No.: D287., 2005. US Department of Health and Human Service. http://nccam.nih.gov/health/ayurveda/introduction.htm

12 New Approaches for Foods and Nutrition for the Bottom of the Pyramid (Gandhi's Vision)

Ashok Vaidya

CONTENTS

12.1 INTRODUCTION

Sri Mohandas Karamchand Gandhi, known to millions of Indians as "Mahatma"—the great soul—and father of the nation, experimented in several domains of life. His autobiography—*My Experiments with Truth*—is considered a classic in the history of hagiography.[1] It is a wonder that in spite of his extremely busy life as a nonviolent leader against the British empire, he found time to ponder and work on the problems of all those who were poor, exploited, and hungry. He, from his utter simplicity and sincerity, tuned into their problems—sanitation, nutrition, crowding, social justice, and so on. In our days of intense professional superspecialization, we stand dismayed at his breadth of interest and intensity of concerns. Sometimes, our scientific hubris prevents us from even a study of his lifework and thoughts—so relevant to the global crises in diverse fields of life, including foods and nutrition.

Mahatma Gandhi showed an unusual common sense and followed his intuition, he called that the inner voice, a whisper from God, and even a great scientist like Einstein said, "Ideas come from God!" As Gandhi presaged several later discoveries in the science of nutrition, it may be worthwhile to have a relook at his vision on foods and nutrition for the world population—particularly the bottom of the pyramid of "consumers."[2]

Gandhi used the term "Daridra Narayana"—the God of the poor, God present in the hearts of the poor.[3] Gandhi was deeply religious and—though he denied the epithet—a saint. He had said that people call him Mahatma—a great soul, but he expected people to wait because he believed that if and only if at the time of his death he uttered God's name—Rama—would the "Mahatma" label be justified. His prophecy was fulfilled when his last words were "He Rama," on his assassination.

Gandhi's concern for the bottom of the pyramid population was supreme. He was so impressed with Ruskin's "Unto this Last" that he coined a term "Antyodaya" (the benefits to the most backward), besides revering the term "Daridra Narayana." He said, "I dare not take the message of God before those hungry millions who have no luster in their eyes and whose only God is their bread ... It is good enough to talk of God whilst we are sitting here after a nice breakfast and looking forward to a nicer luncheon, but how am I to talk of God to the millions who have to go without two meals a day?"[3] Recently, Dr. V. Prakash, the president of the Nutrition Society of India and the vice president of the International Union of Nutrition Sciences, said at the 6th Nutra Summit of India, "All the sectors which deal with nutrition and foods should bear in mind that around 130 million children, in India, get one meal in 3 days."[4] Such a reminder, from the director of the Central Food Technology Research Institute (CFTRI), with an evangelical fervor and Gandhian concern, is a wake-up call to all stakeholders in food and nutrition—agriculture, industrial research, academia, and governments.

12.2 GLOBAL HUNGER, UNFAIR TRADE PRACTICES, AND FOOD AVAILABILITY LOCALLY

It is a sad commentary on Gandhi's political heirs that India, after more than 60 years of independence, is still counted among the 29 most hungry countries, with stunted children and malnourished women. India, despite its claims of economic growth, is ranked 67th among 85 countries in terms of access to food.[5] It is an irony that India, the largest producer of milk and edible oils, will have to import these items. The UN goal of reducing the hungry population to half appears to be remote. Asian and African children constitute 90% of the world's stunted children. The grim reality of deaths due to malnutrition and related disorders in children is shocking. And more alarming than that is the massive wastage of foods in the entire chain. The 2011–2012 budget of India has initiated allocations for rural food storage and cold chains. At India's premier Central Food Technology Research Institute—CFTRI—the research council has proposed a program to prevent the waste of prepared foods and evolution of new methods of conserving and recycling the leftover food items, in homes and hotels/restaurants. If efforts succeed in these directions, Gandhi's approach—not to waste food—will be vindicated. The National Food Security Act, if implemented well, would arouse food availability.

Under the garb of globalization and free trade, there are significant imbalances in the agricultural produce, storage, distribution, and marketing. On the one hand, the affluent nations give massive subsidies to their farmers and try and capture the world markets. The local farmer at the bottom of the agriculture is bewildered. Prince Charles claimed that the tall promises offered by the GM commercial propaganda have led to thousands of suicides by Indian farmers. The estimates vary around 250,000 suicides due to "the ruthless drive to use India as a testing ground for genetically modified crops." It has become a major Indian and international ethical problem. The local moneylenders, the powerful politicians, and major agro-companies are responsible for the humanitarian crises.[6] Gandhi would have started a major Satyagraha for fighting this tragedy. Vandana Shiva, a conscientious activist, has given an analysis of why Indian farmers commit suicide and how the tragedy can be stopped.[7] She writes that Monsanto's GMO Bt cotton seeds created a suicide economy. Gandhi encouraged Rishi-Kheti and organic farming. He would have fasted to protest against the unfair trade practices. The rigged prices of agriculture trade have robbed the poor farmers of around $26 billion annually in India.

Gandhi's vision for the adequacy of food supply involved a grassroot approach to produce and use locally the essential food grains and crops. No nation should rig up the prices of essential foods. Any shortage due to draught, floods, and other calamities should be met with by the international community or organizations by preventive measures, rather than on a fire-fighting basis. Gandhi's holistic vision on agro-economy, environment, resource conservation, and energy restriction is very relevant to the current scenario.[8,9]

Swadeshi, or local self-sufficiency, was proposed as a vital stance for the communities. He said, "My definition of Swadeshi is well-known. I must not serve my distant neighbour at the expense of the nearest ... Swadeshi is that spirit in us which restricts us to use and service of our immediate surroundings to the exclusion of the more remote." He had visualized every village (~7 lakhs) to be a socioeconomic unit that is self-supporting, viable, and only exchanging selected commodities needed by other villages. This is still a feasible path for the bottom of the pyramid populations in Asia and Africa. Of course, it demands due diligence of the local bodies on food/agro needs and a district-level coordination to make Anna (food)-Swadeshi functional. There can be intense focused food programs for the most vulnerable groups among those below the poverty line (BPL). Pregnant women, growing children, and elderly citizens need to be carefully monitored for their adequate nutrition and health.

All the communities—rural, semiurban, urban, and of megapolis—need to ensure that Gandhi's vision of Sarvodaya is implemented. The classical food pyramid items will have to be investigated as to the alternatives or food concentrates or nutraceuticals. The emphasis has to be on low-margin and high-volume foods and nutrients for the bottom of the pyramid population. For example, the major problem of iron deficiency can be taken up on a war footing by a well-coordinated campaign and its execution. Just as smallpox was eradicated, iron deficiency too can be drastically reduced. There has to be transparency, accountability, and responsibility of the local self-government bodies as to both adequate food supply and nutritional health.

12.3   FOOD PROCESSING AND THE IMPACT ON NUTRIENTS

In the year 1935, Gandhi said, "We eat mill-ground flour, and even the poor villager walks with a head-load of half a mound of grain to have it ground in the nearest flour-mill. Do you know that in spite of the plenty of foodstuff we produce we import wheat from outside and we eat the 'superfine' flour? We do not use our hand-ground flours and the poor villager also foolishly copies us. We then turn our wealth into waste, nectar into poison. But we will not exert ourselves to produce which we must eat fresh every day, and will pay for less nutritious things and purchase ill-health in the bargain. The same is the case with rice, gur (jaggery), and oil. We will eat white rice, polished of its substance and eat less nutritious sugar and pay more for it than most nutritious gur."

Now, it is well known that the flour from even fresh ground wheat has a short half-life due to the rancidity of the wheat germ oil.[10] In most of the countries, for the bottom of the population pyramid, the good practices and the standard operative procedures are inadequate or nonexistent. Many gaps exist at various stages of the food chain—harvesting, storage, transport, distribution, and usage. Grinding one's own daily wheat flour was a norm earlier. Besides the nutrient value of the fresh flour, early morning grinding with the stone-mill at home added to the requisite exercise. Several of Gandhi's followers preserved this practice for a lifetime. Instead of the treadmill, such a household hand-mill would induce better cardiopulmonary reserve.

We sometimes forget that cooking on fire too is a form of food processing. Gandhi recommended the use of soaked cereals and pulses without cooking in his advocacy of nature cure. Gandhi was in good company, viz. that of Jesus Christ, who also recommended avoidance of fire in cooking.

Jesus Christ has been cited in the old Aramaic and Slavonic texts of the Bible (first century AD), "Let the angels of God prepare your bread. Moisten your wheat, that the angel of water may enter it, then set it in the air, that the angel of air also embrace it. And leave it from the morning to the evening beneath the sun, that the angel of sunshine may descend upon it. And the blessing of the three angels will soon make the germ of life to sprout in your wheat. Then crush your grain and make thin wafers, as did your forefathers, when they departed out of Egypt, the house of bondage. Put these back again beneath the sun from its appearing, and when its seen to its highest in the heaven, turn them over on the other side that they be embraced there until the sun be set. For the angels of water, of air and of sunshine fed and ripened the wheat in the field, and they, likewise, must prepare also your bread. And the same sun which, with the fire of life, made the wheat to grow and ripen, must cook your bread with the same fire. For the fires of the sun gives life to wheat, to the bread and to the body. But the fire of death kills the wheat, to the bread and the body."[11] He further emphasized in the same gospel, "Cook not, neither mix all things one with another, lest your bowels become as steaming bogs. For I tell you truly, this is abominable in the eyes of the Lord."[12]

Gandhi's views on polished and unpolished rice are worth citing even after more than 70 years, "If rice can be pounded in the villages after the old fashion the wages will fill the pockets of the rice pounding sisters and the rice eating millions will get some sustenance from the unpolished rice instead of pure starch which the polished rice provides. Human greed, which takes no count of the health or the wealth of the people who come under its heels, is responsible for the hideous rice-mills one sees in all the rice-producing tracts. If public opinion was strong, it will make rice-mills an impossibility by simply insisting on unpolished rice and appealing to the owners of rice-mills to stop a traffic that undermines the health of a whole nation and robs the poor people of an honest means of livelihood."[13] He had also insisted earlier that the villagers and others who eat whole-wheat flour ground in their own chakkis save their money and, what is more important, their health. He insisted also on closure of the wheat-mills and revive village and home grinding.

As recently as in 2010, a chapter on "Nutraceuticals: Possible Future Ingredients and Food Safety Aspects" by Prakash et al. have noted, "There are various regions in the world where local ethnic knowledge is of potential interest ... One example is that of the loss of nutritional value of rice bran resulting from the rice polishing process." The very ingredients which are lost are looked as components for nutraceuticals for adding value.[14] Gandhi would have objected to this dual cheating—first, remove the essential ingredients by polishing rice and then isolate the ingredients from the bran and sell these, at high price, as dietary supplements.

Gandhi was prescient when he recognized the hazards due to a lot of white sugar consumption instead of gur (jaggery) by Indians. Today, India has earned a dubious title of "the diabetic capital of world" besides being "the most iron-deficient nation." This could have been avoided had India listened to Gandhi in 1935, "According to the medical testimony ... gur is any day superior to refined sugar in food value, and if the villagers cease to make gur as they are beginning to do, they will be deprived of an important food adjunct for their children ... Retention of gur and its use by the people in general, means several crores of rupees retained by the villager." Indian children and adolescents are getting overweight and obese at a fast rate. The weight problem is further compounded by iron deficiency. Gandhi's leadership emerged as he led the Dandi march to object against salt tax. Were he alive, he would have led a campaign for a heavy tax on sugar.

The jaggery is rich with antioxidants, micronutrients like minerals and vitamins, and so on. India's most glaring health problem is iron deficiency. Around 60–70% of adolescent girls have iron deficiency anemia. Jaggery contains 2.65 mg of iron per 100 g whereas sugar contains 0.15 mg/100 g. At all the schools, colleges, and institutional canteens, food items (like gurpapdi) containing whole-wheat flour, jaggery, and ghee should be available free or heavily subsidized. This would take care of the big burden of iron deficiency.

12.4   GANDHI'S EXPERIMENTS WITH LIFESTYLE, DIET, AND VEGETARIAN FOODS

Gandhi's philosophy and faith deeply influenced his approach to health, nutrition, and disease. In his writings on constructive program, he said, "Mens sana in corpora sano is perhaps the first law for humanity. A healthy mind in a healthy body is self-evident truth. There is an inevitable connection between mind and body. If we were in possession of healthy minds, we would shed all violence and naturally obeying the laws of health, we would have healthy bodies without an effort."[15] He advocated some basic laws of health and hygiene:

1. Think of the purest thoughts, avoiding idle and random wandering mind.
2. Breathe the freshest air day and night; avoid polluted air.
3. Establish a balance between bodily labor and mental work.
4. Your water, food, and air must be clean. Besides personal cleanliness, your surroundings must be daily kept clean.
5. Eat to live for service of fellow men. Do not live for indulging yourselves.

6. Stand erect, sit erect, and be economical and perceive in all your acts.
7. Your inner calm and chanting Rama's name should get reflected in all your interaction and expression.

Gandhi's family background and his inclination to put to test any ideas, compatible to his creed, made him an unusual experimenter with his diet and of those around him. He carried his experience and views to the public through his speeches and articles. It is difficult to cover his lifetime of nutritional search in such a review. But his diverse statements can be summarized as follows[16]:

1. Sweet dishes should be eliminated altogether. Instead, he advised a small quantity of "gur" (jaggery) with milk.
2. He advised the use of one type of grain at a time. He did not like the common habit of an average household to use chapatti, rice, pulses milk, ghee, gur, and oil together with vegetables and fruits.
3. He, a believer in the needs of the poorest, advocated that those who get high animal protein should eschew pulses and let the vegetarian high-quality protein be available to the poor.
4. He advocated the use of raw salads, instead of cooked vegetables, in the daily meals. He recommended onions, carrot, radish, tomatoes, and salad leaves.
5. He felt that fresh fruit is good to tone the system. But he suggested small quantities of fruits, eaten apart from the meal.
6. He did not regard flesh food as necessary for humans at any stage and under any climate. He held flesh food as unsuited to human species. He realized that the milk is needed by the vegetarians.
7. Avoid fried foods.

He considered vegetarianism as one of the priceless gifts of Hinduism. Once again he was in good company of Jesus Christ, an advice given by him but neglected later by the organized Christianity. In the Aramaic text of the bible it is cited, "Kill not, neither eat the flesh of your innocent prey, lest you become slaves of satan. For that is the path of sufferings, and it leads unto death. But do the will of God ... Obey, therefore the words of God, behold, I have given you every herb bearing seed, which is upon the face of all the earth, and every tree, in which is the fruit of a tree yielding seeds; to you, it shall be for meat ... Also the milk of every thing that moreth and that liveth upon the earth shall be meat for you ... But flesh, and the blood which quickens it shall ye not eat ... For if you eat living food, the same will quicken you, but if you kill for your food, the dead food will kill you also."[17]

Jesus and Gandhi both believed and expressed that the nature of the diet influences the body, the mind, and the soul. There is a paucity of research on what substrates in diet influence the neurobiology of violence. Wurtman initiated the studies on how nutrients can modify the brain function by influencing the neurotransmitters.[18] Wurtmans—the husband and wife team—conducted research at the Massachusetts Institute of Technology showing a relationship of carbohydrate craving at characteristic times of the day with obesity and depression.[19] The appetite for more carbohydrates—particularly sweet items with monosaccharides—is regulated by serotonin (5-hydroxytryptamine). Seasonal mood disorders too have been related to melatonin, particularly the depression during dark winters. Phototherapy in winter depression has been shown to be effective.[20] Gandhi advocated sunbathing in his regimes of nature cure.

The fact that the carbohydrate craving occurred more in the afternoon shows the importance of matching the regularity of meals with the circadian rhythm of the body. He emphasized that there is no need to take more than three meals in a day. His own meal times were fixed like his timing of prayers.[21] On the last day of his life, it is recorded at 9.30 am, his morning meal time, he took the meal which contained cooked vegetables, 12 ounces of goat's milk, four tomatoes, four oranges, carrot juice, and a decoction of ginger, sour limes, and aloes.[22]

Gandhi's book on health, diet, and lifestyles holds interesting views. For example, he stated the amount of various foods (raw) required for a sedentary person, which appears not supported by any studies or analysis: cow's milk 2 lbs, cereals (wheat, rice, bajra in all) 6 oz, leafy vegetables 1 oz, ghee 1.5 oz, butter 2 oz, and white sugar (preferably gur) 1.5 oz and he has stated fresh fruits according to one's taste and purchasing power![21] The dietary guidelines for Indians provided by the National Institute of Nutrition (ICMR) are quite at variance from Gandhi's recommendation.[23] Fresh vegetables and fruits are advised in plenty and low fat has been advised for the adults. The scenario has changed in India as we have on one hand the problem of malnutrition/starvation and stunted children and on the other hand the obesity of the affluent. Gandhi would have given a different recipe for the current problem.

12.5 FASTING, NATURE CURE, AND SYSTEMS OF MEDICINE

Gandhi firmly believed that nature has provided the body with a mechanism to cleanse impurities. The latter when being cleansed manifests as illness. He promoted fasting, enema hydropathy, and mud packs as modalities of nature cure. He was also critical of other systems of medicine. He said, "I found that our Ayurveda and Unani Physicians lack sanity. They lack the humility. Instead that I found in them an arrogance that they knew everything that there was no disease they could not cure." He himself claimed a significant success of his use of naturally curative substances. But 2 years before his death, he stated, "My love of nature cure and the indigenous systems does not blind me to the advance that Western medicine has made inspite of the fact that I have stigmatized it as black magic. I have used the harsh term and I do not withdraw it. I cling to nature cure inspite of its great limitations and inspite of the lazy pretensions of nature-curists. Above all, in nature cure, everybody can be his or her own doctor, not so in various systems of medicine." He was a great believer in prevention of disease through proper diet, lifestyle, prayers, sanitation, and environmental care[24] and he asserted that the name of God was, of course, the hub around which the nature cure system revolved. For India's villages, he insisted that nature cure clinics and education be major steps to health.

12.6 NEO-GANDHIAN VISION ON FOODS AND NUTRITION

Notwithstanding Gandhi's dietary preoccupation and certain well-entrenched views, we must go to the fundamentals of his vision. Only then we may be guided to neo-Gandhian effective approaches to foods and nutrition. Tarlok Singh has well summarized that "Sarvodaya" and "Antyodaya" are Gandhi's pragmatic vision.[25]

Gandhi's repeated emphasis was on truth, nonviolence, and trusteeship. His idea of Sarvodaya (benefit to all) was actualized by incorporation of these three foundations of his life. About 1 year after his death, his leading constructive workers, including Vinoba Bhave, Kishor Mashruwala, and Kaka Kalelkar, met at Sevagram and agreed to form Sarvodaya Samaj. The aim was stated "to strive towards a society based on truth and non-violece in which there will be no distinction of class or creed, no opportunity for exploitation and full scope in the development of both individuals and groups." That was a tall ideal. And lot has happened since then in the world to negate the stated values. This vision when applied to the domains of food and nutrition would lead to the following approaches:

1. Truth demands that fraud on the farmers of the third world under the garb of globalization be terminated. The highly pegged-up prices of foods under the pretence of free trade and heavy subsidies constitute untruth and evil.
2. Nonviolence as a basic value demands that vegetarian and dairy/cow-care be promoted actively. Enough evidence exists that the massive intake of nonvegetarian foods has created eco-imbalance, metabolic disorders, and violent behaviors. Vegetarianism must be inculcated during education.

3. The trusteeship principle of Gandhi, though given much lip service, has not found enlightened corporate leadership to pursue it. Recently, Mukesh Ambani, the chief of Reliance, reiterated this holding wealth and assets as societal trust during his address to the industry and business leaders.[26] Vinoba stressed the importance of nonpossession and to remove "possessiveness." Agro-business is not only for the profit motive but also the larger societal needs, viz. hunger-free children, should be the benchmarks of success. All the food processes, products, and profits must be subjected to social audit.

Lastly, the Western hegemony of the rich nations has made exploitative global commerce a holy dogma. The dogma engulfs the entire sector of foods and nutrition. The burden of around 250,000 Indians farmers' suicides, 5000 malnourished children dying every day, and the cardiovascular hazards of colas and fast foods should be matters of major concerns for mankind. Gandhi had warned us. The wake-up call is there not to let any child sleep hungry.

12.7 "THE FORTUNE AT THE BOTTOM OF THE PYRAMID" AND AYURCEUTICALS

When C. K. Prahalad proposed the humongous potential of fortune from more than four billion at the bottom of the pyramid, the corporation, the management schools, and agro-industrial complex drooled with greed. The basic approach to poverty and its eradication of hunger and its relief, and diseases and their cure were brushed aside. Even the so-called poor can pay and let us dip into their torn pockets became a mantra. But the results of the gold rush were not all that rosy.

Karamchandani et al. critically questioned, "Is the bottom of the pyramid really for you?" In an interesting article in the *Harvard Business Review*,[27] they found that "only minority of corporations that engaged with poor population have created business worth 100,000 or more customers in Africa or one million in India." They gave an example of PUR, a water purification powder. Proctor and Gamble invested more than $10 million in the product for the bottom of the pyramid market. It was quite a noble gesture! Clean and pure water would prevent thousands of deaths! The company was compelled to shift the product to its philanthropic activity because the market capture was so low.

In contrast to the aforesaid example, in the earlier incarnation of Novartis, viz. Ciba-Geigy, there was the top management decision for social marketing in leprosy with the help of the World Health Organization and national leprosy programs. It has been an unsung story of a massive success; leprosy got practically wiped out.[28]

To wipe out hunger and to create health through proper foods and nutrients, we need Gandhi's vision that could be quite disruptive to modern multinational corporate mad quest for profits and more profits. What could be a nonviolent disruptive force that we may resort to for the aforesaid goals? Gandhi's weapons of Satyagraha couple with Rachanatmak Karya (constructive work) which led to India's freedom can be redeployed in our war on hunger. A new world economic order based on truth, nonviolence, and trusteeship may emerge by these weapons of mass mobilization. One major path that can be taken up, as a priority for the bottom of the pyramid, is to revive, revitalize, and redeploy the traditional wisdom of local foods for health.[28]

For India, Ayurveda offers a very rich heritage of health and seasonal foods. Almost 70% of Indians still use Ayurveda, and many medicinal plants and foods have evidence of preventive and curative value.[29] At the grassroot level, farmers can add value to their agro-products by generating a new class of nutraceuticals called Ayurceuticals.[30] Recently, Prakash et al. have listed some of these sources and observed a paradigm shift from the "Food Guide Pyramid" to today's "Phytochemical complex ladders" of nutrients and bioactives. Table 12.1 lists the plants with much potential for health and diseases. The model of Amul milk cooperative can be adopted for Ayurceuticals from villages. This may turn out to be a major disruptive business model for foods and nutrients. The current model of agro-business has failed to deliver, despite the prosperity of the few.

TABLE 12.1
Phytochemical Paths to Ayurceuticals

Common Name	Technical Name	Uses and Indications
Amla	*Phyllanthus emblica*	Immunity and aging
Haldi	*Curcuma longa*	Cancer preventive
Amrita	*Tinospora cordifolia*	Hepatoprotective, anticancer
Arjuna	*Terminalia arjuna*	Cardioprotective
Adarakh	*Zingiber officinale*	Antinausea, arthritis
Vasa	*Adhatoda zeylanicum*	Cough, asthma
Kutki	*Picrorrhiza kurroa*	Hepatitis, asthma
Kumari	*Aloe vera*	Skin blemishes
Asoka	*Saraca asoca*	Menorrhagia
Nagajihwa	*Enicostemma littorale*	Diabetes mellitus
Bakuchi	*Psorulea corylifolia*	Leukoderma, psoriasis
Isapgul	*Plantago ovata*	Constipation, colitis
Haritaks	*Terminalia chebula*	Memory loss, aging
Guggulu	*Commiphora wightii*	Arthritis, high cholesterol
Lasun	*Allium sativum*	Aging, atherosclerosis
Methi	*Trigonella foenum-graecum*	Obesity, diabetes
Khair	*Acacia catechu*	Sore throat, wound healing
Bilwa	*Aegle marmelos*	Diabetes mellitus, colitis
Musli	*Asparagus adscendens*	Weakness, libido
Shatavari	*Asparagus racemosus*	Lactation, aging,
Punarnava	*Boerhavia diffusa*	Edema, hepatitis
Palasha	*Butea frondosa*	Aging, helminths
Ajowan	*Carum copticum*	Flatulence, urticaria
Mandukparni	*Centella asiatica*	Anxiety, memory loss
Hadjod	*Cissus quadrangularis*	Fractures, weakness
Kulith	*Dolichos biflorus*	Kidney stones, piles
Vata	*Ficus benghalenis*	Wound healing, weakness

12.8   CONCLUSION

Gandhi's vision of incorporating truth, nonviolence, and trusteeship principles in daily life offers a novel value-based approach to meet our challenges in foods and nutrition. His emphasis on resources-sparing, energy-conserving, and nonexploitative processes in the entire food chain would be a major challenge to agricultural domain and corporate bodies concerned merely with profits. There is a need to evolve a farmer-centric, decentralized, and cost-effective path to empower the bottom of the pyramid population. The bottom—more than four billion people—are not to be perceived merely as consumers. They have to be and also are producers of food. They are holding a stake—social, economic, and technical—in the grassroot generation of genuine wealth, not only currency notes. The adult people below the poverty line must earn their bread as part of wages by their sweat and not be provided free rations. Only malnourished children, women, and aged persons have to be supervised and given proper nutrition; whole-wheat flour (hand-ground), unpolished rice, leafy vegetables, oil, and milk should be produced and made locally available. The major exploiters of the food chain need to be contained. If they do not fall in line, Gandhian Satyagraha is a must.

With rich flora in many developing countries, special nutrient-value-added Ayurceuticals must be produced by the village cooperatives on the Amul model. There must be special technology evolved to save cooked and unused foods to create nutritive products. Attempts to use agro-biotech to create nutrients from the agricultural "wastes" need to be taken up on a war footing (Tuli, S., The Vision of National Agro-Biotechnology Institute, personal communication). The enlightened business and agro-industries can be engaged actively for fighting hunger and malnutrition. Gandhi-type leadership would be impossible to have. But a mass mobilization is needed against the unfair trade practices, violent animal food usage, and farmer suicides. The leaders of industry, business, academia, regulatory bodies, farmers, and retailers need to come together and deliberate on Gandhi's vision vis-à-vis the global situation of hunger and malnutrition.

REFERENCES

1. Gandhi, M.K. 1927. *Satyana Prayogo Athava Atma-Katha.* Ahmedabad: Navajivan Trust.
2. Prahalad, C.K. 2004. *The Fortune at the Bottom of the Pyramid.* Philadelphia: Wharton School Publishing.
3. Gandhi, M.K. 1929. Daridranarayana. *Young India.* 4 April.
4. Prakash, V. 2011. Presidential address, 6th Nutra Summit, Mumbai.
5. Zia Haq. 2010. Hunger haunts India. *Hindustan Times.* http://www.hindustantimes.com/Hunger-haunts-India/Article-611546.aspx.
6. Malone, A. 2008. The GM genocide: Thousands of Indian farmers are committing suicide after using genetically modified foods. www.dailymail.co.uk/news/worldnews/article-1082559.html.
7. Shiva, V. 2009. Why are Indian farmers committing suicide and how can we stop this tragedy? www.voltairnet.org/article-159305.html.
8. Kumarappa, J.C. 2003. Gandhian economy and the way to realize it. In *Aspects of Gandhian Thoughts,* ed. Himmat Jhaveri. Mumbai: Manibhavan Gandhi Sangrahalaya.
9. Gandhi, M.K. 1947. *India of My Dreams.* Ahmedabad: Navjivan Publishing House.
10. Fresh-milled flour vs shelved whole wheat flour http://www.healthbanquet.com/fresh-milled-flour.html.
11. Szekely, E. 1937. *Translation of the Gospel of Peace of Jesus Christ by the Disciple John (The Aramaic and Old Slavonic Texts—First Century AD).* Washington: C.W. Daniel, pp. 50–51.
12. Szekely, E. 1937. *Translation of the Gospel of Peace of Jesus Christ by the Disciple John (The Aramaic and Old Slavonic Texts—First Century AD).* Washington: C.W. Daniel, pp. 52–53.
13. Gandhi, M.K. 1944. Polished vs unpolished rice. *Harijan,* 26 October.
14. Prakash, V. and van Bockel M.A.J.S. 1910. Nutraceuticals: Possible future ingredients and food safety aspects. In *Ensuring Global Food Safety: Exploring Global Harmonization,* eds. Christine Boisrobert, Sangsvikoh, Alexandra Stjepanobic, Huub Lelieveld, Chapter 19. New York: Academia Press, pp. 333–338.
15. Gandhi, M.K. 1941. *Constructive Programme.* Ahmedabad: Navajivan Mudranalaya, pp. 18–19.
16. Gandhi, M.K. 1942. Minimum diet. *Harijan,* 25 January.
17. Szekely, E. 1937. *Translation of the Gospel of Peace of Jesus Christ by the Disciple John (The Aramaic and Old Slavonic Texts—First Century AD).* Washington: C.W. Daniel, pp. 42–46.
18. Wurthman, R.J. 1982. Nutrients that modify brain function. *Scientific American,* 246(April):50–59.
19. Wurtman, R.J. and Wurtman Jane J. 1989. Carbohydrates and depression. *Scientific American,* 253:68–75.
20. Terman, M. 1988. On the questions of mechanism in phytotherapy for seasonal affective disorders: Considerations of clinical efficacy and epidemiology. *Journal of Biological Rhythms,* 3:155–172.
21. Gandhi, M.K. Diet and diet programme. http://www.gandhi-manibhavan.org/gandhiphilosophy/philosophy-health-dictprogramme.htm.
22. Murphy, S. The last hours of Mahatma Gandhi. http://www.mkgandhi.org/last%20days/last%20hours.htm.
23. CDAC, 2010. Dietary guidelines for Indians—National Institute of Nutrition (ICMR). http:///www.indg.in/health/nutrition/dietary-guidelines-forIndians.
24. Gandhi, M.K., Views on environment: Nature cure and holistic treatment. http://www.gandhi-manibhavan.org/gandhiphilosophy.htm.
25. Singh, T., 1997. Sarvodaya and Antyodaya in Gandhian thought and practice. *IASSI Quarterly,* 15:3.
26. Ambani, M. 2011. Business must care for society. http://www.ndtv.com/vodeo.player/news/business-must-care-for-society-mukesh-ambani/1923hg.
27. Karamchandani A., Kubzansky M., and Lalwani N., 2011. The Glove: Is the bottom of the pyramid really for you? *Harvard Business Review,* March :107–111.

28. Action Programme for the Elimination of Leprosy: Status Report 1998. Geneva: World Health Organization (document WHO/Lep/98.2).

29. Patwardhan B., Vaidya A.B., and Chorghade M., Ayurveda and natural products drug discovery. *Current Science*, 86:789–799.

30. Bhavan's SPARC, 1992. *Selected Medicinal Plants of India (A Monograph of Identity, Safety and Clinical Usage)*. Mumbai: CHEMEXCIL.

13 Consumer Reactions to Health Claims on Food Products

Klaus G. Grunert and Lisa Lähteenmäki

CONTENTS

13.1 HEALTH CLAIMS FROM A CONSUMER PERSPECTIVE

Healthiness is one of the major quality attributes that consumers look for in food products, second only to taste (Grunert 2005). However, in contrast with taste, healthiness cannot be perceived directly by the human senses; it is what is called a *credence attribute*. Health needs to be communicated, and this communication may be more or less credible and convincing. It may be understood correctly, or lead to different kinds of inferences in the mind of the consumer.

Communication promising that a food product has positive health effects is called a health claim. Health claims have become a major issue in the development and marketing of healthy food products, and especially functional foods. There has been widespread concern that consumers could be misled by health claims to believe that food products have health properties that they in fact do not possess. As a result, the use of health claims has been regulated. In the EU (EU Regulation 1924/2006), health claims are allowed on food products if they are based on scientific evidence. The strength of this evidence is assessed by the European Food Safety Authority (EFSA) with its expert groups, and based on their advice the European Commission makes decisions on which claims are allowed. EFSA has been following a strict practice with regard to the evaluation of health claims, and as a result, few products with health claims are found on the European market at present. But even if health claims are based on sufficient scientific evidence so that they can pass the legal hurdles and in fact be used on food products, the questions remain how consumers will perceive them, and how they will affect their purchasing and eating behavior.

Health claims have been the subject of a good deal of consumer research (for overviews see Pothoulaki and Chryssochoidis 2009; Williams 2005). Issues addressed have been the effects of health claims on overall product evaluations and purchase intentions (e.g., Garretson and Burton 2000; Lyly et al. 2007), on product sales (e.g., Ippolito and Mathios 1991, 1994), and on inferences about other product attributes (e.g., Andrews et al. 1998; Mitra et al. 1999; Roe et al. 1999). Also, the possible reciprocal impact of health claims and nutrition information has been analyzed (e.g., Ford et al. 1996; Mazis and Raymond 1997; Kozup et al. 2003). Despite this stream of research, we still have a rather fragmented view of the factors that influence how consumers react to health claims. In the following, we will first present a theoretical framework that is useful for distinguishing different questions that can be posed on how consumers react to health claims on food products. We will then go into more depth with regard to three of these questions:

1. What determines whether a health claim is regarded as convincing by consumers?
2. Are consumers able to understand health claims correctly, and are some consumers more apt to misunderstand health claims than others?
3. How does the presence of the health claim affect the overall perception of the product?

In answering these questions, we will draw on research undertaken to shed light on these issues, drawing especially on a consumer study carried out in the Nordic countries (Grunert et al. 2009; Lähteenmäki et al. 2010) and a study carried out together with Danone in Germany (Grunert et al. 2011).

13.2 ROLE OF HEALTH CLAIMS IN THE PROCESS OF QUALITY PERCEPTION

We argue that the effect of health claims on consumers can be understood best by regarding health claims as *quality cues*. To illustrate this, we draw on the work on consumer food quality perception done within the framework of the Total Food Quality Model (Grunert 2005). A simplified version of this model is shown in Figure 13.1. Consumers evaluate food quality on some key dimensions—typically taste, healthiness, convenience, and production process. All of these are uncertain before the purchase, and consumers therefore need to use quality cues to make (uncertain) inferences about the expected quality. Two types of cues are distinguished in the quality perception literature: intrinsic cues (physical characteristics of the product) and extrinsic cues (everything else, including all communicational

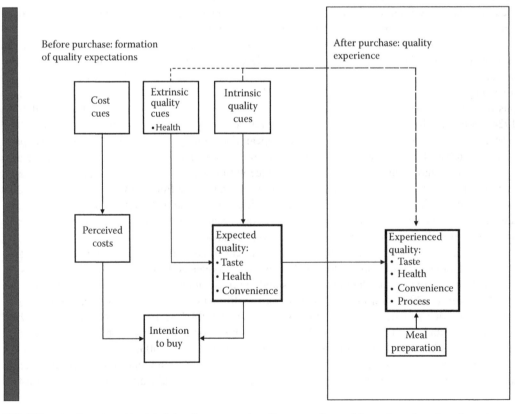

FIGURE 13.1   Function of health claims in process of quality perception and formation of purchase intentions.

cues). After the purchase, some dimensions of quality—taste, convenience—become amenable to experience, so that expectations can become confirmed or disconfirmed, whereas others—healthiness, production process—remain a question of communication also after the purchase.

A health claim is an extrinsic quality cue. Looking at the possible role of health claims as extrinsic quality cues in the quality perception process, the following questions can be asked:

1. Are health claims used as extrinsic cues when buying food?
   This refers to the question whether health claims on food products are indeed noticed, read, and further processed, with a possible impact on purchase decisions made.
2. Which types of health claims are regarded as more convincing?
   Health claims come in several variations, combining information about active ingredients, their physiological function and the resulting health benefit. They can also be formulated in different ways, for example by positive/negative framing of the message or the use or non-use of qualifiers. We will address this question in more detail below.
3. Does presence of health claims affect use of other cues?
   Some cues have a summary function in the quality perception process and make, when present, the processing of other cues redundant. The major example of such a summary cue is the brand name, which consumers may view as summarizing information on various aspects of the product. Health claims may likewise be used as summary cues, and may for example lead consumers to believe that the processing of information about the nutritional content of the product is not necessary.
4. Do consumers understand the health claim correctly?
   Understanding means assigning meaning to the message. Understanding is always a constructive process and there is no one-to-one correspondence between message and perceived meaning; but in the case of health claims there is a concern about whether what the consumer understands is within the realms of the scientific dossier on the health claim. We will deal more with this question below.
5. What are the inferences from the health claim?
   It is common in the quality perception process that consumers make inferences beyond the manifest meaning of a message. This also goes for health claims, even when they are "correctly" understood. Two types of inferences have been discussed in the literature: the "magic bullet effect" and the "halo effect." The "magic bullet effect" implies that consumers may believe that if a product has a certain specific health benefit, as indicated by the health claim, then the product as a whole is also healthier than comparable products without a health claim. The "halo effect" implies that the positive evaluation that a consumer attaches to a health claim may spread to the overall evaluation of the product, so that the product is regarded as generally superior to other products without this health claim. These questions will be dealt with in more detail below.
6. How will health claims affect purchase intention?
   This refers to the question whether health claims indeed move purchases. Healthiness is almost never the only criterion when buying food, and any healthiness inferred from the health claim will be traded off against other criteria, notably taste, convenience, and production process.
7. Will the effect of health claims build up or wear off over repeated purchases?
   Since health qualities are not reinforced by immediate gratification like taste and convenience qualities are, there is the possibility that over time health-related qualities diminish in importance compared with the experience qualities (especially) taste and convenience. Continuous communication would then be necessary to remind the consumers about the health-related qualities. On the other hand, purchase of the product bearing the health claim may become habitualized and no wear-off will occur. Little is known about these longitudinal effects of health information on food products.

In the following, we will present some examples of studies shedding light on which health claims are regarded as convincing, on whether health claims are understood, and on the inferences made form health claims.

13.3   WHICH TYPE OF HEALTH CLAIM IS MOST CONVINCING?

What makes health claims convincing? Three issues have dominated the discussion on this issue. The first refers to the architecture of the health claim. Health claims usually contain one, two, or all three of the following components: information about a functional ingredient, information about the physiological function of the ingredient, and information about the health benefit. These components can occur by themselves—for example the claim "This product contains omega-3" contains only information about the active ingredient, whereas the claim "This product promotes cardiovascular health" contains only information about the health benefit. Or they can occur together—the claim "This product contains omega-3 which reduces blocking of arteries" contains information about the ingredient and about the physiological function. The claim "This product contains omega-3 which may help to keep arteries clean and therefore promote cardiovascular health" contains both ingredients, physiological function, and health benefit. Research on which combination of elements is most convincing to consumers (Bech-Larsen and Grunert 2003; van Trijp and van der Lans 2007; Verbeke et al. 2009) has not led to conclusive evidence, but failed to take into account that consumers may differ in their ability to interpret health claims, which may be related to the diverging effects. The second issue refers to whether a health claim is framed positively or negatively. The claim "This product contains omega-3 which reduces blocking of arteries" is negatively framed, whereas the claim "This product contains omega-3 which may help to keep arteries clean" is positively framed. Also research findings are not conclusive here, suggesting that whether positive or negative framing works best may depend on the type of health benefit (Svederberg 2002; van Kleef et al. 2005). Finally, the third issue refers to the use of qualifiers, like "this product *may* reduce . . .," which may make a claim less convincing because of the weaker formulation, but at the same time may increase credibility of the claim (Kapsak et al. 2008).

A recent study conducted in the five Nordic countries (Grunert et al. 2009) investigated all the above three issues by constructing claims that included all logically possible combinations of the three elements ingredient/physiological function/health benefit, which were then tested both with positive and negative framing, and with and without the use of qualifiers. Two active ingredients were used—omega-3 and bioactive peptides—and three benefits were used as examples: cardiovascular health, memory functions, and weight management, as these represent the three kinds of functions allowed in the new EU legislation (Regulation, 1924/2006).

A total of 4612 respondents filled out a survey on the web in the five Nordic countries. Claims were presented in pairs, and respondents had to decide which of the two claims in a pair was more convincing. The active ingredient and structure of the claim had the most impact on whether the claim was found convincing, whereas framing and qualifier had only a minor role. Claims containing omega-3 were found much more convincing than claims about bioactive peptides, which can be interpreted as a familiarity effect. When the active ingredient was familiar omega-3, the claim on cardiovascular health and dementia was perceived to be more convincing than claims with no ingredient or with bioactive peptides. For weight management, the ingredient did not add convincingness: not mentioning the ingredient was as convincing as having omega-3 as a functional component, the unfamiliar bioactive peptides were less convincing than not mentioning the ingredient at all. Consumers use their existing knowledge when assessing the claims and familiarity seems to be crucial for finding the claim convincing.

As regards claim architecture—the combination of information on ingredient, physiological function, and health benefit—the respondents could be divided into two groups according to the way they perceived the convincingness of the claims (Figure 13.2). The "benefit only" group (46%)

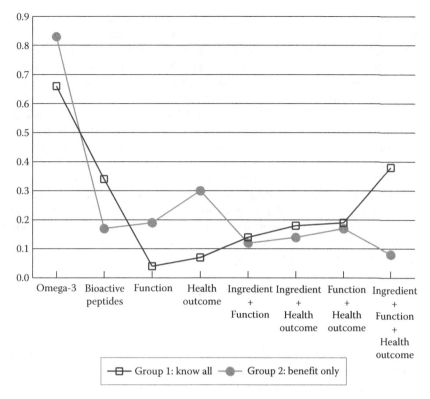

FIGURE 13.2 Effect of active ingredient and claim architecture on likelihood of finding a claim more convincing (paired comparisons). (From Grunert, K.G. et al. 2009. *Journal of Consumer Policy*, 32, 269–287.)

thought that short claims describing the function or the health outcome only were most convincing, whereas longer claims were less convincing. The other half of respondents, the "know all" group (54%), found the longest claim having the whole chain of information from ingredient via function to health outcome as most convincing. Previous exposure to health claims seems to facilitate the ability to process the information in long claims. When the shares of individuals belonging to the "benefit only" and "know all" groups were compared among the five Nordic countries, the size of "know all" people was clearly higher in Finland and Sweden, where health claims have been allowed even before EU-legislation. There were also a higher proportion of "know all" respondents among women than among men.

These results suggest that consumers' previous knowledge and experience play a major role in the perception of health claims, and that their effects therefore need to be seen in a dynamic perspective. Certain ingredients, like omega-3, can achieve brand-like status and just mentioning them, even without any information on their function and associated benefits, can be a convincing selling argument to consumers. And while consumers unfamiliar with health claims may easily be overwhelmed by excessive information and technical language, repeated exposure and processing of this type of information result in greater proficiency and may also result in a preference for more informative claims.

13.4 CONSUMER UNDERSTANDING OF HEALTH CLAIMS

If consumers do not understand the health claims that are attached on the product, the health claim has at best no effect on consumer behavior and in the worst cases misleads the consumer into believing that the product has some characteristics which it in fact does not have. Formulating health claims in a way that consumers will understand, and understand correctly, is required both by legislation and by corporate social responsibility. Health claims should therefore be tested for consumer understanding, and such testing should include a comparison of different types of potential customers, such that groups of consumers who may be especially vulnerable with regard to misunderstanding a claim can be identified. Such testing calls for a standardized methodology (Leathwood et al. 2007a). However, studies on understanding of health claims have been rather sparse. Qualitative studies showed considerable potential for consumer confusion and misunderstanding (Food Standards Agency 2002; Svederberg 2002). A few studies have related understanding to demographic criteria (low-educated consumers understand less, Fullmer et al. 1991) and previous knowledge (knowledgeable consumers understand better, Andrews et al. 2000). No standardized methodology has become adopted in the consumer research community.

A promising methodology for measuring consumer understanding of health claims is the consumer understanding test (CUT) developed by Danone (see Rogeaux 2010). CUT is a web-based approach, where the health claim is presented to respondents in the context of the packaging and/or the TV commercial in which it appears; for the packaging, respondents have the possibility to view all faces of the product. After exposure, respondents are asked two questions:

After seeing this pack and commercial, if you had to tell a friend what XXX does, what would you say?
And if you had to tell a friend how it works?

These are open questions, and respondents type their answers into a screen window. The use of open questions does not preclude any type of answer. Answers are content analyzed into a hierarchical coding scheme, and each resulting code is then categorized as follows:

- *Safe*: the statement is in line with the scientific dossier.
- *Risky*: the statement is not in line with the scientific dossier.
- *Vague*: the statement expresses a vague notion (e.g., a healthy product) or an expression that is irrelevant with regard to the health claim (e.g., the product is easy to eat).

The CUT methodology was developed according to the principles recommended by ILSI (Leathwood et al. 2007b; see also Leathwood et al., 2007a). It combines a qualitative and a quantitative approach, and it investigates how the health claim is understood in the context in which it appears in a real-life exposure situation.

As an example, a health claim for the Danone product Actimel was studied with a sample of 720 respondents in Germany (Grunert et al. 2011). The health claim was "Actimel helps strengthens the body's natural defenses" (in German: Actimel aktiviert Abwehrkräfte). Answers to the open questions on understanding of the health claim were coded and, according to the scientific dossier on the health claim, classified as *safe*, *risky*, or *vague* (where vague answers could be benefit-related or not). Depending on their coded answers, respondents were classified into three categories: respondents with answers categorized only as safe, and respondents with answers classified partly as safe and partly as vague were categorized as *safe*. Respondents with at least one answer classified as risky, or with answers that were only vague but at least partly benefit-related, were classified as *risky*. Respondents giving no answer or respondents whose answers were all vague and not benefit-related were classified as *other*.

Of the potential determinants of understanding measured, only *attitude to functional foods* emerged as a direct predictor of respondent membership in the three categories of claim understanding. The other latent constructs—interest in healthy eating and subjective knowledge on food and health—as well as the demographic characteristics of the respondent had no predictive power with regard to respondent membership in the three categories of claim understanding. Figure 13.3 shows how membership probability of the three categories of understanding is related to membership in the

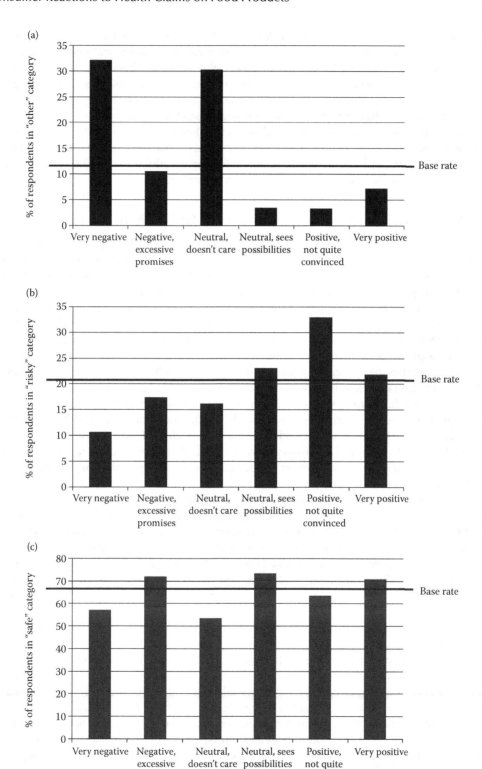

FIGURE 13.3 Relationship of attitude to functional foods to categories of claim understanding. (a) Other; (b) risky; and (c) safe. (From Grunert, K.G., Scholderer, J., and Rogeaux, M. 2011. *Appetite*, 56, 269–277.)

six categories of attitude to functional foods. We can see that respondents in the *other* category either have a very negative attitude to functional foods or do not care about functional foods. We can also see that the probability of being in the *risky* group is higher for respondents with a positive attitude to functional foods. The picture is not quite as clear with regard to membership in the *safe* category, where differences between the six categories of attitude to functional foods are less pronounced.

The study illustrates the use of the CUT methodology to study consumer understanding of health claims, and it gives an indication of which consumers may be most apt to misunderstand the health claim: those that are most enthusiastic about functional foods. Since standard measures for measuring attitude to functional foods exist (Urala and Lähteenmäki 2007), conducting tests of understanding that focus on this group of consumers is easy to implement.

13.5   WHAT ARE THE INFERENCES FROM HEALTH CLAIMS?

One specific concern about health claims has been that consumers may think that foods with health-related claims offer a "magic bullet" against all health problems or that these products are perceived as generally superior (a "halo effect"). A "magic bullet" effect occurs if a consumer associates the product with inappropriate health benefits (Roe et al. 1999). For example, from a low cholesterol claim it might be inferred that the product will automatically help against cardio-vascular disease. A "halo effect" occurs if the consumer generalizes positive perceptions to other product attributes (Roe et al. 1999). For example, a low cholesterol claim may lead to assume that the product is low in fat even though this is not mentioned in the claim.

In previous studies, health-related claims have resulted in higher ratings of perceived healthiness, but the increase has been small or moderate (Urala et al. 2003; Lyly et al. 2007; van Trijp and van der Lans 2007). Inferences to other product-quality attributes have been studied less in products with health claims, but there are suggestions that health and taste can sometime be regarded as opposite attributes so that increasing healthiness results in decreased palatability (Hamilton et al. 2000). Adding health claims to food products may on one hand increase health value by adding new health benefits, but, may on the other result in inferences on less eating quality and naturalness and thus decrease their appeal.

Effects of health claims on the perception of other product attributes (attractiveness, healthiness, naturalness, and tastiness) were studied in the Nordic investigation referred to above (Lähteenmäki et al. 2010). Respondents had to rate product descriptions (yogurt, bread, or pork chops) with different health claims according to expected tastiness, healthiness, naturalness, and overall attractiveness, and these ratings were compared with ratings of the same products without any claim. On average, putting a health claim on the product resulted in lower ratings on all attributes compared with the same product without a health claim (Figure 13.4), suggesting that negative inferences were elicited by the health claim. Also here, the familiarity of the active ingredient (omega-3 or bioactive peptides) made a big difference on how the health claims affected the perception of other attributes. With the familiar omega-3, the perceived healthiness did not change compared with the base product and decrease in perceived tastiness, attractiveness, and naturalness was clearly lower than for the unfamiliar bioactive peptides. The ingredient also had a different effect depending on the carrier product. Omega-3, was perceived positively when added to bread, but negatively when added to pork. Bioactive peptides were perceived less negatively when added to bread and yogurt than to pork. Regardless of the familiarity, both ingredients caused a major decrease in perceived naturalness. This was especially steep for pork chops and may be due to people's beliefs that adding things to raw meat requires more drastic methods than adding things to processed foods, such as yogurt and bread, although enhancement can be achieved through animal feeding. Furthermore, yogurt and bread products already are common carriers of health claims whereas meat is not.

The amount of information in the claim had an impact on how the product characteristics were perceived. Claims that contained, in addition to ingredient, information about the function and the outcome of the claim reduced the negative responses to the unfamiliar bioactive peptides, whereas

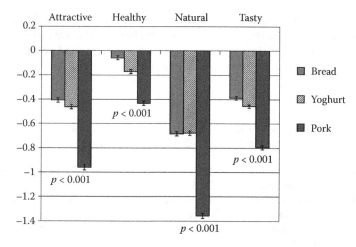

FIGURE 13.4 Effect of adding a health claim to evaluation of products on several quality dimensions (means and standard errors). (From Lähteenmäki, L. et al. 2010. *Food Policy*, 35(3), 230–239.)

for omega-3 the additional information had a mild negative impact. The former can be explained by more information increasing the awareness of the component, but the responses to omega-3 are more difficult to explain. Perhaps omega-3 elicits a number of positive associations in people's minds and specifying them to specific functions and outcomes limits these associations. However, whether the promised outcome was improving one's health or avoiding a possible disease had no impact on the perception of product characteristics. The country-wise differences among Denmark, Finland, Norway, and Sweden reflect the earlier exposure to health claims. The negative influences were the clearest in Denmark and smallest in Finland with Norway and Sweden somewhere in between.

While the average inference effects of the health claims were thus predominantly negative, there was a minority of respondents where the effects were in fact the opposite, that is, the claims did lead to positive inferences. This underlines the role of food products bearing health claims as niche products.

13.6 FUTURE OF HEALTH CLAIMS FROM A CONSUMER PERSPECTIVE

The discussion about legal restrictions of health claims, the requirements with regard to the documentation of scientific evidence, and, in Europe, the restrictive practice of the European Food Safety Authority has to a large degree masked the discussion about how consumers will react to health claims. But being allowed to put a health claim on a product is only the first step. Whether it will have any effect on the sales of a food product will depend on whether the health claim is perceived as convincing and is understood. It will also depend on which other inferences are made from the health claim, and the role it will play in the overall evaluation of a food product. Along that road, numerous pitfalls exist, resulting in health claims that may be ignored, misunderstood, or result in negative effects on overall product evaluation.

In addition, health claims are only one of many indicators that consumers use when forming opinions about the healthiness of a food product. Other product-related information that can have an impact on the evaluation of healthiness include nutrition information, ingredients, use of additives, the degree of processing, whether the product is artisanal or industrial, origin, and whether the product is organic. This is complemented by information that consumers obtain from the media and from word-of-mouth.

For food manufacturers trying to develop and market products based on health benefits, this implies that health claims have to be seen in the context of market communication. Consumers form opinions about food products, including their healthiness and health benefits, based on the totality of information that is available on these products. Health claims will always only be a part of this, albeit an important one. Health claims are not a panacea for modern food production, but just one element in the process of developing and marketing healthy food products.

REFERENCES

Andrews, J.C., Burton, S., and Netemeyer, R.G. 2000. Are some comparative nutrition claims misleading? The role of nutrition knowledge, and claim type and disclosure conditions. *Journal of Advertising*, 29(3), 29–42.

Andrews, J.C., Netemeyer, R.G., and Burton, S. 1998. Consumer generalization of nutrient content claims in advertising. *Journal of Marketing*, 62(4), 62–75.

Bech-Larsen, T. and Grunert, K.G. 2003. The perceived healthiness of functional foods. A conjoint study of Danish, Finnish and American consumers' perception of functional foods. *Appetite*, 40, 9–14.

Food Standards Agency. 2002. *Health Claims and Food Packaging—Consumer-Related Qualitative Research.* London: Food Standards Agency.

Ford, G.T., Hastak, M., Mitra, A., and Ringold, D.J. 1996. Can consumers interpret nutrition information in the presence of a health claim? *Journal of Public Policy & Marketing*, 15, 16–27.

Fullmer, S., Geiger, C.J., and Parent, C.R. 1991. Consumers' knowledge, understanding, and attitudes toward health claims on food labels. *Journal of the American Dietetic Association*, 91, 166–171.

Garretson, J.A. and Burton, S. 2000. Effects of nutrition facts panel values, nutrition claims, and health claims on consumer attitudes, perceptions of disease-related risks, and trust. *Journal of Public Policy & Marketing*, 19, 213–227.

Grunert, K.G. 2005. Food quality and safety: Consumer perception and demand. *European Review of Agricultural Economics*, 32(3), 369–391.

Grunert, K.G., Lähteenmäki, L., Boztug, Y., Martinsdottir, E., Ueland, O., Åström, A., and Lampila, P. 2009. Perception of health claims among Nordic consumers. *Journal of Consumer Policy*, 32, 269–287.

Grunert, K.G., Scholderer, J., and Rogeaux, M. 2011. Determinants of consumer understanding of health claims. *Appetite*, 56, 269–277.

Hamilton, J., Knox, B., Hill, D., and Parr, H. 2000. Reduced fat products. Consumer perceptions and preferences. *British Food Journal*, 102, 494–506.

Ippolito, P.M. and Mathios, A.D. 1991, Health claims in food marketing: Evidence on knowledge and behaviour in the cereal market. *Journal of Public Policy & Marketing*, 10, 15–32.

Ippolito, P.M. and Mathios, A.D. 1994. Information, policy, and the sources of fat and cholesterol in the U.S. diet. *Journal of Public Policy & Marketing*, 13, 200–217.

Kapsak, W.R., Schmidt, D., Childs, N.M., Meunier, J., and White, C. 2008. Consumer perception of graded, graphic and text label presentations for qualified health claims. *Critical Reviews in Food Science and Nutrition*, 48, 248–256.

Kozup, J.C., Creyer, E.H., and Burton, S. 2003. Making healthful food choices: The influence of health claims and nutrition information on consumers' evaluations of packaged food products and restaurant menu items. *Journal of Marketing*, 67(2), 19–34.

Lähteenmäki, L., Lampila, P., Grunert, K.G., Boztug, Y., Ueland, Ø., Åström, A., and Martinsdottir, E. 2010. Impact of health-related claims on the perception of other product attributes. *Food Policy*, 35(3), 230–239.

Leathwood, P.D., Richardson, D.P., Sträter, P., Todd, P.M., and van Trijp, H.C.M. 2007a. Consumer understanding of nutrition and health claims: Sources of evidence. *British Journal of Nutrition*, 98, 474–484.

Leathwood, P.D., MacFie, H., and van Trijp, Hans 2007b. *Consumer Understanding of Health Claims.* Summary report of a workshop held in May 2006. Brussels: ILSI Europe.

Lyly, M., Roininen, K., Honkapää, K., and Lähteenmäki, L. 2007. Factors influencing consumers willingness to use beverages and ready-to-eat frozen soups containing oat ß-glucan in Finland, France and Sweden. *Food Quality and Preference,* 18, 242–255.

Mazis, M.B. and Raymond, M.A. 1997. Consumer perceptions of health claims in advertisements and on food labels. *Journal of Consumer Affairs*, 31, 10–26.

Mitra, A., Hastak, M., Ford, G.T., and Ringold, D.J. 1999. Can the educationally disadvantaged interpret the FDA-mandated nutrition fact panels in the presence of an implied health claim? *Journal of Public Policy & Marketing*, 18, 106–117.

Pothoulaki, M. and Chryssochoidis, G. 2009. Health claims: Consumers' matters. *Journal of Functional Foods*, 1, 222–228.

Roe, B., Levy, A.S., and Derby, B.M. 1999. The impact of health claims on consumer search and product evaluation outcomes: Results from FDA experimental data. *Journal of Public Policy & Marketing*, 18, 89–105.

Rogeaux, M. 2010. Consumer understanding and reaction to health claims: Insights and methodology. In: S.R. Jaeger and H. MacFie (Eds.), *Consumer-Driven Innovation in Food and Personal Care Products* (pp. 277–302). Cambridge: Woodhead.

Svederberg, E. 2002. *Consumers Views Regarding Health Claims on Two Food Packages*. Lund: Department of Education, Lund University.

Urala, N., Arvola, A., and Lähteenmäki, L. 2003. Strength of health-related claims and their perceived advantage. *International Journal of Food Science and Technology*, 38, 815–826.

Urala, N. and Lähteenmäki, L. 2007. Consumers' changing attitudes towards functional foods. *Food Quality and Preference*, 18, 1–12.

Van Kleef, E., van Trijp, H.C.M., and Luning, P. 2005. Functional foods: Health claim—Food product compatibility and the impact of health claim framing on consumer evaluation. *Appetite*, 44, 299–308.

Van Trijp, H.C.M. and van der Lans, I.A. 2007. Consumer perceptions of nutrition and health claims. *Appetite*, 48, 305–324.

Verbeke, W., Scholderer, J., and Lähteenmäki, L. 2009. Consumer appeal of nutrition and health claims in three existing product concepts. *Appetite*, 52, 684–692.

Williams, P. 2005. Consumer understanding and use of health claims for foods. *Nutrition Reviews*, 63, 256–264.

Section IV

Technological Development on Healthy and Functional Foods

14 Effect of Processing on Nutrients in Foods

Fanbin Kong and R. Paul Singh

CONTENTS

A major aim of food processing and preservation is to extend the shelf life of food products by eliminating pathogenic microorganisms and inactivating spoilage bacteria and enzymes. Meanwhile, processing can improve digestibility, quality, and the availability of nutrients, and offer desirable sensory quality attributes. Food processing impacts nutritional properties of food by modifying macro- and micronutrients. For example, protein is denatured by heat; nonenzymatic browning reactions occur between amino acids and sugars in food during heating that influence protein bioavailability. Lipid oxidation takes place causing rancidity problems. Food processing can also cause degradation and loss of vitamins and minerals, especially water-soluble vitamins (vitamin B and C) due to mass transfer, thermal breakdown, and enzymatic oxidation. The extent of losses depends on the type of nutrients, pH and water content of food, the type of food, especially the structure of food matrix, and the processing conditions such as temperature, light, and oxygen.

This chapter discusses the impact of some of the major food-processing techniques on the nutritional components with a particular focus on vitamins. Processing approaches discussed include heating, drying, freezing, and newly developed processing technologies, such as high-pressure processing (HPP) and use of pulsed electric field (PEF). Vitamins are the most sensitive nutrients in foods. Food processing also affects minerals, fiber, and phytochemicals; however, the effect is generally minimal compared to vitamins (Dewanto et al. 2002; Rickman et al. 2007a,b) and is not covered in this chapter. The rate kinetics of vitamin loss during food processing is briefly reviewed.

14.1 STABILITY OF VITAMINS

Vitamins can be categorized into water- and fat-soluble vitamins. Water-soluble vitamins, including vitamin B-group and C, are generally more unstable than fat-soluble vitamins (including vitamins K, A, D, and E). Vitamin C (ascorbic acid), B1 (thiamin), and B3 (folate) are among the most unstable vitamins. High levels of heat, light, and/or oxygen promote nutrient loss. Thiamin is extremely sensitive to heat. Vitamin A and C are sensitive to oxidative degradation. Riboflavin is highly light sensitive. B-group vitamins are generally sensitive to neutral and alkaline pH. Some vitamins are relatively stabler during processing and storage, including niacin (vitamin B3), vitamin K, vitamin D, biotin (vitamin B7), and pantothenic acid (vitamin B5). Table 14.1 is a summary of the sensitivity of vitamins to heat, light, oxygen, and pH conditions.

Ascorbic acid (vitamin C) is one of the least stable vitamins. It is often used as an indicator to evaluate the influence of food processing and preservation on vitamin content. The extent of vitamin C loss is dependent on temperature, presence of oxygen, light, pH (stable in acidic environment), and metal ions (copper). Leaching causes the most loss of vitamin C. The water-soluble nature of vitamin C renders it prone to leaching into the surrounding medium when large amount of water is combined into the process. Especially, boiling can cause up to 80–90% loss of vitamin C in vegetables. Oxidation is another important cause. The highly unsaturated structure of ascorbic acid makes it easily oxidized during heating, where ascorbic acid is oxidized into dehydroascorbic acid (DHA). The DHA further degrades into 3-hydroxy-2-pyrone (3H2P) at pH 2–5, 2-furoic acid (2FA) at pH < 2 and 2,5-dimethyl-4-hydroxy-3(2H)-furanone (DMHF) at pH > 5. Vitamin C is stable in the absence of oxygen. The typical large surface area of vegetables causes high cooking loss due to the easy accessibility to water and oxygen.

Thiamin is degraded by thermal breakdown and oxidation. The presence of heat, air, or oxygen enhances the degradation. Sulfites, SO_2, and alkali contribute to the loss of thiamin. Thiamin loss in salmon fillet during canning can be up to 80% (Kong et al. 2007). Leaching is also a major cause of thiamin loss due to its water-soluble nature.

Riboflavin (vitamin B2) is stable against heat and oxidation. However, riboflavin is highly light sensitive and easily decays under UV and visible light especially with alkaline condition. Milk can lose half of the vitamin B2 after exposure to sunlight for 2 h.

Loss of folates is due to thermal degradation and leaching. A typical cooking process of spinach can cause up to 50% loss of folates (McKillop et al. 2002). It is more resistant to heat in natural and basic solutions. Oxygen, pH, and metal ion concentrations such as copper all affect its degradation. The presence of reducing agents such as ascorbic acid can increase folate retention.

TABLE 14.1
Stability of Vitamins

	Heat	Light	Oxygen	Acid	Alkali
Fat Soluble					
Vitamin A	O	OO	OO	O	X
Vitamin D	O	OO	OO	O	O
Vitamin E	O	O	O	X	O
Vitamin K	X	OO	O	X	OO
Water Soluble					
Vitamin C	O	X	OO	O	OO
B-complex					OO
Thiamin	OO	O	X	X	OO
Riboflavin	X	OO	X	X	OO
Niacin	X	X	X	X	X
Vitamin B6	X	O	X	O	O
Vitamin B12	X	O	X	OO	OO
Pantothenic acid	O	X	X	OO	OO
Folic acid	X	O	OO	O	O
Biotin	X	X	X	O	O

Note: OO, very sensitive; O, sensitive; X, not sensitive.

Niacin is the stablest vitamin resistant to heat and oxygen. The major reason of niacin loss is leaching into cooking water. Similarly, biotin is stable during heat treatment. About 70–90% of biotin survives through thermal processing in fruits and vegetables, legumes, milk, and meat.

For fat-soluble vitamins, vitamin A, such as retinol and carotenoids, is susceptible to heat, oxygen, and light degradation due to its unsaturated structure. Oxidation is the major cause of carotenoid degradation (Achir et al. 2010). The presence of oxygen, metals, enzymes, unsaturated lipids, and other prooxidant molecules promote oxidation. Also, isomerization of carotenoids can occur in which *trans*-carotenoid is converted to *cis*-carotenoid that reduces the nutritive value of vegetables.

Vitamin D is mostly stable but can be oxidized when exposed to heat and light. It is also leached into the liquid medium, for example, due to fat drip in meats. Vitamin E (tocopherol) can be easily oxidized. For example, boiling of rabbit meat at 100°C for 8 min caused 39% loss of α-tocopherol (Dal Bosco et al. 2001).

14.2 EFFECT OF PROCESSING ON THE LOSS OF VITAMINS

14.2.1 HEATING

Heat treatment is the most common method of food processing, including canning, blanching, pasteurization, baking, frying, extrusion, steaming, microwave heating, ohmic heating, and infrared heating. Canning is one of the severest heating processes aimed to removing all pathogenic and spoilage microorganisms and destroying enzymes, with long time (up to 1 h) heating at high temperatures (e.g., 121°C). Vitamin loss occurs mainly in water-soluble vitamin C and B due to heat degradation, oxidization, and leaching into the liquid medium. On average, canned vegetables retain 60% of the water-soluble vitamins, with 20% dispersed in liquid and 40% in the solids. More vitamin loss occurs in the outer layer of food receiving more heat than the core area. Blanching is a mild heating condition in which fruits and vegetables are heated in boiling water, steam, or hot air for a few minutes. It is frequently used before freezing to inactivate enzymes, and before canning to remove air. Pasteurization is used for fruit juice and milk to inactivate pathogenic and food spoilage microorganisms. The less severe heating in blanching and pasteurization helps retain more vitamins than canning. Słupski (2011) reported vitamin C retention in flageolet bean after blanching, cooking, and sterilization being 71–82%, 56–63%, and 29–44%, respectively. In milk, pasteurization caused about 20% loss of ascorbic acid and 10% loss of vitamin B1, while sterilization and evaporation caused about 60% loss of vitamin C and 50% of vitamin B1.

Leaching of vitamins into the cooking medium (water) is usually the largest portion of the loss. Boiling causes the largest vitamin loss, especially water-soluble vitamin C, thiamin, and riboflavin. Golaszewska and Zalewski (2001) reported that potato can retain 83–92% of vitamin C by dry methods, and 60–80% by wet methods of heating. Approaches that involve less water can improve vitamin retention. Steam blanching results in less leaching loss than boiling. The retention of vitamin C can be up to 99% in steaming as compared to 25% for boiling (Lešková et al. 2006). Similarly, minerals present in foods may leach into the liquid medium although they are usually stable in heat.

Boiling also results in higher loss of carotenoids than stewing, steaming, microwave cooking, and pressure steaming. Stir-frying vegetables with oil leads to a greater retention of β-carotene than those stir-fried with water (Masrizal et al. 1997). Cooking has a complicated effect on β-carotene. It can lead to oxidation and isomerization of *trans*-β-carotene, reducing the nutritional value, but on the other hand it can increase the release of β-carotene by disruption of the plant cell wall that improves its extractability (Bernhardt and Schlich 2006). Dewanto et al. (2002) reported higher total antioxidant activity in tomatoes after heating at 88°C up to 30 min, despite vitamin C loss, due to increased extractability of lycopene.

Pretreatment may affect vitamin loss during heat treatment. Xue et al. (2011) reported that soaking strongly affected the reduction of folate in navy beans cooked in distilled water for 10–40 min.

The folate loss was 16.3–64% in nonsoaked beans, 25.8–79% in beans presoaked for 6 h, and 33.1–84.9% in 12 h soaked beans. Soaking weakens the matrix structure, facilitating release and diffusion of nutrients into the cooking medium.

Reducing heating time and using lower temperature improves nutrient retention. Chen et al. (1995) reported that canning of carrot juice resulted in the highest destruction of vitamin A (55.7%), followed by 120°C heating (48.8%) and 110°C heating (45.2%). In canning, container size and shape affect heating time thereby affecting the degradation of vitamins. When pouches are used to replace cans, the heating time is reduced with improved retention of nutrients. High-temperature short-time processing (HTST) is preferred due to the high retention of nutrient quality. The use of this principle is preferred due to the greater sensitivity of bacteria to temperature than nutrient (Singh and Heldman 2009).

New technologies are emerging such as electromagnetic heating, including ohmic heating, microwave heating, and infrared heating. These technologies have the advantage of rapid heating that improves retention of nutrients. Vikram et al. (2005) compared the retention of vitamin C during thermal treatment of orange juice heated by electromagnetic heating (infrared, ohmic, and microwave heating) in comparison with conventional heating. Ohmic heating generates heat the fastest, followed by microwave, and infrared heating. Correspondingly, ohmic heating also retained the most vitamin C.

Table 14.2 summarizes the literature about thermal effects on nutrient loss. Readers may also refer to recent review papers by Singh et al. (2007) and Ruiz-Rodriguez et al. (2008).

14.2.2 Drying (Dehydration)

Drying is one of the most ancient food preservation technologies, and it is used for a large range of food materials such as fruits, vegetables, dairy products, and cereals. Various drying technologies are available, including solar and sun drying, hot air drying, microwave drying, freezing drying, and osmotic dehydration. Hot air drying is the most commonly used method in the food industry to dry fruit and vegetables, grains, and other products. The operating conditions employed for convective drying range from 40°C to 110°C in air temperature, and 0.1–5 m/s in air velocity. The drying time varies depending upon product formulation, dimension, and final moisture of the product.

Vitamin C and carotenoids are among the vitamins with most loss during drying. The level of nutrient loss is mostly dependent upon drying temperature, duration, and exposure to oxygen. Hot air drying at 80°C can cause 92% loss of vitamin C in blueberries (López et al. 2010). Nutrient retention is improved when low temperatures are used. Inert gas drying and vacuum drying decrease nutrient loss. Also, the shape and size of product, final moisture, and air velocity affect vitamin retention through influencing drying time. Small size (thickness) can reduce drying time thus increasing vitamin retention.

Blanching is often used prior to drying to inactivate enzymes and reduce microbial load. Unblanched vegetables can lose 80% of carotene while blanched products have losses to <5% depending on the product (Ramesh et al. 2001). Blanching in sulfite solution can improve the retention of vitamin C due to the protective effect on ascorbic acid degradation as well as oxidation.

Microwave drying, commonly used in the drying of pasta and postbaking of biscuits, can greatly reduce the drying time than hot air drying due to the fast volumetric heating, which favors nutrient retention. The vitamin loss is also dependent on the microwave power (Santos and Silva 2008). Khraisheh et al. (2004) compared retention of vitamin C in potatoes during microwave drying and air drying. Air drying (30°C) caused 70% reduction of vitamin C, while the loss of vitamin C in the samples dried by microwaves (10.5 W) was <25%. However, when higher microwave power (38 W) was used, vitamin C loss increased to 55%. Microwave–vacuum (MWV) drying, a combination of vacuum and microwave drying, further reduces drying time and lowers drying temperature, which is advantageous for drying bulk products with poor thermal conductivity, and thermal-sensitive

TABLE 14.2

Effect of Heat Treatment on Nutrient Loss

Food Item	Analyzed Nutrient	Treatment and Conditions	Nutrient Retention/Loss	Reference
Broccoli	Vitamin C	Conventional cooking 5 min	72.8% retention in conventional cooking	Vallejo et al. (2002)
		High-pressure cooking 3 min	74.5% in high pressure cooking	
		Steam cooking 3.5 min	99.7% in steaming cooking	
		Microwave 5 min	54% in microwave	
Brinjal, bitter gourd, colocasia, and tomato	Ascorbic acid	Boiling	61.45% loss in brinjal, 53.42% in bitter gourd, 49.92% in colocasia, 89.12% in tomato	Alvi et al. (2003)
Pork loin	Thiamin, vitamin B_2, vitamin B_6	Traditional cooking	72% retention of thiamin, 90% retention of vitamin B_2, 82% retention of vitamin B_6	Lassen et al. (2002)
Orange juice	Vitamin C	Thermal pasteurization (90°C, 1 min)	82.4% retention	Elez-Martínez and Martín-Belloso (2007)
Milk	Vitamin B1 Vitamin B6 (pyridoxamine pyridoxal)	Continuous-flow microwave and conventional heating	Vitamin B1 content unchanged; pyridoxamine increased by 4–5% in microwave and 9–11% in conventional heating, respectively; pyridoxal decreased by 5–6% in microwave and 9–12% in conventional heating, respectively	Sierra and Vidal-Valverde (2001)
Flageolet bean	Vitamin C	Blanching, cooking, sterilizing	71–82% retention for blanching, 56–63% for cooking, 29–44% for sterilization	Słupski (2011)
Carrot slices	Vitamin C β-carotene	Boiling 1 min	Vitamin C: 80% retention β-Carotene: 92% retention	Frias et al. (2010)
Oil (vegetaline and palm olein)	*Trans*-β-carotene	Deep-fat frying at 120°C/120 min, 140°C/90 min, 160°C/60 min and 180°C/30 min	Retention of *trans*-β-carotene for vegetaline and palm olein: 52% and 20% at 120°C/120 min; 38% and 2% at 140°C/90 min, 13% and 7% at 160°C/60 min. No difference in the two oils at 180°C 30 min.	Achir et al. (2010)
Tomato puree	Carotenoids, total polyphenols, vitamin C	Heated for 10 min at 92°C, concentration, sterilization	No significant effect for carotenoids. Loss of total polyphenols: 28–43%. Loss of vitamin C: 80%	Georgé et al. (2011)
Pepper	Ascorbic acid	Boiling; steaming; microwave; pressure steaming; stewing	Maximum loss: 30% in boiling	Bernhardt and Schlich (2006)
Carrot	Vitamin C, β-carotene	Boiling for 1 min	80% retention for vitamin C and 92% for β-Carotene	Frias et al. (2010)

continued

TABLE 14.2　(continued)
Effect of Heat Treatment on Nutrient Loss

Food Item	Analyzed Nutrient	Treatment and Conditions	Nutrient Retention/Loss	Reference
Chickpea	B-vitamin	Boiling, autoclaving, microwave cooking	48–59% retention of riboflavin, 33–43% thiamin, 4–14% niacin, 57–81% pyridoxine. Loss: microwave < autoclaving < boiling	Alajaji and El-Adawy (2006)
Spinach, broccoli	Folate	Boiling for typical time periods; steaming 5 min; grilling 16 min	49% retention of folate in spinach and 44% in broccoli after boiling; no significant decrease in folate content after steaming; 95% retention of folate after grilling	McKillop et al. (2002)
Milk	Vitamin B12	Sterilization	Loss: 20%	Ottaway (2002)
Carrot juice	Vitamin A	Canning (121°C, 30 min) HTST heating (120°C for 30 s) and 110°C for 30 s	Canning causes the highest destruction of vitamin A (55.7%), followed by 120°C heating (48.8%), and 110°C heating (45.2%)	Chen et al. (1995)
Amaranth leaves, drumstick leaves, carrot, and pumpkin	β-Carotene	Pressure cooking (10 min at 15 psi) boiling for 10 min	Loss of 27–71% after pressure cooking and 16–67% after boiling	Gayathri et al. (2004)
Navy beans	Saponins B	Autoclaving	Destroy most of saponins B	Shi et al. (2009)
Tomato juice	Total carotenoids and lycopene contents	Thermal treatment hot break (92°C; 2 min) or cold break (60°C; 2 min)	Loss: insignificantly decreased about 1%	Hsu (2008)
Salmon fillet	Thiamin	Canning (100–131°C)	Loss: 68%, 83%, 91%, and 93% after heating at 100°C/180 min, 111.1°C/150 min, 121.1°C/120 min, and 131.1°C/90 min	Kong et al. (2007)
Palm and soy oils	Vitamin E content	Repeated heating (5 times)	Up to 98% of the three most abundant vitamin E fractions in the palm oil (α-tf, α-tt, and γ-tt) were destroyed	Adam et al. (2007)
Flageolet beans	Vitamin C L-ascorbic acid	Blanching cooking	Retention: 71–82% of vitamin C and 63–84% of ascorbic acid after blanching; 56–63% of vitamin C and 52–69% of ascorbic acid after cooking	Słupski (2011)
Rabbit meat	α-Tocopherol	Boiling (100°C/8 min), frying (175°C/3 min, and roasting 200°C/15 min)	Loss of 39% after boiling, 12% after frying and 14% after roasting	Dal Bosco et al. (2001)

products such as fruits and vegetables. Clary et al. (2008) compared MWV drying and sun drying in grape dehydration. Microwave-dried raisins contained 378 IU/100 g vitamin A, while in sun-dried raisins vitamin A was not detectable. Vitamin C was 12.5 mg/100 g in microwave-dried raisins as compared to 8.83 mg/100 g in sun-dried raisins. Thiamin and riboflavin were about twice the contents in microwave-dried raisins as in the sun-dried raisins.

Osmotic dehydration involves soaking fruits and vegetables in hypertonic solution (i.e., sucrose, salt), and water in the food moves out of the food into the solution. The process is driven by the difference between osmotic pressures of osmotic agent and plant tissue. It is energy efficient and may offer dried food better quality without shrinkage. Substantial amount of nutrients can also leach into the solution causing vitamin loss. Chemical deterioration of vitamins also occurs especially at high temperature. Cao et al. (2006) analyzed vitamin C loss in sliced kiwifruit (8 mm thickness) and reported 12–30.4% ascorbic acid loss when dehydrated in 60% sucrose concentration, at 30–40°C temperatures for 150 min. It was found that temperature of the osmotic solution was the most significant factor affecting the loss of ascorbic acid, followed by slice thickness and duration of treatment. Alam et al. (2010) reported 68.4–91.1% vitamin C loss in aonla slices during dehydration in 50–70° Brix of sugar concentration at 30–60°C solution temperature for 60–180 min.

Freeze drying is considered to be one of the best methods for heat-sensitive materials to maintain product quality due to the use of low temperature during drying. However, it is the most expensive process and more time consuming. In addition, freeze-dried products are generally more porous. The high porosity facilitates oxygen transfer that promotes rapid oxidation of vitamin C and carotenoids. Also, when freeze-dried products are cooked, more cooking loss can occur. Freeze drying can be combined with other drying technologies to save energy. Cui et al. (2008) evaluated combination of MWV drying and freeze drying to process carrots and apples. The retention of vitamin C in apples was 91.8%, 97%, 89%, and 63.7%, respectively, for MWV drying + freeze drying, freeze drying alone, MWV drying alone, and hot air drying, and the retention of carotene in carrots was 94.9%, 95.4%, 94.7%, and 70.6%, respectively, for the four different methods. Compared with freeze drying, combined MWV and freeze drying obtained comparable high-quality products with shorter drying time and less energy consumption.

Ultrasound drying is another novel drying technique in which ultrasound wave travels through the food materials leading to rapid compressions and expansions and producing cavitation in the food matrix, facilitating moisture removal without significantly heating the product. The minimal thermal effect preserves heat-sensitive food constituents improving the retention of vitamin C and β-carotene. Frias et al. (2010) reported 82–92% of vitamin C retention for ultrasound-dried carrots (blanched), as compared to <50% of air-dried products.

A summary of the literature on the effects of various drying techniques on vitamins is shown in Table 14.3.

14.2.3 FREEZE PRESERVATION

Freezing and frozen storage extend shelf life of food products while maintaining sensory and nutrient characteristics. The influence of freezing on vitamin C is generally minimal (Ancos et al. 2000; Gonçalves et al. 2009). However, during frozen storage, the loss of vitamin C can be significant due to oxidation. Ancos et al. (2000) reported loss of 33–55% vitamin C in raspberry after frozen storage for 12 months. Gonçalves et al. (2009) reported that after 400 days frozen storage at temperatures of −7°C, −15°C, and −30°C, the ascorbic acid content in watercress decreased by 95%, 93%, and 76%, respectively. Degradation of carotenoids through enzymatic oxidation is another major vitamin loss. The loss of carotenoids in pumpkin pieces was 35–40% at 0°C, 15–20% at −18°C, and 25–30% at −40°C (Dutta et al. 2009).

In spite of the loss of nutrients during blanching of food products, blanching inhibits further vitamin loss by inactivating enzyme activity during storage. Patras et al. (2011) reported a greater stability of nutritional parameters for blanched frozen carrots and broccoli during storage compared

TABLE 14.3

Effect of Drying on Nutrient Loss

Food	Nutrients	Treatment Conditions	Nutrient Retention/Loss (%)	Reference
Unblanched and blanched carrots	Vitamin C and β-carotene	Convective air drying (40°C and 65°C; air flow rate 2–6 × 10⁻¹ m/s); ultrasound drying (20°C, 40°C, and 60°C for 120, 90, and 75 min)	Retention: 32–50% for vitamin C and 73–90% for β-carotene after blanching + convective air drying; 55% for vitamin C and 88% for β-carotene after blanching + ultrasound drying	Frias et al. (2010)
Blueberry	Vitamin C	Hot air drying (80°C)	92% loss	López et al. (2010)
Grapes	Vitamin A, C, thiamin, riboflavin, and niacin	Microwave–vacuum drying; sun drying	Vitamin A: 378 IU/100 g after microwave–vacuum drying and undetectable after sun drying; vitamin C: 12.5 mg/100 g after microwave–vacuum drying and 8.83 mg/100 g after sun drying; thiamin and riboflavin twice in microwave–vacuum-dried raisins as in the sun-dried raisins	Clary et al. (2008)
Carrot, apple	Carotene in carrot; vitamin C in apple	Freeze drying: frozen at −25°C for 205 min + freeze drying; MWV + freeze drying: MWV to remove moisture to 48% for carrot slices, and 37% for apple slices + freeze drying; Microwave–vacuum drying and conventional hot air (60–65°C, 0.5 m/s velocity) were used too	The retention of vitamin C in apple was 91.8%, 97%, 89%, 63.7%, respectively, for MWV drying + freeze drying, freeze drying alone, MWV drying alone, and hot air drying; and the retention of carotene in carrots was 94.9%, 95.4%, 94.7%, and 70.6%, respectively.	Cui et al. (2008)
Kiwifruit	Vitamin C	Osmotic dehydration (60% sucrose concentration, 30–40°C temperatures, 150 min time, and 8 mm thickness)	12–30.4% loss	Cao et al. (2006)
Aonla	Vitamin C	Osmotic dehydration (sugar concentration 50–70° Brix, solution temperature 30–60°C, solution to fruit ratio (4:1–8:1) and immersion time 60–180 min	68.4–91.1% loss	Alam et al. (2010)
Carrot	Vitamin C and β-carotene	Convective air drying (40 and 65°C, air flow rate 0.2–0.6 m/s), and power ultrasound drying (20, 40, and 60°C for 120, 90, and 75 min)	Retention of 32–50% vitamin C and 73–90% β-carotene, respectively, for blanching + air drying; 82–92% and 96–98%, respectively, for blanching + ultrasound drying	Frias et al. (2010)

TABLE 14.3 (continued)
Effect of Drying on Nutrient Loss

Food	Nutrients	Treatment Conditions	Nutrient Retention/Loss (%)	Reference
Red and yellow tomatoes	β-Carotene, polyphenol, vitamin C	One-week lyophilization (freezing at −20°C, followed by two successive drying steps at 0.5 and 0.1 mbar, respectively, at 10°C). The samples were then stored at −20°C for a maximum of 3 months	Loss of β-carotene was 14% (red tomato) and 11% (yellow tomato) The total polyphenol content in red tomato was not affected by lyophilization The vitamin C content was not affected by lyophilization in both varieties	Georgé et al. (2011)
Tomato	Lycopene	Freeze drying	Loss: 33–48%	Chang et al. (2006)
Potato	Vitamin C	Microwave (10.5 W) and convective drying (30°C)	Microwave- and air-dried samples retained 75% and 30% of vitamin C, respectively	Khraisheh et al. (2004)

to unblanched frozen samples, including a lower rate of degradation in ascorbic acid and a higher antioxidant activity.

In practice, normal storage temperature for frozen foods is between −25°C and −18°C. However, temperature fluctuation can occur where temperature could rise by −2°C to −10°C (Giannakourou and Taoukis 2003). The temperature abuse can greatly enhance oxidation of vitamin C. Therefore, it is important to maintain proper storage conditions, especially temperature. In addition, large surface area of food increases oxygen accessibility, contributing to vitamin loss during frozen storage. For example, spinach leaf is more prone to vitamin C degradation than peas partly due to its high surface area (Giannakourou and Taoukis 2003). Subsequent thawing will cause more vitamin loss for frozen foods. The drip loss during thawing of frozen meat can cause loss of 10% of the water-soluble vitamins. It is recommended that frozen vegetables should not be thawed before cooking (Nursal and Yücecan 2000). Table 14.4 is a summary of the literature on nutrient loss caused by freezing and frozen storage.

14.2.4 HIGH-PRESSURE PROCESSING

HPP of foods involves application of high hydrostatic pressure (100–1000 MPa) to inactivate microorganisms. The processing temperature is often between 0°C to above 100°C, and processing time ranges from a few seconds to over 20 min. HPP can work on food uniformly and instantaneously throughout the food despite the irregular geometry, which is a unique feature distinguishing it from other preservation technologies such as canning.

Due to the limited effect of pressure on covalent bonds, HPP at moderate pressure and temperatures cause minimal or no major degradation of vitamins and tend to produce nutritious and fresh-like food products. Patras et al. (2009) found no significant changes in ascorbic acid and anthocyanin content in strawberry and blackberry purees treated by pressures of 400, 500, or 600 MPa for 15 min at room temperature. Also, higher stability of carotenes of carrot juice during pressure treatment up to 300 MPa was observed than heat treatment (105°C, 30 s) (Kim et al. 2001).

Vitamin loss can increase significantly at high pressure and temperature, such as in pressure-assisted thermal processing (PATP), referring to simultaneous application of high pressure (600–700 MPa) and thermal treatments (90–120°C) to pasteurize and sterilize foods. A higher loss of

TABLE 14.4
Effect of Freezing on Nutrient Loss

Food	Nutrients	Treatment Conditions	Nutrient Retention/ Loss (%)	Reference
Watercress	Vitamin C	Frozen storage for 400 days	Loss of vitamin C: 95%, 93%, and 76%, respectively, at temperatures of −7, −15, and −30°C	Gonçalves et al. (2009)
Chicken liver	Retinol	−18°C for 90 days	Loss: 44.1%	Santos et al. (2009)
Rye breads	Folate	−18°C for 2, 5, 16 weeks	No significant loss after 2 weeks; loss was 14% after 5 weeks and 25–38% after 16 weeks	Gujska et al. (2009)
Okra, potatoes, green beans, broccoli, spinach, and peas	Vitamin C	−18°C, 6 month	Loss: 27.6–57.9%	Tosun and Yücecan (2008)
Broccoli, carrots	Vitamin C	Blanching (95°C for 3 min)/ unblanching + blast freezing + chilled storage (7 days)	Reaction rate constant (k) increased from 1.06×10^{-1} day^{-1} to 1.17×10^{-1} day^{-1} for blanched and unblanched broccoli florets and from 4.6×10^{-3} to 1.98×10^{-1} day^{-1} for blanched and unblanched carrots	Patras et al. (2011)
Raspberry fruit	Ellagic acid, vitamin C, total phenolics	Frozen at −80°C in liquid nitrogen for 15 min, then stored at −20°C for 12 months	No significant change of total phenolic content. Loss of 14–21% in ellagic acid and 33–55% in vitamin C	Ancos et al. (2000)
Pumpkin pieces	Carotenoids	Thermally treated pumpkin pieces stored at 0, −18°C and −40°C for 80 days	Loss: 35–40% at 0°C, 15–20% at −18°C and 25–30% at −40°C	Dutta et al. (2009)
Homogenates of collard greens, clementines, and russet potatoes	Vitamin C	Stored at −60°C and analyzed at time points up to 49 weeks	Stable in clementines, loss in collard greens and potatoes was 13.7% and 26.0%, respectively.	Phillips et al. (2010)

β-carotenes in carrot juice under PATP conditions (300–500 MPa and 50–70°C, for 10 min) than under pressure alone was observed by Kim et al. (2001). Doblado et al. (2007) reported that the loss of vitamin C in HPP-processed germinated cowpeas increased from 9% to 41% when pressure was increased from 300 to 500 MPa and the loss increased with pressure. Pressure and temperature have synergistic effect on the nutrient loss, for example, loss of 5-ethyltetrahydrofolate was significantly increased with increasing pressure at temperature >40°C, while below 40°C it is pressure stable (Ramirez et al. 2009). It is also noted that nutrients are different in their sensitivity of reactions toward pressure (activation volume) and temperature (activation energy) which cause a varying effect on nutrient loss (Oey et al. 2008). Oxygen enhances the oxidation of ascorbic acid during HPP. Eliminating oxygen in packaging inhibits degradation of vitamin C during processing and subsequent storage (Ramirez et al. 2009). Food matrix and composition can have significant effect; the ascorbic acid degradation is severer in orange juice than in tomato juice (van den Broeck et al. 1998). The presence of antioxidant improves nutrient retention. Addition of ascorbic acid significantly reduced the oxidation of folates (Oey et al. 2008).

Several researchers have reported that the HPP process increases the contents of total lycopene and carotenoids as well as the antioxidant capacity in tomato puree. This effect was attributed to the fact that high pressure can rupture the tissue of tomato puree that increases the extractability of extractable carotenoids and lycopene (Krebbers et al. 2003; Qiu et al. 2006; Hsu 2008).

Table 14.5 lists vitamin retention information on HPP-processed foods from the literature. Recent reviews on HPP are published by Ramirez et al. (2009), Norton and Sun (2008), and Oey et al. (2008).

14.2.5 Pulsed Electric Field

PEF inactivates microbial cells by electroporation of their membranes, which is caused by placing fluid foods (e.g., milk and juice) between two electrodes and applying pulses of high voltage (typically 20–80 kV/cm). The treatment time is only a few microseconds, therefore minimal heat is generated thus minimizing the thermal effect on nutrients (Kong and Singh 2009).

PEF treatment is reported to cause less change in vitamin content than conventional processing treatments in different products such as tomato juice (Odriozola-Serrano et al. 2007), watermelon juice (Oms-Oliu et al. 2009), orange juice (Elez-Martínez and Martín-Belloso 2007), and strawberry juice (Odriozola-Serrano et al. 2009). Riener et al. (2008) reported milk subjected to PEF treatment (electric field strengths ranging from 15 to 35 kV/cm, treatment times of 12.5 to 75 μs) showed no change in the levels of thiamin, riboflavin, retinol, and α-tocopherol. Odriozola-Serrano et al. (2009) studied PEF-treated strawberry juice at electric field strength at 35 kV/cm, frequencies from 50 to 250 Hz, pulse width from 1 to 7 ms, with treatment time 1000 ms, and reported >95% vitamin C retention, >83% anthocyanin, >75% antioxidant capacity retention. Elez-Martínez and Martín-Belloso (2007) reported that high-intensity PEF (HIPEF)-treated orange juice and gazpacho always showed higher vitamin C retention than that of the heat-pasteurized products. Orange juice and gazpacho retained 87.5–98.2% and 84.3–97.1% of vitamin C, respectively, after HIPEF treatments. The antioxidant capacity was not affected by HIPEF treatment.

Processing parameters in PEF treatment affecting nutrient retention include pulse polarity, electric field strength, pulse frequency, pulse width, and treatment time. Lower electric field strength, short treatment time, low pulse frequency and pulse width, and pulses applied in bipolar mode favor retention of vitamins C (Elez-Martínez and Martín-Belloso 2007; Odriozola-Serrano et al. 2007; Odriozola-Serrano et al. 2009). Watermelon juice treated at 25 kV/cm for 50 μs at 50 Hz exhibited vitamin C retention of 96.4–99.9%, while vitamin C loss was higher than 50% after HIPEF treatment at 35 kV/cm for 2050 μs at 250 Hz when applying mono- or bipolar 7 μs pulses (Oms-Oliu et al. 2009).

In addition, PEF treatment has been shown to improve extraction of vitamin A as well as antioxidant capacity of the juice. Odriozola-Serrano et al. (2007) found that the lycopene content increased by 31.8% in tomato juice after PEF treatment at 35 kV/cm for 1000 μs using squared wave pulses, with frequencies from 50 to 250 Hz, and a pulse width from 1 to 7 μs. Similar result was also reported by Oms-Oliu et al. (2009) in watermelon juice, where 13% increase in lycopene content was observed after treatment under electric field strength (35 kV/cm), pulse frequency (200 Hz), and treatment time (50 μs). The increased amount of lycopene extracted also improved the antioxidant capacity of HIPEF-treated watermelon juice. Torregrosa et al. (2005) also reported a 58.2% increase of carotenoids when a field of 30 kV/cm was used in orange–carrot juice mixture for 220 μs. Table 14.6 is a summary of literature about vitamin changes in PEF-processed foods. For more information, authors are referred to recently published review papers by Soliva-Fortuny et al. (2009) and Aguiló-Aguayo et al. (2011).

TABLE 14.5
Effect of HPP on Nutrient Loss

Food	Nutrients	Process and Condition	Nutrient Retention/Loss (%)	Reference
Germinated cowpea seeds	Vitamin C	300, 400, and 500 MPa/15 min/room temperature	Loss: 9–41%	Doblado et al. (2007)
Tomato juice	Total carotenoids and lycopene contents	Pressure beyond 300 MPa at 4°C and 25°C	Retention: both total carotenoids and lycopene contents significantly increased up to 62% and 56%	Hsu (2008)
Pork	Thiamin and riboflavin	600 MPa/20 to 100°C/45 min	Retention: 78% thiamin at 100°C, 600 MPa, 45 min. Riboflavin increased by 30%	Butz et al. (2007)
Strawberry and blackberry purees	Antioxidant activity, phenolic, ascorbic acid, anthocyanin content	400, 500, or 600 MPa/15 min/ambient temperature	No significant changes in ascorbic acid and anthocyanin content Antioxidant activities of pressure-treated strawberry and blackberry purees were significantly higher ($p < 0.05$) than in thermally processed samples	Patras et al. (2009)
Blueberry juice	Total anthocyanins	40°C/600 MPa/15 min	4% loss	Buckow et al. (2010)
Sprouted alfalfa	Ascorbic acid	500 MPa/room temperature/10 min	77% loss	Gabrovska et al. (2005)
Tomato puree	Ascorbic acid	400 MPa/25°C/15 min	40% loss	Sanchez-Moreno et al. (2006)
Orange juice	Vitamin C	400 MPa/40°C/1 min	<9% loss	Sanchez-Moreno et al. (2005)
Strawberry coulis	Ascorbic acid	400 MPa/20°C/30 min	88.68% retention	Sancho et al. (1999)
Green pea	Ascorbic acid	Two pulses of 75°C/1000 MPa/80 s	76% retention	Krebbers et al. (2002)
Orange juice	Carotenoids	400 MPa/40°C/1 min	53.88% increase	Sanchez-Moreno et al. (2005)

14.2.6 DEGRADATION KINETIC OF NUTRIENTS IN FOODS

Kinetic modeling has been used to characterize the changes in vitamins in foods during processing and storage. The rate of chemical reactions is an important determinant of food quality changes and shelf life. Chemical kinetics involves the study of the rates and mechanisms by which a chemical species converts to another, which can be characterized by the rate constant and the order of the reaction. The rate of a chemical reaction (or deterioration of a quality

TABLE 14.6
Effect of PEF on Nutrient Loss

Food	Nutrient	Process and Condition	Nutrient Retention/ Loss (%)	Reference
Tomato juice	Lycopene, vitamin C, and antioxidant capacity	35 kV/cm, 1000 μs, squared wave pulses, frequencies 50–250 Hz, pulse width from 1 to 7 μs, monopolar or bipolar mode	Lycopene content increased by 31.8%, retention of vitamin C and antioxidant capacity content 90.2% and 89.4%, respectively	Odriozola-Serrano et al. (2007)
Watermelon juice	Lycopene, vitamin C, and antioxidant capacity	35 kV/cm, 200 Hz, 50 ms, bipolar pulses	Lycopene content increased by 13%, retention of vitamin C and antioxidant capacity: 72% and 100%, respectively	Oms-Oliu et al. (2009)
Orange–carrot juice mixture	Carotenoids	HIPEF (30 kV/cm/220 μs); pasteurization (98°C, 21 s)	HIPEF: 58.2% increase; pasteurization: 7.8% increase	Torregrosa et al. (2005)
Orange juice	Vitamin C	35 kV/cm, 1000 ms, 200 Hz, bipolar pulses of 4 ms	Retention: 87.5–98.2%	Elez-Martínez and Martín-Belloso (2007)
Strawberry juice	Vitamin C, anthocyanins, and antioxidant capacity	35 kV/cm, 1000 ms, 50–250 Hz, pulse width 1–7 ms, monopolar or bipolar mode	Retention: vitamin C >95% anthocyanin >83% antioxidant capacity retention >75%	Odriozola-Serrano et al. (2009)
Bovine raw milk	Thiamine, riboflavin, tocopherol, retinol	15–35 kV/cm, 12.5–75 μs	No significant differences ($p > 0.05$)	Riener et al. (2008)
Milk	Vitamin D	18-3-27.1 kV/cm, up to 400 μs	Very low or negligible reductions	Bendicho et al. (2002)

indicator) is defined as the change of concentration of a reactant (or quality factor) (C) at a given time (t):

$$-\frac{dC}{dt} = kC^n \tag{14.1}$$

where k is the rate constant in appropriate units and n is the order of the chemical reaction of the quality factor. Solutions of Equation 14.1 for zero-, first-, or second-order reactions are shown in Equations 14.2 through 14.4:

$$C = C_0 - kt \tag{14.2}$$

$$C = C_0 e^{-kt} \tag{14.3}$$

$$\frac{1}{C} = \frac{1}{C_0} + kt \tag{14.4}$$

where C_0 is the initial concentration. First-order reactions are frequently reported for vitamin losses in foods, such as vitamin C in tomato during hot air drying (Marfil et al. 2008), orange juice during sonication (Tiwari et al. 2009a), watermelon juice during HIPEFs (Oms-Oliu et al. 2009), citrus juice during heat treatment (Dhuique-Mayer et al. 2007), and watercress during frozen storage (Gonçalves et al. 2009). Second- and third-order reactions are relatively less common. Kong et al. (2007) used second-order reaction to describe the decay of thiamin during heating. Achir et al. (2010) used third-order equation to describe the loss of *trans*-β-carotene during deep-fat frying. The processing condition affects the reaction rate and order. For example, the thermal degradation of 5-methyltetrahydrofolate is a first-order reaction with high-oxygen accessibility and a second-order reaction at low-oxygen environment (Ruddick et al. 1980).

The Weibull model is also used to describe the degradation kinetics of vitamins during processing:

$$C_t = C_0 \times e^{-(kt)^\beta} \tag{14.5}$$

where β is the shape constant. When β = 1, it becomes a first-order equation. The inclusion of a shape constant in addition to the rate constant improves the flexibility of the Weibull model. Odriozola-Serrano et al. (2008) used the Weibull model to describe the changes in anthocyanins, vitamin C, and antioxidant capacity in strawberry juice during HIPEF treatment.

Arrhenius equation is derived from thermodynamic laws and statistical mechanics principles, and it is the most prevalent and widely used model describing the temperature dependence of the rate of chemical reactions (Equation 14.5):

$$k = Ae^{-\frac{E_a}{RT}} \tag{14.6}$$

where A is the so-called preexponential factor, E_a the activation energy, R the gas constant, and T the absolute temperature. High activation energy implies that the reaction is strongly temperature dependent, that is, accelerate greatly with increase in temperature.

Table 14.7 shows some of the kinetic parameters describing vitamin degradation during processing.

14.3   EFFECT OF PROCESSING ON THE BIOAVAILABILITY OF VITAMINS

The nutrient bioavailability is another critical criterion for evaluating the effect of processing. Bioavailability describes the fraction of ingested nutrient that is available for utilization in normal physiologic functions and for storage in the human body. Food processing and preparation methods may enhance the bioavailability of nutrients in the diet. For example, mechanical processing of vegetables such as homogenization destroys the subcellular membranes that makes carotenoids more extractable for micellarization and improves its bioavailability (Hotz and Gibson 2007). Cooking improves *in vitro* protein digestibility, protein efficiency ratio, and essential amino acid index (Alajaji and El-Adawy 2006). Heating can enhance the bioavailability of vitamins, including vitamin B6, niacin, folate, and carotenoids by releasing them from entrapment in the plant tissue matrix. Carotenoids in raw carrots can be hardly released due to the rigid cell structure. Cooking can dramatically enhance both carrot digestibility and absorption of carotenoids by disruption of the metrics structure (Thane and Reddy 1997; Kong and Singh 2009). Alajaji and El-Adawy (2006) found that microwave cooking of chickpea, compared to conventional cooking process, not only reduced cooking time but also reduced the level of antinutritional and flatulence factors, increased *in vitro* protein digestibility, and improved the retention of both B-vitamins and minerals. Evidence also indicates that HPP results in higher folate bioaccessibility due to depolymerization of folates to shorter chains induced by pressure (Oey et al. 2008). Similarly, *in vivo* tests have indicated that the vitamin C content in human plasma increased more significantly

TABLE 14.7
Kinetic Parameters

Food	Nutrient	Process	Reaction Order or β	EA (kJ mol^{-1})	k_0 (min^{-1})	Reference
Watercress	Vitamin C	Thermosonication 0.4–2 min/82.5–92.5°C,	First order	136.20 ± 60.97		Cruz et al. (2008)
Citrus juice	Ascorbic acid, carotenoids	Thermal treatment 50–100°C up to 300 min	First order	35.9 (vitamin C) 110–156 (carotenoids)		Dhuique-Mayer et al. (2007)
Orange juice	Ascorbic acid	Microwave processing (100–125°C), infrared, ohmic heating, conventional heating (50–90°C)	First order	64.78 (microwave processing), 47.27 (ohmic heating), 39.84 (conventional heating), and 37.12 (infrared heating)		Vikram et al. (2005)
Orange, blackberry, and roselle	Anthocyanins	Thermal treatment, 30–90°C, 300 min	First order	66 (blood orange), 37 (blackberry), 47–61 (roselle extracts)	19.44 (blood orange), 0.02–2.65 (roselle extracts)	Cisse et al. (2009)
Apple slices	Ascorbic acid	Infrared drying, 40–70°C, 400 min		14.8		Timoumi et al. (2007)
Palm oil and vegetaline	*Trans-β-carotene*	Deep-fat frying 120°C/120 min 140°C/90 min 160°C/60 min 180°C/30 min	Third order	86 (palm olein) and 90 (vegetaline)		Achir et al. (2010)
Watercress	Vitamin C	400 days frozen storage (−7°C, −15°C, and −30°C)	First order	24.73 ± 4.52		Gonçalves et al. (2009)
Salmon fillet	Thiamin	Canning (100–131°C)	Second order	105.23	3.47 × 10^{12}	Kong et al. (2007)
Green peas, spinach, green beans, and okra	Vitamin C	Frozen storage (−3°C to −20°C)	First order	98–112		Giannakourou and Taoukis (2003)

after consumption of HP-treated orange juice and gazpacho compared to control (Sanchez-Moreno 2006).

The effect of food material properties such as the food matrix structure holding the nutrient together on nutrient availability is being recognized in the recent years. Artificial GI models are available to test the breakdown kinetics of food matrix as affected by various types of processing. For example, Kong and Singh (2010) have developed artificial stomach models to evaluate how peanuts processed in different ways, including roasting, boiling, and frying, disintegrate in the stomach model. They found that fried peanuts and roasted peanuts possess faster disintegration rates, which should lead to a more rapid release of nutrients from the fried and roasted peanuts than raw and boiled peanuts. This effect has been linked to the structural changes in the peanuts during processing. High temperature employed in frying and roasting caused severer degradation of the cell wall in the peanuts that facilitated the leaching of nutrients, and the voids and channels were created in the cells during high-temperature heat treatment enabling a faster diffusion of gastric juice into the food matrix, promoting acidic and enzymatic reactions. Furthermore, they found that the texture of peanuts after absorbing the gastric juice is a representative indicator for predicting the disintegration rate. Therefore, it is important to understand how processing affects the food material properties and subsequently digestion kinetics in order to fully understand the effect of processing on the bioavailability of nutrients.

14.4 FURTHER CONSIDERATIONS

This chapter discussed some of the major processing techniques commonly used in the food industry. Many other food technologies are also used, such as irradiation, ultrasound processing, and ozone processing. For example, food irradiation is the process of exposing food to a controlled source of ionizing radiation to reduce microbial load and destroy pathogens. Whereas a substantial level of activity can be retained after irradiation, significant degradation was found in vitamin C when high levels of irradiation were used (Girennavar et al. 2008). Ultrasound processing is used to inactivate microorganisms due to the cavitation and mechanical effects, and/or chemical reactions including formation of free radicals. It has been used to process orange juices with minimal loss of ascorbic acid during processing and improved stability during storage due to the removal of oxygen. Tiwari et al. (2009a) reported <5% loss of ascorbic acid in orange juice when sonicated at 0.81 W/mL for 10 min. On the other hand, a combination of heat and ultrasound processing, also called thermosonication, caused 40–60% loss of vitamin C in watercress after treatment for 0.4–2 min at 82.5–92.5°C (Cruz et al. 2008). Ozone processing is also used to destroy microorganisms. Strawberry juice treated by ozone at a concentration of 7.8% for 10 min caused significant reduction of anthocyanin content (98.2%) and ascorbic acid (85.8%) (Tiwari et al. 2009b). For more details of these technologies, authors may find related published information in the literature. It is generally found that nonthermal processing can improve the nutrient retention due to the low temperature and short time involved. However, it can be reasonably concluded that all the available food-processing technologies will affect the nutrients at a different level, depending on the severity of the processing conditions.

USDA (2007) has published a table of nutrition retention factors. The nutrients, including vitamins, in cooked food can be calculated by multiplying the initial content by the retention factor. The data set contains factors for calculating retention of 26 vitamins, minerals, and alcohol during food preparation. This is a simple way to estimate the nutrient content in the cooked foods. In addition, Bognar's *Tables of Weight Yield and Recommended Average Nutrient Retention Factors during Preparation of Food and Dishes by Cooking* (Bognar 2002) are commonly used in European countries to evaluate the nutrient retention, covering a more complete list of components, including protein, fat, carbohydrate, vitamins, and minerals. These databases provide useful information in estimating the processing effect on nutritive properties of foods.

The effect of processing on nutritive properties of foods is complicated; thus, a comprehensive approach is needed to reach reasonable conclusions. The consideration should include the changes of nutrients during harvest, processing, storage, and food preparation, and it should extend to digestion in the GI tract. Rickman et al. (2007a,b) compared the nutritive properties of fresh, frozen, and canned vegetables. It is generally accepted that fresh and frozen vegetables are more nutritious than canned vegetables. However, it may not be always true when considering the whole food distribution chain. Canning may cause 10–90% loss of vitamin C but the loss of nutrients will be minimal during storage of canned products due to absence of oxygen in the can, and minimal amount of nutrients will be lost during cooking (reheating) as the required heating time is short. On the contrary, fresh vegetables can lose vitamin C very rapidly during storage. For example, green beans may lose up to 77% of the nutrients in 7 days storage at 4°C. Similarly, for frozen vegetables, they may lose fewer nutrients during blanching, but much higher loss will occur during storage due to oxidation. Rickman et al. (2007a,b) pointed out that by the time they are consumed, fresh, frozen, and canned fruits and vegetables may be similar in the concentration of nutrients.

As mentioned before, food material properties may strongly affect the bioavailability of nutrients. Previous reviews have noted that processing can increase the extractability of vitamins and bioactives by disrupting food matrix and enabling the release of bioactives, such as lycopene and carotenoids (Qiu et al. 2006; Odriozola-Serrano et al. 2007; Hsu 2008). Canned tomato products have been reported to have higher levels of β-carotene and lycopene content than fresh tomato, due to the heat-induced release of this nutrient from its cellular matrix. It is important to understand how processing alters the material properties of food and subsequently affects the release and absorption of nutrients in the human GI tract. Processing loosens the food matrix, reducing rigidity and hardness in the texture of foods, contributing to an improved breakdown rate of food matrix in the GI tract facilitating the release of the nutrients. Severe processing conditions may lead to more vitamin loss, but at the same time the high level of disruption in the food matrix may lead to faster disintegration and digestion, thus improving the bioaccessibility and bioavailability of nutrients. An in-depth understanding of the link between food processing, microstructure, and digestion will enhance our ability to produce foods for health. A comprehensive approach is needed to study systematically the effect of food processing, including the change of food properties during digestion, to provide more accurate and in-depth understanding of the influence of food processing on nutritive components. This is an interdisciplinary area requiring the participation of experts from different areas such as human physiology, nutrition, food chemistry, and food engineering. Numerous opportunities are available in this new and important area calling for more research. The outcome of this research will help the food industry to serve consumers with food with better health benefits.

REFERENCES

Achir, N., Randrianatoandro, V.A., Bohuon, P., Laffargue, A., and Avallone, S. 2010. Kinetic study of beta-carotene and lutein degradation in oils during heat treatment. *Eur. J. Lipid Sci. Technol.* 112: 349–361.

Adam, S.K., Sulaiman, N.A., Md Top, A.G., and Jaarin, K. 2007. Heating reduces vitamin E content in palm and soy oils. *Malaysian J. Biochem. Mol. Biol.* 15(2): 76–79.

Aguiló-Aguayo, I., Soliva-Fortuny, R., Elez-Martínez, P., and Martín-Belloso, O. 2011. Pulsed electric fields to obtain safe and healthy shelf-stable liquid foods. Advances in food protection. *NATO Sci. Peace Security Ser. Chem. Biol.* 205–222.

Alajaji, S. and El-Adawy, T. 2006. Nutritional composition of chickpea (*Cicer arietinum* L.) as affected by microwave cooking and other traditional cooking methods. *J. Food Comp. Anal.* 19: 806–812.

Alam, M.S., Amarjit, S., and Sawhney, B.K. 2010. Response surface optimization of osmotic dehydration process for aonla slices. *J. Food Sci. Technol.* 47(1): 47–54.

Alvi, S., Khan, K.M., Sheikh, M.A., and Shadid, M. 2003. Effect of peeling and cooking on nutrients in vegetables. *Pakistan J. Nutr.* 2(3): 189–191.

Ancos, B., Gonzalez, E.M., and Cano, M.P. 2000. Ellagic acid, vitamin C, and total phenolic contents and radical scavenging capacity affected by freezing and frozen storage in raspberry fruit. *J. Agric. Food Chem.* 48(10): 4565–4570.

Bendicho, S., Espachs, A., Arántegui, J., and Martín, O. 2002. Effect of high intensity pulsed electric fields and heat treatments on vitamins of milk. *J. Dairy Res.* 69: 113–123.

Bernhardt, S. and Schlich, E. 2006. Impact of different cooking methods on food quality: Retention of lipophilic vitamins in fresh and frozen vegetables. *J. Food Eng.* 77: 327–333.

Bognar, A. 2002. *Tables on Weight Yield of Food and Retention Factors of Food Constituents for the Calculation of Nutrient Composition of Cooked Foods (Dishes)*, Berichte der Bundesforschungsanstalt fur Ernahrung (BFE), Karlsruhe.

Butz, P., Bognar, A., Dieterich, S., and Tauscher, B. 2007. Effect of high-pressure processing at elevated temperatures on thiamin and riboflavin in pork and model systems. *J. Agric. Food Chem.* 55(4): 1289–1294.

Buckow, R., Kastell, A., Terefe, N.S., and Versteeg, C. 2010. Pressure and temperature effects on degradation kinetics and storage stability of total anthocyanins in blueberry juice. *J. Agric. Food Chem.* 58: 10076–10084.

Cao, H., Zhang, M., Mujumdar, A.S., Du, W., and Sun, J. 2006. Optimization of osmotic dehydration of Kiwifruit. *Dry. Technol.* 24: 1: 89–94.

Chang, C.H., Lin, H.Y., Chang, C.Y., and Liu, Y.C., 2006. Comparisons on the antioxidant properties of fresh, freeze-dried and hot-air-dried tomatoes. *J. Food Eng.* 77: 478–485.

Chen, B.H., Peng, H.Y., and Chen, H.E. 1995. Changes of carotenoids, color, and vitamin A contents during processing of carrot juice. *J. Agric. Food Chem.* 43(7): 1912–1918.

Cisse, M., Vaillant, F., Acosta, O., Dhuique-Mayer, C., and Dornier, M. 2009. Thermal degradation kinetics of anthocyanins from blood orange, blackberry, and roselle using the arrhenius, eyring, and ball models. *J. Agric. Food Chem.* 57: 6285–6291.

Clary, C.D., Mejia, M.E. , Wang, S., and Petrucci, V.E. 2007. Improving grape quality using microwave vacuum drying associated with temperature control. *J. Food Sci.,* 72(1): E23–E28.

Cruz, R.M.S., Vieira, M.C., and Silva, C.L.M. 2008. Effect of heat and thermosonication treatments on watercress (*Nasturtium officinale*) vitamin C degradation kinetics. *Innovat. Food Sci. Emerg. Technol.* 9: 483–488.

Cui, Z., Li, C., Song, C., and Song, Y. 2008. Combined microwave-vacuum and freeze drying of carrot and apple chips. *Dry. Technol.* 26(12): 1517–1523.

Dal Bosco, A., Castellini, C., and Bernardini, M. 2001. Nutritional quality of rabbit meat as affected by cooking procedure and dietary vitamin E. *J. Food Sci.* 66(7): 1047–1050.

Dewanto, V., Wu, X., Adom, K., and Liu, R. 2002. Thermal processing enhances the nutritional value of tomatoes by increasing total antioxidant activity. *J. Agric. Food Chem.* 50(10): 3010–3014.

Dhuique-Mayer, C., Tbatou, M., Carail, M., Caris-Veyrat, C., Dornier, M., and Amiot, M. J. 2007. Thermal degradation of antioxidant micronutrients in citrus juice: Kinetics and newly formed compounds. *J. Agric. Food Chem.* 55: 4209–4216.

Doblado, R., Frías, J., and Vidal-Valverde, C. 2007. Changes in vitamin C content and antioxidant capacity of raw and germinated cowpea (*Vigna sinensis* var. *carilla*) seeds induced by high pressure treatment. *Food Chem.* 101: 918–923.

Dutta, D., Chaudhuri, U.R., and Chakraborty, R. 2009. Degradation of total carotenoids and texture in frozen pumpkins when kept for storage under varying conditions of time and temperature. *Int. J. Food Sci. Nutr.* 60(s1): 17–26.

Elez-Martínez, P. and Martín-Belloso, O. 2007. Effects of high intensity pulsed electric field processing conditions on vitamin C and antioxidant capacity of orange juice and gazpacho, a cold vegetable soup. *Food Chem.* 102(2007): 201–209.

Frias, J., Peñas, E., Ullate, M., and Vidal-Valverde, C. 2010. Influence of drying by convective air dryer or power ultrasound on the vitamin C and β-Carotene content of carrots. *J. Agric. Food Chem.* 58: 10539–10544.

Gabrovska, D., Paulickova, I., Maskova, E., Fiedlerova, V., Kocurova, K., Pruchova, J. et al. 2005. Changes in selected vitamins, microorganism counts and sensory quality during storage of pressurized sprouted seed of alfalfa (Medicago sativa L.). *Czech J. Food Sci.* 23(6): 246–250.

Gayathri, G.N., Platel, K., Prakash, J., and Srinivasan, K. 2004. Influence of antioxidant spices on the retention of β-carotene in vegetables during domestic cooking processes. *Food Chem.* 84(1): 35–48.

Georgé, S., Tourniaire, F., Gautier, H., Goupy, P., Rock, E., and Caris-Veyrat, C. 2011. Changes in the contents of carotenoids, phenolic compounds and vitamin C during technical processing and lyophilisation of red and yellow tomatoes. *Food Chem.* 124(4): 1603–1611.

Golaszewska, B. and Zalewski, S. 2001. Optimization of potato quality in culinary process. *J. Food Nutr. Sci.,* 10(1): 59–63.

Gujska, E., Michalak, J., and Klepacka, J. 2009. Folates stability in two types of rye breads during processing and frozen storage. *Plant Foods Hum. Nutr.* 64(2): 129–134.

Giannakourou, M.C. and Taoukis, P.S. 2003. Kinetic modelling of vitamin C loss in frozen green vegetables under variable storage conditions. *Food Chem.* 83(1): 33–41.

Girennavar, B., Jayaprakasha, G.K., Mclin, S.E., Maxim, J., Yoo, K.S., and Patil, B.S. 2008. Influence of electron-beam irradiation on bioactive compounds in grapefruits (*Citrus paradisi* Macf.). *J. Agric. Food Chem.* 56(22): 10941–10946.

Gonçalves, E.M., Cruz, R.M.S., Abreu, M., Brandão, T.R.S., and Silva, C.L.M. 2009. Biochemical and colour changes of watercress (*Nasturtium officinale* R. Br.) during freezing and frozen storage. *J. Food Eng.* 93(1): 32–39.

Hotz, C. and Gibson, R. 2007. Traditional food-processing and preparation practices to enhance the bioavailability of micronutrients in plant-based diets. *J. Nutr.* 137: 1097–1100.

Hsu, G. 2008. Evaluation of processing qualities of tomato juice induced by thermal and pressure processing. *LWT—Food Sci. Technol.* 41: 450–459.

Khraisheh, M.A.M., McMinn, W.A.M., and Magee, T.R.A. 2004 Quality and structural changes in starchy foods during microwave and convective drying. *Food Res. Int.* 37(5): 497–503.

Kim, Y.S., Park, S.J., Cho, Y.H., and Park, J. 2001. Effects of combined treatment of high hydrostatic pressure and mild heat on the quality of carrot juice. *J. Food Sci.* 66(9): 1355–1360.

Kong, F. and Singh, R.P. 2010. A human gastric simulator (HGS) to study food digestion in human stomach. *J. Food Sci.* 75(9): E627–635.

Kong, F. and Singh, R.P. 2009. Emerging food technologies, in: Stadler, RH, Lineback, DR (Eds.), *Process-Induced Food Toxicants: Occurrence, Formation, Mitigation, and Health Risk*, John Wiley & sons, New Jersey, USA, pp. 621–644.

Kong, F., Tang, J., Rasco, B., and Crapo, C. 2007. Kinetics of salmon quality changes during thermal processing. *J. Food Eng.* 83(4): 510–520.

Krebbers, B., Matser, A.M., Koets, M., Bartels, P., and van den Berg, R. 2002. Quality and storage-stability of high-pressure preserved green beans. *J. Food Eng.* 54: 27–33.

Krebbers, B., Matser, A.M., Hoogerwerf, S.W., Moezelaar, R., Tomassen, M.M.M., and Berg van den, R.W. 2003. Combined high pressure and thermal treatments for processing of tomato puree: Evaluation of microbial inactivation and quality parameters. *Innovat. Food Sci. Emerg. Technol.* 4(4): 377–385.

Lassen, A., Kall, M., Hansen, K., and Ovesen, L. 2002. A comparison of the retention of vitamins B1, B2 and B6, and cooking yield in pork loin with conventional and enhanced meal-service systems. *Eur. Food Res. Technol.* 215: 194–199.

Lešková, E., Kubíková, J., Kovácikóvá, E., Košická, M., Porubská, P., and Holcíková, K. 2006. Vitamin losses: Retention during heat treatment and continual changes expressed by mathematical models. *J. Food Compos. Anal.,* 19(4): 252–276.

López, J., Uribe, E., Vega-Gálvez, A., Miranda, M., Vergara, J., Gonzalez, E. et al. 2010. Effect of air temperature on drying kinetics, vitamin C, antioxidant activity, total phenolic content, non-enzymatic browning and firmness of blueberries variety O'Neil. *Food Bioprocess Technol.* 3: 772–777.

Marfil, P.H.M., Santos, E.M., and Telis, V.R.N. 2008. Ascorbic acid degradation kinetics in tomatoes at different drying conditions. *LWT—Food Sci. Technol.* 41: 1642–1647.

Masrizal, M.A., Giraud, D.W., and Driskell, J.A. 1997. Retention of vitamin C, iron, and beta-carotene in vegetables prepared using different cooking methods. *J. Food Quality* 20: 403–418.

McKillop, D.J., Pentieva, K., Daly, D., McPartlin, J.M., Hughes, J., Strain, J.J., Scott, J.M., and McNulty, H. 2002. The effect of different cooking methods on folate retention in various foods that are amongst the major contributors to folate intake in the UK diet. *Br. J. Nutr.* 88: 681–688.

Norton, T. and Sun, D.W. 2008. Recent advances in the use of high pressure as an effective processing technique in the food industry. *Food Bioprocess Technol.* 1(1): 2–34.

Nursal, B. and Yücecan, S. 2000. Vitamin C losses in some frozen vegetables due to various cooking methods. *Nahrung* 44: 451–453.

Odriozola-Serrano, I., Soliva-Fortuny, R., Gimeno-Añó, V., and Martín-Belloso, O. 2008. Kinetic study of anthocyanins, vitamin C, and antioxidant capacity in strawberry juices treated by high-intensity pulsed electric fields. *J. Agric. Food Chem.* 56: 8387–8393.

Odriozola-serrano, I., Aguiló-aguayo, I., Soliva-fortuny, R., Gimeno-añó, V., and Martín-belloso, O. 2007. Lycopene, vitamin C, and antioxidant capacity of tomato juice as affected by high-intensity pulsed electric fields critical parameters. *J. Agric. Food Chem.* 55: 9036–9042.

Odriozola-Serrano, I., Soliva-Fortuny, R., and Martín-Belloso, O. 2009. Impact of high-intensity pulsed electric fields variables on vitamin C, anthocyanins and antioxidant capacity of strawberry juice. *LWT–Food Sci. Technol.* 42: 93–100.

Oey, I., Van der Plancken, I., Van Loey, A., and Hendrickx, M. 2008. Does high pressure processing influence nutritional aspects of plant based food systems? *Trends Food Sci. Technol.* 19(6): 300–308.

Oms-Oliu, G., Odriozola-Serrano, I., Soliva-Fortuny, R., and Martín-Belloso, O. 2009. Effects of high-intensity pulsed electric field processing conditions on lycopene, vitamin C and antioxidant capacity of watermelon juice. *Food Chem.* 115: 1312–1319.

Ottaway, P.B. 2002. The stability of vitamins during food processing: Vitamin K. In: C.J.K. Henry and C. Chapman, editors, *The Nutrition Handbook for Food Processors*. CRC Press, Boca Raton, FL, pp. 247–264.

Patras, A., Brunton, N.P., Da Pieve, S., and Butler, F. 2009. Impact of high pressure processing on total antioxidant activity, phenolic, ascorbic acid, anthocyanin content and colour of strawberry and black-berry purees. *Innovat. Food Sci. Emerg. Technol.* 10: 308–313.

Patras, A., Tiwari, B.K., and Brunton, N.P. 2011. Influence of blanching and low temperature preservation strategies on antioxidant activity and phytochemical content of carrots, green beans and broccoli. *LWT–Food Sci. Technol.* 44(1): 299–306.

Phillips, K.M., Tarragó-Trani, M.T., Gebhardt, S.E., Exler, J., Patterson, K.Y., Haytowitz, D.B., Pehrsson, P.R., and Holden, J.M. 2010. Stability of vitamin C in frozen raw fruit and vegetable homogenates. *J. Food Comp. Anal.* 23: 253–259.

Qiu, W., Jiang, H., Wang, H., and Gao, Y. 2006. Effect of high hydrostatic pressure on lycopene stability. *Food Chem.* 97: 516–523.

Ramesh, M.N., Wolf, T.D., and Jung, G. 2001. Influence of processing parameters on the drying of spice paprika. *J. Food Eng.* 49: 63–72.

Ramirez, R., Saraiva, J., Pérez Lamela, C., and Antonio Torres, J. 2009. Reaction kinetics analysis of chemical changes in pressure-assisted thermal processing. *Food Eng. Rev.* 1: 16–30.

Rickman, J., Barrett, D., and Bruhn, C. 2007a. Nutritional comparison of fresh, frozen and canned fruits and vegetables: Part 1. Vitamins C and B and phenolic compounds. *J. Sci. Food Agric.* 87: 930–944.

Rickman, J., Bruhn, C., and Barrett, D. 2007b. Nutritional comparison of fresh, frozen, and canned fruits and vegetables II. Vitamin A and carotenoids, vitamin E, minerals and fiber. *J. Sci. Food Agric.* 87(7): 1185–1196.

Ruiz-Rodriguez, A., Marin, F.R., Ocana, A., and Soler-Rivas, C. 2008. Effect of domestic processing on bioac-tive compounds. *Phytochem. Review.* 7: 345–384.

Riener, J., Noci, J., Cronin, F., Morgan, D.A., and Lyng, D.J. 2008. Effect of high intensity pulsed electric fields on enzymes and vitamins in bovine raw milk. *Int. J. Dairy Technol.* 62: 1–6.

Ruddick, J.E., Vanderstoep, J., and Richards, J.F. 1980. Kinetics of thermal degradation of methyltetrahydrofolic acid. *J. Food Sci.* 45(4): 1019–1022.

Sánchez-Moreno, C., Plaza, L., Elez-Martínez, P., De Ancos, B., Martín-Belloso, O., and Cano, M.P. 2005. Impact of high-pressure and pulsed electric fields on bioactive compounds and antioxidant activity of orange juice and comparison with traditional thermal processing. *J. Agric. Food Chem.* 53(11): 4403–4409.

Sánchez-Moreno, C., Plaza, L., De Ancos, B., and Cano, M.P. 2006. Impact of high-pressure and traditional thermal processing of tomato puree on carotenoids, vitamin C and antioxidant activity. *J. Sci. Food Agric.* 86(2): 171–179.

Sancho, F., Lambert, Y., Demazeau, G., Largeteau, A., Bouvier, J.M., and Narbonne, J.F. 1999. Effect of ultra-high hydrostatic pressure on hydrosoluble vitamins. *J. Food Eng.* 39: 247–253.

Santos, P.H.S. and Silva, M.A. 2008. Retention of vitamin C in drying processes of fruits and vegetables— A review. *Dry. Technol.* 26(12): 1421–1437.

Santos, V.V., Costa, A.P., Soares, N.K., Pires, J.F., Ramalho, H.M., and Dimenstein, R. 2009. Effect of storage on retinol concentration of Cobb and Ross strain chicken livers. *Int. J. Food Sci. Nutr.* 60(s1): 220–231.

Shi, J., Xue, S., Ma, Y., Li, D., Kakuda, Y., and Lan, Y. 2009. Kinetic study of saponins B stability in navy beans under different processing conditions. *J. Food Eng.* 93(1): 59–65.

Sierra, I. and Vidal-Valverde, C. 2001. Vitamin B1 and B6 retention in milk after continuous-flow microwave and conventional heating at high temperatures. *J. Food Prot.* 64(6): 890–894.

Singh, S., Gamlath, S., and Wakeling, L. 2007. Nutritional aspects of food extrusion: A review. *Int. J. Food Sci. Technol.* 42: 916–929.

Singh, R. and Heldman, D. 2009. *Introduction to Food Engineering*. Academic Press, Amsterdam.

Słupski, J. 2011. Effect of freezing and canning on the content of vitamin c in immature seeds of five cultivars of common bean (*Phaseolus vulgaris* l.). *Acta Sci. Pol., Technol. Aliment.* 10(2): 197–208.

Soliva-Fortuny, R., Ana B., Dietrich K., and Olga M.-B. 2009. Effects of pulsed electric fields on bioactive compounds in foods: A review. *Trends Food Sci. Technol.* 20: 544–556.

Thane, C. and Reddy, S. 1997. Processing of fruit and vegetables: Effect on carotenoids. *Nutr. Food Sci.* 2: 58–65.

Tiwari, B.K., O'Donnell, C.P., Muthukumarappan, K., and Cullen, P.J. 2009a. Ascorbic acid degradation kinetics of sonicated orange juice during storage and comparison with thermally pasteurised juice. *LWT–Food Sci. Technol.* 42: 700–704.

Tiwari, B.K., O'Donnell, C.P., Patras, A., Brunton, N., and Cullen, P.J. 2009. Effect of ozone processing on anthocyanins and ascorbic acid degradation of strawberry juice. *Food Chem.* 113: 1119–1126b.

Timoumi, S., Mihoubi, D., and Zagrouba, F. 2007. Shrinkage, vitamin C degradation and aroma losses during infra-red drying of apple slices. *LWT* 40: 1648–1654.

Tosun, B.N. and Yücecan, S. 2008. Influence of commercial freezing and storage on vitamin C content of some vegetables. *Int. J. Food Sci. Technol.* 43(2): 316–321.

Torregrosa, F., Cortés, C., Esteve, M.J., and Frígola A. 2005. Effect of high intensity pulsed-electric fields processing and conventional heat treatment on orange–carrot juice carotenoids. *J. Agric. Food Chem.* 53(24): 9519–9525.

US Department of Agriculture (USDA), Agricultural Research Service, 2007. USDA Nutrient Database for Standard Reference, Release 6. Retrieved 2011 from the Nutrient Data Laboratory Home Page on the World Wide Web: http://www.ars.usda.gov/Main/docs.htm?docid=9448.

Vikram, V.B., Ramesh, M.N., and Prapulla, S.G. 2005. Thermal degradation kinetics of nutrients in orange juice heated by electromagnetic and conventional methods. *J. Food Eng.* 69: 31–40.

Vallejo, F., Tomás-Barberán, F.A., and García-Viguera, C. 2002. Glucosinolates and vitamin C content in edible parts of broccoli florets after domestic cooking. *Eur. Food Res. Technol.* 215: 310–316.

van den Broeck, I., Ludikhuyze, L., Weemaes, C., Van Loey, A., and Hendrickx, M.E. 1998. Kinetics for isobaric–isothermal degradation for L-ascorbic acid. *J. Agric. Food Chem.* 46: 2001–2006.

Xue, S., Ye, X.Q., Shi, J., Jiang, Y.M., Liu, D.H., Chen, J.C., Shi, A., and Kakuda, Y. 2011. Degradation kinetics of folate (5-methyltetrahydrofolate) in navy beans under various processing conditions. *LWT—Food Sci. Technol.* 44: 231–238.

15 Requirements for Innovative Food Packaging

Kata Galić

CONTENTS

15.1 INTRODUCTION

Changes in the way food products are produced, distributed, stored, and retailed, reflecting the continuing increase in consumer demand for improved safety, quality, and extended shelf life for packaged foods, are placing greater demands on the performance of food packaging. Nowadays, varieties of packaging materials with different properties for different product packaging are available. Thus, the selection of appropriate packaging for particular food product becomes more difficult than ever. Three basic functions (storage, preservation, and protection) of food packaging are still required today for better maintenance of quality and handling of foods. However, following the evolution of modern society and lifestyle, the significance of several functions of packaging is also shifting from one aspect to another (Brody et al. 2008). The key to successful packaging is selection of materials and designs that best balance the competing needs of product characteristics, marketing considerations, including distribution and consumer needs, environmental and waste management issues, and cost (Marsh and Bugusu 2007). Traceability of products through appropriate identification and tracking, tamper indicators, and convenience are also important to provide cost-effective packaging (Marsh and Bugusu 2007). New developments in packaging materials and processing technologies have created the potential for new food products that have more limited shelf life expectations than their traditional shelf-stable or frozen counterparts, but still meet consumer needs.

Developments in packaging include all known materials, plastic, paper, glass, and metal. The glass industry has taken advantage of the microwave transparency of glass and has worked with the food industry in developing new product–package combinations. The glass industry has also improved the way that glass containers are manufactured in order to reduce the cost of glass. The principal developments have been in making glass containers lighter in weight. Metal manufacture has substantially changed over the last decades. Metal cans are no longer manufactured by tin-coated, three-piece (a body and two end pieces), side-soldered techniques. A majority of cans are now made without lead solder or tin. Most modern cans are either made from two pieces (a body and one end piece) or made from three pieces with a welded side seam.

15.2 PACKAGING MATERIALS AND BARRIER REQUIREMENTS

An important requirement in selecting food-packaging systems is the barrier properties of the packaging material. Barrier properties include permeability of gases (such as O_2, CO_2, N_2, and ethylene), water vapor, aroma compounds, and light. Altering film permselectivity (i.e., beta, which is the ratio of CO_2/O_2 permeation coefficients) could be utilized to concurrently optimize levels of both CO_2 and O_2 in packaged systems (Budd and McKeown 2010). These are vital factors for maintaining the quality of foods. Plastic packaging, due to their flexibility, variability in size and shape, thermal stability, and barrier properties, is the fastest growing sector, replacing the traditional materials of glass, metal, paper, and board. In general, the permeability of plastics depends on crystallinity, molecular orientation, chain stiffness, free volume, cohesive energy density, temperature, and moisture sensitivity. The temperature and humidity conditions to which the product is likely to be exposed in the supply chain are vital in calculating the required barrier. It is essential to specify these and check that the data being quoted are applicable to the conditions expected. The gas transmission rate may be measured directly by forming packages with included gas of known composition and sampling changes over time with a commercially available O_2 and/or CO_2 meter. However, accurate data on nitrogen permeabilities are less widely available, and are generally calculated by difference measurement—that is, by measuring that which remains after CO_2 and O_2 have been accounted for. Permeation of noble gases is less well known, but some very good data exist (Nörenberg et al. 2001; Kim et al. 2010; Schowalter et al. 2010).

Haze and gloss are extremely important properties in plastic packages, since many users demand a highly transparent material with a glossy and brilliant appearance. Haze appears as milkiness, which lowers the transparency of the film, and can be measured by determining the amount of light diffused by the test sample as well as the amount transmitted through the material. Gloss relates to the measurement of the amount of light reflected by the film. A light beam is projected against the surface at a known angle and the amount of light reflected is measured by a light meter (Misra et al. 2000; Raj et al. 2004; Ščetar et al. 2010). Food can be adversely affected by prolonged exposure to light. The chemistry of light-catalyzed changes can be quite complex. For instance, light promotes oxidation of fats and oils oxidation of milk and changes in various pigments (Bosset et al. 1993; Saffert et al. 2006; Akhtar et al. 2010). The light transmitted through a given material gives a characteristic spectrum of transmitted light dependent on incident light and the properties of the package (Karel and Lund 2003). It is readily apparent that several of the plastics, while transmitting similar amounts of light in the visible range, offer varying degrees of protection against the damaging ultraviolet wavelengths. The protection against UV light by different packaging materials can often be characterized by a "cutoff" wavelength below which transmission of light becomes negligible, and these wavelengths are sometimes listed in compilation of package properties. The barrier properties with respect to light of a packaging material can be improved by special treatments. Glass is frequently modified by inclusion of color-producing agents or by application of coatings. Modification of plastic materials may be achieved by incorporation of dyes or by application of coatings. As a consequence of the successive absorption of light in both the packaging material and the food, the total energy delivered to different points in the food varies and the spectral characteristics of the light vary as well (Emblem 2000).

Like glass, metal containers (tinplate or aluminum) offer a total barrier to water vapor and gases, subject to the integrity of the closure and the seams. They also offer a total light barrier. Plastics used for packaging vary from the glass-clear transparency of poly(ethylene terephthalate), PET, bottles for soft drinks, to the milky white translucence of high-density polyethylene (PE-HD) bottles used, for example, for milk. If a light barrier is needed for product preservation, pigments are easily incorporated into the mix prior to manufacture of the film or container. Polypropylene (PP) films used for wrapping chocolate confectionery, where a light barrier will help to delay rancidity, can be pigmented or cavitated. This process introduces small voids into one layer of the film, thereby obstructing light transmission. Vacuum deposition of a very thin layer of aluminum also provides a light barrier, as well as improving moisture and oxygen barriers.

Christy et al. (1981) reported that clear polyethylene (PE) pouches transmit light in both UV and visible regions of the spectrum while pouches covered with a black/white PE overwrap transmitted <3% light in the UV and visible regions. However, translucent PE-HD has an advantage over clear PET in that it blocks approximately 40% light between 300 and 700 nm, whereas clear PET only blocks approximately 20% light in the same range (Van Aardt et al. 2001). The effect of storage/display of pizza (unfortified and roselle fortified) under different conditions (day, dark, and direct sunlight) showed that products packaged in transparent film were higher on peroxide values than their corresponding counterparts stored in translucent film (Daramola and Asunni 2006). An adequate light barrier, which did not transmit any wavelength of the spectrum, was shown to avoid the light-induced oxidation in milk samples (Mestdagh et al. 2005). Consequently, oxygen-sensitive foods, high in polyunsaturated fatty acid, therefore, can be protected by reducing the amount of absorbed rays through the use of light-proof packages such as translucent films. Translucent film materials with poor gas barrier are light-proof and their application in packaging of deep-fat-fried product significantly reduces the rate of peroxidation (Daramola and Asunni 2006).

15.2.1 Edible Film

Edible film formulation generally associates a film-forming substance (such as polysaccharides, proteins, etc.) to ensure good matrix cohesion, and a barrier substance composed of lipids or waxes, for their good impermeability to water (Karbowiak et al. 2009; Mishra et al. 2010). Their structure can be homogeneous. In that case, the film is composed of a unique layer of the same material, polysaccharides, proteins, or lipids. A multilayer structure can also combine successive homogeneous layers. In the solid emulsion form, lipid particles are dispersed in the macromolecular network. A solid dispersion can also be encountered in case of chocolate-based coatings, in which sucrose crystals, fibers, and proteins are dispersed in a continuous lipid phase (Debeaufort et al. 2002). In terms of barrier efficiency of this edible packaging, water barrier efficiency is mainly dependent on the nature of the film-forming material that makes the continuous matrix (Table 15.1 shows examples of edible packaging properties and applications). In this respect, plastic films are more efficient than lipid films, which have better efficiency than protein or polysaccharide films (Morillon et al. 2002). The use of plasticizers in order to improve the film deformability also modifies the structure of the system and strongly influences mass transfers (Sobral et al. 2001). Permeability of edible films to aroma compounds (Quezada Gallo et al. 1999), or the diffusion of small molecules in these films, such as antimicrobial agents (Ozdemir and Floros 2001), remains a relatively less studied field.

For the past decade, many research programs have focused on developing more sophisticated edible films and coatings (Sebti et al. 2007; Rojas-Graü et al. 2007a,b, 2008, 2009; Denavi et al. 2009). Among them, polysaccharide polymers such as hydroxypropyl methylcellulose (HPMC) and chitosan (CS) have been particularly studied (Chien et al. 2007; Hernández-Muñoz et al. 2008; de Moura et al. 2009). In the study by No et al. (2007) were discussed the applications of chitosan for improvement of quality and shelf life of various foods. However, the hydrophilic nature of such packaging materials, which produces a loss of barrier properties or even a solubilization into foods with high water activities, prevents their industrial applications (Bertuzzi et al. 2007). A commercial edible coating formulation based on carboxymethylcellulose and sucrose fatty acid esters has been applied to pears (Zhou et al. 2008), cherries (Yaman and Bayoindirli 2002), and asparagus (Tzoumaki et al. 2009). One example of pullulan used as a coating hydrocolloid was for strawberries

TABLE 15.1

Edible Packaging Applications

Food	Packaging Materials/Coatings	Storage Conditions	References
White asparagus	CMC and sucrose fatty acid esters, whey protein isolate alone and in combination with stearic acid, and pullulan and sucrose fatty acid esters Plastic trays + wrapp stretch film (16 μm): $P(O_2) = 583$ $P(CO_2) = 1750$ mL/m^2 h bar, WVTR 14.6 g/m^2 h bar, at 39°C and 90% RH	At 4°C and 95% RH for 11 days	Tzoumaki et al. (2009)
Carrots	CMC + CF CMC CF	25°C and 65% RH for 14 days	Rashidi and Bahri (2009); Bahri and Rashidi (2009)
Fresh-cut papaya	Sodium alginate (2% w/v) or gellan-based (0.5% w/v) coating + formulations: Glycerol formulations: 2% (w/v) glycerol + 1% ascorbic acid or 1% glycerol + 1% ascorbic acid Sunflower oil added to some samples in concentrations of 0.025%, 0.05%, and 0.125% (w/w)	At 4°C for 8 days	Tapia et al. (2008)
Fresh-cut Fuji apples	PP trays + PP film: $P(O_2) = 110$ cm^3/m^2 bar day at 23°C, 0% RH + coating: Coatings: alginate (2 g/100 mL water) or gellan (0.5 g/100 mL water). Glycerol added: at 1.5 g/100 mL alginate solution and 0.6 g/100 mL gellan solution. Emulsified with sunflower oil (0.025 g/100 mL film forming solution). *N*-Acetylcysteine (1 g/100 mL) added to the calcium chloride bath (2 g/100 mL water)	At 4°C for 23 days	Rojas-Graü et al. (2008)
Raisin	PE pouch + coating: gum, high methoxy pectin, wheat starch, corn syrup, and calcium chloride	20–25°C for 6 months	Ghasemzadeh et al. (2008)
Fresh-cut pears	PP trays + sealing film: $P(O_2) = 5.2419 \times 10^{-13}$ mol/m^2 s Pa; $P(CO_2) = 2.3825 \times 10^{-12}$ mol/m^2 s Pa at 23°C and 0% RH + coating: Alginate (2%, w/v), pectin (2%, w/v), and gellan-based (0.5%, w/v) edible coatings containing *N*-acetylcysteine (0.75% w/v) and glutathione (0.75% w/v)	At 4°C for 14 days	Oms-Oliu et al. (2008)
Strawberry	Coatings: a. 1% chitosan acetate b. 1.5% chitosan acetate c. 1% chitosan + 0.5% calcium gluconate d. 1.5% chitosan + 0.75% calcium gluconate solution	At 10°C and 70 ± 5% RH for 1 week	Hernández-Muñoz et al. (2008)
Strawberry	Coatings: starch, starch + calcium chloride, carrageenan, carrageenan + CaCl$_2$, chitosan, chitosan + CaCl$_2$	0–5°C, 85–90% RH for 6 days	Ribeiro et al. (2007)
Strawberry	Coating: cactus mucilage	At 5 ± 0.5°C, 75% RH for 10 days	Del-Valle et al. (2005)
Fresh and frozen strawberries, raspberries	Coating: chitosan, chitosan containing 5% Gluconal CAL, and chitosan containing 0.2% DL-α-tocopheryl acetate Pack: plastic container or PE bag	2°C, 88% RH for 3 weeks; −23°C up to 6 months	Han et al. (2004)
Mushrooms, cauliflowers	Coating: MC + ethanol + PEG + stearic acid (SA), ascorbic acid (AA), and citric acid (CA)	At 25°C and 84% RH	Ayranci and Tunc (2003)

Note: P = permeability; WVTR = water vapor transmission rate; PP = polypropylene; PE = polyethylene; PEG = polyethylene glycol; MC = methyl cellulose; CMC = carboxymethylcellulose; CF = cellophane.

and kiwifruit (Diab et al. 2001). Proteins that can also be used in formulations of edible coatings for fruits and vegetables include those derived from animal sources, such as casein and whey proteins, or obtained from plant sources, such as corn zein, wheat gluten, and soy protein (Vargas et al. 2008). Whey protein has received much attention for its potential use as an edible film and coating because it has been shown to make transparent films and coatings that can act as excellent oxygen barriers and provide certain mechanical properties (Sothornvit and Krochta 2000, 2005). Whey protein-based coatings have been extensively used to extend the shelf life of fruits and vegetables (Lerdthanangkul and Krochta 1996; Cisneros-Zevallos and Krochta 2003).

The use of edible coatings as carriers of antimicrobial compounds is another potential alternative to enhance the safety of fresh-cut produce. Antimicrobial edible coatings may provide increased inhibitory effects against spoilage and pathogenic bacteria by maintaining effective concentrations of the active compounds on the food surfaces. There are several categories of antimicrobials that can be potentially incorporated into edible coatings, including organic acids (acetic, benzoic, lactic, propionic, sorbic), fatty acid esters (glyceryl monolaurate), polypeptides (lysozyme, peroxidase, lactoferrin, nisin), plant essential oils (cinnamon, oregano, lemongrass), nitrites, and sulfites, among others (Franssen and Krochta 2003). Although several types of antimicrobials incorporated into edible coatings have been used for extending the shelf life of fresh commodities, their use in fresh-cut fruits is yet limited. Currently, organic acids and plant essential oils are the main antimicrobial agents incorporated into edible coatings for fresh-cut fruits. Unlike chitosan film, whey protein films have not shown any antimicrobial activity; therefore, incorporation of antimicrobial agents, such as sorbic acid, p-aminobenzoic acid (Cagri et al. 2001), and lysozyme (Min et al. 2008), is needed to impart this property.

Edible coatings are also an excellent vehicle to enhance the nutritional value of fruits and vegetables by carrying basic nutrients that lack or are present in low amounts in fruits and vegetables. Tapia et al. (2008) reported that the addition of ascorbic acid to the alginate edible coating helped to preserve the natural vitamin C content in fresh-cut papaya. Hernández-Muñoz et al. (2006) indicated that chitosan-coated strawberries retained more calcium gluconate than strawberries dipped into calcium solutions. Despite the good results achieved so far with the incorporation of active compounds into edible films and coatings, the use of certain ingredients into formulations may have detrimental consequences on the flavor of the coated product. For instance, the use of some antibrowning agents in edible coatings can yield an unpleasant odor, particularly when high concentrations of sulfur-containing compounds such as N-acetylcysteine and glutathione are used. Finally, many nutraceutical compounds have natural bitter, astringent, or other off-flavors that could lead to rejection of the product by consumers. For this reason, more studies are required in order to develop edible coatings with high sensory performance (Rojas-Graü et al. 2009).

15.2.2 ACTIVE PACKAGING

Packaging systems tend to be designed to perform some specific role other than to provide an inert barrier between the product and its surroundings, resulting in an extension of the shelf life or in improved characteristics of the product. These new packaging systems are called active and intelligent packaging. Active packaging (AP) employs a packaging material that interacts with the internal gas environment to extend the shelf life of a food. Such new technologies continuously modify the gas environment (and may interact with the surface of the food) by removing gases from or adding gases to the headspace inside a package. AP techniques for preservation and improving quality and safety of foods can be divided into three categories: absorbers (i.e., scavengers: remove undesired compounds such as oxygen, carbon dioxide, ethylene, excessive water, taints, and other specific compounds), releasing systems (add or emit compounds to the packaged food or into the head-space of the package such as carbon dioxide, antioxidants, and preservatives), and other systems may have miscellaneous tasks, such as self-heating, self-cooling, and preservation (Vermeiren et al. 1999; Brody et al. 2002; Suppakul et al. 2003). Table 15.2 shows some examples of AP for different food application.

TABLE 15.2

Active and Intelligent Packaging Applications

Food	Packaging Method	Packaging Materials	Storage Conditions	References
Raw ground almond kernels	Under N_2 or with an oxygen absorber (ZPT-type O_2 absorber)	PET/PE-LD, 75 μm; $P(O_2) = 103$ mL/m^2 day bar PE-LD/EVAL/PE-LD, 75 μm: $P(O_2) = 2$ mL/m^2 day bar at 75% RH, 20°C	(a) Fluorescent light (825 ± 50 lux) (b) Dark at 4 or 20°C for 12 months	Mexis et al. (2009)
Chicken meat	Nisin and EDTA + MAP (%): 65 CO_2/30 N_2/5 O_2	PE-LD/PA/PE-LD pouches (75 μm): $P(O_2) = 52.2$ cm^3/m^2 day bar at 75% RH, 25°C; WVP = 2.4 g/m^2 day at 100% RH 25°C	At 4°C for 24 days	Economou et al. (2009)
Cheese (Fior di Latte)	Active + MAP (%): 30 CO_2/5 O_2/65 N_2	Pack: PA/polyolefin: OTR = 50 mL/ m^2 day bar, at 23°C, 75% RH Coating: sodium alginate (8% wt/ vol) + lysozyme (0.25 mg/ mL) + EDTA, disodium salt (Na_2-EDTA, 50 mM)	At 10°C for 8 days	Conte et al. (2009a)
Beef	Vacuum MAPs (%): 80 O_2/20 CO_2; 0.4 CO/35 CO_2/64.6N_2 +O_2-s; 0.4CO/99.6 CO_2 + O_2-s; 0.4 CO/99.6 N_2+ O_2-s; 0.4 CO/99.6 Ar+ O_2-s	Plastic tray + barrier wrapp: OTR < 20.0 mL/m^2 day at 4.4°C, 100% RH; WVTR < 0.1 g/day per 645.2 cm^2 at 4.4°C, 100% RH	At 2°C for 7 days At 2°C for 4 days dark storage at 2°C for 14 days	Grobbel et al. (2008)
Pork sausages	Vacuum MAPs (%): 0 O_2/20 CO_2/80 N_2; 0 O_2/20 CO_2/80 N_2 + O_2-s; 20 O_2/20 CO_2/60 N_2; 40 O_2/20 CO_2/40 N_2; 60 O_2/20 CO_2/20 N_2	Tray: PS foam, Wrapp: (a) PE, (b) PE/PA, WVP = 5–7 g/m^2 day at 23°C, $P(O_2) = 40$–50 mL/m^2 day at 23°C	At 2 ± 1°C for 20 days	Martínez et al. (2006)
Beef ribs	MAPs (%): 80 O_2/20 CO_2; 100 N_2+ O_2-s	Tray: PP/EVAL, Wrapp: barrier film: $P(O_2) = 0.02$ cm^3/645.16 cm^2 day at 10°C, 80% RH, WVP = 0.92 g/645.16 cm^2/day at 37.8°C, 100% RH	At 1°C for 7 days	Mancini et al. (2005)
Beef short loins	MAPs (%): 80 N_2/20 CO_2; 0.4CO/30 CO_2/69.6 N_2; 80 O_2/20 CO_2		At 4°C for 6 weeks	
Pork steak, ground beef, hamburgers		Bacteriocin-activated (soaking, spraying, and coating) PE-OPA	At room temperature for 3 months, after 24 h at 4°C	Mauriello et al. (2004)
Tomatoes	Air: with/without absorbers	Pack: PE-LD (50 μm) Oxygen absorbers (ATCO LH100)	At 20°C	Charles et al. (2003)
Bags filled with: air, air/N_2, CO_2	Oxygen scavengers: Ageless FX-100; FreshPax M-100, R-300, and R-2000, Bioka S-75 and S-100	Pack: laminate of polyester, OPA, EVAL/EVAC; OTR = 0.55 mL/m^2 day at 23°C 70% RH	At 25, 12, 2 or −1.5°C,	Tewari et al. (2002a)

TABLE 15.2   (continued)
Active and Intelligent Packaging Applications

Food	Packaging Method	Packaging Materials	Storage Conditions	References
Beef and pork cuts	N_2 atmosphere Ageless FX-100 O_2-s + absorbent pad	Pack1: PS tray + shrink film: OTR = 8000 mL/m^2 day at 23°C 70% RH Pack2: plastic cafeteria tray + bimetalized, plastic laminate bag: OTR = 0.55 mL/m^2 day at 23°C 70% RH	At 2°C for 1–3 weeks	Tewari et al. (2002b)
Fresh beef	Air Vacuum MAPs (%): 40 CO_2/30 N_2/30 O_2; 100 CO_2; 80 CO_2/20 air Acitve pack: with/without oregano essential oil	PE bags: $P(O_2)$ = 1.7 cm^3/m^2 day at 23°C 75% RH	At 0°C, 5°C, 10°C, and 15°C for 65 days	Skandamis and Nychas (2002)
Fresh beef steaks	MAP (%): 70 O_2/20 CO_2/10 N_2 Antioxidants: vitamin C (500 ppm), taurine (50 mM), rosemary (1000 ppm) and vitamin E (100 ppm)	Tray: PS, Wrapp: PE/PA: WVTR = 5–7 g/m^2 day at 23°C; $P(O_2)$ = 40–50 mL/m^2 day at 23°C	At 1°C for 29 days	Djenane et al. (2002)
Fresh beef	N_2 atmosphere O_2-s: Ageless FX-100, FreshPax R-2000	Tray: PS, Wrapp: film OTR = 8000 mL/m^2 day at 23°C 70% RH, perforated	At 1°C for 8 days	Tewari et al. (2001)
Beef	O_2-s: Ageless SS-200 MAP: 50% CO_2/50% N_2 + Ageless Z-2000	Tray: plastic, Wrapp: film $P(O_2)$ = 20000 cm^3/m^2 day bar Mother pack: film $P(O_2)$ = 35 m^3/m^2 day bar	At 0°C for 6 weeks	Isdell et al. (1999)
Fish	Sensors (pH-sensitive dye): bromocresol green or BCG (sodium salt), cellulose acetate and ammonium bromide salts	Substrate: optically clear PET (175 μm) + hydrophobic gas-permeable membrane	19–21.5°C for 70 h	Pacquit et al. (2007)
Broiler chicken cuts	TTI: Vitsab, Fresh-Check, 3 M TTIs MAP: 80% CO_2/20% N_2	Tray: PE-HD + lid	At +3°C to +22°C for 12 days	Smolander et al. (2004)
Fresh seafood	Commercial TTIs: Vistab M2-10, C2-10, and Fresh-check TJ2 3 TTIs prototype	Hermetically sealed package, ROP	At 0°C, 5°C, 10°C, 15°C for 450 h	Mendoza et al. (2004)
Frozen green peas Frozen white mushrooms	TTI (enzymatic)	BOPP/PE	From –3°C to –20°C for 163 days	Giannakourou and Taoukis (2002)

Note: EDTA = ethylenediaminetetraacetic acid; PE = polyethylene; PET = poly(ethylene terephthalate); PE-LD = low-density polyethylene; PE-HD = high-density polyethylene; EVAL = ethylene/vinyl alcohol; PA = polyamide; OPA = oriented polyamide; EVAC = ethylene/vinyl acetate; PS = polystyrene; BOPP = biaxially oriented polypropylene; WVP = water vapor permeability; WVTR = water vapor transmission rate; OTR = oxygen transmission rate; P = permeability; O_2-s = O_2-scavenger; ROP = reduced oxygen packaging.

When active materials are placed inside the package, they actively modify the headspace and reduce the O_2 levels within 1–4 day at room temperature (Smith et al. 1986). The majority of currently commercially available O_2 scavengers work on the basis of iron. The iron under appropriate humidity conditions uses up residual O_2 to form nontoxic iron oxide (Smith et al. 1986; Smith et al. 1990). Salminen et al. (1996) reported that the microbial shelf life of sliced bread was extended considerably by packaging with ATCO O_2 absorbers (with an O_2 absorbing capacity of 100 mL). They detected that the O_2 concentration decreased to below 0.1% within a few days of packaging. Absorbers did not seem to have any effect on sensory quality of bread during storage. In various countries, AP is already successfully applied. For the moment, the applications of AP are found more often at the product distribution chain than at the retail market (Fernández-Alvarez 2000).

Different types of absorbents are now available on the market. These include Freshilizer and FreshPax absorbents which act in a similar manner to Ageless (Smith and Simpson 1995). Oxygen absorbents must meet specific criteria to be accepted scientifically and succeed commercially. These are (a) the ingredients should be nontoxic; (b) they should absorb oxygen at an appropriate rate; (c) there should not be any unfavorable side reactions; (d) they should be of uniform quality; and (e) they must be compact and uniform in size. Several factors influence the choice of oxygen absorbents including (a) the nature of the food, that is, size, shape, and weight; (b) the a_w of the food; (c) the amount of dissolved oxygen in the food; (d) the desired shelf life of the product; (e) the initial level of oxygen in the package headspace; and (f) the oxygen permeability of the packaging material (Smith and Simpson 1995). Absorption kinetics of two commercial O_2 and CO_2 scavengers, used in active modified atmosphere, in poly(vinylidene chloride), PVDC, and pouches, was described by a first-order reaction (Charles et al. 2006). It was shown that oxygen absorbents are three times more effective than gas packaging at increasing the mold-free shelf life of bread rolls. Ageless S and FX were packaged alongside the rolls and the oxygen never increased above 0.05%. The product remained mold-free for over 60 days at ambient storage temperature (Zuckerman and Miltz 1992). Studies have shown that oxygen absorbents can be used to prevent mold growth, rancidity problems, and flavor changes in pasta and pizza crust thereby enhancing consumer appeal for such a product (Smith and Simpson 1995). A similar effect can be obtained by the use of water/moisture absorbers. Research is ongoing in the removal of other undesired substances, like bitter-tasting components in orange juice, aldehydes, or amines-causing off-flavors, or components, such as lactose and cholesterol (Day 2008).

Despite its widespread use as a germicidal agent, few studies have evaluated ethanol as a preservative for food products. Ethyl alcohol has been shown to increase the shelf life of bread when sprayed onto the surface of the product prior to packaging indicating its potential as a vapor-phase inhibitor (Smith et al. 1987). Another model of atmosphere modification is sold under the name of Ethicap or Antimold 102. Ethicap is a sachet placed alongside food and it releases ethanol vapor into the package headspace. The released ethanol vapor (0.5–2.5% v/v) then condenses on the food surface and acts as a microbial inhibitor (Labuza and Breene 1989). Ethicap consists of food-grade alcohol adsorbed on to silicon dioxide powder and contained in a sachet made up of a copolymer of paper and ethylene/vinyl acetate (EVAC) (Smith and Simpson 1995). Vanilla and other compounds are used to mask the alcohol flavor. Ethicap sachets come in various sizes ranging from 0.6 to 6 g or 0.33 to 3.3 g of ethanol evaporated. The size of the sachet used depends on the weight of the food, the a_w of the food, and the desired shelf life of the product. This sachet is being used for many bakery, cheese, and semidried fish products. The vapor deposits on the food surface, eliminating the growth of molds and pathogens (Shapero et al. 1978). The main disadvantage of using ethanol vapor for shelf life extension of food is its absorption from the package headspace by the product (Smith et al. 1987). Ethanol has been generally regarded as safe (GRAS) in the United States as a direct human food ingredient. It is suggested that ethanol also prevents or delays staling by acting as a plasticizer of the protein network in the bread crumb. The antistaling effect of ethanol has been observed in Japanese confectionary products and in doughnuts (Russell 1991).

The use of "active" (interacts with food to reduce oxygen levels or add flavorings or preservatives) and "intelligent" packaging (monitors the food and transmits information on its quality) is introduced into the EU legislation (Regulation 1935/2004) in 2004.

15.2.3 INTELLIGENT PACKAGING

Intelligent packaging can change color to let the customer know how fresh the food is and show if the food has been spoiled because of a change in temperature during storage or a leak in the packaging.

Various indicators (Table 15.2 shows examples of intelligent packaging for different food application.) have been presented to the producers of packed foodstuffs, such as indicators for temperature, microbial spoilage, package integrity, physical shock, and product authenticity (Giannakourou and Taoukis 2002; Vinci and Antonelli 2002; Mendoza et al. 2004; Smolander et al. 2004; Pacquit et al. 2007). Indicators in or on the food package can give information on the quality of the food product directly, on the package and its headspace gases, as well as on the storage conditions of the package. Some indicators do not need to interact with the product or the headspace, while others do. These indicators are already commercially available, and their uses seem to be increasing. New concepts of leak indicators and freshness indicators are patented, and it can be expected that new commercially available products will be assessable in the near future.

Freshness indicators (Vinci and Antonelli 2002) indicate directly the microbial quality of the product by reacting to the metabolites produced in the growth of microorganisms. Freshness detector concepts have been proposed for, for example, carbon dioxide, diacetyl, amines, ammonia, ethanol, and hydrogen sulfide. A specific indicator material for the detection of *E. coli* O157 enterotoxin has been developed, and the possibility for applying the technology for the detection of other toxins is currently being explored. In addition, other concepts for contamination indicators have been proposed. The indicator could be based on a color change of chromogenic substrates of enzymes produced by contaminating microbes, the consumption of certain nutrients in the product, or on the detection of microorganisms, as such (Ahvenainen 2003).

If perishable food products are stored above the correct storage temperature, a rapid microbial growth takes place. The product is spoiled before the estimated "use by" date. Time–temperature indicators (TTIs) attached to the package surface is intended to integrate the cumulative time–temperature history of the package throughout the whole distribution chain, and hence, gives indirect information on the product quality. The time–temperature history is visualized as a color change or color movement. Commercially available TTIs are based on various reaction mechanisms (polymerization, diffusion, or enzyme reaction). A common feature for all concepts is the temperature-dependent reaction kinetics of the indicator and activation of the indicator at the moment of packaging (Giannakourou and Taoukis 2002; Taoukis and Labuza 2003).

A leak indicator attached into the package gives information on the package integrity throughout the whole distribution chain. For many perishable products, exclusion of oxygen and high concentration of carbon dioxide improves the stability of the product as the growth of aerobic microorganisms is prevented. As a result of package leaks, the protecting atmosphere is deteriorated (Smolander et al. 1997). Package leaks also increase the microbial spoilage by enabling the product contamination with harmful microorganisms. A typical visual O_2 indicator consists of a redox dye (e.g., methylene blue), a reducing compound (e.g., reducing sugars), and an alkaline compound (e.g., sodium hydroxide). Optical oxygen sensors have extensive applications and have attracted significant attention in recent years (Wang et al. 2010).

In addition to these main components, compounds such as a solvent (typically water and/or an alcohol) and bulking agent (e.g., zeolite, silica gel, cellulose materials, and polymers) are added to the indicator. The indicator can be formulated as a tablet, a label, a printed layer, or it can also be laminated in a polymer film.

Fresh-Check Lifelines integrator is supplied as self-adhesive labels, which may be applied to packages of perishable products to assure consumers at point of purchase and at home that the product is still fresh. It is commonly referred to as having a bull's eye configuration. It is a full-history indicator whose working mechanism is based on the color change of a polymer formulated from diacetylene monomers. It consists of a small circle of polymer surrounded by a printed ring for color reference. The polymer, which starts lightly colored, gradually deepens in color to reflect the cumulative exposure to temperature. The polymer changes color at a rate proportional to the rate of food quality loss: the higher the temperature, the more rapidly the polymer changes in color.

Vitsab indicator is a full-history integrator based on an enzymatic reaction. The device consists of a bubble-like dot containing two compartments: one for the enzyme solution, lipase plus a pH-indicating dye compound, and the other for the substrate, consisting primarily of triglycerides. The dot is activated at the beginning of the monitoring period by application of pressure on the plastic bubble, which breaks the seal between compartments. The ingredients are mixed and as the reaction proceeds, a pH change results in a color change. The dot, initially green in color, becomes progressively yellow as product approaches the end of shelf life. The reaction is irreversible and will proceed faster as temperature is increased and slower as temperature is reduced. The integrator, in the format of adhesive labels, is available in two basic configurations: single or triple dot. Single-dot tags are used for transit temperature monitoring of cartons and pallets of product and for consumer packages as well.

RipeSense is the world's first intelligent ripeness indicator label. RipeSense evolved from the simple idea of making a fruit label that is capable of more than just branding product and this has led to the next revolution in fresh produce marketing.

The 3M MonitorMark uses a colored ester and phthalate mix with the desired melting point that is colored with a blue dye. Above its melting point, it diffuses along a wick, and the progress along this wick gives an indication of how long the indicator has been liquid. A polyester strip keeps the liquid away from the wick, until it is pulled by the operator to start the device.

It is believed that tomorrow's food packages will certainly include radio frequency identification (RFID) tags (Yam et al. 2005). RFID tags are an advanced form of data information carrier that can identify and trace a product (Wang et al. 2006).

Nanotechnology can provide solutions for these, for example, modifying the permeation behavior of foils, increasing barrier properties, improving mechanical and heat-resistance properties, developing active antimicrobial and antifungal surfaces, and sensing as well as signaling microbiological and biochemical changes. Whatever the impacts of nanotechnology on the food industry and products entering the market, the safety of food will remain the prime concern. This need will strengthen the adoption of nanotechnology in sensing applications, which will ensure food safety and security, as well as technology which alerts customers and shopkeepers when a food is nearing the end of its shelf life.

15.2.4 Antimicrobial Packaging

Antimicrobial films may incorporate antimicrobial agents into sachets connected to the packaging for release of the volatile bioactive agent during storage, may directly incorporate the agent into the packaging film, or coat the package with a matrix that is a carrier for the antimicrobial agent (Cooksey 2000; Coma 2008). Extrusion of the antimicrobial agent into the film results in less product-to-agent contact than application of the agent to the surface of the film. However, agents bound to the film surface are likely limited to enzymes or other proteins because the molecular structure must be large enough to retain activity on the microorganism cell wall while being bound to the plastic (Quintavalla and Vicini 2002). Another approach is the release of active agents onto the surface of the food. Slow migration of the antimicrobial agents to the product surface improves efficiency and helps maintain high concentrations. Packages with headspace require volatile active substances to migrate through the headspace and gaps between the package and food (Quintavalla

TABLE 15.3

Antimicrobial Packaging Applications

Food	Packaging Materials	Storage Conditions	References
Soft cheese	PE-LD (60 μm) with PVC lacquer; addition of nisin NISAPLIN (5% w/w) and/or natamycin DELVOCID (10% w/w)	4°C and 23°C for 23 days	Hanušová et al. (2009)
Raw chicken meat	CF + incorporated lactic acid CF + incorporated sodium lactate With lacquer layer + nisin Film without antimicrobial agents (blank)	4°C for 7 days	
Semiskimmed milk; pasteurized apple juice	2.5% (w/v) chitosans dispersed in 1.0% (v/v) acetic acid solution; pH adjusted to 5.8 with 10 M NaOH 2.5% (w/v) chitooligosaccharide (COS) in deionized water; pH adjusted to 5.8 with 10 M NaOH	At 37°C for 120 h	Fernandes et al. (2008)
Fresh-cut apples	Pack: PP tray + PP film $P(O_2) = 110$ cm^3/m^2 day bar at 23°C and 0% RH Coating: apple puree + Na-alginate + glycerol + N-acetylcysteine + lemongrass, oregano oil, and vanillin	At 4°C for 21 days	Rojas-Graü et al. (2007b)
Mozzarella cheese	Active agent: Lemon extract in gel or solution	At 15°C for 10 days	Conte et al. (2007)

Note: PE-LD = low-density polyethylene; PVC = poly(vinyl chloride); CF = cellophane; PP = polypropylene.

and Vicini 2002). Potential antimicrobial agents for use in food-packaging systems are organic acids, acid salts, acid anhydrides, parabenzoic acids, alcohol, bacteriocins, fatty acids, fatty acid esters, chelating agents, enzymes, metals, antioxidants, antibiotics, fungicides, sterilizing gases, sanitizing agents, polysaccharides, phenolics, plant volatiles, plant and spice extracts, and probiotics (Cleveland et al. 2001; Quintavalla and Vicini 2002; Han 2005; Lee 2010). Comprehensive reviews on antimicrobial food packaging have been published recently (Appendini and Hotchkiss 2002; Suppakul et al. 2003; Burt 2004; Dutta et al. 2009). Some antimicrobial agents for different food application are shown in Table 15.3.

15.2.5 Biodegradable and Bio-Based Materials

One of the limitations with plastic food-packaging materials is that it is meant to be discarded, with very little being recycled. The presence of these types of packaging materials in landfills can be problematic on many fronts. First, if plastic is not recycled, these items end up in landfills, where they can last forever and never degrade. Second, many countries are faced with a decrease in landfill space, especially in densely populated areas. So, finding landfills for consumer and industrial waste may become more difficult in the future. There are increased demands that food-packaging materials be more natural, disposable, potentially biodegradable, and recyclable.

The American Society for Testing of Materials (ASTM) and the International Standards Organization (ISO) define degradable plastics as those which undergo a significant change in chemical structure under specific environmental conditions. These changes result in a loss of physical and mechanical properties, as measured by standard methods. Biodegradable plastics undergo degradation from the action of naturally occurring microorganisms such as bacteria, fungi, and algae. Plastics may also be designated as photodegradable, oxidatively degradable, hydrolytically degradable, or those which may be composted. When examining polymer materials from a scientific standpoint, there are certain ingredients that must be present in order for biodegradation to occur. Most importantly, the active microorganisms (fungi, bacteria, actinomycetes, etc.) must be present in the disposal site. The organism type determines the appropriate degradation temperature, which usually falls between 20°C to 60°C (Huang et al. 1990). The disposal site must be in the presence of oxygen, moisture, and mineral nutrients, while the site pH must be neutral or slightly acidic (pH 5–8) (Kolybaba et al. 2003; Krzan et al. 2006).

One of the challenges for the successful use of biodegradable polymer products is to achieve controlled lifetime. Products must remain stable and function properly during storage and intended use, but after that they should biodegrade efficiently. Biodegradable polymers suffer a change in their properties during time, aging, which make them not suitable for commercial applications. The aging of a biodegradable film can be due to physical (migration of additives) or chemical reactions (oxidation) in the polymer matrix. Thus, bilayer and multicomponent films resembling synthetic packaging materials with excellent barrier and mechanical properties need to be developed. The attempts to improve the properties of biopolymer films include their modifications as "pretreatments" (the changes occur in the film-forming solution) or "posttreatments" (applied on the film). Cross-linking, either chemically or enzymatically, of the various biomolecules is one of the approaches in composite biodegradable film developments (Van de Velde and Kiekens 2002). Sustained multidisciplinary research efforts by chemists, polymer technologists, microbiologists, chemical engineers, environmental scientists, and bureaucrats are needed for a successful implementation and commercialization of biopolymer-based ecofriendly packaging materials. Undoubtedly, biodegradation offers an attractive route to environmental waste management.

Bio-based food-packaging materials are materials derived from renewable sources. Bio-based polymers may be divided into three main categories based on their origin and production:

Category 1. Polymers directly extracted/removed from biomass. Examples are polysaccharides such as starch and cellulose and proteins such as casein and gluten (Jbilou et al. 2010).

Category 2. Polymers produced by classical chemical synthesis using renewable bio-based monomers. A good example is polylactic acid (PLA), a biopolyester polymerized from lactic acid monomers. The monomers themselves may be produced via fermentation of carbohydrate feedstock. PLA has gained much interest in recent years because it is being commercially produced in a large scale at a reasonable price and it has some unique properties such as high modulus, excellent flavor, and aroma barrier capabilities, and good heat sealability. However, broader application of PLA is hindered by its brittleness (Yang et al. 2008). Table 15.4 shows bio-based packaging used for food application.

Category 3. Polymers produced by microorganisms or genetically modified bacteria. To date, this group of bio-based polymers consists mainly of the polyhydroxyalkonoates (PHAs), but developments with bacterial cellulose are in progress (Tharanathan 2003; Ruban 2009; Koller et al. 2010).

Bio-based materials will most likely be applied to foods requiring short-term chill storage, such as fruits and vegetables, since bio-based materials present opportunities for producing films with variable CO_2/O_2 selectivity and moisture permeability. However, to succeed, bio-based packaging of foods must be in compliance with the quality and safety requirements of the food product and meet legal standards. Additionally, the bio-based materials should preferably preserve the quality of the product better and longer to justify any extra material cost (Webber 2000).

15.2.6 NANOCOMPOSITE PACKAGING

In gas separation membranes, nanotechnology is often employed to develop new classes of materials with improved permselectivity preserving the productivity levels already achieved by pure polymer membranes. In this concern, the combination of nano-sized ceramic materials with the polymer matrix has received much attention in recent years (Mark 1996; Alexandre and Dubois 2000; Jordan

TABLE 15.4

Bio-Based Packaging Applications

Food	Packaging Method	Packaging Materials	Storage Conditions	References
Zucchini	Passive MAP Active MAPs (%) $N_2/CO_2/O_2$: 90/5/5; 75/10/15	1: OPP bag; 2: biopolymeric film (COEX)	At 5°C for 8–9 days	Lucera et al. (2010)
Black currant	Air	PP trays sealed with laminated PET/PP; inserted in PLA pouches (25 and 40 µm; holes area 7.9 cm^2); OPP (40 µm) + cardboard boxes placed in PLA film pouches (25 and 40 µm; holes area 7.9 cm^2)	At 4 ± 1°C for 24 days	Seglina et al. (2009)
Grape	Air	Biodegradable monolayer films: NVT-100 (100 µm) NVT-50 (50 µm) Multilayer PET-based coextruded film: NVT-35 (35 µm) OPP (20 µm) PA layer with a polyolefin-based film (95 µm) Alu/PE (133 µm)	At 5°C for 35 days	Del Nobile et al. (2009a)
Lettuce	Air	Biodegradable: PE-HD (51 µm); PP (61 µm); with or without antifog treatment PE/OPP (58 µm)	At 4.4°C, 80% RH for 14 days	Brown et al. (2009)
Strawberries, black currents, raspberries		PP/OPP PP/carton PLA pouches (25 and 40 µm) PP/PLA Carton/PLA	At 5 ± 2°C for 25 days	Dukalska et al. (2008)
Lettuce (Iceberg)		OPP Monolayer: blend of biodegradable polyesters (NVT1) Multilayer: coextruded film based on a blend of biodegradable polyesters (NVT2) Multilayer: film made by laminating an aluminum foil with a polyethylene film (Alu/PE)	At 4°C for 9 days	Del Nobile et al. (2008)
Beef steaks		Tray: PS Wrapp 1: starch + PET (60 µm) Wrapp 2: three biodegradable polyesters (50 µm) Wrapp 3: PVC (12 µm)	At 4°C and 15°C for 6 days	Cannarsi et al. (2005)
Sweet cherries	Air MAP: 10%O_2/4% CO_2/86%N_2	OPP (20 µm) Biodegradable coextruded polyesters (COEX, 35 µm)	At 0°C for 30–36 days	Conte et al. (2009b)

continued

TABLE 15.4 (continued)
Bio-Based Packaging Applications

Food	Packaging Method	Packaging Materials	Storage Conditions	References
Fresh-cut "Gold" pineapple	HiO$_2$: 38–40%; LoO$_2$: 10–12%O$_2$/1%CO$_2$	Trays: PP, Wrapp: PP (64 µm), P(O$_2$) = 110 cm^3/m^2 day bar, P(CO$_2$) = 550 cm^3/m^2 day bar at 23°C 0% RH	At 5°C for 20 days	Montero-Calderón et al. (2008)
	Air: passive MAP	PP/PP		
	Air	PP/PP + coat: 1% w/v alginate + glycerol + sunflower oil + CaCl$_2$		

Note: OPP = oriented polypropylene; PP = polypropylene; PET = poly(ethylene terephthalate); PLA = polylactide; PA = polyamide; Alu = aluminum; PE = polyethylene; PE-HD = high-density polyethylene; PS = polystyrene; PVC = poly(vinyl chloride); P = permeability.

et al. 2005; Paul and Robeson 2008). Although the barrier performance of materials has perhaps never attracted so much industrial attention as over the recent decades, when it started to be associated with some modern food and beverage-packaging technologies making use of plastic materials, it became an important issue associated with food commercialization, food shelf life extension, quality, and safety (Weiss et al. 2006; de Azeredo 2009; Arora and Padua 2010; Emamifar et al. 2010).

Many different types of commercial plastics (Powell and Beall 2006), flexible and rigid, are utilized for nanocomposite structures, including PP, polyamide (PA), PET, and PE. Table 15.5 shows analyses performed on different nanocomposite films. Different types of fillers are utilized, the

TABLE 15.5
Nanocomposite Films Analyses for Food-Packaging Applications

Packaging Type	Packaging Materials	Analyses	References
Antimicrobial nanocomposite	Whey protein isolate (WPI)-based composite films with nanoclays: Cloisite Na+, Cloisite 20A, and Cloisite 30B	Physical and antimicrobial properties	Sothornvit et al. (2009)
Antimicrobial nanocomposite	PLA-based composite films with nanoclays: Cloisite Na+, Cloisite 30B, and Cloisite 20A,	Tensile, water vapor barrier and antimicrobial properties	Rhim et al. (2009)
Edible nanocomposite	Chitosan/tripolyphosphate nanoparticles incorporated in hydroxypropyl methylcellulose (HPMC)	Mechanical properties, water vapor permeability, thermal stability, scanning electron microscopy	de Moura et al. (2009)
Edible nanocomposite	Cellulose nanoreinforcement to mango puree-based edible films	Tensile properties, water vapor permeability, and glass transition temperature	Azeredo et al. (2009)
Nanocomposite	PA(6) Organically modified montmorillonite (OMMT) PA(6) nanocomposite containing: 0.08, 0.1, 0.2, 0.3, and 0.5wt.% OMMT	Morphology, thermal properties, barrier	Jiang et al. (2005)
Nanocomposites	Zeolite/PE blends	Film structure	Nur et al. (2003)

most common is a nanoclay material called montmorillonite (MMT). Clays, in a natural state, are hydrophilic while polymers are hydrophobic. To make the two compatible, the clay's polarity must be modified to be more "organic" to interact successfully with polymers (Kim and White 2006). One way to modify clay is by exchanging organic ammonium cations for inorganic cations from the clay's surface (Shabestary et al. 2007). The effects of nanoclay in polymers are increased stiffness, strength, nucleating agent in foams, smaller cell size, higher cell density, and flame retardant (Gacitua et al. 2005; Golzar and Khalighi 2010). For true nanocomposites, the clay nanolayers must be uniformly dispersed (exfoliated) in the polymer matrix, as opposed to being aggregated as tactoids or simply intercalated. Once nanolayer exfoliation has been achieved, the improvement in properties can be manifested as an increase in tensile properties, as well as enhanced barrier properties, decreased solvent uptake, increased thermal stability, and flame retardance (LeBaron et al. 1999; Meneghetti and Qutubuddin 2006; Sorrentino et al. 2007; Yeh et al. 2009). In particular, these nanocomposites have excellent barrier properties because the presence of clay layers delays the diffusing molecule pathway due to tortuosity (Bharadwaj 2001; Sorrentino et al. 2007; Sothornvit et al. 2009). Additional nanofillers include carbon nanotubes, graphite platelets, carbon nanofibers, as well as other fillers being investigated such as synthetic clays, natural fibers (hemp or flax), and polyhedral oligomeric silsesquioxane (POSS) (Stefanescu et al. 2009). Carbon nanotubes, a more expensive material than nanoclay fillers which are more readily available, offer superb electrical and thermal conductivity properties.

In order to modify the properties of the polymeric materials, thin layers of inorganic coatings can be deposited by plasma techniques on the substrate surface. These coatings are expected to provide properties such as hydrophilicity, hardness, good barriers, good biocomparability, and good adhesive coatings to paints. Plasma-enhanced chemical vapor deposition (PECVD) of silicon oxide (SiO_x) films is widely used for several applications. These films are particularly well suited as gas diffusion barriers for food and pharmaceutical-packaging applications due to their optical transparency, recyclability, and suitability for microwaving. The deposition of SiO_x on polyesters, for example, PET, is extensively explored (Roberts et al. 2002; Lewis and Weaver 2004). More than PET, PP shows interesting properties for packaging applications, such as a high mechanical strength at elevated temperatures, an inherent water vapor barrier, and a low density at extremely low costs. Other properties of PP, its low glass transition temperature, and its high thermal expansion, pose a challenge for the deposition process. Significantly enhanced barrier properties, toward gas and water vapor, for various polymer-coated papers and paperboards are achieved by coating them with a thin Al_2O_3 or SiO_x layer (Howells et al. 2008). Good barrier properties were afforded by the presence of uniform and densely packed SiO_x grains because of the lower number of defects and longer diffusion path of water vapor (Chatham 1996; Galić and Ciković 2003; Kim et al. 2010).

The introduction of TiO_2 nanoparticles can provide antibacterial effect to PE-LLD/PE-LD (linear low-density polyethylene/low-density polyethylene) composite films. However, the relatively large particles or aggregates of TiO_2 in PE-LLD/PE-LD/TiO_2 composite films may lead to inferior transparency, and even opaque. Thus, the transparency of final thin films becomes the first problem encountered in the application of TiO_2 (Wang et al. 2005).

The application of nanocomposites promises to expand the use of edible and biodegradable films (Lagarón et al. 2005; Sorrentino et al. 2007). Some of the works done with biopolymer-based nanocomposites were based on starch or polysaccharides, such as wheat and maize starch (McGlashan and Halley 2003), thermoplastic starch (Park et al. 2003), and chitosan (Lin et al. 2005; Rhim et al. 2006; Xu et al. 2006; Gunister et al. 2007). A few studies on protein-based nanocomposites have been published, including soy protein (Dean and Yu 2005; Rhim et al. 2005), whey protein (Hedenqvist et al. 2006), and wheat gluten (Olabarrieta et al. 2006). Most of the biopolymer-based nanocomposites have shown appreciable improvements in mechanical and barrier properties compared to the counterpart biopolymer films. Recently, Rhim et al. (2006) found that chitosan-based nanocomposite films blended with some organically modified MMT, such as Cloisite 30B, exhibited antimicrobial activity against Gram-positive bacteria. They postulated that the antimicrobial action came from the quaternary ammonium salt of the organically modified nanoclay.

Nanoparticle films with embedded sensors in packaging, in order to detect pathogens, will be able to detect and alert the consumers if the food is contaminated by triggering a color change in the packaging (Yam et al. 2005).

Polymer nanocomposites are the future for the global packaging industry. Once production and materials cost are less, companies will be using this technology to increase the product's stability and survivability through the supply chain to deliver higher quality to the customers while saving money. Research continues into other types of nanofillers, allowing new nanocomposite structures with different improved properties that will further advance nanocomposite use in many diverse packaging applications.

15.3 FOOD PROCESSING AND PACKAGING MATERIALS

Processing and packaging are the two important phases of operations in the food industry (Mahalik and Nambiar 2010). Processing also includes preprocessing and cleaning which sometimes is referred to as postharvesting processes. The final phase is the packaging stage. A great deal of automation strategies are constantly being utilized in every phase of processing and packaging. Traditional processing principles are based on thermal processing where the combination of temperature and time plays a significant role in eliminating the desired number of microorganisms from the food product without compromising its quality. Optimization of thermal techniques (e.g., aseptic processing and ohmic and air impingement heating) is a measure of effectiveness and efficiency. Nonthermal-processing methods such as PEF (pulsed electric field), UV (ultraviolet), and ozone yield products with more "fresh-like" flavor than those produced by traditional thermal processes due to fewer chemical and physical changes although they are not completely effective in reducing the activity of bacterial spores (Dunne and Kluter 2001). Furthermore, hurdle technology (HT) is the term often applied when foods are preserved by a combination of processes. In general, hurdle technology is now widely used for food design in making new products according to the needs of processors and consumers (Álvarez 2007; Siripatrawan and Jantawat 2008). The most important hurdles used in food preservation are temperature (high or low), water activity (a_w), acidity (pH), redox potential (Eh), preservatives (e.g., nitrite, sorbate, sulfite), and competitive microorganisms (e.g., lactic acid bacteria). However, more than 60 potential hurdles for foods, which improve the stability and/or quality of the products, have been described, and the list of possible hurdles for food preservation is by no means complete. Generally, biopreservation and natural antimicrobials provide an excellent opportunity for such combined preservation systems. For example, oregano essential oil, combined with modified atmosphere packaging (MAP), was studied as hurdle in the storage of fresh meat and a longer shelf life was observed over that of the same packaging alone (Skandamis and Nychas 2002; Chouliara et al. 2007). These low-temperature treatments widen the selection of packaging materials and system does not require high melting temperature for heat seal. These methods produce far less volatile odor of plastics, additives, and printing solvent. This is very beneficial to high-fat foods and frozen/refrigerated foods. Since some of these techniques might require the processing of foods inside their package, it is important to understand the interaction between the package and the process itself (Clough 2001; Ozen and Floros 2001; Devlieghere et al. 2004). Proper selection and optimizing of packaging are of major importance to food manufacturers due to aspects such as economy, marketing, logistics, and distribution (Trienekens et al. 2003; Min and Zhang 2005; Lelieveld 2007). After packaging, nonthermal processing generally requires hermetic closure before processing and maintenance of hermetic closure throughout the process and distribution. Nonthermal process may also be conducted while in package prior to hermetic closure. The packaging for nonthermally processed foods may necessitate extra functions of packaging for successful commercialization. Packaging materials should have strong physical and mechanical resistance to the nonthermal process mechanisms. Critical protective barrier properties of packaging materials must be preserved to prevent chemical, physical, or microbial degradation of contents after nonthermal processing. Therefore, it is necessary to understand the process parameters and mechanisms/kinetics of the nonthermal process and their effects on packaging material properties (Min and Zhang 2005; Galić et al. 2010).

15.3.1 Modified Atmosphere Packaging

MAP relies on the modification of the atmosphere inside a package, achieved by the natural interplay between the respiration of the product and the transfer of gases through the package. Polymeric films are the most usual packaging material but because of the increase in the consumption of fresh-cut products with a higher respiration rate and higher tolerance to CO_2, alternative materials are being investigated. The perforation-mediated package is one of those alternatives, where the regulation of the gas exchange is achieved by single or multiple tubes that perforate an otherwise impermeable packaging material. From an engineering point of view, the transport of gases through perforations is a complex phenomenon that involves diffusion gradients together with cocurrent transport of multiple species, with oxygen entering the package and carbon dioxide leaving it. A mathematical model considering the cocurrent effect of CO_2 flux on the gas exchange rate for O_2 was developed. These results suggest that there is a significant drag effect in the gas exchange process that should be taken into consideration when designing perforation-mediated MAP. A lot of work has been reported on MAP using different types of films (Barth and Zhuang 1996; Hong and Kim 2004; Jacobsson et al. 2004). Films using microperforations can attain very high rates of gas transmission (Alique et al. 2003). The diameter of microperforation generally ranges from 40 to 200 µm and by altering the size and thickness of microperforations, gas permeability through a package can be altered to meet well-defined product requirements. Based on the rates of respiration and gas transmission through the microperforations and the base film, packages have been developed that maintain desired levels of O_2 and moisture for high-respiring mushrooms (Ares et al. 2007). Microperforated films have also been used to extend the storability of strawberries and nectarines, leeks, asparagus, parsnips, cherry tomatoes, sweet corn, and apple (Aharoni et al. 2007, 2008). A procedure permitting the simple determination of O_2 and CO_2 permeance of microperforated films used to pack respiring foods under real conditions has been evaluated (Ozdemir et al. 2005). Macroperforated films have also been used to improve the keeping quality of strawberries and raspberries by combining high O_2 atmospheres with low-oxygen MAP (Van der Steen et al. 2002). However, commercial microperforated films are relatively expensive, permit moisture and odor loss, and may allow for the ingress of microorganisms into sealed packs during wet handling situations. It is necessary to continue on searching for alternative packaging for minimally processed collard greens, and to associate it with storage at low temperatures, but mimicking distribution and commercialization conditions of the cold chain (Simões et al. 2009).

Metabolic processes such as respiration and ripening rates are sensitive to temperature. Biological reactions generally increase two- to threefold for every 10°C rise in temperature. Therefore, temperature control is vitally important in order for a MAP system to work effectively. Film permeability also increases as temperature increases, with CO_2 permeability responding more than O_2 permeability. Low relative humidity (RH) can increase transpiration damage and lead to desiccation, increased respiration, and ultimately an unmarketable product. One serious problem associated with high in-package humidity is condensation on the film that is driven by temperature fluctuations. A mathematical model was developed for estimating the changes in the atmosphere and humidity within perforated packages of fresh produce (Lee et al. 2000; Montanez et al. 2010a,b). The model was based on the mass balances of O_2, CO_2, N_2, and H_2O vapors in the package.

By placing a modified atmosphere (MA) package inside a controlled atmosphere (CA) environment, it is possible to maintain a desired atmosphere inside the package when this package is exposed to two different temperatures (Silva et al. 1999). The effect of superatmospheric O_2 and MAP on plant metabolism, organoleptic quality, and microbial growth of minimally processed baby spinach was also studied (Allende et al. 2004). Packaging film O_2 transmission rate and initial levels of superatmospheric O_2 in the packages significantly affected the changes of in-package atmospheres during storage and consequently quality of baby spinach leaves. The optimum gas composition of MAP for strawberry is 2.5% O_2/16% CO_2 (Zhang et al. 2003). The MAP combined with ozone and edible coating films were used for improving the effect of preservation of strawberry (Zhang et al. 2005). It was observed that the quality of SO_2-free "superior seedless" table grapes was preserved in MAP (Artes-Hernandez et al. 2006). The improvement of the overall quality of table grapes stored under MAP in combination with natural antimicrobial compounds had also been studied (Guillen et al. 2007). The effect of MA on the quality of many fresh-cut products has been studied (Table 15.6 shows MAP conditions and packaging materials for different food application). Successful applications include mushroom (Simon et al. 2005), apples (Soliva-Fortuny et al. 2005), tomato (Gil et al. 2002; Aguayo et al. 2004), pineapple (Marrero and Kader 2006), butterhead lettuce (Escalona et al. 2006), kiwifruit (Rocculi et al. 2005), salad savoy (Kim et al. 2004), honeydew (Bai et al. 2003), mangoes (Beaulieu and Lea 2003), and carrot (Barry-Ryan and O'Beirne 2000).

15.4 FOOD-PACKAGING INTERACTION

The mass transfer of components, between and within food and packaging, leads to the loss of volatile flavors and aromas from food. The most common methods of mass transfer food-packaging systems are migration, flavor scalping, selective permeation, and ingredient transfer between heterogeneous parts of the food.

Scalping refers to the absorption of one or more compounds from the food into the packaging material (Sajilata et al. 2007; Iglesias et al. 2011). This process has been observed primarily in plastic containers. Even though it is generally accepted that volatile composition is altered as a result of scalping, there were conflicting reports as to whether the loss of certain volatile compounds influenced taste or aroma of the packaged product.

Current food-packaging plastics have been used for decades, but there are some material–food interactions that have been discovered that can cause additives within materials to migrate into the food (Figge and Koch 1973). Migration refers to the transfer of compounds from the container into the food. This can be caused by residual monomers, plasticizers, processing aids, and solvents from printing inks and adhesives (Begley et al. 2005; Kerry et al. 2006; Grob et al. 2009). This can be toxic in many cases, causing harm to whoever consumes the food as well as allowing the food to become contaminated with bacteria if the barrier and mechanical properties are lost because of the leaching (Hourston 2010).

When the polymer is heated, or in some cases is exposed to UV radiation, the matrix can loosen or distort. This can cause some of the additives to be released and migrate out of the matrix bond that was holding it (Birley 1982). These additives, though usually inert and nontoxic when bound by the matrix of the polymer, can interact with food and become harmful in large doses (Kerry et al. 2006). Most commonly, additives are able to latch on well to fats and oils because they are very easily solvable into them and can then be consumed and be toxic (Figge and Koch 1973).

Though this problem is not commonly seen in PET or PE-HD, plastics like PVC (poly(vinyl chloride)) that are used in plastic wrap are often heated in the microwave and are capable of leaching chemicals as well as PP which is used in baby bottles and is sometimes put in the microwave or heated in hot water (Figge and Koch 1973; Atek and Belhaneche-Bensemra 2005). One study found the migration of PVC chemicals and additives with change in temperature. Though the study did not test food specifically, it found that when PVC polymers reached temperatures greater than 100°C, chemicals would migrate from the plastic (Wong et al. 1988). Another study found additives migration into water from polystyrene (PS) cups along with styrene particles which are toxic (Ahmad and Ahmad 2007). Studies have also been conducted on the reuse of plastic containers. When PET bottles are reused and sanitized using solar water disinfection, exposure to UV for 6–9 h while filled with water, the plastic leaches additives (Schmid et al. 2008). Authors also found an increase in

TABLE 15.6
MAP Packaging Applications

Food	Packaging Method	Packaging Materials and Properties	Storage Conditions	References
Beef quadriceps	Vacuum	Bag: $P(O_2) = 3$–6 mL/m^2 day bar at 4.4°C 0% RH; WVP = 0.5–0.6 g/64.516 cm^2 day at 37.8°C 100% RH	Stored in the dark at -0.4 ± 0.8°C for 21 days	Seyfert et al. (2005)
	MAP1: 80% O_2/20% CO_2	PP trays: $P(O_2) = 0.1$ mL/tray day at 22.7°C 0% RH; WVP = 2.0 g/64.516 cm^2 day at 37.8°C 100% RH Wrapp: EVAL/PE-LLD (25 μm); $P(O_2) = 6$ mL/m^2 day at 4.4°C 0% RH; WVP = 0.10 g/64.516 cm^2 day at 4.4°C 100% RH		
	MAP2: 80% N_2/20% CO_2	Tray: $P(O_2) = 0.1$ mL/tray day at 22.7°C 0% RH; WVP = 2.0 g/64.516 cm^2 day at 37.8°C 100% RH, Wrapp (outer): EVAL/PE-LLD film (3.25 mil); $P(O_2) = 4.2$ mL/m^2 day bar; WVP = 0.24 g/64.516 cm^2 day at 37.8°C 100% RH. Wrapp (inner): EVAL/PE-LLD (0.7 mil); $P(O_2) > 300\,000$ mL/m^2 day bar; WVP = 0.24g/64.516 cm^2 day at 37.8°C 100% RH		
Dry-cured Iberian ham slices	MAPs (%): 60 N_2/40 CO_2; 70 N_2/30 CO_2; 80 N_2/20 CO_2; 70 Ar/30 CO_2 Vacuum	PA/PE; OTR = 38 cm^3/m^2 day bar	Stored in dark at 4 ± 1°C for 120 days	Parra et al. (2010)
Beef product (meatball)	MAPs: 21%O_2/33%CO_2, 21%O_2/66%CO_2, 1%O_2/0%CO_2, 1%O_2/33%CO_2, 1%O_2/66%CO_2, 0%O_2/0%CO_2, 0%O_2/33%CO_2, 0%O_2/66%CO_2, 0%O_2/100%CO_2 gas mixtures completed to %100 with N_2 when needed	PET/PE/EVAL/PE (62 μm); OTR = 1.2 cm^3/m^2 day bar at 0°C 0% RH, PE-LD (50 μm); OTR of 3800 cm^3/m^2 day bar at 0°C 0% RH	Storage at 3°C for 3 weeks	Ozturk et al. (2010)
	Air Vacuum	PE-LD High-barrier packaging film		
Cooked ground beef patties ±2.5% lactate (w/w)	Vacuum Air MAPs (%): 80 O_2/20 CO_2; 0.4 CO/19.6 CO_2/80 N_2	Cryovac food-packaging Trays: Styrofoam, Wrapp: PVC, $P(O_2) = 15.500$–16.275 cm^3/m^2 day at 23°C Prime source pouches (4 mil)	Stored for 0, 2, or 4 days at 2°C	Mancini et al. (2010)

continued

TABLE 15.6 (continued)
MAP Packaging Applications

Food	Packaging Method	Packaging Materials and Properties	Storage Conditions	References
Atlantic salmon fillets	Air MAPs (%): 25 CO_2/75 N_2; 40 CO_2/60 N_2; 75 CO_2/25 N_2 MAPs (%): 60 CO_2/40 N_2; 75 CO_2/25 N_2; 90 CO_2/10 N_2	PVC PA/PP PA/PE	At 2°C for 28 days	Fernández et al. (2010)
Broccoli	Passive MAP	PE (40 μm)—no holes PE—two microholes (750 μm in diameter, one on each side of the bag) PE—four microholes (8.8 mm in diameter, two on each side of the bag)	23 days of dark storage at 4°C or 5 days of dark storage at 20°C	Jia et al. (2009)
Peach, cauliflower, truffle	Passive MAP	Tray: PP, Wrapp: PE + film film:PE-LD/ PET + microperforations of different sizes (40 μm)	At 4°C for 9 days	González-Buesa et al. (2009)
Ricotta	MAPs (%): 50 CO_2/50 N_2; 70 CO_2/30 N_2; 95 CO_2/5 N_2	PA-based high-barrier multilayer plastic bags (200 μm); OTR = 30 cm³/m² day bar at 23°C 75% RH; WVTR = 1 g/m² day at 23°C 85% RH	4°C for 8 days	Del Nobile et al. (2009b)
Beef steaks	MAPs (%): (O_2/N_2/CO_2) 0/80/20; 10/70/20; 20/60/20; 50/30/20; 80/0/20	Trays: PS/EVAL/PE, Wrapp: heat-sealed laminated barrier film (polyolefin), OTR = 3 cm³/m² day bar	At 4°C under fluorescent light (616 lux) for 15 days	Zakrys et al. (2008)
Smoked fish	MAP (%): 60 N_2/35 CO_2/5 O_2 Vacuum	PA/PE	4 ± 1°C for 8 weeks	Ibrahim et al. (2008)
Broccoli	MAP	PP bags sealed with a 90 μm microperforated film	At 4°C for 9 days	Granado-Lorencio et al. (2008)
Poultry meat with addition of vegetables	Air MAP (%): 30 CO_2/70 N_2	Tray: EPS; Wrapp: PE	At 1 ± 1°C for 16 days	Cegielska-Radziejewska et al. (2008)
Shiitake mushrooms	Air Active MAP: 15% and 25% O_2 Passive MAP	PE-LD (30 μm); P (O_2) = 6.8×10^{-7} to 8.0×10^{-7} mL/m² s Pa, P (CO_2) = 1.8×10^{-7} to 3.4×10^{-7} mL/m² s Pa (both at 25°C and 101.325 kPa), WVTR = 2.8×10^{-5} to 6.5×10^{-5} g/m² s at 37°C 90% RH PE-LD (30 μm) macroperforated: A: 9×10^3 perforations/m², 0.1 mm² surface, B: 17 perforations/m², 0.1 mm² surface	At 5 ± 0.5°C, 80–85% RH for 18 days	Antmann et al. (2008)

TABLE 15.6 (continued)
MAP Packaging Applications

Food	Packaging Method	Packaging Materials and Properties	Storage Conditions	References
Mediterranean chub mackerel	Air Vacuum MAP (%): 50 CO_2/50 N_2	PA laminate bags (90 μm), P (CO_2) = 25, P(O_2) = 90, P(N_2) = 6 cm^3/m^2 day bar at 20°C 50% RH	At 3 ± 0.5 and 6 ± 0.5°C for 15 days.	Stamatis and Arkoudelos (2007)
Dry-fermented sausage	Vacuum	Tray: PS, Bags: PA/PE, OTR = 30–40 cm^3/m^2 day bar at 23°C 50% RH, WVTR = 2.5 g/m^2 day at 23°C 50% RH	At 6°C for 210 days	Rubio et al. (2007)
	MAP (%): 20 CO_2/80 N_2	High-barrier film, OTR = 5 cm^3/m^2 day bar at 23°C 50% RH, WVTR = 19 g/m^2day at 23°C 90% RH		
Cod	Distilled water	PE-HD semirigid tray, OTR = 3.2 cm^3 day bar, P(CO_2) = 14.0 cm^3 day bar, at 23°C, 0% RH	At 1°C, 4°C, and 7°C for 15 min	Rotabakk et al. (2007)
	MAPs (%): 25 CO_2/75 N_2, 50 CO_2/50 N_2, 75 CO_2/25 N_2 Gas: 100% N_2	PA/PE-LMD (15/70 μm), OTR = 30 cm^3/m^2 day bar		
Pork sausages	MAP: 80% O_2/20% CO_2 with/without antioxidants	Tray: PP, pouch: PA/PE (80/20 μm); WVP = 5–7 g/m^2 day at 23°C, P(O_2) = 40–50 mL/m^2day at 23°C	At 2 ± 1°C for 16 days	Martínez et al. (2007)
Kiwifruit	MAPs (%): 90 N_2/5 O_2/5 CO_2; 90 Ar/5 O_2/5 CO_2; 90 N_2O/5 O_2/5 CO_2	Tray: PP, Wrapp: PP, WVTR = 1.9×10^{-18} to 3.8×10^{-18} mol/s mm^2 Pa; OTR: 2.5×10^{-19} to 3.6×10^{-19} mol/s mm^2 Pa; CO_2TR: 7.6×10^{-20} to 1.3×10^{-19} mol/s mm^2 Pa	At 4°C for 12 days	Rocculi et al. (2005)
Cod	Air Vacuum MAPs (%): 65 N_2/30 CO_2/5 O_2, 20 CO_2/80 O_2	PA/PE (102 μm), P(CO_2) = 3.26×10^{-19} mol m/m^2 s Pa, P(O_2) = 9.23×10^{-19} mol m/m^2 s Pa, WVTR = 1.62×10^{-10} kg/m^2 s	At 4°C, 8°C, and 12°C for 9 days	Corbo et al. (2005)

Note: EVAL = ethylene/vinyl alcohol; PE = polyethylene; PE-LLD = linear low-density polyethylene; PE-LD = low-density polyethylene; PE-LMD = linear medium-density polyethylene; PA = polyamide; PVC = poly(vinyl chloride); PP = polypropylene; PET = poly(ethylene terephthalate); PE-LD = low-density polyethylene; PS = polystyrene; EPS = expanded polystyrene; P = permeability; WVP = water vapor permeability; OTR = oxygen transmission rate; WVTR = water vapor transmission rate.

migration when the bottles were exposed to UV light and heated to 60°C (Schmid et al. 2008). Though additives may help obtain some mechanical and barrier properties that are necessary for food packaging, they can also be dangerous if they interact with food and leach harmful chemicals (Hourston 2010). It is important then to have a method for measuring additive migration. This, however, is difficult due to the measurement of migration and the various values for diffusivity that are calculated (Rosca and Vergnaud 2006). Studies have found variations in diffusivity on the order of two times the magnitude in PE-LD (Brandsch et al. 1999; Begley et al. 2005) and 10 times in PET (Pennarun et al. 2004).

Accelerated migration tests apply severer test conditions by using volatile solvents with strong interactions toward the plastic to enhance the migration rate from the plastic. Thus, the extraction test is based on an accelerated mass transport mechanism where the diffusion coefficients of migrants are increased by several orders of magnitude compared to the original migration test (Piringer and Baner 2008).

15.5 PACKAGED FOOD SHELF LIFE

Packaging considerations are critical to shelf life testing; thus, it is of great importance to understand the requirements of the product, to understand package alternatives, and then to select suitable candidate packages. An understanding of the intrinsic and extrinsic stability of a food product can have an important influence on packaging considerations for shelf life.

Specific approaches and procedures for shelf life testing and prediction have been described thoroughly by numerous authors (Del Nobile et al. 2003; Mizrahi 2004; Achour 2006). In general, the key approach to shelf life testing is to first identify the major failure modes or mechanisms for a product. Shelf life prediction becomes very complex when a food system has several modes of deterioration, which may each have its own temperature sensitivity. However, shelf life at any given temperature will be determined by that mechanism which proceeds most rapidly and thus causes the shortest life. Traditional approaches to shelf life testing generally involve storage tests where products are maintained under a set of controlled (specific temperature and relative humidity) or uncontrolled (i.e., warehouse) conditions. However, an overestimation of shelf life is likely when only some of the conditions a product may encounter during distribution are taken into account. Environmental conditions can also be accelerated by a known factor so that the product deteriorates at a faster than normal rate. However, accelerated shelf life conditions may also influence the barrier properties of packaging materials and thereby introduce additional degradation reactions that do not occur under normal storage conditions (Hough et al. 2006; Corradini and Peleg 2007).

15.6 FOOD-PACKAGING LEGISLATION

The European Union (EU) legislation (Regulation 1935/2004) covers in general terms all requirements for all food contact materials (FCMs). It governs specific legislation, but so far only a minority of the FCMs is specifically regulated, that is, materials and articles exclusively consisting of plastic, ceramics, and regenerated cellulose (Baughan and Montfort 2001). Specific legislation on all other FCMs only exists as nonharmonized national regulation or is absent. The Council of Europe passed resolutions on numerous types of FCMs, but most of these have not been transposed into national legislation. Recently, the EU Commission introduced legislation insisting on production by good manufacturing practice (GMP) as required by Regulation 1935/2004 (and previous legislation) and requested compliance declarations as well as supporting documentation rendering compliance work traceable. It gives no detailed instructions but provides the grounds for a promising new approach to solve several of the basic problems in this industry (Grob et al. 2009). Even though the EU Regulation 2023/2006 has been in place since 2008, these major changes, primarily the involvement of the producers of the starting and intermediate materials, still need to be implemented. The difficulty of the system results from the protected confidentiality for the documentation supporting the declaration provided to the customer. Only the competent authorities have legal access, which means that intense control of the supporting documentation by authorities is a prerequisite to build up trust within the industry.

Active and intelligent packaging introduces new perspectives for the packaging of food, such as the concept of intentional migration of substances, like, for example, preservatives and antioxidants from the package into the food. Thus, the general requirements in food packaging legislation will have to be considered together with requirements in other relevant parts of the food legislation. Seen from this legislative viewpoint, active and intelligent packaging does raise series of questions.

The EU directive on plastic materials has a general limit on the maximum, overall migration of the total transfer of substances from food packaging materials of 60 mg/kg, which is of importance to consider. The overall migration limit was established before the development and use of active and intelligent packaging was extended. This limit is based on general considerations on both hygiene and health, but the overall migration limit in some cases will also have implications on the possibility to make use of active and intelligent packaging.

Specific regulations for nanomaterials and nano-related products are still rare, and, consequently, these applications fall under the scope of existing regulatory schemes. However, the regulation of nanotechnologies is becoming a key issue, pressing governments, regulatory agencies, industry, and other stakeholders to take a position and become proactive in defining adequate regulation and risk management structures that address the responsible development of these technologies and their applications.

Quality assurance of the packaged product and therefore the guarantee of consumer safety will always have priority and must remain the most important criterion for optimization. The fulfillment of these requirements assumes complete knowledge of possible interactions between packaging and product during their contact time. In this respect, the properties of both parts of package, the packaging material and the product, must be coordinated with one another. Here, possible interactions between the two parts play an important role in the quality assurance of the product.

15.7 CONCLUSIONS

It is self-evident that these novel materials should have proper permeability properties, good appearance, and good mechanical properties, and they must be reasonable in price, suitable for packaging machines already used in the food industry, and suitable for normal sealing procedures. In other words, they must have all those properties that traditional packaging materials have.

It is very probable that in the future the management of the food supply chain will be based on wireless communication and active, intelligent, and communicating packages. The packages will protect the food without additives, inform about the product quality and history in every stage of the logistic chain, guide the journey of the package, reduce product loss, and will give real-time information to the consumer about the properties/quality/use of the product.

REFERENCES

Achour M. 2006. A new method to assess the quality degradation of food products during storage, *J. Food Eng.*, 75, 560–564.

Aguayo E., Escalona V., Artes F. 2004. Quality of fresh-cut tomato as affected by type of cut, packaging, temperature and storage time, *Eur. Food Res. Technol.*, 219, 492–499.

Aharoni N., Rodov V., Fallik E., Afek U., Chalupowicz D., Aharon Z., Maurer D., Orenstein J. 2007. Modified atmosphere packaging for vegetable crops using highwater-vapor-permeable films. In: C. Wilson (ed.), *Intelligent and Active Packaging for Fruits and Vegetables*, Boca Raton, FL: CRC Press, pp. 73–112.

Aharoni N., Rodov V., Fallik E., Porat R., Pesis E., Lurie S. 2008. Controlling humidity improves efficacy of modified atmosphere packaging of fruits and vegetables, *Acta Hort.*, ISHS 804, 121–128.

Ahmad M., Ahmad S.B. 2007. Leaching of styrene and other aromatic compounds in drinking water from PS bottles, *J. Environ. Sci.*, 19, 421–426.

Ahvenainen R. 2003. Active and intelligent packaging: an introduction. In: R. Ahvenainen (ed.), *Novel Food Packaging Techniques*, Cambridge, U.K.: Woodhead Publishing Limited, pp. 5–19.

Akhtar M.J., Jacquot M., Arab-Tehrany E., Caiani C., Linder M., Desorby S. 2010. Control of salmon oil photo-oxidation during storage in HPMC packaging film: Influence of film colour, *Food Chem.*, 20, 395–401.

Alexandre M., Dubois P. 2000. Polymer-layered silicate nanocomposites: Preparation, properties and uses of a new class of materials, *Mater. Sci. Eng.*, 28, 1–63.

Alique R., Martinez M.A., Alonso J. 2003. Influence of the modified atmosphere packaging on shelf life and quality of Navalinda sweet cherry, *Eur. Food Res. Technol.*, 217, 416–420.

Allende A., Luo Y., McEvoy J.L., Artes F., Wang C.Y. 2004. Microbial and quality changes in minimally processed baby spinach leaves stored under super atmospheric oxygen and modified atmosphere conditions, *Postharvest Biol. Tec.*, 33, 51–59.

Álvarez I. 2007. Hurdle technology and the preservation of food by pulsed electric fields. In: H.L.M. Lelieveld, S. Notermans, and S.W.H. de Haan (eds.), *Food Preservation by Pulsed Electric Fields*, Boca Raton, FL: CRC Press, pp. 165–178.

Antmann G., Ares G., Lema P., Lare C. 2008. Influence of modified atmosphere packaging on sensory quality of shiitake mushrooms, *Postharvest Biol. Tec.*, 49, 164–170.

Appendini P., Hotchkiss J.H. 2002. Review of antimicrobial food packaging, *Innov. Food Sci. Emerg.*, 3, 113–126.

Ares G., Lareo C., Lema P. 2007. Modified atmosphere packaging for postharvest storage of mushrooms: A review, *Fresh Produce Global Sci. Books*, 1(1), 32–40.

Arora A., Padua G.W. 2010. Review: Nanocomposites in food packaging, *J. Food Sci.*, 75, R43–R49.

Artes-Hernandez F., Tomas-Barberan F.A., Artes F. 2006. Modified atmosphere packaging preserves quality of SO_2-free 'Superior seedless' table grapes, *Postharvest Biol. Tec.*, 39, 146–154.

Atek D., Belhaneche-Bensemra N. 2005. FTIR investigation of the specific migration of additives from rigid poly(vinyl chloride), *Eur. Polym. J.*, 41, 707–714.

Ayranci E., Tunc S. 2003. A method for the measurement of the oxygen permeability and the development of edible films to reduce the rate of oxidative reactions in fresh foods, *Food Chem.*, 80, 423–431.

Azeredo H.M.C., Mattoso L.H.C., Wood D., Williams T.G., Avena-Bustillos R.J., McHugh T.H. 2009. Nanocomposite edible films from mango puree reinforced with cellulose nanofibers, *J. Food Sci.*, 74, N31–N35.

Bahri M.H., Rashidi M. 2009. Effects of coating methods and storage periods on some qualitative characteristics of carrot during ambient storage, *Int. J. Agric. Biol.*, 11, 443–447.

Bai J., Saftner R.A., Watada A.E. 2003. Characteristics of fresh-cut honeydew (*Cucumis xmelo* L.) available to processors in winter and summer and its quality maintenance by modified atmosphere packaging, *Postharvest Biol. Tec.*, 28, 349–359.

Barry-Ryan C., O'Beirne D. 2000. Effects of peeling methods on the quality of ready-to-use carrot slices, *Int. J. Food Sci. Tech.*, 35, 243–254.

Barth M.M., Zhuang H. 1996. Packaging design affects antioxidant vitamin retention and quality of broccoli florets during postharvest storage, *Postharvest Biol. Tec.*, 9, 141–150.

Baughan J.S., Montfort J-P. 2001. Food contact materials. In: K. Goodburn (ed.), *EU Food Law: A Practical Guide*, Cambridge: CRC Press, Woodhead Publishing Limited, Chapter 6.

Beaulieu J.C., Lea J.M. 2003. Volatile and quality changes in fresh-cut mangoes prepared from firm-ripe and soft-ripe fruit, stored in clamshell containers and passive MAP, *Postharvest Biol. Tec.*, 30, 15–28.

Begley T., Castle L., Feigenbaum A. et al. 2005. Evaluation of migration models that might be used in support of regulations for food-contact plastics, *Food Addit. Contamin.*, 22, 73–90.

Bertuzzi M.A., Armada M., Gottifredi J.C. 2007. Physicochemical characterization of starch based films, *J. Food Eng.*, 82, 17–25.

Bharadwaj R.K. 2001. Modeling the barrier properties of polymer-layered silicate nanocomposites, *Macromolecules*, 34, 9189–9192.

Birley A.W. 1982. Plastics used in food packaging and the rôle of additives. *Food Chem.*, 8, 81–84.

Bosset J.O., Gallmann P.U., Sieber R. 1993. Influence of light transmittance of packaging materials on the shelf-life of milk and dairy products, a review, *Le Lait.*, 73, 3–49.

Brandsch J., Mercea P., Piringer O. 1999. Modeling of additives diffusion coefficients in polyolefins. In: S.J. Risch (ed.), *ACS Symposium Series Vol. 753, Food Packaging: Testing Methods and Applications*, Washington, D.C: ACS, Chapter 4, pp. 27–37.

Brody A., Bugusu B., Han J.H., Sand C.K., McHough T.H. 2008. Innovative food packaging solutions, *J. Food Sci.*, 73, R107–R116.

Brody A.L., Strupinsky E.R., Kline L.R. 2002. *Active Packaging for Food Applications*, Boca Raton, FL: CRC Press LLC.

Brown J.W., Vorst K., Palmer S., Singh J. 2009. Performance of pre-cut lettuce packaged in biodegradable film formed on commercial vertical-form-fill-and-seal machines, *J. Appl. Packag. Res.*, 3, 1–14.

Burt S. 2004. Essential oils: Their antibacterial properties and potential applications in foods—A review, *Int. J. Food Microbiol.*, 94, 223–253.

Budd P.M, N.B. McKeown. 2010. Highly permeable polymers for gas separation membranes, *Polym. Chem.*, 1, 63–68.

Cagri A., Ustunol Z., Ryser E.T. 2001. Antimicrobial, mechanical, and moisture barrier properties of low pH whey protein based edible films containing *p*-aminobenzoic or sorbic acids, *J. Food Sci.*, 66, 865–870.

Cannarsi M., Baiano A., Marino R., Sinigaglia M., Del Nobile M.A. 2005. Use of biodegradable films for fresh cut beef steaks packaging, *Meat Sci.*, 70, 259–265.

Cegielska-Radziejewska R., Tycner B., Kijowski J., Zabielski J., Szablewski T. 2008. Quality and shelf life of chilled, pretreated MAP poultry meat products, *B. Vet. I. Pulawy*, 52, 603–609.

Charles F., Sancherz J., Gontard N. 2006. Absorption kinetics of oxygen and carbon dioxide scavengers as part of active modified atmosphere packaging. *J. Food Eng.*, 72, 1–7.

Charles F., Sanchez J., Gontard N. 2003. Active modified atmosphere packaging of fresh fruits and vegetables: Modeling with tomatoes and oxygen absorber, *J. Food Sci.*, 68, 1736–1742.

Chatham H. 1996. Review oxygen diffusion barrier properties of transparent oxide coatings on polymeric substrates, *Surf. Coat. Tech.*, 78, 1–9.

Chien P.J., Sheu F., Yang F.H. 2007. Effects of edible chitosan coating on quality and shelf life of sliced mango fruit, *J. Food Eng.*, 78, 225–229.

Chouliara E., Badeka A., Savvaidis I., Kontominas M.G. 2007. Combined effect of irradiation and modiffed atmosphere packaging on shelf-life extension of chicken breast meat: Microbiological, chemical and sensory changes, *Eur. Food Res. Technol.*, 226, 877–888.

Christy G.E., Amantea G.F., Irwin R.E.T. 1981. Evaluation of effectiveness of polyethylene over-wraps in preventing light-induced oxidation of milk in pouches. *Can. I. Food Sc. Tech. J.*, 14, 135–138.

Cisneros-Zevallos L., Krochta J.M. 2003. Whey protein coatings for fresh fruits and relative humidity effects, *J. Food Sci.*, 68, 176–181.

Cleveland J., Montville T.J., Nes I.F., Chikindas M.L. 2001. Bacteriocins: Safe, natural antimicrobials for food preservation, *Int. J. Food Microbiol.*, 71, 1–20.

Clough, R.L. 2001. High energy radiation and polymers: A review of commercial processes and emerging applications, *Nucl. Instr. Meth. Phys. Res. B*, 185, 8–33.

Coma V. 2008. Review—Bioactive packaging technologies for extended shelf life of meat-based products, *Meat Sci.*, 78, 90–103.

Conte A., Gammariello D., Di Giulio S., Attanasio M., Del Nobile M.A. 2009a. Active coating and modified-atmosphere packaging to extend the shelf life of Fior di Latte cheese, *J. Dairy Sci.*, 92, 887–894.

Conte A., Scrocco C., Lecce L., Mastromatteo M., Del Nobile M.A. 2009b. Ready-to-eat sweet cherries: Study on different packaging systems, *Innov. Food Sci. Emerg.*, 10, 564–571.

Conte A., Scrocco C., Sinigaglia M., Del Nobile M.A. 2007. Innovative active packaging systems to prolong the shelf life of Mozzarella cheese, *J. Dairy Sci.*, 90, 2126–2131.

Cooksey K. 2000. Utilization of antimicrobial packaging films for inhibition of selected microorganism. In: S.J. Risch (ed.), *Food Packaging: Testing Methods and Applications*, Washington, DC: American Chemical Society, pp. 17–25.

Corbo M.R., Altieri C., Bevilacqua A., Campaniello D., D'Amato D., Sinigaglia M. 2005. Estimating packaging atmosphere—Temperature effects on the shelf life of cod fillets, *Eur. Food Res. Technol.*, 220, 509–513.

Corradini M.G., Peleg M. 2007. Shelf-life estimation from accelerated storage data, *Trends Food Sci. Technol.*, 18, 37–47.

Daramola B., Asunni O.A. 2006. Nutrient composition and storage studies on roselle extract enriched deep-fat-fried snack food, *Afr. J. Biotechnol.*, 5, 1803–1807.

Day B.P.F. 2008. Active packaging of food, In: J. Kerry and P. Butler (eds.), *Smart Packaging Technologies for Fast Moving Consumer Goods*, Chichester: John Wiley & Sons, Ltd.

de Azeredo H.M.C. 2009. Nanocomposites for food packaging applications, *Food Res. Int.*, 42, 1240–1253.

de Moura M.R., Aouada F.A., Avena-Bustillos R.J., McHugh T.H., Krochta J.M., Mattoso L.H.C. 2009. Improved barrier and mechanical properties of novel hydroxypropyl methylcellulose edible films with chitosan/tripolyphosphate nanoparticles, *J. Food Eng.*, 92, 448–453.

Dean K., Yu L. 2005. Biodegradable protein-nanocomposites. In: R. Smith (ed.), *Biodegradable Polymers for Industrial Application*, Boca Raton, FL: CRC Press, pp. 289–309.

Debeaufort F., Voilley A., Guilbert S. 2002. Procédés de stabilisation des produits alimentaires par les films "barrière." In: M. Le Meste, D. Lorient, and D. Simatos (eds.), *L'Eau dans les Aliments*, Paris: Tec & Doc-Lavoisier, pp. 549–600.

Del Nobile M.A., Conte A., Cannarsi M., Sinigaglia M. 2008. Use of biodegradable films for prolonging the shelf life of minimally processed lettuce, *J. Food Eng.*, 85, 317–325.

Del Nobile M.A., Conte A., Scrocco C. et al. 2009a. A study on quality loss of minimally processed grapes as affected by film packaging, *Postharvest Biol. Tec.*, 51, 21–26.

Del Nobile, M.A., Conte, A., Incoronato, A.L., Panza, O. 2009b. Modified atmosphere packaging to improve the microbial stability of Ricotta, *Afr. J. Microbiol. Res.*, 3, 137–142.

Del Nobile, M.A., Buonocor, G.G., Limbo, S., Fava, P. 2003. Shelf life prediction of cereal-based dry foods packed in moisture-sensitive films, *J. Food Sci*, 68, 1292–1300.

Del-Valle V., Hernández-Muñoz P., Guarda A., Galotto M.J. 2005. Development of a cactus-mucilage edible coating (*Opuntia ficus indica*) and its application to extend strawberry (*Fragaria ananassa*) shelf-life, *Food Chem.*, 91, 751–756.

Denavi, G., Tapia-Blácido, D.R., Añón, M.C., Sobral, P.J.A., Mauri, A.N., Menegalli, F.C. 2009. Effects of drying conditions on some physical properties of soy protein films, *J. Food Eng.*, 90, 341–349.

Devlieghere F., Vermeiren L., Debevere J. 2004. New preservation technologies: Possibilities and limitations, *Int. Dairy J.*, 14, 273–285.

Diab T., Biliaderis C., Gerasopoulos D., Sfakiotakis E. 2001. Physicochemical properties and application of pullulan edible films and coatings in fruit preservation, *J. Sci. Food Agric.*, 81, 988–1000.

Djenane D., Sánchez-Escalante A., Beltrán J.A., Roncalés P. 2002. Ability of a-tocopherol, taurine and rosemary, in combination with vitamin C, to increase the oxidative stability of beef steaks packaged in modified atmosphere, *Food Chem.*, 76, 407–415.

Dukalska L., Muizniece-Brasava S., Kampuse S., Seglina D., Straumite E., Galoburda R. et al. 2008. Studies of biodegradable polymer material suitability for food packaging applications, *3rd Baltic Conference on Food Science and Technology FOODBALT–2008*, pp. 64–68.

Dunne C.P., Kluter R.A. 2001. Emerging non-thermal processing technologies: Criteria for success, *Aust. J. Dairy Technol.*, 56, 109–112.

Dutta P.K., Tripathi S., Mehrotra G.K., Dutta J. 2009. Perspectives for chitosan based antimicrobial films in food applications, *Food Chem.*, 114, 1173–1182.

Economou T., Pournis N., Ntzimani A., Savvaidis I.N. 2009. Nisin–EDTA treatments and modified atmosphere packaging to increase fresh chicken meat shelf-life, *Food Chem.*, 114, 1470–1476.

Emamifar A., Kadivar M., Shahedi M., Soleimanian-Zad S. 2010. Evaluation of nanocomposite packaging containing Ag and ZnO on shelf life of fresh orange juice, *Innov. Food Sci. Emerg.*, 11, 742–748.

Emblem A. 2000. Predicting packaging characteristics to improve shelf-life. In: D. Kilcast, P. Subramaniam (eds.), *The Stability and Shelf-life of Food*, Cambridge: CRC Press, Woodhead Publishing Limited.

Escalona V.H., Verlinden B.E., Geysen S., Nicolai B.M. 2006. Changes in respiration of fresh-cut butter head lettuce under controlled atmospheres using low and super atmospheric oxygen conditions with different carbon dioxide levels, *Postharvest Biol. Tec.*, 39, 48–55.

Fernandes J.C., Tavaria F.K., Soares J.C., Ramos S., Monteiro M.J., Pintado M.E. et al. 2008. Antimicrobial effects of chitosans and chitooligosaccharides, upon *Staphylococcus aureus* and *Escherichia coli*, in food model systems, *Food Microbiol.*, 25, 922–928.

Fernández K., Aspé E., Roeckel M. 2010. Scaling up parameters for shelf-life extension of Atlantic Salmon (*Salmo salar*) fillets using superchilling and modified atmosphere packaging, *Food Control*, 21, 857–862.

Fernández-Álvarez M. 2000. Review: Active food packaging, *Food Sci. Tech. Int.*, 6, 97–108.

Figge K., Koch J. 1973. Effect of some variables on the migration of additives from plastics into edible fats, *Food Cosmet. Toxicol.*, 11, 975–988.

Franssen L.R., Krochta J.M. 2003. Edible coatings containing natural antimicrobials for processed foods. In: S. Roller (ed.), *Natural Antimicrobials for the Minimal Processing of Foods*, Boca Raton, FL: CRC Press.

Gacitua W.E., Ballerini A.A., Zhang J. 2005. Polymer nanocomposites: Synthetic and natural fillers—A review, *Maderas. Ciencia y tecnología*, 7, 159–178.

Galić K., Ciković N. 2003. The effect of liquid absorption on gas barrier properties of triplex film coated with silicon oxide, *Food Technol. Biotechnol.*, 41, 247–251.

Galić K., Ščetar M., Kurek M. 2010. The benefits of processing and packaging, *Trends Food Sci. Tech.*, 22(2–3), 127–137, doi:10.1016/j.tifs.2010.04.001.

Ghasemzadeh R., Karbassi A., Ghoddousi H.B. 2008. Application of edible coating for improvement of quality and shelf-life of raisins, *World Appl. Sci. J.*, 3, 82–87.

Giannakourou M.C., Taoukis P.S. 2002. Systematic application of time temperature integrators as tools for control of frozen vegetable quality, *J. Food Sci.*, 67, 2221–2228.

Gil M.I., Conesa M.A., Artes F. 2002. Quality changes in fresh cut tomato as affected by modified atmosphere packaging, *Postharvest Biol. Tec.*, 25, 199–207.

Golzar M., Khalighi A.R. 2010. Tensile and relaxation properties of PA6/nanoclay nanocomposites, *Proceedings of the World Congress on Engineering and Computer Science 2010 Vol II, WCECS 2010, October 20–22, 2010*, San Francisco, USA.

González-Buesa J., Ferrer-Mairal A., Oria R., Salvador M.L. 2009. A mathematical model for packaging with microperforated films of fresh-cut fruits and vegetables, *J. Food Eng.*, 95, 158–165.

Granado-Lorencio F., Olmedilla-Alonso B., Herrero-Barbudo C. et al. 2008. Modified-atmosphere packaging (MAP) does not affect the bioavailability of tocopherols and carotenoids from broccoli in humans: A cross-over study, *Food Chem.*, 106, 1070–1076.

Grob K., Stocker J., Colwell R. 2009. Assurance of compliance within the production chain of food contact materials by good manufacturing practice and documentation—Part 1: Legal background in Europe and compliance challenges, *Food Control*, 20, 476–482.

Grobbel J.P., Dikeman M.E., Hunt M.C., Milliken G.A. 2008. Effects of packaging atmospheres on beef instrumental tenderness, fresh color stability, and internal cooked color, *J. Anim. Sci.*, 86, 1191–1199.

Guillen F., Zapata P.J., Martinez-Romero D., Castillo S., Serrano M., Valero, D. 2007. Improvement of the overall quality of table grapes stored under modified atmosphere packaging in combination with natural antimicrobial compounds, *J. Food Sci.*, 72(3), 185–190.

Gunister E., Pestreli D., Unlu C.H., Atici O., Gungor N. 2007. Synthesis and characterization of chitosan-MMT biocomposite systems, *Carbohyd. Polym.*, 67, 358–365.

Han C., Zhao Y., Leonard S.W., Traber M.G. 2004. Edible coatings to improve storability and enhance nutritional value of fresh and frozen strawberries (*Fragaria × ananassa*) and raspberries (*Rubus ideaus*), *Postharvest Biol. Tec.*, 33, 67–78.

Han J.H. 2005. New technologies in food packaging overview. In: J.H. Han (ed.), *Innovations in Food Packaging*, London: Elsevier Academic Press., pp. 3–10.

Hanušová K., Dobiáš J., Klaudisová K. 2009. Effect of packaging films releasing antimicrobial agents on stability of food products, *Czech J. Food Sci.*, 27, 347–349.

Hedenqvist M.S., Backman A., Gallstedt M., Boyd R.H., Gedde U.W. 2006. Morphology and diffusion properties of whey/montmorillonite nanocomposites, *Compos. Sci. Technol.*, 66, 2350–2359.

Hernández-Muñoz P., Almenar E., Del Valle V., Velez D., Gavara R. 2008. Effect of chitosan coating combined with postharvest calcium treatment on strawberry (*Fragaria × ananassa*) quality during refrigerated storage, *Food Chem.*, 110, 428–435.

Hernández-Muñoz P., Almenar E., Ocio M.J., Gavara R. 2006. Effect of calcium dips and chitosan coatings on postharvest life of strawberries (*Fragaria × ananassa*), *Postharv. Biol. Technol.*, 39, 247–253.

Hong S., Kim D. 2004. The effect of packaging treatment on the storage quality of minimally processed bunched onions, *Int. J. Food Sci. Tech.*, 39, 1033–1041.

Hough G., Garitta L., Gómez G. 2006. Sensory shelf-life predictions by survival analysis accelerated storage models, *Food Qual. Prefer.*, 17, 468–473.

Hourston, D.J., 2010. Degradation of plastics and polymers, *Shreir's Corrosion*, 3, 2369–2386.

Howells D.G., Henry B.M., Leterrier Y., Månson J.-A.E., Madocks J., Assender H.E. 2008. Mechanical properties of SiO_x gas barrier coatings on polyester films, *Surf. Coat. Tech.*, 202, 3529–3537.

Huang J.C., Shetty A.S., Wang M.S. 1990. Biodegradable plastics: A review. *Adv. Polym. Tech.*, 10, 23–30.

Ibrahim S.M., Nassar A.G., El-Badry N. 2008. Effect of modified atmosphere packaging and vacuum packaging methods on some quality aspects of smoked mullet (*Mugil cephalus*), *Global Veterinaria*, 2, 296–300.

Iglesias M.M., Peyron S., Chalier P., Gontard N. 2011. Scalping of four aroma compounds by one common (LDPE) and one biosourced (PLA) packaging materials during high pressure treatments, *J. Food Eng.*, 102, 9–15.

Isdell E., Allen P., Doherty A.M., Butler F. 1999. Colour stability of six beef muscles stored in a modified atmosphere mother pack system with oxygen scavengers, *Int. J. Food Sci. Tech.*, 34, 71–80.

Jacobsson A., Nielsen T., Sjoholm I. 2004. Influence of temperature, modified atmosphere packaging and heat treatment on aroma compounds in broccoli, *J. Agric. Food Chem.*, 52, 1607–1614.

Jbilou F., Galland S., Ayadi F. et al. 2010. Biodegradation of corn flour-based materials assessed by enzymatic, aerobic, and anaerobic tests: Influence of specific surface area, *Polym. Test.*, 30, 131–139.

Jia C-G., Xu C-J., Wei J., Yuan J., Yuan G-F., Wang B-L. et al. 2009. Effect of modified atmosphere packaging on visual quality and glucosinolates of broccoli florets, *Food Chem.*, 114, 28–37.

Jiang T., Wang Y-H., Yeh J-T., Fan Z-Q. 2005. Study on solvent permeation resistance properties of nylon6/clay nanocomposite, *Eur. Poly. J.*, 41, 459–466.

Jordan J., Jacob K.I., Tannenbaum R., Sharaf M.A., Jasiuk I. 2005. Experimental trends in polymer nanocomposites—A review, *Mater. Sci. Eng.*, 393, 1–11.

Karbowiak T., Debeaufort F., Voilley A., Trystram G. 2009. From macroscopic to molecular scale investigations of mass transfer of small molecules through edible packaging applied at interfaces of multiphase food products, *Innov. Food Sci. Emerg.*, 10, 116–127.

Karel M., Lund D. 2003. *Physical Principles of Food Preservation*, 2nd edn, Cambridge: CRC Press, Woodhead Publishing Limited, Chapter 12.

Kerry J.P., O'Grady M.N., Hogan S.A. 2006. Past, current and potential utilisation of active and intelligent packaging systems for meat and muscle-based products: A review. *Meat Sci.*, 74, 113–130.

Kim J.G., Luo Y., Gross K.C. 2004. Effect of package film on the quality of freshcut salad savoy, *Postharvest Biol. Tec.*, 32, 99–107.

Kim S-R., Choudhury M.H., Kim W-H., Kim G-H. 2010. Effects of argon and oxygen flow rate on water vapor barrier properties of silicon oxide coatings deposited on polyethylene terephthalate by plasma enhanced chemical vapor deposition, *Thin Solid Films*, 518, 1929–1934.

Kim Y., White J.L. 2006. Modeling of polymer/clay nanocomposite formation, *J. Appl. Poly. Sci.*, 101, 1657–1663.

Koller M., Salerno A., Dias M., Reiterer A., Braunegg G. 2010. Modern biotechnological polymer synthesis: A review, *Food Technol. Biotechnol.*, 48, 255–269.

Kolybaba M., Tabil L.G., Panigrahi S., Crerar W.J., Powell T., Wang B. 2003. Biodegradable polymers: Past, present, and future, Paper number: RRV03–0007, An ASAE Meeting Presentation.

Krzan A., Hemjinda S., Miertus S., Corti A., Chiellini E. 2006. Review article—Standardization and certification in the area of environmentally degradable plastics, *Polym. Degrad. Stabil.*, 91, 2819–2833.

Labuza, T.P., Breene, W.M. 1989. Application of active packaging for improvement of shelf-life and nutritional quality of fresh and extended shelf-life foods, *J. Food Process. Preserv.*, 13, 1–69.

Lagarón J.M., Cabedo L., Cava D., Feijoo J.L., Gavara R., Gimenez E. 2005. Improving packaged food quality and safety. Part 2: Nanocomposites. *Food Addit. Contam.*, 22, 994–998.

LeBaron P.C., Wang Z., Pinnavaia T.J. 1999. Polymer-layered silicate nanocomposites: An overview, *Appl. Clay Sci.*, 15, 11–29.

Lee C.H., An D.S., Lee S.C., Park H.J., Lee D.S. 2004. A coating for use as an antimicrobial and antioxidative packaging material incorporating nisin and α-tocopherol, *J. Food Eng.*, 62, 323–329.

Lee D.S., Kang J.S., Renault P. 2000. Dynamics of internal atmosphere and humidity in perforated packages of peeled garlic cloves, *Int. J. Food Sci. Tech.*, 35, 455–464.

Lee K.T. 2010. Quality and safety aspects of meat products as affected by various physical manipulations of packaging materials, *Meat Sci.*, 86, 138–150.

Lelieveld, H.L.M. 2007. Pitfalls of pulsed electric filed processing. In: H.L.M. Lelieveld, S. Notermans, and S.W.H. de Haan (eds.), *Food Preservation byPulsed Electric Fields*, Boca Raton, FL: CRC Press, pp. 294–300.

Lerdthanangkul S., Krochta J.M. 1996. Edible coating effects on post harvest quality of green bell peppers, *J. Food Sci.*, 61, 176–179.

Lewis J.S., Weaver M.S. 2004. Thin-film permeation-barrier technology for flexible organic light-emitting devices, *IEEE J. Sel. Top. Quant.*, 10, 45–57.

Lin K.F., Hsu C.Y., Huang T.S., Chiu W.Y.M., Lee Y.H., Young T.H. 2005. A novel method to prepare chitosan/montmorillonite nanocomposites, *J. Appl. Polym. Sci.*, 98, 2042–2047.

Lucera A., Costa C., Mastromatteo M., Conte A., Del Nobile M.A. 2010. Influence of different packaging systems on fresh-cut zucchini (*Cucurbita pepo*), *Innov. Food Sci. Emerg.*, 11, 361–368.

Mahalik N.P., Nambiar A.N. 2010. Trends in food packaging and manufacturing systems and technology, *Trends Food Sci. Tech.*, 21, 117–128.

Mancini R.A., Hunt M.C., Hachmeister K.A., Kropf D.H., Johnson D.E. 2005. Exclusion of oxygen from modified atmosphere packages limits beef rib and lumbar vertebrae marrow discoloration during display and storage, *Meat Sci.*, 69, 493–500.

Mancini R.A., Ramanathan R., Suman S.P. et al. 2010. Effects of lactate and modified atmospheric packaging on premature browning in cooked ground beef patties, *Meat Sci.*, 85, 339–346.

Mark J.E. 1996. Ceramic-reinforced polymers and polymer-modified ceramics, *Polym. Eng. Sci.*, 36, 2905–2920.

Marrero A., Kader A.A. 2006. Optimal temperature and modified atmosphere for keeping quality of fresh-cut pineapples, *Postharvest Biol. Tec.*, 39, 163–168.

Marsh K., Bugusu B. 2007. Food packaging—Roles, materials,and environmental issues, *J. Food Sci.*, 72(3), R39–R55.

Martínez L., Cilla I., Beltrán J.A., Roncalés P. 2007. Effect of illumination on the display life of fresh pork sausages packaged in modified atmosphere. Influence of the addition of rosemary, ascorbic acid and black pepper, *Meat Sci.*, 75, 443–450.

Martínez L., Djenane D., Cilla I., Beltrán J.A, Roncalés P. 2006. Effect of varying oxygen concentrations on the shelf-life of fresh pork sausages packaged in modified atmosphere, *Food Chem.*, 94, 219–225.

Martino V.P., Ruseckaite R.A., Jiménez A. 2005. Processing and Mechanical characterization of plasticized Poly (lactide acid) films for food packaging, *Proceeding of the 8th Polymers for Advanced Technologies International Symposium*, Budapest, Hungary, 13–16 September.

Mauriello G., Ercolini D., La Storia A., Casaburi A., Villani F. 2004. Development of polythene films for food packaging activated with an antilisterial bacteriocin from *Lactobacillus curvatus* 32Y, *J. Appl. Microbiol.*, 97, 314–322.

McGlashan S.A., Halley P.J. 2003. Preparation and characterization of biodegradable starch-based nanocomposite materials, *Polym. Int.*, 52, 1767–1773.

Mendoza T.F., Welt B.A., Otwell S., Teixeira A.A., Kristonsson H., Balaban M.O. 2004. Kinetic parameter estimation of time-temperature integrators intended for use with packaged fresh seafood, *J. Food Sci.*, 69, FMS90–FMS96.

Meneghetti P., Qutubuddin S. 2006. Synthesis, thermal properties and applications of polymer-clay nanocomposites, *Thermochim. Acta*, 442, 74–77.

Mestdagh F., De Meulenaer B., De Clippeleer J., Devlieghere F., Huyghebaert A. 2005. Protective influence of several packaging materials on light oxidation of milk, *J. Dairy Sci.*, 88, 499–510.

Mexis S.F., Badeka A.V., Kontominas M.G. 2009. Quality evaluation of raw ground almond kernels (*Prunus dulcis*): Effect of active and modified atmosphere packaging, container oxygen barrier and storage conditions, *Innov. Food Sci. Emerg.*, 10, 580–589.

Min S., Rumsey T.R., Krochta J.M. 2008. Diffusion of the antimicrobial lysozyme from a whey protein coating on smoked salmon, *J. Food Eng.*, 84, 39–47.

Min S., Zhang Q.H. 2005. Packaging for non-thermal food processing. In: J.H. Han (ed.), *Innovations in Food Packaging*, Oxford: Elsevier Academic Press, pp. 482–500.

Mishra B., Khatkar B.S., Garg M.K., Wilson L.A. 2010. Permeability of edible coatings, *J. Food Sci. Technol.*, 47, 109–113.

Misra E., Basavarajaiah S., Kumar K. R., Ravi P. 2000. Effect of recycling on the properties of poly(ethylene terephthalate) films, *Polym. Int.*, 49, 1636–1640.

Mizrahi S. 2004. Accelerated shelf life tests. In: R. Steele (ed.), *Understanding and Measuring the Shelf-Life of Food*, Cambridge, UK: Woodhead Publishing.

Montanez J.C., Rodriguez F.A.S., Mahajan P.V., Frias J.M. 2010a. Modelling the gas exchange rate in perforation-mediated modified atmosphere packaging: Effect of the external air movement and tube dimensions, *J. Food Eng.*, 97, 79–86.

Montanez J.C., Rodriguez F.A.S., Mahajan P.V., Frias J.M. 2010b. Modelling the effect of gas composition on the gas exchange rate in perforation-mediated modified atmosphere packaging, *J. Food Eng.*, 96, 348–355.

Montero-Calderón M., Rojas-Graü M.A., Martín-Belloso O. 2008. Effect of packaging conditions on quality and shelf-life of fresh-cut pineapple (*Ananas comosus*), *Postharvest Biol. Tec.*, 50, 182–189.

Morillon V., Debeaufort F., Bond G., Capelle M., Voilley A. 2002. Factors affecting the moisture permeability of lipid-based edible films: A review. *Crit. Rev. Food Sci.*, 42, 67 – 89.

No H.K., Meyers S.P., Prinyawiwatkul W., Xu Z. 2007. Applications of chitosan for improvement of quality and shelf life of foods: A review, *J. Food Sci.*, 72, 87–100.

Nörenberg H., Burlakov V.M., Kosmella H.-J., Smith G.D.W., Briggs G.A.D., Miyamoto T. et al. 2001. Pressure-dependent permeation of noble gases (He, Ne, Ar, Kr, Xe) through thin membranes of oriented polypropylene (OPP) studied by mass spectrometry, *Polymer*, 42, 10021–10026.

Nur S. (Aktaş), Dirim, Esin, A. Bayindirli, A. 2003. A new protective polyethylene based film containing zeolites for the packaging of fruits and vegetables: Film preparation, *Turkish J. Eng. Env. Sci.*, 27, 1–9.

Olabarrieta I., Gallistedl M., Ispizua I., Sarasua J.-R., Hedenqvist M.S. 2006. Properties of aged montmorillonite-wheat gluten composite films, *J. Agric. Food Chem.*, 54, 1283–1288.

Oms-Oliu G., Soliva-Fortuny R., Martín-Belloso O. 2008. Edible coatings with antibrowning agents to maintain sensory quality and antioxidant properties of fresh-cut pears, *Postharvest Biol. Tec.*, 50, 87–94.

Ozdemir I., Monnet F., Gouble B. 2005. Simple determination of the O_2 and CO_2 permeances of micro perforated pouches for modified atmosphere packaging of respiring foods, *Postharvest Biol. Tec.*, 36, 209–213.

Ozdemir M., Floros J.D. 2001. Analysis and modeling of potassium sorbate diffusion through edible whey protein films, *J. Food Eng.*, 47, 149–155.

Ozen B.F., Floros J.D. 2001. Effects of emerging food processing techniques on the packaging materials, *Trends Food Sci. Tech.*, 12, 60–67.

Ozturk A., Yilmaz N., Gunes G. 2010. Effect of different modified atmosphere packaging on microbial quality, oxidation and colour of a seasoned ground beef product (meatball). *Packag. Technol. Sci.*, 23, 19–25.

Pacquit A., Frisby J., Diamond D., Lau K.T., Farrell A., Quilty B. et al. 2007. Development of a smart packaging for the monitoring of fish spoilage, *Food Chem.*, 102, 466–470.

Park H.M., Lee W.K., Park C.Y., Cho W.J., Ha C.S. 2003. Environmentally friendly polymer hybrids. Part I Mechanical, thermal, and barrier properties of thermoplastic starch/clay nanocomposites, *J. Mater. Sci.*, 38, 909–915.

Parra V., Viguera J., Sánchez J., Peinado J., Espárrago F., Gutierrez J.I. et al. 2010. Modified atmosphere packaging and vacuum packaging for long period chilled storage of dry-cured Iberian ham, *Meat Sci.*, 84, 760–768.

Paul D.R., Robeson L.M. 2008. Polymer nanotechnology: Nanocomposites, *Polymer*, 49, 3187–3204.

Paz H.M., Guillard V., Reynes M., Gontard N. 2005. Ethylene permeability of wheat gluten film as a function of temperature and relative humidity, *J. Membrane Sci.*, 256, 108–115.

Pennarun P.Y., Dole P., Feigenbaum A. 2004. Functional barriers in PET recycled bottles. Part I. Determination of diffusion coefficients in bi-oriented PET with and without contact with Food Stimulants, *J. Appl. Polym. Sci.*, 92, 2845–2858.

Piringer O.G., Baner A.L. 2008. *Plastic Packaging, Interactions with Food and Pharmaceuticals*, 2nd edn, Weinheim: Wiley-VCH Verlag GmbH & Co KGaA.

Powell C.E., Beall G.W. 2006. Physical properties of polymer/clay nanocomposites, *Curr. Opin. Solid St. M.*, 10, 73–80.

Quezada Gallo, J.A., Debeaufort, F., Voilley, A. 1999. Interactions between aroma and edible films. 1. Permeability of methylcellulose and low density polyethylene films to methylketones, *J. Agric. Food Chem.*, 47, 108 – 113.

Quintavalla S., Vicini L. 2002. Antimicrobial food packaging in meat industry, *Meat Sci.*, 62, 373–380.

Raj B., Sankar U.K., Siddaramaiah. 2004. Low density polyethylene/starch blend films for food packaging applications, *Adv. Polym. Tech.*, 23, 32–45.

Rashidi M., Bahri M.H. 2009. Interactive effects of coating method and storage period on quality of carrot (cv. Nantes) during ambient storage, *ARPN J. Agric. Biol. Sci.*, 4, 29–35.

Regulation 2023/2006 (EC) of 22 December 2006 on good manufacturing practice for materials and articles intended to come into contact with food (OJ L 384/75, 29.12.2006).

Regulation 1935/2004 Regulation (EC) of the European parliament and of the council of 27 October 2004 on materials and articles intended to come into contact with food and repealing Directives 80/590/EEC and 89/109/EEC (1) OJ C 117, 30.4.2004, p. 1. 2004. OJ L 284, 31.10.2003, p. 1.

Rhim J.W., Hong S.I., Park H.M., Ng P.K.W. 2006. Preparation and characterization of chitosan-based nanocomposite films with antimicrobial activity, *J. Agric. Food Chem.*, 54, 5814–5822.

Rhim J.W., Hong S.I., Ha C.S. 2009. Tensile, water vapor barrier and antimicrobial properties of PLA/nanoclay composite films, *Lebensm-Wiss Technol.*, 42, 612–617.

Rhim J.W., Lee J.H., Kwak H.S. 2005. Mechanical and barrier properties of soy protein and clay mineral composite films, *Food Sci. Biotechnol.*, 14, 112–116.

Ribeiro C., Vicente A.A., Teixeira J.A., Miranda C. 2007. Optimization of edible coating composition to retard strawberry fruit senescence, *Postharvest Biol. Tec.*, 44, 63–70.

Roberts A.P., Henry B.M., Sutton A.P. et al. 2002. Gas permeation in silicon-oxide/polymer (SiO$_x$/PET) barrier films:role of the oxide lattice, nano-defects and macro-defects, *J. Membrane Sci.*, 208, 75–88.

Rocculi P., Romani S., Dalla Rosa M. 2005. Effect of MAP with argon and nitrous oxide on quality maintenance of minimally processed kiwifruit, *Postharvest Biol. Tec.*, 35, 319–328.

Rojas-Graü M.A., Avena-Bustillos R.J., Olsen C. et al. 2007a. Effects of plant essential oils and oil compounds on mechanical, barrier and antimicrobial properties of alginate–apple puree edible films, *J. Food Eng.*, 81, 634–641.

Rojas-Graü M.A., Raybaudi-Massilia R.M., Soliva-Fortuny R.C., Avena-Bustillos R.J., McHugh T.H., Martín-Belloso O. 2007b. Apple puree-alginate edible coating as carrier of antimicrobial agents to prolong shelf-life of fresh-cut apples, *Postharvest Biol. Tec.*, 45, 254–264.

Rojas-Graü M.A., Soliva-Fortuny R.C., Martín-Belloso O. 2009. Edible coatings to incorporate active ingredients to fresh-cut fruits: A review, *Trends Food Sci. Tech.*, 20, 438–447.

Rojas-Graü M.A., Tapia M.S., Martín-Belloso O. 2008. Using polysaccharide-based edible coatings to maintain quality of fresh-cut Fuji apples, *Lebensm-Wiss Technol.*, 41, 139–147.

Rosca I.D., Vergnaud J-M. 2006. Approach for a testing system to evaluate food safety with polymer packages, *Polym. Test.*, 25, 532–543.

Rotabakk B.T., Lekang O.I., Sivertsvik M. 2007. Volumetric method to determine carbon dioxide solubility and absorption rate in foods packaged in flexible or semi rigid package, *J. Food Eng.*, 82, 43–50.

Ruban S.W. 2009. Biobased packaging—Application in meat industry, *Veterinary World*, 2, 79–82.

Rubio B., Martínez B., Sánchez M.J., García-Cachán M.D., Rovira J., Jaime I. 2007. Study of the shelf life of a dry fermented sausage "salchichon" made from raw material enriched in monounsaturated and polyunsaturated fatty acids and stored under modiffied atmospheres, *Meat Sci.*, 76, 128–137.

Russell A.D. 1991. Mechanisms of bacterial resistance to non-antibiotics: Food additives and food and pharmaceutical preservatives, *J. Appl. Bacteriol.*, 71, 191–201.

Saffert A., Pieper G., Jetten J. 2006. Effect of package light transmittance on the vitamin content of pasteurized whole milk, *Packag. Technol. Sci.*, 19, 211–218.

Sajilata M.G., Savitha K., Singhal R.S., Kanetkar V.R. 2007. Scalping of flavors in packaged foods, *Compr. Rev. Food Sci. F.*, 6, 17–23.

Salleh E., Muhamad I.I., Khairuddin N. 2009. Structural characterization and physical properties of antimicrobial (AM) starch-based films, *World Acad. Sci. Eng. Technol.*, 55, 432–440.

Salminen A., Latva-Kala K., Randell K., Hurme E., Linko P., Ahvenainen R. 1996. The effect of ethanol and oxygen absorption on the shelf-life of packaged slice rye bread, *Packag. Technol. Sci.*, 9, 29–42.

Ščetar M., Kurek M., Galić K. 2010. Trends in meat and meat products packaging—A review, *Croat. J. Food Sci. Technol.*, 2, 32–48.

Schmid P., Kohler M., Meierhofer R., Luzi S., Wegelin M. 2008. Does the reuse of PET bottles during solar water disinfection pose a health risk due to the migration of plasticisers and other chemicals into the water? *Water Res.*, 42, 5054–5060.

Schowalter S.J., Connolly C.B., Doyle J.M. 2010. Permeability of noble gases through Kapton, butyl, nylon, and "SilverShield", *Nucl. Instrum. Methods*, 615, 267–271.

Sebti I., Chollet E., Degraeve P., Noel C., Peyrol E. 2007. Water sensitivity, antimicrobial, and physicochemical analyses of edible films based on HPMC and/or chitosan, *J. Agric. Food Chem.*, 55, 693–699.

Seglina D., Krasnova I., Heidemane G., Kampuse S., Dukalska L., Muizniece-Brasava S. 2009. Influence of packaging materials and technologies on the shelf-life of fresh black currant, *Cheminè Technologija*, 3, 43–49.

Seyfert M., Hunt M.C., Mancini R.A., Hachmeister K.A., Kropf D.H., Unruh J.A. et al. 2005. Beef quadriceps hot boning and modified-atmosphere packaging influence properties of injection-enhanced beef round muscles, *J. Anim. Sci.*, 83, 686–693.

Shabestary N., Khazaeli S., Dutko D., Cutts B.L. 2007. Clay-supported quaternary ammonium and phosphonium cations in triphase catalysis and the effect of cosolvent in catalytic activity, *Scientia Iranica*, 14, 297–302.

Shapero M., Nelson D., Labuza T.P. 1978. Ethanol inhibition of *Staphylococcus aureus* at limited water activity, *J. Food Sci.*, 43, 1467–1469.

Silva F.M., Chau K.V., Brecht J.K., Sargent S.A. 1999. Modified atmosphere packaging for mixed loads of horticultural commodities exposed to two postharvest temperatures, *Postharvest Biol. Tec.*, 17, 1–9.

Simões A.N., Puiatti M., Salomão L.C.C., Mosquim P.R., Puschmann R. 2009. Effect in the quality of intact and minimally processed leaves of collard greens stored at different temperatures, *Hortic. Bras.*, 28, 81–86.

Simon A., Gonzalez-Fandos E., Tobar V. 2005. The sensory and microbiological quality of fresh sliced mushroom (*Agaricus bisporus* L.) packaged in modified atmospheres, *Int. J. Food Sci. Tech.*, 40, 943–952.

Siripatrawan U., Jantawat P. 2008. A novel method for shelf life prediction of a packaged moisture sensitive snack using multilayer perception neural network, *Expert Syst. Appl.*, 34, 1562–1567.

Skandamis P.N., Nychas G-J.E. 2002. Preservation of fresh meat with active and modified atmosphere packaging conditions, *Int. J. Food Microbiol.*, 79, 35–45.

Smith J.P., Ooraikul B., Koersen W.J., Van der Voort F.R., Jackson E.D., Lawrence, R.A. 1987. Shelf-life extension of a bakery product using ethanol vapor, *Food Microbiol.*, 4, 329–337.

Smith J.P., Ramaswamy H.S., Simpson B.K. 1990. Developments in food packaging technology. Part II: Storage aspects, *Trends Food Sci. Technol.*, 5, 111–118.

Smith J.P., Simpson B.K. 1995. Modified atmosphere packaging of bakery and pasta products. In: J.M. Farber, K.L. Dodds (eds.), *Principles of Modified Atmosphere Packaging and Sous-Vide Processing*, Lancaster: Technomic Publishing Company, pp. 207–242.

Smith, J.P., Ooraikul, B., Koersen, W.J., Jackson, E.D., Lawrence, R.A. 1986. Novel approach to oxygen control in modified atmosphere packaging of bakery products, *Food Microbiol.*, 3, 315–20.

Smolander M., Alakomi H-L., Ritvanen T., Vainionpää J., Ahvenainen R. 2004. Monitoring of the quality of modified atmosphere packaged broiler chicken cuts stored in different temperature conditions. A. Time–temperature indicators as quality-indicating tools, *Food Control*, 15, 217–229.

Smolander M., Hurme E., Ahvenainen R. 1997. Leak indicators for modified-atmosphere packages. *Trends Food Sci. Tech.*, 8, 101–106.

Sobral P.J.A., Menegalli F.C., Hubinger M.D., Roques M.A. 2001. Mechanical, water vapor barrier and thermal properties of gelatin based edible films, *Food Hydrocolloid.*, 15, 423 – 432.

Soliva-Fortuny R.C., Ricart-Coll M., Martin-Belloso O. 2005. Sensory quality and internal atmosphere of fresh-cut Golden Delicious apples, *Int. J. Food Sci. Tech.*, 40, 369–375.

Sorrentino A., Gorrasi G., Vittoria V. 2007. Potential perspectives of bio-nanocomposites for food packaging applications, *Trends Food Sci. Tech.*, 18, 84–95.

Sothornvit R., Krochta J.M. 2000. Oxygen permeability and mechanical properties of films from hydrolyzed whey protein, *J. Agric. Food Chem.*, 48, 3913–3916.

Sothornvit R., Krochta J.M. 2005. Plasticizers in edible films and coatings. In: J.H. Han (ed.), *Innovations in Food Packaging*, London, UK: Elsevier Academic Press, pp. 403–433.

Sothornvit R., Rhim J.W., Hong S.I. 2009. Effect of nano-clay type on the physical and antimicrobial properties of whey protein isolate/clay composite films, *J. Food Eng.*, 91, 468–473.

Stamatis N., Arkoudelos J. 2007. Quality assessment of *Scomber colias japonicus* under modified atmosphere and vacuum packaging, *Food Control*, 18, 292–300.

Stefanescu E.A., Daranga C., Stefanescu C. 2009. Insight into the broad field of polymer nanocomposites: From carbon nanotubes to clay nanoplatelets, via metal nanoparticles, *Materials*, 2, 2095–2153.

Suppakul, P., Miltz, J., Bigger, S.W. 2003. Active packaging technologies with an emphasis on antimicrobial packaging and its applications, *J. Food Sci.*, 68, 408–420.

Taoukis P.S., Labuza T.P. 2003. Time-temperature indicators (TTIs). In: R. Ahvenainen (ed.), *Novel Food Packaging Techniques*, Cambridge UK: Woodhead Publishing Limited, pp. 103–126.

Tapia M.S., Rojas-Graü M.A., Carmonac A., Rodríguez F.J., Soliva-Fortuny R., Martín-Belloso O. 2008. Use of alginate- and gellan-based coatings for improving barrier, texture and nutritional properties of fresh-cut papaya, *Food Hydrocolloid.*, 22, 1493–1503.

Tewari G., Jayas D.S., Jeremiah L.E., Holley R.A. 2001. Prevention of transient discoloration of beef, *J. Food Sci.*, 66, 506–510.

Tewari G., Jayas D.S., Jeremiah L.E., Holley R.A. 2002a. Absorption kinetics of oxygen scavengers, *Int. J. Food Sci. Tech.*, 37, 209–217.

Tewari G., Jeremiah L.E., Jayas D.S., Holley R.A. 2002b. Improved use of oxygen scavengers to stabilize the colour of retail-ready meat cuts stored in modified atmospheres, *Int. J. Food Sci. Tech.*, 37, 199–207.

Tharanathan R.N. 2003. Biodegradable films and composite coatings: Past, present and future, *Trends Food Sci. Tech.*, 14, 71–78.

Trienekens J.H., Hagen J.M., Beulensc A.J.M., Omta S.W.F. 2003. Innovation through (international) food supply chain development: A research agenda, *Int. Food Agribusiness Manage. Rev.*, 6, 1–15.

Tzoumaki M.V., Biliaderis C.G., Vasilakakis M. 2009. Impact of edible coatings and packaging on quality of white asparagus (*Asparagus officinalis*, L.) during cold storage, *Food Chem.*, 117, 55–63.

Van Aardt M., Duncan S.E., Marcy J.E., Long T.E., Hackney C.R. 2001. Effectiveness of poly(ethylene terephthalate) and high-density polyethylene in protection of milk flavor, *J. Dairy Sci.*, 84, 1341–1347.

Van de Velde K., Kiekens P. 2002. Biopolymers: Overview of several properties and consequences on their applications, *Polym. Test.*, 21, 433–442.

Van der Steen C., Jacxsens L., Devlieghere F., Debevere J. 2002. Combining high oxygen atmospheres with low oxygen modified atmosphere packaging to improve the keeping quality of strawberries and raspberries, *Postharvest Biol. Tec.*, 26, 49–58.

Vargas M., Pastor C., Chiralt A., McClements D.J., Gonzalez-Martinez C. 2008. Recent advances in edible coatings for fresh and minimally processed fruits, *Crit. Rev. Food Sci.*, 48, 496–511.

Vermeiren L., Devlieghere F., van Beest M., de Kruijf N., Debevere J. 1999. Developments in the active packaging of foods, *Trends Food Sci. Technol.*, 10, 77–86.

Vinci G., Antonelli M.L. 2002. Biogenic amines: Quality index of freshness in red and white meat, *Food Control*, 13, 519–524.

Wang N., Zhang N., Wang M. 2006. Wireless sensors in agriculture and food industry—Recent development and future perspective, *Computers Electron. Agric.*, 50, 1–14.

Wang X.D., Chen H.X., Zhao Y., Chen X., Wang X.R. 2010. Optical oxygen sensors move towards colorimetric determination, *Trends Anal. Chem.*, 29, 319–338.

Wang Z., Li G., Xie G., Zhang Z. 2005. Dispersion behavior of TiO2 nanoparticles in LLDPE/LDPE/TiO2 nanocomposites, *Macromol. Chem. Phys.*, 206, 258–262.

Weber C.J. 2000. Biobased Packaging Materials for the Food Industry: Status and Perspectives, Food Biopack Project, EU Directorate 12, November 2000.

Weiss J., Takhistov P., McClements D.J. 2006. Functional materials in food nanotechnology, *J. Food Sci.*, 71, R107–R116.

Wong M.K., Gan L.M., Koh L.L. 1988. Temperature effects on the leaching of lead from unplasticized poly(vinyl chloride) pipes, *Water Res.*, 22, 1399–1403.

Xu Y., Ren X., Hanna M.A. 2006. Chitosan/clay nanocomposite film preparation and characterization, *J. Appl. Polym. Sci.*, 99, 1684–1691.

Yam K.L., Takhistov P.T., Miltz J. 2005. Intelligent packaging: Concepts and applications, *J. Food Sci.*, 70, R1-R10.

Yaman O., Bayoindirli L. 2002. Effects of an edible coating and cold storage on shelf-life and quality of cherries, *Lebensm.-Wiss. Technol.*, 35, 146–150.

Yang S.L., Wu Z.H., Yang W., Yang M.B. 2008. Thermal and mechanical properties of chemical crosslinked polylactide (PLA), *Polym. Test.*, 27, 957–963.

Yeh J.T., Chang C.J., Tsai F.C., Chen K.N., Huang K.S. 2009. Oxygen barrier and blending properties of blown films of blends of modified polyamide and polyamide-6 clay mineral nanocomposites, *Appl. Clay Sci.*, 45, 1–7.

Zakrys P.I., Hogan S.A., O'Sullivan M.G., Allen P., Kerry J.P. 2008. Effects of oxygen concentration on the sensory evaluation and quality indicators of beef muscle packed under modified atmosphere, *Meat Sci.*, 79, 648–655.

Zhang M., Xiao G., Peng J., Salokhe V.M. 2003. Effects of modified atmosphere package on preservation of strawberries, *Int. Agrophysics*, 17, 143–148.

Zhang M., Xiao G., Peng J., Salokhe V.M. 2005. Effects of single and combined atmosphere packages on preservation of strawberries, *Int. J. Food Eng.*, 1, 141–148.

Zhou R., Mo Y., Li Y.F., Zhao Y.Y., Zhang G.X., Hu Y.S. 2008. Quality and internal characteristics of Huanghua pears (*Pyrus pyrifolia Nakai*, cv. *Huanghua*) treated with different kinds of coatings during storage, *Postharvest Biol. Tec.*, 49, 171–179.

Zuckerman, H., Miltz, J. 1992. Characterization of thin layer susceptors for the microwave oven, *J. Food Proc. Preserv.*, 16, 193–204.

16 Innovation in Iron Fortification
Is the Future in Iron-Binding Milk Proteins?

Ashling Ellis, Vikas Mittal, and Maya Sugiarto

CONTENTS

16.1 INTRODUCTION

Iron deficiency is a phenomenon affecting populations both in developed and in developing countries worldwide. It is the most common type of nutrient deficiency recognized by the World Health Organization (WHO), with almost 1.62 billion people (24.2% of world population) estimated to be suffering from anemia (McLean et al., 2009). Affected populations are concentrated mainly in the poor and developing nations, with the highest proportion (47.5–67.6%) being in the African continent, and the largest number (315 million) in South East Asia. Although there are various reasons for anemia (infections, inflammations, etc.), nutritional deficiency of iron (Fe) is at least a contributing factor in all cases.

Iron is essential for optimally functioning red blood cells which carry oxygen throughout the body. Lack of iron can result in a range of health issues, with the most severe being iron deficiency anemia (IDA). Some of the main symptoms associated with iron deficiency are fatigue, general weakness, shortness of breath, hair loss, and restless leg syndrome. Iron deficiency has been shown to affect people of all ages; however, those most at risk are predominantly preschool children, adolescent females, pregnant women, and the unborn fetus (Benoist et al., 2008). Statistics from the WHO Global Database showed that iron deficiency anemia in young infants of preschool age affected approximately 47% of this population. High rates of anemia were also seen in pregnant women, with up to 42% being affected (Benoist et al., 2008). This may have an effect on fetal growth, with many iron-deficient mothers giving birth to preterm, low-weight infants. Children of school-going age with iron deficiencies have shown decreased concentration spans and performance in comparison to their counterparts (Falkingham et al., 2010). Overall, it is obvious that deficiency in iron has extensive global implications. The WHO feels that the most startling consequences are to be found in the statistics relating to the death tolls, reduced productivity of the workforce as well as deaths/hemorrhaging occurring during child birth. It is felt that all of these statistics could be minimized if further steps could be taken to reduce iron deficiency worldwide.

The bioavailability of heme iron versus nonheme iron in the human body is discussed in greater detail in the next section; however, it is well known that nonheme iron from plants is not as easily absorbed in the body. This is partially due to the presence of inhibitors or antinutrients present in plant-based foods containing nonheme sources of iron (Lynch, 2000). Phytic acid (myoinositol hexaphosphate) has the ability to chelate some micronutrients such as iron, calcium, and zinc, therefore making it insoluble and unavailable for absorption by the body. The level of phytate present in a range of foods (indigenous to poorer countries) was recently investigated (Gibson et al., 2010). Phytate was found to be present in highest amounts in grains and legumes which were unrefined. The processing and soaking/germination of cereal grains and seeds prior to food manufacture have been shown to release phytase, an enzyme, which has the ability to remove phosphorus from phytate (Hurrell et al., 2003). It should also be mentioned that in undeveloped countries, meat (source of heme iron) is less widely available to the population due to various socioeconomic conditions. These are some of the reasons why the statistics of iron deficiency in countries such as Africa are significantly worse than the United States and Europe.

The bottomline is that iron is a key component in human metabolism the deficiency of which can have a severe effect on human health and efficiency. As well as the transfer of oxygen to tissues via hemoglobin; energy metabolism, activation of enzymes, and synthesis of DNA are some of its other vital functions. The issue of iron deficiency is still very real, even with advances and innovations in the area over recent years. This point was reinforced recently in a review article (Milman, 2011) which stated that while we have more modern tools and have seen success with some of the iron fortification programs around the world, IDA is still an issue affecting billions.

In the next sections, the types of iron available to the human body and how it is distributed will be discussed in further detail. Later sections will go on to examine how fortification of food has impacted on iron deficiency, the type of fortificants currently on the market, where improvements can still be made, and the areas which may hold the key to solving this global problem.

16.1.1 DISTRIBUTION AND ABSORPTION OF IRON IN HUMAN BODY

A normal person contains approximately 2.5–4 g of iron, depending on gender, body weight, and age. Of this, the majority (65–70%) is present in the red blood cells as hemoglobin. At least 15% of iron is stored in muscles as myoglobin, with the remaining portion stored in the liver, spleen, and bone marrow as ferritin. Most of the iron in the human body is recycled through the process of phagocytosis of red blood cells. Even though women have less iron (approximately 3.0 g) than men, they have a higher requirement for iron due to menstrual blood loss and increased requirement during pregnancy. Of the total amount of iron in the body, only 0.5–2 mg enters and leaves the human body on a daily basis (Andrews, 2000). Regular consumption of minor but important quantities of iron is required to maintain these small losses on a daily basis and makeup for higher demands during pregnancy, growth, and blood loss.

Absorption of iron in the human body is highly regulated with only 10–15% of the total ingested iron being absorbed (Lynch, 2000). The low bioavailability of nonheme iron sources may be a blessing in disguise, as if it were more bioavailable it could lead to excess iron in the body, with serious repercussions to health. Absorption of iron in the human body is affected by multiple factors, including its form (heme or nonheme), oxidation state (+2 or +3), properties of the food matrix, inhibitory substances present in the food, iron status of individual, and health of individual. Multiple dynamic equilibrium adjustments and regulation mechanisms determine the iron homeostasis (balance) in human body, which depends on the ability of the digestive and absorptive processes to extract iron from the ingested food (Lynch, 2000). Iron absorption occurs predominantly in the duodenum and upper jejunum (Crichton, 1991, Conrad et al., 1999). The absorption of iron rather than its excretion is considered the most important determinant of iron balance (Finch, 1981).

Dietary iron is available either as a relatively easily absorbed heme iron or as nonheme iron which is considered less bioavailable. Heme iron is primarily available via a nonvegetarian diet rich in meat, fish, and poultry as a constituent of hemoglobin present in flesh. This high bioavailability of heme iron is attributed mainly to its solubility in alkaline conditions present in the duodenum and jejunum (West and Oates, 2008). Nonheme sources of iron are available mainly from plant sources as ferrous or ferric iron. The low bioavailability of nonheme sources of iron is owing to their low solubility at intestinal pH. The ferrous form of iron can be easily oxidized to its ferric state in the presence of oxygen commonly encountered under processing conditions. The fact that ferric salts of iron are precipitated as ferric hydroxide above pH 3 makes them unavailable for absorption in the duodenum (Conrad and Umbreit, 2002). The availability of nonheme iron in the duodenum is governed by the ability of dietary and intestinal-derived substances to chelate the mineral, which keeps iron in the solution. The role of amino acids released during gastric digestion is to bind this solubilized iron and deliver it in a soluble form in the duodenum, therefore aiding its absorption. Inhibition of iron absorption by the presence of phytate, tannin, oxalate, and polyphenols in diet is due to their ability to precipitate and form insoluble complexes (Conrad and Umbreit, 2002).

Once the iron is delivered to the duodenum in a soluble state, irrespective of its form (heme or nonheme), absorption of iron follows different pathways for entry into a common pool of iron. Two pathways demonstrated for heme iron absorption include the direct absorption of intact metalloporphyrin receptor and presence of heme transporter which carries heme from the small intestinal lumen directly into the cytoplasm (West and Oates, 2008). Whatever the mode of heme iron absorption may be, it is eventually cleaved by oxygenase to release iron into the common pool (Grasbeck et al., 1979). Nonheme iron which reaches the duodenum in a soluble state in the ferric form is first acted upon by ferric reductase which converts it to the ferrous form before it is transported across the membrane by divalent metal transporter 1 (DMT1) (Nancy, 1999).

16.1.2 IRON-FORTIFIED FOODS

There are various solutions to solving the worldwide problem of iron deficiency anemia. This may involve further education to ensure that people understand the benefits of eating a varied diet, or through the supplementation/fortification of food products with iron. It is generally agreed that fortification of food is the most promising way to reduce the prevalence of iron deficiency as a medium to long-term strategy. In certain cases (less privileged populations), the cost or availability of eating a varied diet may not be possible. By fortifying basic foods eaten in these populations such flour, breads, cereals, and dairy products, there is a greater chance that micronutrients such as iron will be delivered (Horton et al., 2011).

One of the issues with iron fortification is whether it should be directed toward a targeted group or aimed at the general population. There is also the option of self-supplementation where iron could be added to foods as a condiment or similar by the consumer at home. As noted in the previous section, the male population of the world tends to be less affected by iron deficiency. Therefore, the mass fortification of food products could easily lead to iron toxicity in this population, which has as many detrimental health effects as being iron deficient. While adding up the advantages and disadvantages in relation to the scale on which fortification should be implemented, the real problems lie in the type of food product and type of fortificants that can be used. As we will see in the next section, there are many different types of iron fortifiers present on the commercial market for placement in food.

16.1.2.1 Fortificants

Fortification of foods is a common method used to deliver nutritionally important minerals in required quantities to the consumer. Many technological problems can occur in fortified foods due to the chemical reactivity of minerals. These problems are reflected as changes in color, flavor, and functional properties of the product. The solubility and chemical reactivity of the added mineral salt/fortifier determines the kind and extent of reactions that may occur within a food system. The following factors are considered important when choosing a mineral for fortification of foods: (1) relative bioavailability of the mineral, (2) reactivity of the mineral, (3) stability of the mineral under processing and storage conditions, and (4) compatibility with other food components. In the past, one of the main conflicts which has arisen surrounding iron fortification is delivering bioavailability while maintaining the product characteristics that the consumer is used to. The general consensus is that greater bioavailability is found in iron ingredients which have increased solubility at the duodenal pH of 6–6.5, with ferrous sulfate seen as having the ideal properties. In Table 16.1, a list of the common fortifiers that are used for food applications can be seen, along with the main properties of each fortifier. Probably the most commonly used iron fortificants within the food industry are ferrous sulfate, ferrous fumarate, NaFeETDA, and elemental iron. Ferrous sulfate is freely water soluble, highly bioavailable (100%), and cheap to buy, therefore making it a popular choice with many food manufacturers. However, its solubility means that it is likely to interact with other ingredients in the food matrix and cause oxidation of fats and discoloration, and deteriorate in terms of organoleptic properties over long-term storage. Less soluble iron fortificants such as those mentioned in Table 16.1 can be incorporated into food products relatively easily, with their reduced solubility meaning that there are fewer side effects experienced with the product. Ferrous fumarate has a similar bioavailability to ferrous sulfate and works well in most food products; however, issues have arisen when acid conditions in food products caused complete dissolution of the fumarate affecting both product color and taste. Chelated forms of iron are also a convenient choice with solubility occurring at high pHs which render it available for absorption within the body. As the iron is bound to a ligand, it is prevented from interacting with various inhibitors present in the food matrix. The inclusion of these fortificants is dependent on product characteristics such as pH like most other fortificants. NaFeEDTA is an example of one such chelated iron product which is widely used in both the food and animal feed industries, at a higher cost to the producer and therefore consumer. Another example of an iron fortificant which is used frequently in the food industry is ferrous glycinate which while stable in most conditions is not stable at low pH (Ding et al., 2011).

As mentioned previously, many compounds present in or added to foods can act as antinutrients or inhibitors to iron absorption. On the other hand, there are also substances that enhance iron absorption in the body. Addition of substances such as ascorbic acid to a food product has been shown to help as it (1) can reduce ferric iron to its ferrous form making it available for absorption and (2) has the ability to chelate Fe, making it a soluble complex at the pH experienced in the duodenum. An increase in iron absorption due to ascorbic acid has been documented in numerous *in vitro* and *in vivo* trials to date (Kim et al., 2011, Cook and Reddy, 2001, Siegenberg et al., 1991, Forbes et al., 1989). Other substances which may play a role in iron absorption are cysteine-containing amino acids (Taylor et al., 1986).

16.1.3 LATEST INNOVATIONS IN IRON FORTIFICATION

Though there has been a surge of review articles and book chapters on the topic of mineral or iron fortification in recent years, very few have mentioned the latest technologies and exactly what food companies for one are doing in terms of research and product development to provide products with a bioavailable source of iron or other minerals. The past decade has seen a substantial amount of patents filed in relation to the manufacture of ingredients containing iron. These ingredients, aimed at fortifying of foods with essential minerals, come from some of the major food manufacturing

TABLE 16.1

Characteristics and Application of Common Iron Fortificants

Fortificants	Characteristics	Iron (%)	Relative Bioavailability in Humans	Application
Ferrous sulfate · 7H$_2$O	Bluish green crystals, water soluble, saline styptic taste, off flavor generation, pH-3.7, easily oxidized in moist air	20	100	Powdered milk, infant formula, wheat flour products
Ferrous gluconate	Yellowish gray to yellowish green powder, caramel odor, water soluble	12	89	Powdered milk, infant formula, wheat flour products
Ferrous lactate	Yellow to green powder, sweet taste, water soluble	19	106	Cereals, milk
Ferric ammonium citrate	Reddish brown granular powder, water soluble	16.5–18.5	—	Powdered milk, infant formula, wheat flour products
Ferrous fumarate	Reddish brown powder, slightly soluble in water, odorless and tasteless	33	100	Infant cereals, corn meal, wheat flour, salt, semolina bread flour
Ferric citrate	Brown granular powder, slowly soluble in water	16.5–18.5	—	Infant cereals, corn meal, wheat flour, salt
Ferric pyrophosphate	Yellowish to white, odorless, insoluble in water	24–26%	21–74	Infant cereals, rice, salt
Electrolytic iron	Grayish black colored irregularly shaped powder, insoluble in water	>97	75	Infant cereals, wheat flour, cake flour, semolina
Carbonyl iron	Gray colored, water insoluble	>98	5–20	Wheat flour
NaFeEDTA	Yellowish to brown crystalline powder, odorless, pH 3.5–5.5 (1% w/w)	12.5–13.5	>100	Cereals, condiments, sugar, soy sauce, fish sauce

Source: Modified from Richard, H. 1999. *The Mineral Fortification of Foods.* First ed. Surrey: Leatherhead Food RA; Penelope, N. and Nalubola, R. 2002. *Technical Brief on Iron Compounds for Fortification of Staple Foods.* Washington, DC 20005 USA: INACG.

companies in the world (Mead Johnson, Nestle, etc.). This section will therefore examine some of the more recent innovations and technologies that have been employed or examined in order to overcome iron deficiency.

While the chelated products that were mentioned earlier such as NaFeEDTA have been on the commercial market for a considerable length of time, encapsulated iron products are relatively new. Microencapsulation forms a barrier between the reactive iron atom and the surrounding environment, therefore reducing its ability to interact with the other ingredients. In most cases ferrous sulfate is the iron source, with liposome technologies used to protect the core element. One study investigated the use of liposomes to protect ferrous glycinate, which in a previous work was found to be unstable at low pH (gastric juice). The liposomes were prepared using reverse phase evaporation along with a mixture of egg phosphatidycholine, lecithin, and cholesterol (Ding et al., 2009, 2011). Results showed that release from the liposomes protected a high percentage of the ferrous glycinate during 4 h in simulated gastric juice, whereas the nonencapsulated iron was either partially or fully dissociated from the glycine complex under the same conditions. A company called "Lipofoods" has commercialized a liposome product on the market called "LipoFer." While results seem to be positive for this iron ingredient, it remains to be seen if the production of liposomes can be achieved on an industrial scale within the tight money constraints of food companies, and also with higher iron loading than those presently available. Other microencapsulation techniques that have been used to protect iron include spray cooling techniques (Lee et al., 2004, Biebinger et al., 2009) with various matrix ingredients used. Spray drying/cooling techniques are more industrial-scale friendly in terms of feasibility and readily available equipment. Spray cooling of ferric pyrophosphate and ferrous sulfate within a matrix of hydrogenated palm oil has been previously investigated by Biebinger et al. (2009) and Wegmüller et al. (2004). Hydrogenated fats provide a barrier around the iron particles embedded within the matrix and prevent the transfer of oxygen which can cause deterioration. Ingredients such as hydrogenated fats can cause problems in other areas of health and so may not be ideal encapsulation matrices.

The liposome particles previously discussed are on the nano scale and this seems to be the way forward in some respects. Other particle size-associated technologies include micronization of compounds such as ferric chloride and sodium pyrophosphate to form ferric pyrophosphate. Studies have shown that decreasing the particle size of iron powders toward the nano size improves absorption of iron in rats. The bioavailability of ferric phosphate ($FePO_4$) nanoparticles has been investigated (Rohner et al., 2007). $FePO_4$ is a poorly water-soluble compound; however, after micronisation to nanoparticles, the Fe was more soluble *in vivo*, leading to an increase in bioavailability. The increase in surface area means that the Fe can be more readily absorbed. Micronisation also renders ferric pyrophosphate soluble in aqueous solutions and in the same bioavailability range as ferrous sulphate (Zimmermann et al., 2004).

Unilever filed a patent application in 2009 describing an iron-containing nano ingredient (Marshman, 2009). The patent describes a method for producing nanoparticles in the range of 5–1000 nm which contain an iron salt stabilized by biopolymers (in particular dairy-based proteins and amino acids). Due to the size of the particles, the iron is said to be very stable in terms of reactivity within a food product and does not sediment in liquid preparations. Nestle has examined the effect of iron addition to casein, and claims to have an iron casein complex which is stable in a food system while the iron remaining bioavailable to the body (Sher et al., 2006). This complex is formed by the addition of iron to a casein solution and adjustment of the pH to between 5.8 and 6.2 before addition of the ferric iron solution. The complexes formed which are insoluble but dispersible in water can be either used in a liquid form or can be spray dried to form an iron-fortified ingredient. Another patent recently filed along the theme of iron binding to milk protein was from the Fonterra Co-operative. Here, a process for preparing an iron–lactoferrin complex was detailed in which lactoferrin is separated from milk (or other sources). Lactoferrin is a cationic glycoprotein which in this case was concentrated using ion exchange before saturating the lactoferrin pockets with iron (Palmano et al., 2008). The efficiency of lactoferrin in comparison to ferrous sulfate (orally administered) was investigated recently by Paesano et al. (2010). They found that lactoferrin saturated with 30% Fe positively influenced hematological parameters such as serum IL-6, hemoglobin, serum ferritin, and prohepcidin levels in pregnant women in comparison to ferrous sulfate.

After reviewing the literature in this area, it is obvious to the authors that the main focus in the last couple of years has been in relation to iron-binding proteins, especially those derived from milk. These patents claim that binding of iron to protein renders the iron unreactive in the presence of polyphenols and fat, but remains completely bioavailable. Therefore, it would be worthwhile examining the binding of iron to milk proteins on a deeper level as the next section will do. Another factor which complicates the fortification of food products is the need to use a range of fortifiers for different types of food systems (i.e., liquid, dairy, etc.). The ideal solution would be to find a fortifier which can be used in the majority of food products irrelevant of type therefore reducing the costs to both the manufacturer and the consumer.

16.2   IRON-BINDING MILK PROTEINS

Milk is a poor source of iron and contributes only 0.2–0.5 mg/L to the daily nutritional requirements of the human body (Flynn and Cashman, 1997). Of this minor quantity of iron in cow's milk, 14% is associated with the fat globule membrane, 24% is bound to casein, 29% to whey proteins, and the rest (32%) is associated with the low-molecular-weight fraction. However, when externally added to milk, iron binds strongly to proteins, especially caseins (Carmichael et al., 1975). In order to achieve a greater understanding of how milk proteins are involved in iron binding, the physicochemical aspects of the proteins involved need to be investigated. The interaction of calcium (Ca) with the proteins in milk forms a platform from which a greater understanding of iron binding can be achieved. Therefore, in this section of the chapter, we will try to provide the reader with a basic understanding of this binding.

Milk proteins fall majorly into two principal categories, caseins which represent 80% of the proteins and whey proteins with the remaining 20%. In Table 16.2, the composition and chemical characteristics of these major milk proteins are outlined. For a more in-depth look at milk proteins, the following reviews may prove to be beneficial (Holt, 1992, Holt and Horne, 1996, McMahon and Brown, 1984, Dalgleish et al., 2004, Horne, 2006, 1998, Fox and Brodkorb, 2008, McMahon and Oommen, 2008). As mentioned previously, caseins represent a major portion of milk proteins (80–90%) and bind externally added iron more strongly than whey proteins; hence, the major part of the following discussion will be focused on the interactions with iron with casein.

Casein is a general name given to a group of phosphoproteins (α_{s1}, α_{s2}, β, κ caseins) present in milk. One of the principal roles of these caseins is recognized as its ability to transport calcium and phosphorus in a readily bioavailable form to the site of assimilation in the mother to the young (Holt, 1992). Specificity of caseins to bind Ca as colloidal calcium phosphate prevents precipitation of Ca which is in a supersaturated state in milk. Synergistically, the calcium phosphate in milk plays an important role in stability and structure of casein micelles. The specificity of casein is principally related to the clustered phosphoserine residues distributed in varying numbers on individual caseins

TABLE 16.2
Characteristics of Milk Proteins

	Whey			Caseins			
	β-lg	α-lac	BSA	α_{S1}	α_{S2}	β	κ
Molecular weight	18,362	14,194	65,000	23,612	25,228	23,980	19,005
Total residues	162	123	581	199	207	209	169
Apolar residues (%)	34.6	36	28	36	40	33	33
Isoionic point	5.2	4.2–4.5	5.3	4.96	5.27	5.2	5.54
Proline residues	8	2	28	17	10	35	20
Phosphoserine groups	0	0	0	8–9	10–13	5	1

Source: Adapted from Kinsella, J. E. et al. 1989. In: P. F. Fox (ed.) *Developments in Dairy Chemistry*. London, England: Elsevier Applied Science.

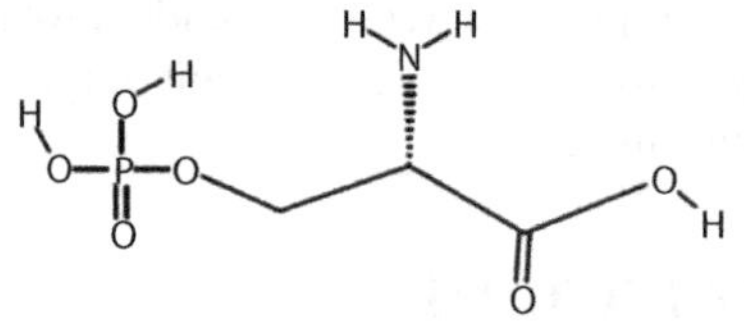

FIGURE 16.1   Phosphoserine structure.

and follows the order $\alpha_{s2} > \alpha_{s1} > \beta > \kappa$. It is postulated that the amount of Ca which is directly bound to the phosphoseryl residues is 300 mg/L of milk and rest of Ca is associated with the casein micelles as colloidal calcium phosphate (Fox and McSweeney, 1998). The clustering of phosphoserine residues is particularly apparent and has a marked influence on the metal-binding properties of caseins. The structure of phosphoserine is given in Figure 16.1.

The affinity of caseins is not limited to Ca and is highest for Fe^{3+}, with the succeeding affinities of different cations in descending order $Fe^{3+} > Zn^{2+} > Ca^{2+} > Cu^{2+} > Mg^{2+}$ (Philippe et al., 2005). Addition of iron to milk or its individual components (casein, whey powders) in liquid form is always accompanied by a drop in pH, change in color, modifications of salt balance between the soluble and colloidal phase, and casein structure (Raouche et al., 2009b). The severity of the effect depends on the amount of iron added and the type of salts used for iron addition. Table 16.3 provides a list of iron binding studies involving milk, model systems (caseinate, phospho-caseinate), and pure milk proteins. Added iron principally binds via coordination bonds with oxygen atoms of phosphoseryl residues on individual caseins, although similar bonds are formed with aspartic acid and glutamic acid residues available for bonding (Hegenauer et al., 1979).

Similar studies to determine the interactions of iron with whey proteins are lacking in the literature, although binding of iron to whey proteins has been demonstrated and the complex formed has

TABLE 16.3
Summary of Proteins Used for Various Iron-Binding Studies

Author	Iron Salts/Chelates	Quantity	Protein Source
Baumy and Brule (1988)	Ferrous chloride	6.64 mol/mol	β-Casein
Carmichael et al. (1975)	Ferric nitrilotriacetate, ferric casein complex, ferric fructose	10–15 mg/kg	Casein and skim milk
Demott and Dincer (1976)	Ferric chloride	10.6 mg/L	Milk
Hegenauer et al. (1979)	Ferric nitrilotriacetate, ferric fructose, ferric lactobionate, ferrous sulfate, ferric polyphosphates	1 mmol/L	Skim milk
Potter and Nelson (1979)	Ferrous sulfate, ferric pyrophosphate	0–20 mg/g protein	Casein
Gaucheron et al. (1996)	Ferric chloride	1.5 mmol/L	Sodium caseinate
Gaucheron et al. (1997)	Ferrous chloride, Ferric chloride	1.5 mmol/L	Skim milk
Hekmat and McMahon (1998)	Ferric chloride	100 mg/L	Acidified milk, yoghurt
Philippe et al. (2005)	Ferric chloride	0–8 mmol/kg	Phosphocaseinate powder
Sugiarto et al. (2009)	Ferrous sulfate	0–20 mmol/kg	1% Sodium caseinate, 1% whey protein isolate
Raouche et al. (2009)	Ferrous chloride, ferric chloride	0–20 mmol/kg	Skim milk

been used for experimental purposes (Wp–Fe complex) (Douglas et al., 1981, Zhang and Mahoney, 1989a, Rice and McMahon, 1998). Inorganic Fe salts in ferrous or ferric form have always been used to study the binding of iron to milk proteins, in either milk or its extracted components.

A recent study has demonstrated that there are eight binding sites on whey protein isolates, although these numbers and affinities were lower than that for sodium caseinate which contained 14 binding sites (Sugiarto et al., 2009). The lower ability of whey proteins to bind iron might be due to their compact structure as opposed to the open structure of casein. This binding of iron to milk proteins is influenced by pH, ionic strength, holding time, temperature, and type of salt. The binding of a ferrous ion to casein induces oxygen-catalyzed oxidation of iron from the ferrous to the ferric state (Emery, 1992). An incomplete oxidation occurs during the binding of ferrous ion to casein which undergoes complete oxidation upon storage or carbonation (Raouche et al., 2009b).

Early studies on iron addition to milk were done to determine the extent and mechanism of iron binding to caseins and whey proteins using purified fractions. Though initial studies were done using low (0.06% of proteins) to moderate (0.25% of proteins) amounts of iron, a greater understanding of this binding has helped recent researchers study the effect of higher (3% of proteins) iron additions (Raouche et al., 2009a). While earlier studies in this area were based on idea of iron fortification to milk, recent studies that attempt higher iron binding to proteins have envisaged developing these iron–protein complexes as food additives or functional ingredients.

16.2.1 Physicochemical Aspects of Iron Binding in Milk

16.2.1.1 Distribution of Iron

In milk, iron binding to caseins may be different than in model solutions (sodium caseinate or individual caseins) because the phosphoserine interacts with calcium phosphate salts (Gaucheron, 2000). Some of the added iron is also bound to inorganic phosphate in both serum and colloidal phase (Jackson and Lee, 1992a, Philippe et al., 2005, Raouche et al., 2009a). Almost all of these studies use ultracentrifugation to separate casein micelles from whey proteins and solubilized caseins (5% of total caseins). These researchers found that approximately 90% of iron was bound to caseins and the rest to whey proteins and low-molecular-weight fractions. This higher proportion of iron binding to caseins is owing to their higher concentration, binding sites, and affinity for added iron. However, there is a limit to the amount of iron that can be incorporated in milk without protein precipitation. This precipitation is attributed to partial neutralization of charges on the surface of κ-casein, which occurs at higher levels of iron fortification. The concentration at which this precipitation occurs is influenced by iron addition process, amount of proteins, temperature of iron addition and type of iron salts used. Added iron interacts directly with phosphoserine residues on caseins as well as with inorganic calcium, phosphate, and citrate in the colloidal phase of milk. The highest level of iron fortification in milk (approximately 1100 mg/L) is almost equal to the mass of calcium present in milk. Ferric chloride binds more efficiently than ferrous chloride (Raouche et al., 2009a).

16.2.1.2 Protein Modifications

Modifications to protein structure can be brought about by iron salts, which easily donate iron for interactions with milk proteins (Gaucheron, 2000). The extent of this is directly related to the concentration of ferrous or ferric iron which is added. Higher modifications are observed in individual caseins containing more phosphoserine groups (as in α_{s1} casein). Structural modifications to the proteins have been deduced using chromatography, fluorescence spectroscopy, zeta potential, and by measuring the average size of casein micelles. The greatest influences of iron binding have been found by examining the reduction in intrinsic fluorescence intensities of tryptophan (Gaucheron et al., 1996). Tryptophan fluorescence intensities are very sensitive to their localized environment and have been used as a tool to measure the change in three-dimensional structures of milk proteins upon processing and storage. A reduction in fluorescence intensities along with a shift in λ_{max}

(wavelength of maximum intensity) is considered as a true measure of change in the three-dimensional structure of the caseins. λ_{max} of tryptophan fluorescence has been classified into various categories depending on their wavelengths which generally range from 308 to 355 nm. If the tryptophan fluorescence λ_{max} is <330 nm, it is assigned a nonpolar environment and those above 330 nm a polar environment (Vivian and Callis). Since λ_{max} for milk is always reported above 330 nm (342–343 nm), tryptophan is basically located in a polar environment, due to the open structure of the casein micelles. The reduction in intensities of tryptophan fluorescence is mainly because of ligand binding to amino acids in the immediate environment of tryptophan residues. However, a structural change cannot be ruled out as reduction in intensity has been observed when extrinsic flouropores (ANS) were used to study the changes in the hydrophobic segments on the surface of caseins upon iron fortification of milk (Gaucheron et al., 1997). Modification of proteins upon iron additions has also been confirmed by RP-HPLC, wherein differences in the retention times and areas of α_{s1}-casein and β-casein were also observed (Gaucheron et al., 1996, 1997). The size of casein micelles remains relatively constant irrespective of the oxidation state or concentration of added iron. Both the reduction in zeta potential and hydration of casein micelles is due to neutralization of negative charges on casein micelle (Gaucheron et al., 1997, Philippe et al., 2005, Raouche et al., 2009a).

16.2.1.3 Salt Balance

Salts in milk are in a state of dynamic equilibrium. One-third of calcium, half of phosphorus, and a major portion of magnesium and citrate are in the soluble phase of milk. About 300 mg of calcium in milk is bound directly to the phosphoserine residues in caseins as calcium caseinate and remaining as colloidal calcium phosphate. Minerals in the soluble phase play an important role in the stability of casein micelle structure; hence, any change occurring in the micelle will directly affect the balance of minerals in the colloidal phase. Iron binding to milk proteins causes substantial changes in the distribution of cations and anions between the colloidal and soluble phases. Addition of iron to milk, irrespective of its concentration and oxidation state, has been shown to cause a reduction in both citrate and phosphate content in the soluble phase (Gaucheron et al., 1997, Philippe et al., 2005, Raouche et al., 2009a). A twofold increase in ionic calcium upon fortification with 1100 mg of iron/L of skim milk has been reported (Raouche et al., 2009a). Magnesium content remains fairly constant upon iron addition in both the phases of milk. Though different interactions of iron with milk proteins and its effect on salt balance have been suggested, a consensus on the exact mechanism of iron binding to different proteins in milk is still elusive and further discussion would be speculation at this stage. However, the role of calcium, phosphorus, and citrate in this binding has been confirmed.

16.2.1.4 Effect of pH and Ionic Strength on Iron Binding

An iron–protein complex will prove to be important in food fortification only if it can withstand the changes in temperature, pH, and ionic strength commonly associated with food processing and formulations. The effect of decreasing pH on the release of iron from these types of complexes has been studied by almost all researchers who have worked on this topic. Although there are differences in opinion over the release of iron from the complex at lower pH values (5.0–3.8), in general, the complexes formed are very stable under the most commercially important pH conditions (5.0–7.5). The fact that these complexes are stable even after complete solubilization of colloidal calcium phosphate at pH 5.2 (Hekmat and McMahon, 1998) infers that stability is owing to coordination bonds between the phosphoserine, glutamic acid, and aspartic acid residues on caseins. These studies have been done for low levels of iron fortification (<200 mg/L) wherein the Fe is expected to bind strongly with the phosphoserine residues similar to calcium bound in the casein micelle. However, to date no studies on the effect of pH have been conducted on milk fortified with higher concentrations of iron (>500 mg/L). Ionic strength is important for stability and conformation of proteins. Any change in the ionic strength caused by processing or addition of food additives to products can affect the binding of iron to casein. However, no effect on the release of iron from the iron–casein has been observed under experimental conditions (Baumy and Brule, 1988b, Gaucheron et al., 1997). In contrast to the above, a reduction in pH and increased ionic strength have caused reduced binding of Fe to α-lactalbumin and β-lactoglobulin (Baumy and Brule, 1988a). Decreasing the pH, which reduces the ionization of carboxylic residues associated with aspartic and glutamic acid, was related to the lower-binding ability for Fe, indicating that ionic bonds were majorly involved in binding. Furthermore, they showed that 6 and 3.5 mol of Fe could be bound to α-lactalbumin and β-lactoglobulin, respectively, at pH 6.6.

16.2.1.5 Application of Iron–Protein Complex

As mentioned previously, iron fortificants should not cause any adverse physicochemical changes in the food fortified during manufacture and storage. Complexation of iron with protein will be of technological and physiological importance only if it is stable within the above-mentioned parameters. An iron–protein complex is formed when the iron salts donate an ion to casein or whey protein. This feature has been implemented knowingly or unknowingly during iron fortification experiments and dairy-based Fe fortification programs over many decades. The ability of a complex to prevent any detrimental change in a product depends on the type of salts (ferrous or ferric), the stability constant of the chelating ligand vis-à-vis protein, processing conditions, and the iron salt introduction step to the food matrix.

On careful examination, research shows that iron has been successfully incorporated in most of the dairy products, when this complex was stabilized. The ferric form has almost always been found to be better than ferrous in this respect, owing to oxidation of ferrous to ferric state in the presence of oxygen. The earliest example of ferrous oxidation by oxygen in milk leading to flavor and color change was reported for pasteurized whole milk, wherein deaeration of milk was recommended before addition of ferrous sulfate at only 10 mg/L concentration (Edmondson et al., 1971). The importance of protein concentration on the binding of ferric compounds was observed during preparation of iron-fortified nonfat milk powder. Addition of iron to concentrated milks, which contain more proteins, was recommended to prevent oxidized flavor (Kurtz et al., 1973). Cocoa and chocolate-containing foods have been recommended for iron fortification owing to the presence of antioxidants, masking of color if any, and greater acceptability with children (Kinder et al., 1942, Douglas et al., 1981). Among the nine different fortificants evaluated for effect on organoleptic quality of prepared and stored samples, ferric-polyphosphate–whey protein complex produced the least changes.

Iron fortification to different cheeses has been achieved successfully without affecting their consumer acceptability. The highest fortification level reported is 140 mg/kg of iron for Harvati cheese (Jackson and Lee, 1992b). It is interesting to note that higher retention (90%) was observed upon direct ferric chloride addition to milk than with microencapsulated ferric chloride (70%), thereby indicating the formation of iron–protein complexes and the stability of the complex at the low pH encountered. Cheddar and mozzarella cheeses have been fortified with approximately 40 mg/kg of iron. Fortification of cheese milk was done with preformed Fe–protein complexes (Fe–casein, Fe–whey protein) or by forming the complex upon addition of ferric chloride to milk (Zhang and Mahoney, 1990, Rice and McMahon, 1998) without altering cheese quality. Formation of iron–protein complexes by adding ferric chloride to milk was considered a commercially viable option due to ease of incorporation during mozzarella cheese manufacture. Better organoleptic qualities were observed for white soft cheese and Harvati cheese upon iron fortification at 80 and 140 mg/kg levels with ferric chloride.

Iron–protein complexation is stable to changes in temperature, pH, and ionic strength, and the structure of various dairy products makes it a novel approach to provide a sustainable solution not only for iron fortification to the dairy industry, but also for a range of canned and processed food products. The application of these complexes with even higher iron loading has recently been envisaged (Sher et al., 2006, Raouche et al., 2009a). However, the suitability of such high iron-bound milk-based ingredients and their stability under processing conditions still remains to be seen. Temperature is the most important processing encountered by all food products. Destabilization of iron–protein complex upon heat treatment is dependent on the concentration of added iron bound to caseins. No effect of severe heat treatment (90°C for 15 min) was observed under experimental conditions (Gaucheron et al., 1997).

16.2.1.6 Bioavailability

The mechanism of iron absorption was discussed very briefly earlier in the chapter; however, of the total iron consumed, 5–15% of iron is generally available for absorption depending on individual iron status and requirement (Bothwell et al., 1979, Hallberg and Rossander-Hulten, 1991). Availability of iron from milk and milk products depends on the form of iron incorporated (encapsulated, iron chelates, Fe salts), interactions of added iron source with milk components (fat, protein, and minerals), structure, health/iron status of individual, and the degree of digestion of the ingested food. Research outcomes concerning the accessibility of iron from dairy products is often contradictory, mainly because of differences in the methodologies followed such as single or multiple meal cohort studies, higher amounts of calcium employed during study, and so on.

Among the most important reasons cited for lower bioavailability of iron from milk products is the inhibitory effect of calcium and casein in milk (Hurrell et al., 1989, Lynch, 2000, Bosscher et al., 2001) and milk products. The inhibitory effect of caseins on absorption of iron has been shown via *in vitro* analysis (Hurrell et al., 1989, Bosscher et al., 2001), wherein hydrolysis of proteins (casein, whey protein) was positively correlated to the proportion of dialyzable Fe. However, statistically, an insignificant effect on iron absorption from standardized liquid meal (containing egg white and casein) in human subjects was seen in the same experiment (Hurrell et al., 1989). An understanding of absorption of iron indicates that solubility of iron at the luminal surface is the first step for absorption. Absorption of iron after this solubilization is determined by the action of enzymes and uptake of iron by carrier molecules. A number of current (Ait-Oukhatar et al., 2002, Wall et al., 2005) and past studies (Douglas et al., 1981, Zhang and Mahoney, 1989b, Kim et al., 1995) on milk products demonstrate a very positive effect of caseins and whey protein on iron absorption, in fact Fe–whey protein complex has been found to be better absorbed than heme iron in one of these studies (Nakano et al., 2007). A recent study has rated oral iron medicine at par with iron-fortified follow-on formula and cow's milk (Wall et al., 2005). Addition of milk to an iron-fortified fruit beverages improved Fe retention, transport, and uptake (Garcia-Nebot et al., 2010), the positive effect being seen as an increase in ferritin synthesis due to the presence of milk (Cilla et al., 2008). The positive effect of milk proteins on iron absorption has also been observed in studies done on cheese and chocolate milk. The higher level of iron absorption observed in chocolate milk and cheese indicates that calcium may have a smaller role when it comes to absorption of iron from Fe–milk protein complexes. Calcium is absorbed throughout the intestine and follows an independent absorption pathway than Fe. Lynch (2000) has suggested an interaction of Ca with food components leading to reduction in Fe bioavailability or effect of calcium on luminal surface receptors rather than competition for the transport mechanisms. A thorough survey on effect of calcium on iron absorption (Lynch, 2000) clearly indicated a minimal effect of calcium on iron absorption in multiple meal cohort studies. An exaggerated effect of factors affecting iron bioavailability on iron absorption has been reported, especially in single meal studies (Cook et al., 1991).

16.2.1.7 Caseinophosphopeptide

Hydrolysis of whole caseins has been shown to improve absorption of bound Fe (Hurrell et al., 1989), although the effect is seen less in the *in vivo* study conducted as compared to the *in vitro* model in the same study. Caseinophosphopeptides (CPP) correspond to different phosphorylated regions of the caseins (Fitzgerald, 1998). Caseinophosphopeptides are derived from the tryptic digestion of the protein in milk *in vivo* (Naito and Suzuki, 1974) and fermented dairy products like cheese (Roudot-Algaron and Le Bars, 1994). Cation binding and the solubilization capacity of these CPPs have been a topic of immense research in the last few years. Commercial applications for these peptides have been found in the remineralization of tooth enamel (Cai et al., 2007, Manton et al., 2008) and the area of bone health (Goto, 1996, Hansen et al., 1997, Kerstetter et al., 2005, Sheng et al., 2006). The capacity of CPP to bind cations has been attributed to the presence of phosphoserine residues in clusters which bind cations via coordination bonding with oxygen group phosphorus (West, 1986, Baumy et al., 1989, Meisel and Frister, 1989, Gaucheron et al., 1997). Strong binding of Fe to phosphoseryl residues is because of covalent bonds which are approximately 100 times stronger than for zinc or calcium (Scanff et al., 1991, Emery, 1992). Although all CCP fractions have been demonstrated to bind Fe, the bioavailability of a β-casein-derived CPP fraction on iron uptake and net absorption is higher than α_{S1}-derived CCPs (Miquel et al., 2005). The lower efficiency of α_{S1}-derived CCP has been attributed to a changed conformation because of very strong binding of Fe to the phosphoseryl residues involved and high electronegativity leading to lower bioavailability (Kibangou et al., 2005). In a study using rats as model systems, experiments have shown that β-CN (1–25) CCP can remain soluble and escape gastric enzymatic digestion, thereby improving absorption and tissue uptake as compared to inorganic salts (Bouhallab et al., 1999). This improved absorption of Fe has been attributed to additional absorption of intact β-CN–Fe complex by endocytosis over the regulated route of iron absorption. Thus, the ability of CPP to resist further proteolytic degradation (Kasai et al., 1995) helps keep iron in soluble form during the duodenal transit and improve its bioavailability from ingested foods (Yeung et al., 2002).

Though better absorption for CCP–iron complex has been the basis of many studies, a recent study (García-Nebot et al., 2010) has shown significantly higher Fe retention, transport, and uptake from milk-based fruit beverages than samples with or without CCPs added. They concluded that the presence of milk added to fruit beverages showed significantly higher cell uptake of Fe in comparison to fruit beverages with caseinphosphopeptide ingredient added (García-Nebot et al., 2010) Similar positive effects of milk on the bioavailability of iron from another milk-based fruit beverage and a fortified, processed wheat cereal have been reported using Caco-2 cells (Cilla et al., 2008; Wortley et al., 2005). Wortely et al. (2005) have attributed this positive effect to the presence of natural CCPs in milk, which bind Fe and prevent its interaction with inhibitors such as phytates and phenolics.

16.2.1.8 Lactoferrin

A classic example of an iron-binding milk protein, lactoferrin, was identified first as a red fraction in 1939 and isolated from human milk in 1960 (Johanson, 1960). It is an 80 kDa biologically active glycoprotein present in the milk of almost all mammalian species (Masson and Heremans, 1971). Although the iron-binding characteristics of lactoferrin are well recognized, its multifunctional attributes as a bacteriostatic protein (Bullen et al., 1972, Pakkanen and Aalto, 1997, Lee et al., 2004) and an immune modulator (Levay and Viljoen, 1995) have gained precedence. The low concentration of lactoferrin in bovine milk may thwart its prospects as an iron fortificant, while recent clinical studies show orally administered natural lactoferrin containing 30% iron saturation as a safe and effective way of treating iron-deficient pregnant women (Paesano et al., 2010). Further information regarding biological functions of lactoferrin can be obtained from different reviews (Baker and Baker, 2005, Valenti and Antonini, 2005, Wakabayashi et al., 2006). Most, if not all, of its functions are related to its metal-binding capacity.

Structural identity of lactoferrin remains more or less similar (90%) for bovine, buffalo, goat, and sheep lactoferrin. It consists of two globular lobes forming the N and C terminal. These lobes are joined together by short α-helix. These two lobes represent the protein-binding folds in lactoferrin which very strongly but reversibly enclose the Fe^{3+} ions. Binding of ferric ions occurs synergistically with CO_3^{3-} binding to arginine residues in each lobe which functions as an additional ligand for incoming Fe^{3+} ion (Baker and Baker, 2009). Of these two lobes, C lobe binds iron more efficiently than the N lobe (Kilar and Simon, 1985). It exists in two forms: the iron-saturated (holo) form and iron-deficient (apo) form which contains <5% iron saturation (Steijns and van Hooijdonk, 2000). Apo lactoferrin has an open structure for easy access to the incoming ferric ion followed by a conformation change to a more compact structure enclosing the bound ion. This conformation change reflects the higher resistance to proteolytic degradation of holo lactoferring to the apo form (Iyer and Lönnerdal, 1993) in gut. More than 60% of bovine lactoferrin (20% iron saturated) was found to enter the small intestine intact in one of the studies which is significant from the bioavailability point of view (Troost et al., 2001).

On average, only 10–30% of bovine lactoferrin in milk is saturated with iron, giving a slightly pink appearance to the powder which deepens its color upon further saturation (Steijns and van Hooijdonk, 2000). A study determining the solubilizing effect of lactoferrin on insoluble ferric ions at neutral pH in the presence of phosphate and bicarbonate demonstrated that lactoferrin and digested lactoferrin (pepsin and trypsin) could solubilize 70-fold molar equivalent of iron (Kawakami et al., 1993). The iron-binding capacity of CCP was found to be 1/10th that of lactoferrin in the same experiment. The above-mentioned process has been modified to increase this ratio to 200 (Uchida et al., 2006). This solubilized lactoferrin was found to have better bioavailability and safety vis-à-vis ferrous sulfate and citrate.

16.3 CONCLUSION

Iron is the most abundant metal found on earth, but ironically is the cause for the largest and most widely distributed mineral deficiency in human population. Iron, being a member of the transition metal series, is highly reactive and poses numerous challenges with respect to physicochemical stability of fortified foods, formation of insoluble complex during gastrointestinal transit, and during its absorption in duodenum. Although there are a range of food fortificants available on the market, the "one-size-fits-all" solution is still elusive. Iron absorption in the human body requires it to be made available in a soluble form in the duodenum. Those fortificants which satisfy these requirements are generally incompatible with the food matrix (ferrous sulfate) or are too costly (ferrous bisglycinate, sodium feredetate) to make them attractive for mass fortification programs. Numerous new technologies (microencapsulation, superdispersed Fe, micronization, liposomal delivery) are presently being made available but with limited application due to cost implications that both the food companies and in turn consumer take on. Among the various technologies explored, iron binding to milk proteins have long been understood and applied; however, recently its prospect as an iron fortificant has been gaining increased attention. Methods for the production of ferric caseinate complex and iron-saturated lactoferrin have recently been patented, with the main focus being on their potential application to food products. Though such fortificants are low in their iron concentration, they do seem to satisfy most requirements as an ideal food fortificant. The next challenge therefore lies in greater exploration of techniques that may be used to increase the iron load of these protein–iron complexes while keeping manufacturing and cost implications at the forefront of the mind.

REFERENCES

Ait-oukhatar, N., Peres, J. M., Bouhallab, S., Neuville, D., Bureau, F., Bouevard, G., Arhan, P., and Bougle, D. 2002. Bioavailability of caseinophosphopeptide-bound iron. *Journal of Laboratory & Clinical Medicine*, 140, 290–294.

Andrews, N. C. 2000. Iron homeostasis: Insights from genetics and animal models. *Nature Reviews. Genetics*, 1, 208–217.

Baker, E. and Baker, H. 2005. Lactoferrin. *Cellular and Molecular Life Sciences*, 62, 2531–2539.

Baker, E. N. and Baker, H. M. 2009. A structural framework for understanding the multifunctional character of lactoferrin. *Biochimie*, 91, 3–10.

Baumy, J. J. and Brule, G. 1988a. Binding of bivalent-cations to alpha-lactalbumin and beta-lactoglobulin— Effect of pH and ionic-strength. *Lait*, 68, 33–48.

Baumy, J. J. and Brule, G. 1988b. Effect of pH and ionic-strength on the binding of bivalent-cations to beta-casein. *Lait*, 68, 409–417.

Baumy, J. J., Guenot, P., Sinbandhit, S., and Brule, G. 1989. Study of calcium-binding to phosphoserine residues of beta-casein and its phosphopeptide (1–25) by P-31 NMR. *Journal of Dairy Research*, 56, 403–409.

Benoist, B. D., Erin, M., Egli, I., and Cogswell, M. 2008. Worldwide prevalence of anaemia 1993–2005. In: B. de Benoist, Erin, M., Egli, I. and Cogswell, M. (eds.) *WHO Global Database on Anaemia*. Geneva: World Health Organisation.

Biebinger, R., Zimmermann, M. B., Al-Hooti, S. N., Al-Hamed, N., Al-Salem, E., Zafar, T., Kabir, Y., Al-Obaid, I., Petry, N., and Hurrell, R. F. 2009. Efficacy of wheat-based biscuits fortified with microcapsules containing ferrous sulfate and potassium iodate or a new hydrogen-reduced elemental iron: A randomised, double-blind, controlled trial in Kuwaiti women. *British Journal of Nutrition*, 102, 1362–1369.

Bosscher, D., Van Caillie-Bertrand, M., Robberecht, H., Van Dyck, K., Van Cauwenbergh, R., and Deelstra, H. 2001. *In vitro* availability of calcium, iron, and zinc from first-age infant formulae and human milk. *Journal of Pediatric Gastroenterology and Nutrition*, 32, 54–58.

Bothwell, T.H., Charlton, R.W., Cook, J.D., and Finch, C.A. 1979. *Iron Metabolism in Man*, Oxford, England: Blackwell Scientific, p. 7.

Bouhallab, S., Oukhatar, N. A., Molle, D., Henry, G., Maubois, J. L., Arhan, P., and Bougle, D. L. 1999. Sensitivity of beta-casein phosphopeptide-iron complex to digestive enzymes in ligated segment of rat duodenum. *Journal of Nutritional Biochemistry*, 10, 723–727.

Bullen, J. J., Rogers, H. J., and Leigh, L. 1972. Iron-binding proteins in milk and resistance to *Escherichia coli* infection in infants. *British Medical Journal*, 1, 69–75.

Cai, F., Manton, D. J., Shen, P., Walker, G. D., Cross, K. J., Yuan, Y., Reynolds, C., and Reynolds, E. C. 2007. Effect of addition of citric acid and casein phosphopeptide-amorphous calcium phosphate to a sugar-free chewing gum on enamel remineralization *in situ*. *Caries Research*, 41, 377–383.

Carmichael, D., Christopher, J., Hegenauer, J., and Saltman, P. 1975. Effect of milk and casein on the absorption of supplemental iron in the mouse and chick. *American Journal of Clinical Nutrition*, 28, 487–493.

Cilla, A., Perales, S., Lagarda, M. J., Barbera, R., and Farre, R. 2008. Iron bioavailability in fortified fruit beverages using ferritin synthesis by Caco-2 cells. *Journal of Agricultural and Food Chemistry*, 56, 8699–8703.

Conrad, M. E. and Umbreit, J. N. 2002. Pathways of iron absorption. *Blood Cells Molecules and Diseases*, 29, 336–355.

Conrad, M. E., Umbreit, J. N., and Moore, E. G. 1999. Iron absorption and transport. *The American Journal of the Medical Sciences*, 318, 213–229.

Cook, J., Dassenko, S., and Lynch, S. 1991. Assessment of the role of nonheme-iron availability in iron balance. *The American Journal of Clinical Nutrition*, 54, 717–722.

Cook, J. D. and Reddy, M. B. 2001. Effect of ascorbic acid intake on nonheme-iron absorption from a complete diet. *The American Journal of Clinical Nutrition*, 73, 93–98.

Crichton, R. R. 1991. *Solution Chemistry of Iron in Biological Media*, New York: E. Horwood.

Dalgleish, D. G., Spagnuolo, P. A., and Douglas Goff, H. 2004. A possible structure of the casein micelle based on high-resolution field-emission scanning electron microscopy. *International Dairy Journal*, 14, 1025–1031.

Ding, B., Xia, S., Hayat, K., and Zhang, X. 2009. Preparation and pH stability of ferrous glycinate liposomes. *Journal of Agricultural and Food Chemistry*, 57, 2938–2944.

Ding, B., Zhang, X., Hayat, K., Xia, S., Jia, C., Xie, M., and Liu, C. 2011. Preparation, characterization and the stability of ferrous glycinate nanoliposomes. *Journal of Food Engineering*, 102, 202–208.

Douglas, F. W., Rainey, N. H., Wong, N. P., Edmondson, L. F., and Lacroix, D. E. 1981. Color, flavor, and iron bioavailability in iron-fortified chocolate milk. *Journal of Dairy Science*, 64, 1785–1793.

Edmondson, L. F., Douglas, F. W., and Avants, J. K. 1971. Enrichment of pasteurized whole milk with iron. *Journal of Dairy Science*, 54, 1422–1426.

Emery, T. 1992. Iron oxidation by casein. *Biochemical and Biophysical Research Communications*, 182, 1047–1052.

Falkingham, M., Abdelhamid, A., Curtis, P., Fairweather-Tait, S., Dye, L., and Hooper, L. 2010. The effects of oral iron supplementation on cognition in older children and adults: A systematic review and meta-analysis. *Nutrition Journal*, 9, 4.

Finch, C. A. 1981. Iron nutrition. *Western Journal of Medicine*, 134, 532–533.

Fitzgerald, R. J. 1998. Potential uses of caseinophosphopeptides. *International Dairy Journal*, 8, 451–458.

Flynn, A. and Cashman, K. 1997. Nutritional aspects of minerals in bovine and human milks. *Advanced Dairy Chemistry*, 3, 257–302.

Forbes, A., Arnaud, M., Chichester, C., Cook, J., Harrison, B., Hurrell, R., Kahn, S., Morris, E., Tanner, J., and Whittaker, P. 1989. Comparison of *in vitro*, animal, and clinical determinations of iron bioavailability: International Nutritional Anemia Consultative Group Task Force report on iron bioavailability [published erratum appears in *Am J Clin Nutr* 1989 Jun;49(6):1332]. *The American Journal of Clinical Nutrition*, 49, 225–238.

Fox, P. F. and Brodkorb, A. 2008. The casein micelle: Historical aspects, current concepts and significance. *International Dairy Journal*, 18, 677–684.

Fox, P. F. and Mcsweeney, P. L. H. 1998. Salts of milk. *Dairy Chemistry and Biochemistry*. 1st ed. Tullamore: International Thomson Publishing.

García-Nebot, M. J., Alegría, A., Barberá, R., Clemente, G., and Romero, F. 2010. Addition of milk or caseino-phosphopeptides to fruit beverages to improve iron bioavailability? *Food Chemistry*, 119, 141–148.

Gaucheron, F. 2000. Iron fortification in dairy industry. *Trends in Food Science & Technology*, 11, 403–409.

Gaucheron, F., Famelart, M.-H., and Graët, Y. L. 1996. Iron-supplemented caseins: Preparation, physicochemical characterization and stability. *Journal of Dairy Research*, 63, 233–243.

Gaucheron, F., Le Graet, Y., Raulot, K., and Piot, M. 1997. Physicochemical characterization of iron supplemented skim milk. *International Dairy Journal*, 7, 141–148.

Gibson, R. S., Bailey, K. B., Gibbs, M., and Ferguson, E. L. 2010. A review of phytate, iron, zinc, and calcium concentrations in plant-based complementary foods used in low-income countries and implications for bioavailability. *Food & Nutrition Bulletin*, 31, S134.

Goto, T. T. 1996. Dietary casein phosphopeptides prevent bone loss in aged ovariectomized rats. *Journal of Nutrition*, 126, 86.

Grasbeck, R., Kouvonen, I., Lundberg, M., and Tenhunen, R. 1979. An intestinal receptor for heme. *Scandinavian Journal of Haematology*, 23, 5–9.

Hallberg, L. and Rossander-Hulten, L. 1991. Iron requirements in menstruating women. *The American Journal of Clinical Nutrition*, 54, 1047–1058.

Hansen, M., Sandström, B., Jensen, M., and Sørensen, S. S. 1997. Casein phosphopeptides improve zinc and calcium absorption from rice-based but not from whole-grain infant cereal. *Journal of Pediatric Gastroenterology and Nutrition*, 24, 56–62.

Hegenauer, J., Saltman, P., Ludwig, D., Ripley, L., and Ley, A. 1979. Iron-supplemented cow milk. Identification and spectral properties of iron bound to casein micelles. *Journal of Agricultural and Food Chemistry*, 27, 1294–1301.

Hekmat, S. and Mcmahon, D. J. 1998. Distribution of iron between caseins and whey proteins in acidified milk. *Lebensmittel-Wissenschaft und-Technologie*, 31, 632–638.

Holt, C. 1992. Structure and stability of bovine casein micelles. *Advances in Protein Chemistry*, 43, 63–151.

Holt, C. and Horne, D. S. 1996. The hairy casein micelle: Evolution of the concept and its implications for dairy technology. *Netherlands Milk and Dairy Journal*, 50, 85–111.

Horne, D. S. 1998. Casein interactions: Casting light on the black boxes, the structure in dairy products. *International Dairy Journal*, 8, 171–177.

Horne, D. S. 2006. Casein micelle structure: Models and muddles. *Current Opinion in Colloid and Interface Science*, 11, 148–153.

Horton, S., Wesley, A., and Mannar, V. M. G. 2011. Double-fortified salt reduces anemia, benefit: Cost ratio is modestly favorable. *Food Policy*, 36, 581–587.

Hurrell, R. F., Lynch, S. R., Trinidad, T. P., Dassenko, S. A., and Cook, J. D. 1989. Iron-absorption in humans as influenced by bovine-milk proteins. *American Journal of Clinical Nutrition*, 49, 546–552.

Hurrell, R. F., Reddy, M. B., Juillerat, M.-A., and Cook, J. D. 2003. Degradation of phytic acid in cereal porridges improves iron absorption by human subjects. *The American Journal of Clinical Nutrition*, 77, 1213–1219.

Iyer, S. and Lönnerdal, B. 1993. Lactoferrin, lactoferrin receptors and iron metabolism. *European Journal of Clinical Nutrition*, 47, 232–241.

Jackson, L. S. and Lee, K. 1992a. The effect of dairy-products on iron availability. *Critical Reviews in Food Science and Nutrition*, 31, 259–270.

Jackson, L. S. and Lee, K. 1992b. Fortification of cheese with microencapsulated iron. *Cultured Dairy Products Journal*, 27, 4–7.

Johanson, B. 1960. Isolation of an iron-containing red protein from human milk. *Acta Chemica Scandinavica*, 14, 510–512.

Kasai, T., Iwasaki, R., Tanaka, M., and Kiriyama, S. 1995. Caseinphosphopeptides (cpp) in feces and contents in digestive-tract of rats fed casein and cpp preparations. *Bioscience Biotechnology and Biochemistry*, 59, 26–30.

Kawakami, H., Dosako, S., and Nakajima, I. 1993. Effect of lactoferrin on iron solubility under neutral conditions. *Biochemistry,* 57, 1376.

Kerstetter, J. E., O'brien, K. O., Caseria, D. M., Wall, D. E., and Insogna, K. L. 2005. The impact of dietary protein on calcium absorption and kinetic measures of bone turnover in women. *Journal of Clinical Endocrinology and Metabolism,* 90, 26.

Kibangou, I. B., Bouhallab, S., Henry, G., Bureau, F., Allouche, S., Blais, A., Guerin, P., Arhan, P., and Bougle, D. L. 2005. Milk proteins and iron absorption: Contrasting effects of different caseinophosphopeptides. *Pediatric Research,* 58, 731–734.

Kilar, F. and Simon, I. 1985. The effect of iron binding on the conformation of transferrin. *Biophysics Journal,* 48, 799–801.

Kim, E.-Y., Ham, S.-K., Bradke, D., Ma, Q., and Han, O. 2011. Ascorbic acid offsets the inhibitory effect of bioactive dietary polyphenolic compounds on transepithelial iron transport in caco-2 intestinal cells. *The Journal of Nutrition,* 141, 828–834.

Kim, M., Lee, D. T., and Lee, Y. S. 1995. Iron-absorption and intestinal solubility in rats are influenced by dietary proteins. *Nutrition Research,* 15, 1705–1716.

Kinder, F., Mueller, W. S., and Mitchell, H. S. 1942. The availability of the iron of cocoa and of iron-fortified cocoa mixtures. *Journal of Dairy Science,* 25, 401–408.

Kinsella, J. E., Whitehead, D. M., Brady J., and Bringe, N. A. 1989. Milk Proteins: Possible relationships of structure and function. In: P. F. Fox (ed.) *Developments in Dairy Chemistry.* London, England: Elsevier Applied Science.

Kurtz, F. E., Tamsma, A., and Pallansch, M. J. 1973. Effect of fortification with iron on susceptibility of skim milk and nonfat dry milk to oxidation. *Journal of Dairy Science,* 56, 1139–1143.

Lee, N.-Y., Kawai, K., Nakamura, I., Tanaka, T., Kumura, H., and Shimazaki, K.-I. 2004. Susceptibilities against bovine lactoferrin with microorganisms isolated from mastitic milk. *The Journal of Veterinary Medical Science/The Japanese Society of Veterinary Science,* 66, 1267–1269.

Levay, P. and Viljoen, M. 1995. Lactoferrin: A general review. *Haematologica,* 80, 252–267.

Lynch, S. R. 2000. The effect of calcium on iron absorption. *Nutrition Research Reviews,* 13, 141–158.

Manton, D. J., Walker, G. D., Cai, F., Cochrane, N. J., Shen, P., and Reynolds, E. C. 2008. Remineralization of enamel subsurface lesions *in situ* by the use of three commercially available sugar-free gums. *International Journal of Paediatric Dentistry,* 18, 284–290.

Marshman, C. E. 2009. *Iron Fortified Food Product and Additive.* United States of America patent application 11/988771.

Masson, P. L. and Heremans, J. F. 1971. Lactoferrin in milk from different species. *Comparative Biochemistry and Physiology. B, Comparative Biochemistry,* 39, 119–129.

Mclean, E., Cogswell, M., Egli, I., Woidyla, D., and De Benoist, B. 2009. Worldwide prevalence of anaemia, WHO vitamin and mineral nutrition information system, 1993–2005. *Public Health Nutrition,* 12, 444–454.

Mcmahon, D. J. and Brown, R. J. 1984. Composition, structure, and integrity of casein micelles—A review. *Journal of Dairy Science,* 67, 499–512.

Mcmahon, D. J. and Oommen, B. S. 2008. Supramolecular structure of the casein micelle. *Journal of Dairy Science,* 91, 1709–1721.

Meisel, H. and Frister, H. 1989. Chemical characterization of bioactive peptides from invivo digests of casein. *Journal of Dairy Research,* 56, 343–349.

Milman 2011. Anemia—Still a major health problem in many parts of the world! *Annals of Hematology,* 90, 369–377.

Miquel, E., Alegría, A., Barberá, R., and Farré, R. 2005. Speciation analysis of calcium, iron, and zinc in casein phosphopeptide fractions from toddler milk-based formula by anion exchange and reversed-phase high-performance liquid chromatography-mass spectrometry/flame atomic-absorption spectroscopy. *Analytical & Bioanalytical Chemistry,* 381, 1082–1088.

Naito, H. and Suzuki, H. 1974. Further evidence for the formation *in vivo* of phosphopeptide in the intestinal lumen from dietary β casein. *Agricultural and Biological Chemistry,* 38, 1543–1545.

Nakano, T., Goto, T., Nakaji, T., and Aoki, T. 2007. Bioavailability of iron-fortified whey protein concentrate in iron-deficient rats. *Asian-Australian Journal of Animal Science,* 20, 1120–1126.

Nancy, C. A. 1999. The iron transporter DMT1. *The International Journal of Biochemistry; Cell Biology,* 31, 991–994.

Paesano, R., Berlutti, F., Pietropaoli, M., Pantanella, F., Pacifici, E., Goolsbee, W., and Valenti, P. 2010. Lactoferrin efficacy versus ferrous sulfate in curing iron deficiency and iron deficiency anemia in pregnant women. *BioMetals,* 23, 411–417.

Pakkanen, R. and Aalto, J. 1997. Growth factors and antimicrobial factors of bovine colostrum. *International Dairy Journal*, 7, 285–297.

Palmano, K. P., Abusidou, O. M., and Elgar, D. F. 2008. *Preparation of Metal Ion-Lactoferring*. United States of America patent application 11/916,968.

Penelope, N. and Nalubola, R. 2002. *Technical Brief on Iron Compounds for Fortification of Staple Foods*. Washington, DC 20005 USA: INACG.

Philippe, M., Le Graët, Y., and Gaucheron, F. 2005. The effects of different cations on the physicochemical characteristics of casein micelles. *Food Chemistry*, 90, 673–683.

Raouche, S., Dobenesque, M., Bot, A., Lagaude, A., and Marchesseau, S. 2009a. Casein micelles as a vehicle for iron fortification of foods. *European Food Research and Technology*, 229, 929–935.

Raouche, S., Naille, S., Dobenesque, M., Bot, A., Jumas, J., Cuq, J., and Marchesseau, S. 2009b. Iron fortification of skim milk: Minerals and 57Fe Mössbauer study. *International Dairy Journal*, 19, 56–63.

Rice, W. H. and Mcmahon, D. J. 1998. Chemical, physical, and sensory characteristics of mozzarella cheese fortified using protein-chelated iron or ferric chloride. *Journal of Dairy Science*, 81, 318–326.

Richard, H. 1999. Iron. In: Richard, H. (ed.) *The Mineral Fortification of Foods*. First ed. Surrey: Leatherhead Food RA.

Rohner, F., Ernst, F. O., Arnold, M., Hilbe, M., Biebinger, R., Ehrensperger, F., Pratsinis, S. E., Langhans, W., Hurrell, R. F., and Zimmermann, M. B. 2007. Synthesis, characterization, and bioavailability in rats of ferric phosphate nanoparticles. *The Journal of Nutrition*, 137, 614–619.

Roudot-Algaron, F. and Le Bars, D. 1994. Phosphopeptides from comte cheese: Nature and origin. *Journal of Food Science*, 59, 544.

Scanff, P., Yvon, M., and Pelissier, J. P. 1991. Immobilized Fe3+ affinity chromatographic isolation of phosphopeptides. *Journal of Chromatography*, 539, 425–432.

Sheng, Q. H., Geng, Q., and Qiu, Q. R. 2006. Effects of Casein Phosphopeptides (CPP) on bone mineral density in growing rats. *China Dairy Industry*, 34, 22–25.

Sher, A., Jacobson, M. R., and Vadehra, D. V. 2006. *Ferric Fortification System*. United States of America patent application 09/914,637.

Siegenberg, D., Baynes, R., Bothwell, T., Macfarlane, B., Lamparelli, R., Car, N., Macphail, P., Schmidt, U., Tal, A., and Mayet, F. 1991. Ascorbic acid prevents the dose-dependent inhibitory effects of polyphenols and phytates on nonheme-iron absorption. *The American Journal of Clinical Nutrition*, 53, 537–541.

Steijns, J. M. and Van Hooijdonk, A. C. M. 2000. Occurrence, structure, biochemical properties and technological characteristics of lactoferrin. *British Journal of Nutrition*, 84, S11–S17.

Sugiarto, M., Ye, A., and Singh, H. 2009. Characterisation of binding of iron to sodium caseinate and whey protein isolate. *Food Chemistry*, 114, 1007–1013.

Taylor, P. G., Martínez-Torres, C., Romano, E. L., and Layrisse, M. 1986. The effect of cysteine-containing peptides released during meat digestion on iron absorption in humans. *The American Journal of Clinical Nutrition*, 43, 68–71.

Troost, F. J., Steijns, J., Saris, W. H., and Brummer, R. J. 2001. Gastric digestion of bovine lactoferrin *in vivo* in adults. *The Journal of Nutrition*, 131, 2101–2104.

Uchida, T., Oda, T., Sato, K., and Kawakami, H. 2006. Availability of lactoferrin as a natural solubilizer of iron for food products. *International Dairy Journal*, 16, 95–101.

Valenti, P. and Antonini, G. 2005. Lactoferrin: An important host defence against microbial and viral attack. *Cellular and Molecular Life Sciences*, 62, 2576–2587.

Vivian, J. T. and Callis, P. R. 2001. Mechanisms of tryptophan fluorescence shifts in proteins. *Biophysics Journal*, 80, 2093–2109.

Wakabayashi, H., Yamauchi, K., and Takase, M. 2006. Lactoferrin research, technology and applications. *International Dairy Journal*, 16, 1241–1251.

Wall, C. R., Grant, C. C., Taua, N., Wilson, C., and Thompson, J. M. D. 2005. Milk versus medicine for the treatment of iron deficiency anaemia in hospitalised infants. *Archives of Disease in Childhood*, 90, 1033–1038.

Wegmüller, R., Zimmermann, M. B., Moretti, D., Arnold, M., Langhans, W., and Hurrell, R. F. 2004. Particle size reduction and encapsulation affect the bioavailability of ferric pyrophosphate in Rats. *The Journal of Nutrition*, 134, 3301–3304.

West, A. R. and Oates, P. S. 2008. Mechanisms of heme iron absorption: Current questions and controversies. *World Journal of Gastroenterology*, 14, 4101–4110.

West, D. W. 1986. Structure and function of the phosphorylated residues of casein. *The Journal of Dairy Research*, 53, 333–352.

Wortley, G., Leusner, S., Good, C., Gugger, E., and Glahn, R. 2005. Iron availability of a fortified processed wheat cereal: A comparison of fourteen iron forms using an in vitro digestion/human colonic adenocarcinoma (CaCo-2) cell model. *The British Journal of Nutrition*, 93, 65–71.

Yeung, A. C., Glahn, R. P., and Miller, D. D. 2002. Effects of iron source on iron availability from casein and casein phosphopeptides. *Journal of Food Science—Chicago*, 67, 1271–1275.

Zhang, D. and Mahoney, A. W. 1989a. Bioavailability of iron-milk-protein complexes and fortified cheddar cheese. *Journal of Dairy Science*, 72, 2845–2855.

Zhang, D. and Mahoney, A. W. 1989b. Effect of iron fortification on quality of cheddar cheese. *Journal of Dairy Science*, 72, 322–332.

Zhang, D. and Mahoney, A. W. 1990. Effect of iron fortification on quality of cheddar cheese. 2. Effects of aging and fluorescent light on pilot scale cheeses. *Journal of Dairy Science*, 73, 2252–2258.

Zimmermann, M. B., Wegmueller, R., Zeder, C., Chaouki, N., Rohner, F., Saïssi, M., Torresani, T., and Hurrell, R. F. 2004. Dual fortification of salt with iodine and micronized ferric pyrophosphate: A randomized, double-blind, controlled trial. *The American Journal of Clinical Nutrition*, 80, 952–959.

17 Stabilization of Probiotics for Industrial Application

Devastotra Poddar, Arup Nag, Shantanu Das,
and Harjinder Singh

CONTENTS

17.1 BACKGROUND

17.1.1 DEFINITION OF PROBIOTICS

Probiotic bacteria have been defined in many ways by different people but perhaps the most widely used and accepted definition is proposed by Fuller (1992) according to which probiotics are living microorganisms which when ingested have beneficial effects on the host by improving the physiological functions of the intestinal microflora. Another definition has been provided by Havenaar and Huis In't Veld (1992), which explains probiotics as "a preparation of or a product containing viable, defined microorganisms in sufficient numbers, which alter the microbiota (by implantation or colonization) in a compartment of the host and by that exert beneficial health effects in this host." Probiotics have also been defined as "live microbes which transit the gastro-intestinal tract and in doing so benefit the health of the consumer" (Tannock et al. 2000), which contradicts the earlier definitions focusing only on the interactions between the probiotic organisms and the original intestinal microflora (Fuller 1989). A recent definition can be found in the Food and Agricultural Organization of the United Nations and the World Health Organization's documents which define probiotics as "live microorganisms which when administered in adequate amounts confer a health benefit on the host" (FAO/WHO 2001). But all of these definitions agree in one point that probiotics must deliver some kind of health benefits and should be living in nature, and be able to form colonies on the intestinal wall.

17.1.2 PROBIOTICS AND HEALTH BENEFITS

The health benefits associated with probiotics have been studied extensively over the past century. In early 1900, the Russian Nobel Prize winner, Elie Metchnikoff, observed an increased life expectancy in Bulgarians who consumed fermented milk products. Later, he advanced the theory that the consumption of lactic acid bacteria would minimize intestinal putrefaction and prolong life (Metchnikoff 1907). Overall, cultured milk has become an integral part of diets because of the health-promoting attributes associated with its consumption.

There are several possible modes of action by which probiotic bacteria provide health benefits to the host. These include suppression of pathogenic bacteria by producing antimicrobial compounds and competing for adhesion sites and nutrients and alteration of the microbial metabolism by controlling enzymatic activity in the intestine (Fuller 1991). Further, probiotics stimulate immunity by increasing T-cell production (Anukam et al. 2008; Baron 2009) and modulating cytokines, tumor necrosis factor-α, interleukins, and interferons (Borruel et al. 2002; Bai et al. 2006; Chen et al. 2009a). Moreover, they inhibit the epidermal growth factor receptor and insulin-like growth factors in tumor cells (Chen et al. 2009b). Finally, increased intestinal antibody and macrophage levels enhance the phagocytic capacity of the blood leucocytes (Gill et al. 2001). Thus, probiotics enhance protection against diseases.

Good probiotics should confer health benefits to the host animal. They should also be nontoxic and nonpathogenic in nature. Further, they should be capable of surviving at low pH and in the presence of the high concentration of bile salts in the gastrointestinal system (Fuller 1991). In addition, they should be stable under storage conditions and should be easy to handle for industrial production. Overall, possession of the above properties will make the bacteria suitable for food and pharmaceutical applications.

From the 1990s to the present day, there has been a steady accumulation of scientific evidence that emphasizes the health benefits, including the control of chronic diseases, associated with the consumption of probiotics. Importantly, numerous experimental studies have emphasized the potential protective effects of *Lactobacillus* and *Bifidobacterium* species (Thantsha et al. 2009; Kumar et al. 2010) and their health benefits are summarized in Table 17.1.

17.1.3 APPLICATION OF PROBIOTICS AND THEIR MARKET POTENTIAL

Probiotic bacteria are one of the top functional ingredients and underpin some of the most successful functional food brands in the world. The use of probiotics is limited mainly to foods that are subjected to chilled distribution and storage because there are currently few credible delivery technologies that are able to deliver probiotic bacteria in shelf-stable foods. This establishes "delivery technology for probiotic bacteria in shelf-stable foods" as a significant opportunity of commercial importance because it will expand the current market for probiotics, which is estimated to be approximately US$20 billion (Siró et al. 2008).

Scientists generally agree and FAO/WHO guidelines state that we need to consume between 100 million and 1 billion live probiotic cells per day to realize their health benefits. However, as a significant proportion of the bacterial cells are destroyed during processing, storage, and gastrointestinal transit, "stabilization of probiotic bacteria" is an area of interest for research and development. Some of the established microencapsulation techniques have been able to improve the survival of

TABLE 17.1

Selected Studies Showing the Effectiveness of Various Strains of Probiotic Bacteria against Various Diseases

Probiotic Bacteria	Alleviation of Disease Symptoms	References
Bifidobacterium animalis	Irritable bowel syndrome, dental caries, rotavirus diarrhea, fever, rhinorrhea, colitis	Phuapradit et al. (1999); Çaglar et al. (2005); Rautava et al. (2006); Wildt et al. (2006); Guyonnet et al. (2007); Leyer et al. (2009)
Bifidobacterium bifidus	Necrotizing enterocolitis	Bin-Nun et al. (2005)
Bifidobacterium breve	Irritable bowel syndrome, respiratory infection, refractory enterocolitis, atopic dermatitis	Kanamori et al. (2004); Saggioro (2004); Kukkonen et al. (2008); Yoshida et al. (2010)
Bifidobacterium infantis	Irritable bowel syndrome, necrotizing enterocolitis, diarrhea	Hoyos (1999); Corrêa et al. (2005); Lin et al. (2005); O'Mahony et al. (2005); Whorwell et al. (2006)
Bifidobacterium lactis	Constipation	Puccio et al. (2007)
Bifidobacterium longum	Ulcerative colitis, respiratory tract infection, common cold	de Vrese et al. (2005); Furrie et al. (2005); Puccio et al. (2007)
Lactobacillus acidophilus	Necrotizing enterocolitis, irritable bowel syndrome, bacterial vaginosis, *Helicobacter pylori* therapy, glucose intolerance, hyperglycemia, hyperinsulinemia, dyslipidemia, cancer, fever, rhinorrhea	Hoyos (1999); McLean and Rosenstein (2000); Gaón et al. (2002); Xiao et al. (2003); Johnson-Henry et al. (2004); Saggioro (2004); Lin et al. (2005); Yadav et al. (2007); Leyer et al. (2009); Soltan Dallal et al. (2010)
Lactobacillus bulgaricus	Crohn's disease, inflammatory bowel disease, common cold	Borruel et al. (2002); Şengül et al. (2006); Makino et al. (2010)
Lactobacillus casei	Crohn's disease, constipation, *H. pylori* therapy, arthritis, glucose intolerance, hyperglycemia, hyperinsulinemia, dyslipidemia, diarrhea, atopic eczema	Kato et al. (1998); Tuomola et al. (1999); Gaón et al. (2003); Koebnick et al. (2003); Tursi et al. (2004); Kanazawa et al. (2005); Sýkora et al. (2005); Bu et al. (2007); Yadav et al. (2007); Cukrowska et al. (2010)
Lactobacillus fermentum	Bacterial vaginosis, inflammatory bowel disease, colitis	Peran et al. (2006, 2007); Irvine et al. (2010)
Lactobacillus gasseri	Common cold, *H. pylori* therapy, asthma, allergic rhinitis	Ushiyama et al. (2003); de Vrese et al. (2005); Chen et al. (2010)
Lactobacillus johnsonii	*H. pylori* therapy, cirrhosis, atopic dermatitis	Cruchet et al. (2003); Inoue et al. (2007); Gotteland et al. (2008); Tanaka et al. (2008)
Lactobacillus paracasei	Allergic rhinitis, irritable bowel syndrome, diarrhea, atopic eczema, urogenital infection	Verdú et al. (2004); Wang et al. (2004); Sarker et al. (2005); Zárate et al. (2007); Cukrowska et al. (2008)
Lactobacillus plantarum	Irritable bowel syndrome, colitis	Nobaek et al. (2000); Niedzielin et al. (2001); Schultz et al. (2002)
Lactobacillus reuterii	Colitis, atopic dermatitis, rotavirus diarrhea, *H. pylori* therapy, infantile colic, asthma, gingivitis, HIV/AIDS	Madsen et al. (1999); Mukai et al. (2002); Rosenfeldt et al. (2002, 2004); Forsythe et al. (2007); Anukam et al. (2008); Karimi et al. (2009)
Lactobacillus rhamnosus	Atopic dermatitis, bacterial vaginosis, diarrhea, *H. pylori* therapy, HIV/AIDS	Reid et al. (2001); Urbancsek et al. (2001); Rosenfeldt et al. (2002, 2004); Anukam et al. (2008); Irvine et al. (2010)
Lactobacillus rhamnosus GG	Atopic disease, antibiotic-associated diarrhea, rotavirus gastroenteritis, *H. pylori* therapy, dental caries, ulcerative colitis pouchitis, irritable bowel syndrome, Crohn's disease, cystic fibrosis	Vanderhoof et al. (1999); Armuzzi et al. (2001); Kalliomäki et al. (2001, 2003); Nase et al. (2001); Szajewska et al. (2001); Cremonini et al. (2002); Bruzzese et al. (2004); Montalto et al. (2004); Zocco et al. (2006); Gawrońska et al. (2007)

continued

TABLE 17.1   (continued)

Selected Studies Showing the Effectiveness of Various Strains of Probiotic Bacteria against Various Diseases

Probiotic Bacteria	Alleviation of Disease Symptoms	References
Lactobacillus salivarius	Colitis, arthritis, *H. pylori* therapy	Kabir et al. (1997); McCarthy et al. (2003); Sheil et al. (2004); Peran et al. (2005)
Saccharomyces boulardii	Crohn's disease, *H. pylori* therapy, diarrhea, colitis, amoebiosis	Guslandi et al. (2000, 2003); Cremonini et al. (2002); Gaón et al. (2003); Mansour-Ghanaei et al. (2003); Duman et al. (2005); Gotteland et al. (2005); Kotowska et al. (2005); Kurugöl and Koturoğlu (2005); Villarruel et al. (2007); Hurduc et al. (2009)

probiotic cells in simulated gastric fluid and simulated intestinal fluid, but improvements in their stability during ambient storage have rarely been reported either in academic research or in commercial development. It is the lack of appropriate stabilizing technology that restricts the use of probiotics in shelf-stable foods.

17.2 STABILIZATION OF PROBIOTICS

This review briefly discusses various approaches that are taken to stabilize bacteria. The most commonly used strategy is dehydration and encapsulation in a protective matrix. Optimization of the packaging and the storage conditions is also considered to be vital. Other studies focus on manipulating the cell physiology. These approaches are used independently or in combination to improve the viability of the bacterial cells.

17.2.1 STABILIZATION USING DESICCATION/DEHYDRATION TECHNOLOGIES

Drying is a valuable technology for the long-term preservation of food materials because decreasing the moisture content slows down the action of enzymes. Various drying technologies have therefore been used, with varying success, to improve the stability of bacteria. In particular, freeze drying, spray drying, fluidized bed drying, vacuum drying, and mixed/two-step drying processes for the stabilization of probiotic bacteria have been studied in recent years and are discussed in some detail below.

17.2.1.1 Freeze Drying

Freeze drying is used extensively to preserve biological materials, including bacteria, yeasts, and sporulating fungi, for food and pharmaceutical applications. It is based on the principle of sublimation; the bacteria are frozen, then a vacuum is applied, and the desiccation is carried out by sublimation (Santivarangkna et al. 2007). The advantages of the freeze drying of bacteria include long viability during storage and ease of transportation. Some limitations are the high cost of the operation and difficulties in scaling up and continuous processing (Santivarangkna et al. 2007).

The step in the freeze drying process that most influences viability is the freezing of the bacteria. The rate of cooling is a critical factor. At an optimum rate of cooling, the cells do not lose water and reach the eutectic point in an amorphous state (Berny and Hennebert 1991). If the cooling rate is too slow, water will be lost from the cells by osmosis, dehydrating them and preventing freezing. If the cells do not lose water quickly enough to maintain equilibrium, intracellular formation of ice crystals will occur (Mazur 1977). Significant loss of bacterial cell viability after freeze drying has been attributed to the formation of ice crystals on the cell surface, resulting in an increase in extracellular osmolality, thus leading to dehydration of the cells (Fowler and Toner 2005), loss of membrane integrity, and denaturation of macromolecules (Franks 1995; Thammavongs et al. 1996; De Angelis and Gobbetti 2004). Fonseca et al. (2000) have reported that the size and the shape of the cells are important criteria in their survivability; enterococci (cocci) are more tolerant than lactobacilli (rods) because the membrane damage that is caused by extracellular ice crystal formation during freeze drying is reduced. Loss of viability has also been attributed to peroxidation of the membrane lipids (Brennan et al. 1986; Linders et al. 1997a) and destabilization of the DNA and RNA secondary structures. The recovery rate for freeze-dried cultures can be as low as 0.3% (Abadias et al. 2001).

The technology to protect bacterial cells during freeze drying is known as cryopreservation and the compounds used to achieve this protection are called cryoprotectants or cryoprotecting agents (CPAs). The addition of CPAs prior to fermentation or drying helps the probiotic cells to adapt to the changed environment. The CPA accumulates slowly within the bacterial cells, which helps to reduce the osmotic pressure difference between the inside and the outside of the cells (Kets et al. 1996; Meng et al. 2008). The CPA can be added either to the growth medium or to the drying medium, and its action varies with different bacterial strains. However, certain general compounds, such as nonfat milk solids, lactose, trehalose, glycerol, betaine, adonitol, sucrose, glucose, and dextran, are regarded as being suitable CPAs for many species (Hubálek 2003; Morgan et al. 2006).

The protection mechanism can be better understood by classifying CPAs into two broad groups: (i) amorphous-glass-forming salts and (ii) eutectic-crystallizing salts. The first group, comprising carbohydrates, proteins, and polymers, acts by imparting very high viscosity at the glass transition, thereby restricting the molecular mobility of the cells. Most of the successful CPAs for probiotic bacteria fall into this group. The second group contains certain eutectic salts that tend to crystallize as the temperature approaches the freezing point; however, instead of providing protection, they have sometimes been reported as being detrimental to the cell membranes (Orndorff and MacKenzie 1973; Morgan et al. 2006).

CPAs are sometimes classified in a slightly different manner into three groups: (i) highly permeable compounds such as monovalent alcohols, amides, and sulfoxides, (ii) slowly permeable compounds such as glycerol, and (iii) nonpermeable compounds such as mono-, oligo-, and polysaccharides, sugar alcohols, proteins, and polyalcohols. Permeable CPAs bind the intracellular water and prevent dehydration. Nonpermeable CPAs form a layer on the cell surface, thus allowing partial outflow of water from the cell body, reducing the toxic effect of salts, stopping excessive growth of ice crystals, and maintaining their structures (Hubálek 2003; Saarela et al. 2005).

Trehalose and sucrose have been found to be excellent CPAs against dehydration stress by acting as stabilizers of membranes and proteins and replacers of water from the macromolecular structures (Rudolph and Crowe 1985; Morgan et al. 2006). Conrad et al. (2000) demonstrated the high cryoprotective efficiency of trehalose; a high survival of *Lactobacillus acidophilus* cells during freeze drying was achieved, probably because of the high glass transition temperature (T_g) of trehalose. Compounds with a high T_g can remain relatively immobile at higher temperatures and can help to produce a more stable freeze-dried matrix (Crowe et al. 1996; Sun and Davidson 1998; Morgan et al. 2006). Trehalose is also regarded as a good CPA because it can form dihydrate crystals, which leaves the remaining matrix as a glass and does not reduce the T_g or the stability of the matrix (Crowe et al. 1998). Trehalose and sucrose were shown to be very effective CPAs when *Escherichia coli* DH5 alpha and *Bacillus thuringiensis* HD-1 were subjected to freeze drying (Leslie et al. 1995). In another recent study, trehalose, sucrose, and sorbitol were used as CPAs for lactobacilli, and sucrose was found to be the best agent among the group (Siaterlis et al. 2009). However, in one experiment, trehalose achieved a poorer result than the control sample when used in media prior to air drying (Linders et al. 1997b).

Lactose is another popular CPA, has been shown to be more effective than glycerol (Chavarri et al. 1988), and has been found to be effective for certain species, such as *Lactobacillus lactis*, *Escherichia coli*, *Lactobacillus delbrueckii*, and *Saccharomyces cerevisiae*, moderately effective for *Streptomyces tenebrarius*, and completely ineffective for *Spirulina platensis* (Hubálek 2003). Lactose, and a few other sugar substrates, has been added to the growth medium for *Lactobacillus delbrueckii*, resulting in a marked improvement in postdrying survival, storage stability, and thermotolerance (Carvalho et al. 2004).

17.2.1.2 Spray Drying

In the spray-drying process, the atomized liquid is subjected at high pressure to hot air at temperatures up to 200°C and with an outlet temperature of above 80°C. This results in the evaporation of moisture after a very short exposure. The production of probiotics by spray drying is advantageous because it is cost effective from an operational point of view, is easy to scale up, is less time consuming than freeze drying, and is a continuous operation with a high production rate (Knorr 1998). However, as probiotic bacteria are heat-sensitive microorganisms, they are inactivated if subjected to the high temperatures used in the conventional drying process, which has adverse effects on their viability and, in turn, a negative impact on their viability and stability during storage (Gibbs et al. 1999; Kailasapathy 2002; Madene et al. 2006).

In efforts to reduce cell death during spray drying, Champagne and Fustier (2007) optimized the inlet and outlet temperatures using a combination of spray drying and fluidized bed drying to minimize the heat shock and preadaptation of the bacteria to the heat stress prior to drying. Recent studies to obtain higher viability have focused on controlling the outlet air temperature (Table 17.2). However, lower outlet air temperatures result in powder with a high moisture content, which leads to cell death on storage (O'Riordan et al. 2001). Another major limitation of spray drying is the limited choice of shell materials. The shell material has to be water soluble for spray drying to take place, causing immediate release of the core material in the aqueous medium so that controlled release cannot be achieved.

Success of spray drying for encapsulation of probiotics depends on the bacterial strain used as well as the encapsulating material used. O'Riordan et al. (2001) used spray-drying technology to coat *Bifidobacterium* cells with starch. There was no significant advantage of microencapsulation during acid exposure and storage, but milder spray-drying parameters resulted in less than a 1.0 log reduction in cell viability. Fávaro-Trindade and Grosso (2002) found that *Bifidobacterium lactis* cells were highly resistant to spray-drying conditions, with negligible reduction in viability at an inlet temperature of 130°C and an outlet temperature of 75°C. In contrast, in the same study, *Lactobacillus acidophilus* cells showed a 2.0 log reduction under similar drying conditions. The encapsulating medium used in this study was cellulose acetate phthalate and very good particle morphology with no pores on the surface was achieved. In another study to protect *Lactobacillus paracasei* during spray drying, Desmond et al. (2002) investigated the encapsulating effect of gum acacia. Cells were grown in both 10% gum acacia and 10% reconstituted skim milk as a control. The cells encapsulated in gum acacia survived 10 times better than the controls; even at a high outlet temperature of 95°C, the viability during storage at 4°C was improved 20-fold, and the survival during gastric juice incubation was 100-fold higher. The loss of viability also depends on the type of carrier used. For example, the log reduction in viability was found to be higher in soluble starch than in other carriers, such as gelatin, gum arabic, and skim milk (Lian et al. 2002; Santivarangkna et al. 2007). Picot and Lacroix (2003, 2004) used a modified spray-drying process involving a coating of milk fat and denatured whey protein isolate in an attempt to reduce the loss of viability during spray drying. The micronized freeze-dried cultures were coated during spray drying and it was concluded that this would be a suitable method to scale up industrially and it is also economical.

17.2.1.3 Fluidized Bed Drying

Fluidized bed drying has been widely used in the pharmaceutical industry. It was originally developed for rapid drying but its present applications include granulation, agglomeration, air suspension coating, rotary pelletization, and powder and solution layering. In fluidized bed drying, air travels upward through the bed of particles with sufficient velocity to provide fluid-like behavior, and the freely suspended particles in the air stream are dried by rapid heat exchange and mass transfer. The major advantages of fluidized bed drying are its relatively low operational cost and

TABLE 17.2
Review of Scientific Work Comparing the Viabilities of Probiotic Bacteria When Using Spray Drying

Bacteria	Inlet Air Temperature (°C)	Outlet Air Temperature (°C)	Matrix	Storage Conditions	Study Findings	Reference
Bifidobacterium PL1	60	45 60	Starch	Screw-capped glass bottles at 19–24°C for 20 days	Starch encapsulation did not provide protection during storage. Inlet and outlet temperatures of 100°C/45°C resulted in <1 log reduction after drying	O'Riordan et al. (2001)
	80 100 ≥120					
Bifidobacterium spp. (30 strains)	175	85–90	Skim milk	Polythene bags and aluminum-coated paper bags at 4°C, 15°C, and 25°C for 90 days	High initial survival following spray drying; storage at 4°C maintained viability; increased viability loss at 25°C. The heat and oxygen tolerance varied among closely related species	Simpson et al. (2005)
Lactobacillus bulgaricus	200	70	Skim milk	Hermetically sealed glass bottles, controlled water activity of 0.11 at 20°C	The ratio of unsaturated fatty acids to saturated fatty acids decreased during storage as a consequence of lipid oxidation	Teixeira et al. (1996)
Bifidobacterium longum	100	50–60	Gelatin, starch, skim milk powder, and gum arabic	NA	Increase in outlet air temperature resulted in increased death irrespective of the carrier used	Lian et al. (2002)
Bifidobacterium infantis Bb-02	160	65	Emulsion containing caseinate, fructo-oligo-saccharides, dried glucose syrup, resistant starch	Open containers, 25°C and 50% relative humidity for 5 weeks	Microencapsulation protected the viability of bacteria upon storage (>106-fold) and during simulated gastrointestinal transit	Crittenden et al. (2006)
Bifidobacterium lactis B1-01 and *Lactobacillus acidophilus*	70	47	Pectin and casein	Closed glass vials, 7°C and 37°C, water activity of 0.65	*Lactobacillus acidophilus* was more viable than *Bifidobacterium lactis* at both temperatures	Oliveira et al. (2007)

the high postdrying viability because of the mild-heating conditions. Its major limitations are the irregular particle size, the stickiness, the agglomerated particles, the slow-drying rate (Santivarangkna et al. 2007), and the uneven distribution of cells in the nonliquid food matrix (Santivarangkna et al. 2007). Fluidized bed drying has been used commercially in the production of baker's yeast and wine yeast (Caron 1995).

A limited number of studies on the fluidized bed drying of probiotic bacteria and lactic acid starter cultures have been carried out (Santivarangkna et al. 2007). In most, the bacteria were entrapped or encapsulated in a certain matrix before being dried. Linders et al. (1997c) dried *Lactobacillus plantarum* cells that were granulated to pellets using potato starch as the support material. Selmer-Olsen et al. (1999) immobilized *Lactobacillus helveticus* cells in calcium alginate gel beads, which were then fluidized bed dried. Mille et al. (2004) fluidized bed-dried *Lactobacillus plantarum* and *Lactobacillus bulgaricus*, with the bacteria being uniformly mixed with casein powder before drying. It was found that the bacterial viability was influenced by the water activity of the casein powder; a lower water activity resulted in an increased loss of viability during drying. Strasser et al. (2009) sprayed a concentrated liquid bacterial cell suspension on to fluidized powdered cellulose carrier material. They observed that the addition of protective carbohydrates such as sucrose and trehalose prevented a decline in the cell viability of *Lactobacillus plantarum* and *Enterococcus faecium* during fluidized bed drying.

17.2.1.4 Vacuum Drying

Vacuum drying is used to preserve heat-sensitive functional ingredients such as vitamins, enzymes, and bacteria because the process is carried out at low temperature and under reduced pressure. The major advantages of vacuum drying are the high drying rate, the low drying temperature, and the absence of oxygen. The main disadvantage is the longer-drying time compared with fluidized bed drying (Santivarangkna et al. 2007).

There have been only a few studies on the vacuum drying of probiotic bacteria. Vacuum drying has usually been applied together with other drying processes to increase its effectiveness. King and Su (1994) dried *Lactobacillus acidophilus* using freeze drying, vacuum drying, and the low-temperature vacuum drying. The survival ratio from the vacuum drying (plate temperature, 40–45°C) was too low for the process to be applied in culture preservation. Controlled low-temperature vacuum drying (plate temperature, −2°C to 2°C) resulted in survival ratio close to that from freeze drying. The powder produced from low-temperature vacuum drying had case hardening, shrinkage, and poor rehydration properties.

17.2.1.5 Mixed/Two-Step Drying Systems

In mixed or two-step drying processes, two or more drying systems are combined to minimize cell injury and to improve the bacterial viability. Simpson et al. (2005) found that the combination of spray drying and fluidized bed drying improved the viability of *Bifidobacterium* spp. when powders were stored at 25°C. Wolff et al. (1990) found that a combination of vacuum drying and freeze drying was best suited to the dehydration of concentrated suspensions of *Streptococcus thermophilus*. The survival rate was higher in the vacuum freeze-drying process (3.5×10^{11} cfu/g) than in the atmospheric freeze-drying process (1.7×10^{11} cfu/g).

17.2.2 STABILIZATION BY ENCAPSULATION

Microencapsulation generally refers to the process of stabilizing an active substance (core) by enclosing it within a physical barrier (shell). The shell consists of either a continuous coating film or a solid wall material, which can release the core at a controlled rate under the direction of specific environmental shifts (Dziezak 1988; Anal and Singh 2007). Encapsulation technologies have many useful applications in the food industry, including stabilizing the core material; restraining oxidation; providing prolonged or regulated release; concealing flavors, colors, or odors; improving shelf life; and preventing nutritional loss (Anal and Singh 2007). The technologies have been extended to encapsulate probiotic bacteria successfully, resulting in enhanced viability of the bacteria by providing protection against environmental stresses (oxygen, acidity in the stomach), facilitating the handling of cells, and allowing controlled dosages (Rokka and Rantamäki 2010). Various types of biopolymer materials, such as starch, dextrin, and whey proteins, have been used as the encapsulation matrix for probiotic bacteria.

Table 17.3 summarizes the published research during the last decade on the encapsulation of probiotic bacteria. Selected matrices and encapsulation techniques are discussed in more detail below.

17.2.2.1 Encapsulating Materials

Microencapsulation in tailored carriers composed of nontoxic biopolymers provides mechanical protection and allows probiotic microorganisms to be used in several food products. The encapsulating material serves two major functions: (i) to provide a definite physical structure for delivery in the food systems and (ii) to protect the living cells during harsh processing, during storage, and in the low-pH environment in the stomach (Ding and Shah 2009a,b). The materials that are most commonly used for probiotic encapsulation are (i) polysaccharides—carrageenan and alginate (extracted from marine algae), starch and its derivatives, and bacterial exopolysaccharides such as gellan gum and xanthan gum, (ii) proteins such as casein, whey protein (milk proteins), and gelatin, and (iii) fats and oils such as cocoa butter, sesame oil, and hexaglyceryl-condensed ricinoleate. Brief discussions on each type are presented below.

17.2.2.1.1 Polysaccharides

17.2.2.1.1.1 Carrageenan   κ-Carrageenan is a natural polysaccharide that is made up of repeating sulfated galactose units and 3,6-anhydrogalactose, which are joined together by alternating α-(1,3) and β-(1,4) glycosidic linkages. It is extracted from red marine algae and is commonly used as an emulsifier in food products. The gelation of carrageenan is a temperature-dependent process that is induced by temperature changes. Immobilized beads are formed by dispersing a suspension of cells and a heat-sterilized polymer mix into a warm organic phase (40–45°C) and gelation occurs by cooling to room temperature (Audet et al. 1988). The beads are seasoned by soaking in potassium chloride solution. The potassium ions stabilize the gel and prevent swelling; however, potassium chloride affects the growth of lactic acid bacteria (Audet et al. 1988). Moreover, the addition of locust bean gum to κ-carrageenan, especially at a ratio of 2:1, improves the rigidity (Miles et al. 1984; Audet et al. 1990). There is a synergistic interaction between κ-carrageenan and locust bean gum, which improves the rheological properties of the resulting gel (Miles et al. 1984; Arnaud et al. 1988). Doleyres et al. (2002a, 2004) demonstrated continuous production of a mixed culture (*Bifidobacterium longum* and *Lactococcus diacetylactis*) that was immobilized in κ-carrageenan and locust bean gum gel beads.

17.2.2.1.1.2 Alginate   Alginate is a linear heteropolysaccharide of 1–4-linked β-D-mannuronic acid and α-L-guluronic acid residues, which varies in composition based on the source of extraction (Smidsrod and Skjak-Braek 1990). Microencapsulation in calcium alginate beads for drug delivery systems, enzyme immobilization, and immunoprotective containers in cell transplantation has been investigated. Entrapment with calcium alginate beads has frequently been used for the immobilization of lactic acid bacteria because of the simple method of immobilization and the advantage of being nontoxic to cells. Gel formation occurs when in contact with calcium and multivalent cations (Prevost and Divies 1992; Iyer and Kailasapathy 2005).

Compared with free cells, encapsulating bacteria in alginate beads increased survival during heat treatment, during homogenization, at high sodium chloride concentration, at low pH in simulated gastric juice, at high bile salt concentration in simulated intestinal fluid, and during storage (Song et al. 2003; Mandal et al. 2006; Ross et al. 2008; Mokarram et al. 2009; González-Sánchez et al. 2010;

TABLE 17.3

Summary of Published Research over the Last Decade on the Encapsulation of Probiotic Bacteria

Encapsulating Material	Types of Bacteria Encapsulated	Product Application Studied	Research Findings	Reference
Alginate	*Lactobacillus acidophilus* (ATCC 43121)	NA	Improved survival in artificial gastric juice, artificial intestinal juice, and heat treatment	Kim et al. (2008)
Alginate	*Lactobacillus casei*	Ice cream	Improved survival in ice cream during storage over a 3-month period	Hsiao et al. (2004)
Alginate	*Escherichia coli* GFP +	NA	Showed improved survival of the encapsulated bacteria; also useful in delivering viable bacteria to the intestine	Song et al. (2003)
Alginate	*Lactobacillus acidophilus* CSCC 2400	NA	Effective protection of the bacteria in simulated gastric conditions and bile salt. Increasing the alginate coating increased the bacterial survivability	Chandramouli et al. (2004)
Alginate	*Lactobacillus casei* YIT 9018	NA	Improved viability in simulated gastric acid, intestinal juice, simulated bile conditions, and storage at room temperature, 4°C, and 23°C for 6 weeks	Song et al. (2003)
Alginate	*Lactobacillus reuteri* (ATCC 55730)	Fermented sausages	Improved the viability after processing of the dry fermented sausages	Muthukumarasamy and Holley (2006)
Alginate	*Lactobacillus casei* (NCDC-298)	NA	Increasing the alginate concentration improved the viability of bacteria in simulated gastric pH and intestinal bile salt solution and the survival of encapsulated cells after heat treatment	Mandal et al. (2006)
Alginate	*Lactobacillus acidophilus* LA-5 and *Bifidobacterium bifidum* BB12	White-brined cheese	Microencapsulation increased the viability counts of probiotic bacteria during 90 days of storage in brine solution. However, no significant increase in the proteolytic activity was observed because of the restricted release of proteases and peptidases from the capsules during ripening	Özer and Avni Kirmaci (2009)
Alginate	*Lactobacillus acidophilus* LA-5 and *Bifidobacterium lactis* BB12	Iranian yogurt milk (doogh)	Improved the viability of probiotic bacteria in refrigerated storage for 42 days	Mortazavian et al. (2008)
Alginate	*Lactobacillus acidophilus* 2409 and *Bifidobacterium infantis* 1912 and *Lactobacillus casei* 2603	Yogurt	Improved the viability in simulated high gastric conditions, in high bile salt conditions, and during storage for 8 weeks	Sultana et al. (2000)

Coating material	Probiotic strain	Food matrix	Effect	Reference
Alginate	Lactobacillus acidophilus PTCC 1643, Lactobacillus rhamnosus PTCC 1637	NA	Double coating in alginate improved the viability in simulated gastric juice and simulated intestinal juice	Mokarram et al. (2009)
Alginate	Lactic acid bacteria	NA	Improved the viability in the simulated gastric conditions	Ross et al. (2008)
Alginate	Lactobacillus acidophilus LA-1	NA	Improved the survival of cells after heat treatment, homogenization, high sodium chloride concentration, low pH, and high bile salt concentration	Sabikhi et al. (2010)
Alginate	Bifidobacterium animalis subsp. lactis BB12	NA	Improved the survivability during exposure to nisin and simulated gastric juice; refrigerated storage at 4°C for 28 days	González-Sánchez et al. (2010)
Alginate	Lactobacillus acidophilus LA-5 and Bifidobacterium bifidum BB12	Kasar cheese	Improved the viability during storage for 90 days	Özer et al. (2008)
Alginate	Lactobacillus casei (Lc-01) and Bifidobacterium lactis (BB12)	Ice cream	Improved the survivability during storage at −20°C for 180 days	Homayouni et al. (2008)
Alginate	Lactobacillus acidophilus (ATCC-314)	Yogurt	Encapsulated Lactobacillus acidophilus suppressed the incidence of colon tumor	Urbanska et al. (2007)
Compressed alginate and hydroxypropyl cellulose	Lactobacillus acidophilus (ATCC 4356)	NA	Improved the viability on storage at 25°C for 30 days. The cell viability decreased with the compression pressure	Chan and Zhang (2002)
Alginate and poly-L-lysine and palm oil	Lactobacillus rhamnosus, Bifidobacterium longum, Lactobacillus salivarius, Lactobacillus plantarum, Lactobacillus acidophilus, Lactobacillus paracasei, Bifidobacterium lactis Bl-04, and Bifidobacterium lactis Bi-07	NA	Protected the probiotic bacteria from acid and bile salts. Poly-L-lysine provided better protection than alginate under acidic conditions	Ding and Shah (2009a,b)
Alginate–chitosan	Lactobacillus acidophilus (ATCC-314)	Yogurt	Served as a suitable carrier and protected the bacteria in simulated gastric fluid and simulated intestinal fluid	Urbanska et al. (2007)
Alginate-coated matrix and whey protein	Lactobacillus plantarum (Lp299v, LpA159, Lp800)	NA	Whey protein coating of alginate beads significantly improved the viability of the bacteria in simulated gastric and intestinal fluids	Gbassi et al. (2009)
Alginate–gelatin	Lactobacillus casei ATCC 393	NA	Relative humidity had a minor effect on the characteristics of the microcapsules. Improved viability of the encapsulated cells in simulated gastric fluid and simulated intestinal fluid	Li et al. (2009)

continued

TABLE 17.3 (continued)
Summary of Published Research over the Last Decade on the Encapsulation of Probiotic Bacteria

Encapsulating Material	Types of Bacteria Encapsulated	Product Application Studied	Research Findings	Reference
Alginate–poly-L-lysine–alginate	*Lactobacillus plantarum* 80	NA	Showed the effectiveness of the coating in a simulated human gastrointestinal medium	Lian et al. (2003)
Alginate, N-Tack, N-Lok, and Hylon VII	*Lactobacillus acidophilus*	NA	Improved the viability on refrigerated storage for 4 weeks. Fluidization was found to be the most effective process	Goderska and Czarnecki (2008)
Alginate, poly-L-lysine, chitosan	*Lactobacillus acidophilus* 547, *Lactobacillus casei* 01 and *Bifidobacterium bifidum*	NA	Provided the best protection for *L. acidophilus* and *L. casei* in bile salt solution, simulated gastric juice, and intestinal juice with or without chitosan. *B. bifidum* did not survive in the acidic conditions prevalent in the stomach	Muthukumarasamy and Holley (2006)
Alginate, poly-L-lysine, chitosan, and prebiotics	*Lactobacillus acidophilus* CSCC 2400 or CSCC 2409	Yogurt	Improved the survival of the bacteria *in vitro* under acidic and bile salt conditions and in storage of the yogurt for 6 weeks	Iyer and Kailasapathy (2005)
Alginate, κ-carrageenan	*Bifidobacterium bifidum* and *Lactobacillus acidophilus* LA-5	White-brined cheese	Encapsulation improved the viability of the probiotic cells in the cheese during ripening	Özer et al. (2009)
Alginate/alginate + starch/κ-carrageenan + locust bean gum/xanthan gum + gellan gum	*Lactobacillus reuteri* 1063 (ATCC 53608)	NA	Greater protection in simulated gastric juice and simulated bile juice by both extrusion and phase separation	Muthukumarasamy and Holley (2007)
Alginate–methylcellulose	*Bacillus polyfermenticus* SCD	NA	Improved survival in artificial gastric juices and artificial bile salt	Kim et al. (2006)
Alginate–chitosan	*Bifidobacterium animalis* subsp. *lactis*	NA	Improved the controlled release of bifidobacteria in simulated gastric juice	Liserre et al. (2007)
Alginate–pectin	*Lactobacillus casei* LB C81	Yogurt	Encapsulation of beads with alginate and pectin blends in 1:4 and 1:6 ratios improved the viability in simulated gastric juice, in bile salt solution, and during storage for 20 days at 4°C	Sandoval-Castilla et al. (2010)

Encapsulating material	Organism	Food matrix	Description	Reference
Bacterial cellulose, Nata, calcium alginate, skim milk	*Lactobacillus bulgaricus* NCIM2056, *Lactobacillus plantarum* NCIM 2083, *Lactobacillus delbrueckii* NCIM 2025, *Lactobacillus acidophilus* NCIM 2902, and *Lactobacillus casei* NCIM 2651	NA	Bacterial cellulose as a CPA and immobilization support for probiotic lactic acid bacteria. Storage study at 4°C and 30°C for 60 days	Jagannath et al. (2010)
Chitosan–alginate	*Lactobacillus bulgaricus*	NA	Improved the survival in simulated gastric juice and during refrigerated storage at 4°C	Shima et al. (2006)
Gelatin, gum arabic, soluble starch, and skim milk	*Bifidobacterium longum* B6 and *Bifidobacterium infantis* CCRC 14633	NA	Increased the viability of the microencapsulated cells in simulated gastric juice and bile solution	Lian et al. (2003)
Gellan–alginate	*Bifidobacterium bifidum*	NA	Improved the protection during pasteurization and in simulated gastric juice	Chen et al. (2007)
Genipin–gelatin	*Bifidobacterium lactis* BB12	NA	Increasing the genipin concentration improved the stability in simulated gastric juice. The presence of the gastric enzyme pepsin reduced the bead stability	Annan et al. (2007)
Hexaglyceryl condensed ricinoleate	*Lactobacillus acidophilus* (JCM1132)	NA	The inner phase volume ratio and the median diameter of the oil droplets affected the viability in simulated gastric juice	Shima et al. (2006)
Hydrolyzed potato starch and cocoa butter	*Bifidobacterium longum* 2C, *Bifidobacterium longum* 46, *Bifidobacterium adolescentis* VTT, and *Bifidobacterium lactis* BB12	Fermented and nonfermented oat drink	Encapsulation in cocoa butter improved the culturability whereas hydrolyzed potato starch had no effect when stored for 4 weeks	Lahtinen et al. (2007)
Maize starch	*Bifidobacterium* PL1	Commercial muesli preparation and dry malted beverage powder	Acid tolerance assay and storage in food for 14 days. Advocated that modified starch is not suitable for the encapsulation of probiotic bacteria	O'Riordan et al. (2001)
Pectin starch, gelatin, and starch	*Lactobacillus reuteri* (DSM 20016)	Apple juice	Encapsulated material. Determined the process stability and the storage stability at 5°C for 120 days in simulated gastric juice	Weissbrodt and Kunz (2007)
Rennet-gelled milk protein	*Lactobacillus paracasei* subsp. *paracasei* F19 and *Bifidobacterium lactis* BB12	NA	Improved the bacterial survival in simulated gastric conditions because of the buffering action of the protein	Heidebach et al. (2009a)

continued

TABLE 17.3 (continued)
Summary of Published Research over the Last Decade on the Encapsulation of Probiotic Bacteria

Encapsulating Material	Types of Bacteria Encapsulated	Product Application Studied	Research Findings	Reference
Sesame oil	Lactobacillus delbrueckii subsp. bulgaricus	NA	Improved the viability of the bacteria in simulated high acid gastric conditions and simulated bile salt conditions	Hou et al. (2003)
Sodium alginate and hydroxypropylcellulose	Lactobacillus acidophilus (ATCC 4356)	NA	Improved the survival in simulated gastric fluid	Chan and Zhang (2005)
Supercritical carbon dioxide interpolymer complex	Bifidobacterium longum Bb-46	NA	Improved the survival of bacteria in simulated gastric and intestinal fluids	Thantsha et al. (2009)
Transglutaminase-induced casein gel	Lactobacillus paracasei subsp. paracasei F19 and Bifidobacterium lactis BB12	NA	Provided protection in simulated gastric juice without pepsin	Heidebach et al. (2009b)
Transglutaminase-induced casein gel	Lactobacillus paracasei subsp. paracasei F19 and Bifidobacterium lactis BB12	NA	Improved the viability during storage at 4°C and 25°C for 90 days at 11% and 33% relative humidity	Heidebach et al. (2010)
Whey protein isolate	Lactobacillus rhamnosus R011	Semisweet biscuits, refrigerated vegetable juice, and frozen fruit juice	Protected the cells during a short heat treatment. Storage of the product for 3 weeks	Reid et al. (2007)
Whey protein–pectin and alginate	Bifidobacterium bifidum R071	NA	Improved the viability in simulated gastric conditions and simulated high bile salt conditions	Guérin et al. (2003)

Sabikhi et al. 2010). Furthermore, several researchers have shown improved viability of alginate-encapsulated cells in ice cream (Homayouni et al. 2008), cheese (Özer et al. 2008, 2009; Özer and Avni Kirmaci 2009), yogurt (Sultana et al. 2000; Urbanska et al. 2007), Iranian yogurt milk (doogh) (Mortazavian et al. 2008), and fermented sausages (Muthukumarasamy and Holley 2006).

Gåserød et al. (1999) observed that the presence of calcium-chelating agents such as phosphate, citrate, and lactate or nongelling cations such as sodium and magnesium destabilizes calcium alginate gels. Alginate capsules (or microcapsules) are stable at low pH, but swell in weak basic solutions followed by disintegration and erosion (Lee et al. 2003). Alginate polycation membranes have been used for encapsulation in an attempt to overcome the limitations of uncoated alginate membranes. They provide the added advantage of increased membrane strength and reduced permeability (Gåserød et al. 1999). Liserre et al. (2007) studied alginate–chitosan beads for their controlled release of *Bifidobacterium animalis* in simulated gastric juice. Muthukumarasamy and Holley (2006) found that encapsulation of *Lactobacillus acidophilus* and *Lactobacillus casei* in an alginate–chitosan membrane provided protection against artificial gastric and intestinal juices. Iyer and Kailasapathy (2005) and Urbanska et al. (2007) studied the microencapsulation of *Lactobacillus acidophilus* in an alginate–chitosan membrane and its application in yogurt. They reported that the carrier matrix could protect bacteria in simulated gastric fluid, in simulated intestinal fluid, and under refrigerated storage at 4°C. Other combinations with alginate that have been investigated are alginate–pectin (Sandoval-Castilla et al. 2010), alginate–whey protein (Gbassi et al. 2009), alginate–gelatin (Li et al. 2009), alginate–hydroxypropyl cellulose (Chan and Zhang 2002), and alginate–gellan gum (Chen et al. 2007).

17.2.2.1.1.3 Starch and Its Derivatives   Starch is the storage form of carbohydrate in plants. It is composed of amylose, a linear polysaccharide, and amylopectin, a branched-chain polymer. Amylose consists of D-glucopyranose residues and is joined by α-(1,4) linkages. In native starches, these linkages are resistant to pancreatic α-amylases but are easily degraded by the colonic microflora, which makes them useful for the delivery of bioactive compounds in the colon. Starch also offers the additional advantage of being cheap and readily available.

Native starch can easily be modified to remove some of its unsuitable characteristics that limit its application. Starch is modified by introducing a chemical substituent (hydrophilic or hydrophobic) via a reaction with the hydroxyl groups in the starch molecule. Resistant starch is a type of modified starch that is not digested in the small intestine and reaches the colon, where it is used by the colonic microflora to produce short-chain fatty acids (Goñi et al. 1996; Anal and Singh 2007). High amylose corn starch containing 20% resistant starch has been found to be suitable for enteric delivery (Dimantov et al. 2004) and the addition of resistant starch to an encapsulation matrix has been found to improve the viability of *Lactobacillus casei* (Sultana et al. 2000) and *Bifidobacterium lactis* (Homayouni et al. 2008).

17.2.2.1.1.4 Gellan Gum and Xanthan Gum   Gellan gum is an anionic bacterial exopolysaccharide that is derived from *Sphingomonas elodea*. It is a linear tetrasaccharide, with a 500-kDa backbone of [β1 → 3) Glc (β1 → 4) GlcA (β1 → 4) Glc-(β1 → 4) L-Rha (β1 →], where Glc is glucose, GlcA is glucuronic acid, and Rha is rhamnose, with side groups consisting of O-acetyl and L-glycerate substituents (Pollock 1993). Its functionality depends mostly on the degree of acylation and its constituent ions. Its most unique function is its ability to hold small particles in suspension without increasing its viscosity significantly (Baird and Pettitt 1991). Also, gellan gum is not easily degraded by the action of enzymes (Baird and Pettitt 1991; Lee 1996) and is resistant to an acidic environment (Sun and Griffiths 2000).

Gellan gum forms very firm and brittle gels but melts easily in the mouth, releasing water and any flavor from its gel network (Sun and Griffiths, 2000). Although gellan gum itself is able to form good microcapsules when gelled in the presence of calcium ions, this process needs a preheating of up to 80°C for 1 h (Sanderson 1990), which is not suitable for heat-sensitive core materials such as probiotics. Therefore, for encapsulation purposes, gellan gum has always been used in combination with another gum, such as xanthan gum (Sun and Griffiths 2000; McMaster et al. 2005; Muthukumarasamy et al. 2006), or a few sequestrants, such as sodium citrate, sodium metaphosphate, and EDTA (Camelin et al. 1993).

In several studies, a combination of gellan gum and xanthan gum has been used to encapsulate probiotic bacteria. Norton and Lacroix (1990) reported that the gellan gum–xanthan gum beads were useful for encapsulating *Bifidobacterium* cells and for protecting them from acid injury. Sun and Griffiths (2000) reported improved viability of *Bifidobacterium infantis* cells immobilized with gellan gum–xanthan gum when exposed to simulated gastric juice. Furthermore, they reported improved viability of the encapsulated cells, compared with the free cells, when stored in pasteurized yogurt for 5 weeks at 4°C.

17.2.2.1.2 Proteins

17.2.2.1.2.1 Milk Proteins   Milk proteins provide good functional properties that promote their use as shell or matrix materials for microencapsulation. They are relatively inexpensive, are widely available in nature, possess good sensory properties, are highly soluble, have low viscosity in solution, and have good emulsification and film-forming properties (Forrest et al. 2005; Day et al. 2007; Semo et al. 2007; Sandra et al. 2008; Livney 2010). The protein medium surrounding the bacterial cells provides a very good buffer in comparison with plant hydrocolloid materials. Milk proteins help to increase the pH of gastric juice significantly and, thus, increase the survivability of the encapsulated bacteria (Charteris et al. 1998; Corcoran et al. 2005). Milk proteins have excellent gelation properties, which are appealing to the microencapsulation industry. Their gelation results from the unfolding of the protein and subsequent aggregation. Noncovalent bonds stabilize the gel network, and covalent bonds, such as disulfide bridges, may also participate in the stabilization process (Li et al. 2006).

Casein, in the form of an aqueous solution of sodium caseinate, can be coagulated and gelled by the actions of enzymes, such as rennet and transglutaminase (Heidebach et al. 2009a,b), by crosslinking with glutaraldehyde (Latha et al. 2000), or by slow acidification with glucono-δ-lactone (Lucey et al. 1997). The acid gelation of casein is based on the principle that the net charge on the protein is zero at its isoelectric point. Thus, repulsive forces are minimal, resulting in easy movement and the aggregation of the molecule. Rennet-induced gelation is based on the proteolytic cleavage of the hydrophilic hairy outer layer of κ-casein, resulting in micellar aggregation. Transglutaminase-induced gelation takes place by the catalysis of the acyl-transfer reaction, resulting in the formation of molecular cross-links in the protein (Cho et al. 2003). The functional and physicochemical properties of the transglutaminase-cross-linked proteins depend on factors such as enzyme concentration, incubation time, and the type and concentration of the proteins.

Sodium caseinate appears to offer the ideal physical and functional properties for microencapsulation because of its amphiphilic and emulsifying characteristics (Hogan et al. 2001; Madene et al. 2006). Heidebach et al. (2009b) developed transglutaminase-catalyzed gelation of casein suspensions containing the probiotic cells *Lactobacillus paracasei* and *Bifidobacterium lactis*. The aggregated casein mass was found to protect the microorganisms from damage in simulated gastric conditions. In another study, Heidebach et al. (2009a) used rennet to induce the gelation of skim milk concentrates and determined their potential to encapsulate probiotic bacteria. Nag et al. (2011) used sodium caseinate and gellan gum mixture coagulated by gradually decreasing the pH with glucono-δ-lactone (GDL) to encapsulate *Lactobacillus casei* cells. The capsules provided significant protection to the cells in simulated gastric juice and in the presence of bile salts.

The formation of whey protein gels at above 75°C is mainly due to the gelation of β-lactoglobulin, which comprises 50% of the total whey protein (Kilara and Vaghela 2004) and is the most abundant whey protein in bovine milk. The heat treatment makes this process unsuitable for encapsulating many heat-sensitive materials such as probiotic bacteria (Chen et al. 2006). The cold gelation of whey proteins is a potential solution to this problem (Barbut and Foegeding 1993; Maltais et al.

2005; Heidebach et al. 2009a). As native β-lactoglobulin is resistant to gastric digestion (Miranda and Pelissier 1983), peptic hydrolysis (Guo et al. 1995), and tryptic hydrolysis (Reddy et al. 1988), it is a suitable encapsulating material for probiotic delivery. It also possesses very good oxygen barrier properties (Kim et al. 1996).

An ionotropic gelation technique has been used to encapsulate probiotics with whey protein isolate (Kailasapathy and Sureeta 2004; Ainsley Reid et al. 2005). The addition of cations, in the form of calcium, shields electrostatic charges on the surface of the proteins and allows the molecules to move close together. The resulting aggregation and gelation are due to the absence of electrostatic repulsion. As this method is carried out at room temperature, it is suitable for encapsulating heat-sensitive probiotic microorganisms. Guérin et al. (2003) used a combination of alginate, pectin, and whey protein to encapsulate *Bifidobacterium* cells. The capsules offered much better protection than free cells against the low pH of simulated gastric juice and the bile salts present in simulated intestinal fluid. Gbassi et al. (2009) noted that whey proteins are a convenient, cheap, and efficient material for coating calcium alginate beads loaded with *Lactobacillus plantarum*. The whey protein coating significantly improved bacterial survival in a simulated gastric environment. Picot and Lacroix (2004) observed the potential of immobilized *Bifidobacterium longum* and *Bifidobacterium breve* in whey-protein-based microcapsules to survive the harsh environmental conditions in the stomach and in acidic products such as yogurt.

17.2.2.1.2.2 Gelatin Gelatin is produced from denatured collagen and contains significant amounts of hydroxyproline, proline, and glycine. It is useful as a thermally reversible gelling agent for encapsulation. Gelatin has good membrane-forming ability, has good biocompatibility, and is nontoxic. One limitation of the use of gelatin in the hydrogel matrix is its low network rigidity, but this can be improved by adding cross-linking agents. Lian et al. (2003) reported that the encapsulation of *Bifidobacterium longum* B6 and *Bifidobacterium infantis* CCRC 14633 in gelatin resulted in increased viability of the cells in a simulated gastric juice and bile solution. Li et al. (2009) found that microencapsulation using alginate–gelatin beads improved the survival of *Lactobacillus casei* ATCC 393 during gastrointestinal transit. Annan et al. (2007) encapsulated *Bifidobacterium lactis* BB12 in genipin–gelatin capsules and observed that increasing the genipin concentration improved their stability in simulated gastric juice. Genipin, derived from an iridoid glycoside called geniposide present in the fruit of *Gardenia jasminoides*, is a natural cross-linker for protein.

17.2.2.1.3 Fats and Oils

Fats and oils possess good oxygen and moisture barrier properties. Their presence on a surface increases its hydrophobicity, thus preventing moisture uptake. Lahtinen et al. (2007) observed that encapsulation of *Bifidobacterium longum*, *B. adolescentis*, and *B. lactis* in cocoa butter improved the survivability of the cells when stored for 4 weeks at 4°C in nonfermented oat drink. The average weekly reduction in the plate counts of the encapsulated cells (0.7 log cfu/mL/week) was significantly less than in the free control cells (1.3 log cfu/mL/week). Similarly, Hou et al. (2003) found that the encapsulation of *Lactobacillus delbrueckii* subsp. *bulgaricus* in sesame oil improved its viability under simulated gastric and intestinal conditions.

17.2.2.2 Encapsulation Technologies

Probiotics are most commonly microencapsulated using emulsion and extrusion techniques. In any microencapsulation technique, the size of the capsule beads is important because it influences the sensory properties, governing its use in foods. The extrusion technique results in beads of uniform size (2000–4000 μm), whereas alginate beads made using the emulsion technique vary in size from 20 to 2000 μm but are smaller than extruded alginate beads. Coacervation for probiotic delivery has also been investigated. However, other microencapsulation techniques such as centrifugal extrusion, spray chilling, cocrystallization, and molecular inclusion, which have been utilized to encapsulate food ingredients such as vitamins, flavors, fruit juices, and essential oils, have found limited application with probiotics. The major microencapsulation techniques used for probiotics are discussed in further detail.

17.2.2.2.1 Emulsion Technique

This method involves taking a small volume of cell—polymer suspension (discontinuous phase) and adding it to a large volume of a vegetable oil (continuous phase), such as soybean oil, sunflower oil, canola oil, or corn oil. The mixture is homogenized to form a water-in-oil emulsion. Then, the water-soluble polymer is insolubilized (cross-linked) by slowly adding a solution of calcium chloride, resulting in phase separation. The dispersed phase encapsulates the probiotic bacteria as the core material (Krasaekoopt et al. 2003). Finally, the beads are collected using filtration or mild centrifugation (Sheu and Marshall 1993). One major advantage of the emulsion technique is that it can easily be scaled up for commercial production. Also, the microspheres are smaller in size and of more uniform shape than those produced by the extrusion technique. A major disadvantage is the higher operational cost associated with the use of vegetable oil in the process.

Most studies on the emulsion technique for encapsulation have used sodium alginate as the carrier material. The particle size distribution of the microcapsules is controlled by the speed of agitation, the homogenization parameters, and the type of emulsifier. Song et al. (2003) made an emulsion of sodium alginate in corn salad oil by passing it through a microporous glass membrane; they then used the emulsion to encapsulate *Lactobacillus casei* YIT 9018 cells. The encapsulated cells had a small particle size, and provided increased stability in artificial gastric and bile salt solutions and during storage at different temperatures. Materials other than alginate that are commonly used in the emulsion technique are a mix of κ-carrageenan and locust bean gum (Audet et al. 1988), chitosan (Groboillot et al. 1993), gelatin (Hyndman et al. 1993), and cellulose acetate phthalate (Rao et al. 1989). Adhikari et al. (2000) used 2% κ-carrageenan and 0.9% sodium chloride dispersed into vegetable oil and emulsified the mix with Tween 80, followed by immobilization with potassium chloride. Free and encapsulated *Bifidobacterium longum* cells were tested for their resistance in an acidic yogurt medium during refrigerated storage for 30 days. The encapsulated cells had a significantly better survival rate (>70.5–78%) than the free cells. In another study, Nag et al. (2011) successfully encapsulated *Lactobacillus casei* into a gel matrix (comprising of sodium caseinate and gellan gum) using emulsion technique. The surface-weighted and volume-weighted mean diameters of the capsules were about 287 and 399 μm, respectively. Significant protection against acid, pepsin, and bile salt was achieved.

17.2.2.2.2 Extrusion Technique

Extrusion is the oldest and most common technique for converting hydrocolloids into microcapsules (King 1995). The gelation of hydrocolloids, such as alginate, carrageenan, and pectin, in the presence of minerals such as calcium and potassium has been used successfully to entrap probiotic bacteria using extrusion. The chemical explanation is that the calcium and potassium ions bind to the multiple free carboxylic radicals, thereby forming gels (Champagne and Fustier 2007). Different concentrations of alginate have been used to form tiny gel particles. In this process, the hydrocolloid and the probiotic mixture are dripped into the hardening solution (calcium chloride) through a syringe or nozzle (Eikmeier and Rehm 1987; Champagne et al. 1992; Desai et al. 2005). The viscosity of the sodium alginate solution, the composition of the alginate, the distance between the syringe and the calcium chloride collecting solution, and the orifice diameter of the extruder influence the size and sphericity of the beads (Smidsrod and Skjak-Braek 1990).

Extrusion is the preferred technique for coating volatile flavors and oils. It increases the shelf life of compounds by inhibiting oxygen diffusion through the matrix (Gouin 2004; Desai and Park 2005a,b; Madene et al. 2006). In a recent study, Li et al. (2009) microencapsulated *Lactobacillus casei* cells in a mix of sodium alginate and gelatin using an extrusion process. This combination successfully protected the cells during gastrointestinal transit, but the beads were relatively large in size, with a mean diameter of 1.1 ± 0.2 mm. The encapsulated cells showed increased viability as compared to the free cells. Homayouni et al. (2008) microencapsulated probiotics into calcium alginate beads in the presence of resistant starch and incorporated them into ice cream. After storage for 180 days at −20°C, the survival rate of the encapsulated cells was 30% higher than that of the free cells.

A major advantage of the extrusion process is its shell–core character. The encapsulated material is completely covered and protected by the wall material, and residual or surface core material is removed by a dehydrating liquid, generally isopropyl alcohol (Gibbs et al. 1999; Desai et al. 2005). The cost involved in the production of encapsulated particles is lower for the extrusion technique than for the emulsion technique.

However, it is difficult to scale up the extrusion technique for commercial application. The bead formed by the extrusion technique is larger in size than that produced by the emulsion technique and is not of uniform size and shape.

17.2.3 STABILIZATION BY MANIPULATING THE CELL PHYSIOLOGY

Greater understanding of the physiology of bacterial cells can help to improve the desirable characteristics of bacteria, such as enhanced acid and bile tolerance. Recently, modification of the growth conditions to enhance the stress tolerance level has been used to improve the robustness of probiotic cultures. Optimization of the growth phase medium and the cell-harvesting conditions are also potential ways of improving the stability of the cultures. Intrinsic tolerance of the bacterial strains, bacterial stress adaptation, and growth phase and cell-harvesting conditions as tools for improvement of bacterial stability are discussed below.

17.2.3.1 Intrinsic Tolerance of Culture/Strain Selection

The inherent vulnerability of bacterial cells varies between different genera as well as between distinct species of the same genus. Compared with lactobacilli, streptococci have been found to be more resistant to heat. Consequently, the size and the shape of the cells have become important factors in influencing bacterial viability (Clark and Martin 1994). As example of species to species variation, various species of *Bifidobacterium* show considerable variability in the tolerance to heat and oxygen (Simpson et al. 2005). Moreover, *Bifidobacterium longum* has been found to have high bile salt tolerance, as high as 4% (Clark and Martin 1994), which is notably higher compared to many others *Bifidibacterium* species. However, there is no rational explanation for the variation in viability. The selection of bacterial culture strains based on their ability to resist low pH, bile salt concentrations, heat, desiccation, and oxygen is beneficial for the preservation of viability in food applications.

17.2.3.2 Stress Adaptation Techniques

Bacteria possess an inherent ability to withstand harsh conditions and sudden environmental changes by inducing stress proteins. In particular, bacteria that can withstand an adverse environment can subsequently survive near-fatal conditions. Stress adaptation is defined as an increase in an organism's tolerance to deleterious factors on exposure to sublethal stress (Hendrick and Hartl 1993; Gottesman et al. 1997; Van de Guchte et al. 2002). The resistance offered by a bacterial defense system can be grouped into two categories: (i) a specific system that allows survival against a challenged dose of the same agent, such as heat, osmotic stress, oxygen, and low pH (Desmond et al. 2001; Gouesbet et al. 2001); (ii) preadaptation to a stress condition, which can allow the cells to resist diverse environmental stresses and is known as a cross-adaptive response (Kim et al. 2001). Preadaptation occurs as a result of the convergence of reactive genes to distinct kinds of injury, for example, heat, osmotic stress, oxygen, and low pH (Crawford and Davies 1994). Recent studies have focused on preadaptation to heat, osmotic stress, oxygen, and low pH to improve the stress tolerance level of bacteria. Three of the main stresses are explained below.

17.2.3.2.1 Heat Stress

Heat stress in bacteria results from an abrupt increase in temperature. Cells subjected to high temperatures often show decreased protein stability, and membranes and nucleic acids are affected. High temperature also disturbs the transmembrane proton gradient, which leads to a decrease in intracellular pH (Hecker et al. 1996; Lindquist and Craig 1988). Heat tolerance is a process whereby microorganisms exposed to sublethal heat treatment acquire the ability to withstand subsequent lethal heat challenges (Girgis et al. 2003). Heat-induced thermotolerance has been observed in several *Lactobacillus* species. For example, the application of heat stress resulted in the expression of heat-stress proteins such as GroES, GroEL, htrA, HcrA, GrpE, DnaK, DnaJ, GroEL, and DnaK in *Lactobacillus helveticus* (Hecker et al. 1996; Broadbent et al. 1998; Smeds et al. 1998), *L. acidophilus* (Zink et al. 2000), *L. bulgaricus* (Gouesbet et al. 2001, 2002), *L. sakei* (Schmidt et al. 1999; Stentz et al. 2000), and *L. johnsonii* (Walker et al. 1999; Zink et al. 2000). The stress proteins help to preserve the native conformation of the cellular proteins and minimize denaturation. They also promote proper assembly of the proteins and prevent unfolding and aggregation (Craig et al. 1993). Moreover, in response to heat stress, there is a change in the lipid composition of the bacterial membrane, for example, a substantial increase in the levels of C19:0 cyclopropane fatty acids. A lower ratio of saturated fatty acids to unsaturated fatty acids has been observed (Broadbent and Lin 1999).

17.2.3.2.2 Osmotic Stress

In response to osmotic stress, bacteria accumulate nontoxic low-molecular-weight compounds, called compatible solutes, within their cells. The accumulation of compatible solutes by lactic acid bacteria has been found to be beneficial during drying and osmotic stress (Kets et al. 1996) and to improve the viability on storage. These compatible solutes allow the cell to retain positive turgor pressure by reducing the osmotic pressure difference between the internal environment and the external environment, thereby prolonging the viability of the cells (Kets et al. 1996). They function to balance the osmolality with the extracellular environment, to enhance enzyme stability at low water activity, and to maintain the integrity of the cellular membrane during dissociation (Kets and De Bont 1994).

Microorganisms have been observed to accumulate compatible solutes, such as amino acids, quaternary amines (e.g., glycine, betaine, and carnitine), saccharides, and polyols, to protect them against decreasing water activity, and to help the cell to acclimatize against osmotic stress (Poolman and Glaasker 1998). Glycine betaine is identified as an intracellular osmolyte that protects *Lactobacillus acidophilus* from osmotic stress (Hutkins et al. 1987). Prasad et al. (2003) found that the robustness of *Lactobacillus rhamnosus* HN001 can be enhanced by osmotic stress adaptation to cope with industrial practices such as desiccation and rehydration and the storage environment. They proposed that the process/mechanism associated with the protective osmotic shock effect acquired by dried *L. rhamnosus* HN001 is stress proteins, along with glycolysis-related machinery and other stationary phase proteins and regulatory factors. Desmond et al. (2001) noted the cross-stress tolerance to heat in *Lactobacillus acidophilus* upon exposure to osmotic stress (0.3 mol sodium chloride/L for 30 min). They also observed that the survival rate was 16 times higher after exposure to osmotic stress (0.3 M NaCl for 30 min) than for the untreated control culture each in reconstituted skim milk at 37°C. Exopolysaccharide production acts as a survival approach to safeguard bacteria in damaging environments such as against osmotic stress (Ruas-Madiedo et al. 2002).

17.2.3.2.3 Acid Stress

Acid tolerance and adaptation increase the survival of probiotic bacteria in the gastrointestinal tract. Lactic acid is the major threat to the cell in the low-pH environment in fermented dairy products. The organic acids remain protonated and unchanged and can easily pass into the cell through the cell membrane (Girgis et al. 2003). Bacteria possess several defensive mechanisms, which confer protection against acid injury. These defensive mechanisms perform many functions to maintain viability under low-pH conditions. Some of the important functions are (i) translocation of protons to the environment (Kobayashi et al. 1984, 1986; Nannen and Hutkins 1991); (ii) production of acid-neutralizing ammonia from arginine (Marquis et al. 1987); (iii) amino acid decarboxylation (Molenaar et al. 1993); and (iv) decarboxylation of oxaloacetate (Ramos et al. 1994; Lolkema et al. 1995; MartyTeysset et al. 1996). Shah and Ravula (2000) utilized the acid stress adaptation response of *Lactobacillus acidophilus* to enhance its survival under harsh acid conditions and in yogurt. Fozo et al. (2004) observed that an increased fatty acid length (an increase in the proportion of C19:0 cyclopropane fatty acids and a lower ratio of saturated to unsaturated membrane fatty acids) was an important membrane alteration that increased survival in acidic environments.

17.2.3.3   Growth Phase and Cell-Harvesting Conditions

Bacterial growth occurs in four distinct phases, that is, lag, log, stationary, and death phases. The stress response of the bacterial culture is dependent on the growth phase. For instance, bacteria that enter into the stationary phase develop a general stress resistance. They are more resistant to various types of stress response than bacteria in the log phase because carbon starvation and exhaustion of available food sources trigger responses that allow the survival of the cell population (Van de Guchte et al. 2002). For example, probiotic spray-dried powders containing high numbers of viable cells (over 50% survival; 2.9×10^9 cfu/g) were produced when stationary phase cells of *Lactobacillus rhamnosus* were used while early log phase cultures exhibited only 14% survival (Corcoran et al. 2004). In summary, appropriate growth phase and cell-harvesting conditions are essential for the stabilization of bacteria.

17.2.3.4   Growth Media and Growth Conditions

Bacterial growth media are mainly agar or broth and are designed to support the growth of microbial cells. Specifically, *Lactobacillus* spp. are grown in a De Man, Rogosa, and Sharpe (MRS) medium, which is a selective medium for the growth of lactobacilli. Growth media have been noted to play an important role in cell function. Bâati et al. (2000) observed that variation in the environmental conditions of the growth medium resulted in alteration in the fluidity of the cytoplasmic membrane. Membrane fluidity is responsible for regulation of the flow of nutrients and metabolic products into and out of the cell (Annous et al. 1999). For example, when lactic acid bacteria were grown in the presence of Tween 80, there was an increase in their resistance to freeze drying because of a change in the lipid composition of the membrane (Goldberg and Eschar 1977) and there was an improvement in the bile salt tolerance (Kimoto et al. 2002). Silva et al. (2005) showed that the cells of *Lactobacillus delbrueckii* subsp. *bulgaricus*, when grown under controlled pH conditions, were more sensitive to the stresses encountered during starter culture production/storage and handling. In contrast, the noncontrolled cells showed better viability because of enhanced production of heat-shock proteins. These results indicate the importance of growth media and cell-harvesting conditions in the stabilization of probiotic bacteria.

17.2.4   STABILIZATION BY OPTIMIZING THE STORAGE CONDITIONS

Long-term storage of lactic acid bacteria for use in various products is a common practice in the food industry. It is important to mention factors such as temperature, relative humidity, oxygen content, type of probiotic carrier, and the packaging material during storage. These factors alone or in combination can lead to loss of viability as a result of deteriorative chemical reactions. Overall, optimization of the storage conditions could possibly improve the survival rate of bacteria during storage.

Temperature is an important parameter that influences the viability of probiotic bacteria during storage. Storage at high temperature results in poorer survival rates than storage at lower temperatures (Gardiner et al. 2000; Simpson et al. 2005). For extended periods, storage at −18°C has been found to be more suitable for freeze-dried probiotic bacteria than storage at 20°C (Bruno and

Shah 2003). The loss of viability for *Bifidobacterium* spp. has been found to be lower with storage at 4°C (2%) than with storage at 25°C (40%) for 90 days. Increased survival at low temperature has been associated with a lower rate of fat oxidation (Gunning et al. 1995).

Relative humidity is another variable that controls the viability of probiotic bacteria. During storage, a desiccant enhanced the viability of *Bifidobacterium longum* B6 and *Bifidobacterium infantis* CCRC 14633 by removing moisture (Hsiao et al. 2004). Gunning et al. (1995) observed that a relative humidity of 11% was the optimum to sustain the viability of *Lactobacillus bulgaricus* during storage and that a higher relative humidity resulted in an increased rate of lipid oxidation. During storage at high relative vapor pressure, the crystallization of disaccharides resulted in the loss of viability of freeze-dried *Lactobacillus rhamnosus* GG. The presence of oxygen is detrimental to the survival of bacteria because oxidative damage occurs during long-term storage. Oxygen radicals can damage the polyunsaturated fatty acids present in the phospholipids of the bacterial cell membrane (Halliwell et al. 1993). Oxygen-depleting agents, such as oxygen absorbers and antioxidants, improve the viability of the bacteria by providing a low-oxygen environment and preventing membrane lipid degradation. Nitrogen flushing has been found to improve bacterial viability (Gunning et al. 1995) and vacuum packaging is another alternative technique for the removal of oxygen. Jin et al. (1985) advocated that low oxygen levels are important for the stabilization of bacteria during long-term storage.

Amorphous carbohydrates in probiotic carriers play an important role in storage stability by impeding the detrimental process. They exist as noncrystalline solids (glass) below their glass transition temperature (Miao et al. 2008). Importantly, the formation of a glassy state in a probiotic carrier limits membrane lipid oxidation, protein unfolding, and chemical degradative reactions by providing an effective environmental barrier and, thereby, minimizing the transitional molecular motion (Sun and Leopold 1997; Crowe et al. 1998). The effect of the glassy state on the survival of probiotic bacteria has been studied in spray drying (Ananta et al. 2005) and freeze drying (Miao et al. 2008). Ananta et al. (2005) spray-dried *Lactobacillus rhamnosus* GG in three spraying media, that is, reconstituted skim milk (RSM), RSM with Raftilose 95, and polydextrose. The survival was greater in RSM than in the other media for storage at 37°C and 25°C at 11% relative vapor pressure for 4 weeks. Miao et al. (2008) studied the viability of freeze-dried *Lactobacillus paracasei* and *L. rhamnosus* GG on storage at 22–25°C for 38–40 days at different relative humidities. They also noted the effect of a protective medium consisting of RSM or a cryoprotective disaccharide, that is, lactose, trehalose, sucrose, maltose, and a mixture of disaccharides. Physical changes, such as collapse, crystallization, and stickiness, have been associated with higher relative vapor pressure. A significant loss in viability above a relative vapor pressure of 11.4% was observed and it was concluded that the difference between the storage temperature and the glass transition temperature $(T - T_g)$ influenced the viability.

Packaging materials play an important role in the storage stability of bacteria by providing excellent barriers against gas and water vapor. Hsiao et al. (2004) showed that microencapsulated *Bifidobacterium* cells had better viability when stored in glass bottles than when stored in PET bottles, possibly because of the higher oxygen barrier properties of glass bottles than of PET bottles. As aluminum provides a barrier to both oxygen and moisture, which are injurious to bacteria during long-term storage, a significant improvement in the viability of *Bifidobacterium* spp. was seen during storage in polythene bags within aluminum-coated paper bags (Simpson et al. 2005). Polyester–aluminum–polythene laminate, which has gas and water vapor impermeable properties, provides a superior barrier for stabilizing bacteria (Jin et al. 1985).

Storage time has an inverse relationship with bacterial viability. During storage, there is a change in the ratio of linoleic/palmitic acid (C18:2/C16:0) or linolenic/palmitic acid (C18:3/C16:0), which is linked to the viability of freeze-dried bacteria (Yao et al. 2008; Coulibaly et al. 2009). Other chemical damage mechanisms include the formation of lipid hydroperoxides from free radical reactions, which decompose to secondary products, such as malonic dialdehyde (Raharjo and Sofos 1993). Simpson et al. (2005) has shown that there is a significant loss in the viability (greater than 4 log reduction) in spray-dried *Bifidobacterium* spp. during storage for a period of 3 months at 25°C.

17.3 CONCLUDING REMARKS AND FUTURE PROSPECTS

Probiotics is one of the top functional ingredients for food but the usage is restricted within the products distributed and stored under chilled condition. Application of probiotics in shelf-stable foods has not been possible due to lack of an appropriate probiotics stabilization technology. Scientists both in academia and in industry have been trying to improve the stability of probiotics with varying success. Recently, our team at Riddet Institute developed a novel technique for improving the shelf stability of probiotic cells; it can deliver a viable cell count of 1 billion per gram after 36 weeks of storage and of 100 million per gram after 52 weeks of storage at 25°C (Nag and Das 2011). The probiotic ingredient has been developed in free-flowing powder form using only natural ingredients. The water activity of the probiotic powder is 0.27–0.3 and the average particle size is 125 μm. The initial development was carried out using *Lactobacillus casei* CRL 431 and was later validated with strains of *L. rhamnosus*, *L. plantarum*, *L. acidophilus*, and *Bifidobacterium lactis*. Also, the encapsulation significantly improved the viability of the probiotics in simulated gastric and intestinal fluids.

The encapsulated probiotic ingredient can potentially be applied to a range of shelf-stable formulated foods, including powdered beverages, chocolate, chocolate spread, infant food, cereal bars, and breakfast cereals. We carried out an application trial for some of these food categories, adding 1% of the probiotic ingredient. The products had over 1 million viable cells per gram after 6 months of storage at 25°C. The decline in viable cell count was <1 log over the storage period. An informal sensory test confirmed that the probiotic ingredient did not have any negative impact on the flavor of the product.

Understandably, a technology that enables probiotics to be used in shelf-stable foods will increase the size of the probiotics market significantly by tapping into additional product categories and additional consumers. We believe that this technology will make the benefits of probiotic bacteria available to millions of consumers in developing countries, in which a chilled supply chain is often unavailable.

REFERENCES

Abadias, M., A. Benabarre, N. Teixidó, J. Usall, and I. Vias. 2001. Effect of freeze drying and protectants on viability of the biocontrol yeast *Candida sake*. *International Journal of Food Microbiology* 65(3):173–182.

Adhikari, K., Mustapha, A., Grun, I. U., and Fernando, L. 2000. Viability of microencapsulated bifidobacteria in set yogurt during refrigerated storage. *Journal of Dairy Science* 83:1946–1951.

Ainsley Reid, A., J. C. Vuillemard, M. Britten, Y. Arcand, E. Farnworth, and C. P. Champagne. 2005. Microentrapment of probiotic bacteria in a Ca(2+)-induced whey protein gel and effects on their viability in a dynamic gastro-intestinal model. *Journal of Microencapsulation* 22(6):603–619.

Anal, A. K., and H. Singh. 2007. Recent advances in microencapsulation of probiotics for industrial applications and targeted delivery. *Trends in Food Science and Technology* 18(5):240–251.

Ananta, E., M. Volkert, and D. Knorr. 2005. Cellular injuries and storage stability of spray-dried *Lactobacillus rhamnosus* GG. *International Dairy Journal* 15(4):399–409.

Annan, N. T., A. Borza, D. L. Moreau, P. M. Allan-Wojtas, and L. T. Hansen. 2007. Effect of process variables on particle size and viability of *Bifidobacterium lactis* Bb-12 in genipin-gelatin microspheres. *Journal of Microencapsulation* 24(2):152–162.

Annous, B. A., M. F. Kozempel, and M. J. Kurantz. 1999. Changes in membrane fatty acid composition of *Pediococcus* sp. strain NRRL B-2354 in response to growth conditions and its effect on thermal resistance. *Applied and Environmental Microbiology* 65(7):2857–2862.

Anukam, K. C., E. O. Osazuwa, H. B. Osadolor, A. W. Bruce, and G. Reid. 2008. Yogurt containing probiotic *Lactobacillus rhamnosus* GR-1 and L. reuteri RC-14 helps resolve moderate diarrhea and increases CD4 count in HIV/AIDS patients. *Journal of Clinical Gastroenterology* 42(3):239–243.

Armuzzi, A., F. Cremonini, F. Bartolozzi, et al. 2001. The effect of oral administration of *Lactobacillus* GG on antibiotic-associated gastrointestinal side-effects during *Helicobacter pylori* eradication therapy. *Alimentary Pharmacology and Therapeutics* 15(2):163–169.

Arnaud, J. P., L. Choplin, and C. Lacrox. 1988. Rheological behavior of kappa-carrageenan/locust bean gum mixed gels. *Journal of Texture Studies* 19(4):419–429.

Audet, P., C. Paquin, and C. Lacroix. 1988. Immobilized growing lactic acid bacteria with κ-carrageenan—Locust bean gum gel. *Applied Microbiology and Biotechnology* 29(1):11–18.

Audet, P., C. Paquin, and C. Lacroix. 1990. Batch fermentations with a mixed culture of lactic acid bacteria immobilized separately in κ-carrageenan locust bean gum gel beads. *Applied Microbiology and Biotechnology* 32(6):662–668.

Bâati, L., C. Fabre-Gea, D. Auriol, and P. J. Blanc. 2000. Study of the cryotolerance of *Lactobacillus acidophilus*: Effect of culture and freezing conditions on the viability and cellular protein levels. *International Journal of Food Microbiology* 59(3):241–247.

Bai, A. P., Q. Ouyang, X. R. Xiao, and S. F. Li. 2006. Probiotics modulate inflammatory cytokine secretion from inflamed mucosa in active ulcerative colitis. *International Journal of Clinical Practice* 60(3):284–288.

Baird, J. K. and D. J. Pettitt. 1991. Biogums used in foods and made by fermentation. In *Biotechnology and Food Ingredients*, ed. I. Goldberg, and R. Williams, pp. 223–264. New York, NY: Van Nostrand Reinhold.

Barbut, S. and E. A. Foegeding. 1993. Ca2+-induced gelation of pre-heated whey-protein isolate. *Journal of Food Science* 58(4):867–871.

Baron, M. 2009. Original research: A patented strain of *Bacillus coagulans* increased immune response to viral challenge. *Postgraduate Medicine* 121(2):114–118.

Berny, J. F. and G. L. Hennebert. 1991. Viability and stability of yeast-cells and filamentous fungus spores during freeze-drying—Effects of protectants and cooling rates. *Mycologia* 83(6):805–815.

Bin-Nun, A., R. Bromiker, M. Wilschanski, et al. 2005. Oral probiotics prevent necrotizing enterocolitis in very low birth weight neonates. *Journal of Pediatrics* 147(2):192–196.

Borruel, N., M. Carol, F. Casellas, et al. 2002. Increased mucosal tumour necrosis factor α production in Crohn's disease can be downregulated *ex vivo* by probiotic bacteria. *Gut* 51(5):659–664.

Brennan, M., B. Wanismail, M. C. Johnson, and B. Ray. 1986. Cellular damage in dried *Lactobacillus acidophilus*. *Journal of Food Protection* 49(1):47–53.

Broadbent, J. R. and C. Lin. 1999. Effect of heat shock or cold shock treatment on the resistance of *Lactococcus lactis* to freezing and lyophilization. *Cryobiology* 39(1):88–102.

Broadbent, J. R., C. J. Oberg, and L. Wei. 1998. Characterization of the *Lactobacillus helveticus* groESL operon. *Research in Microbiology* 149(4):247–253.

Bruno, F. A. and N. P. Shah. 2003. Viability of two freeze-dried strains of *Bifidobacterium* and of commercial preparations at various temperatures during prolonged storage. *Journal of Food Science* 68(7):2336–2339.

Bruzzese, E., V. Raia, G. Gaudiello, et al. 2004. Intestinal inflammation is a frequent feature of cystic fibrosis and is reduced by probiotic administration. *Alimentary Pharmacology and Therapeutics* 20(7):813–819.

Bu, L. N., M. H. Chang, Y. H. Ni, H. L. Chen, and C. C. Cheng. 2007. *Lactobacillus casei rhamnosus* Lcr35 in children with chronic constipation. *Pediatrics International* 49(4):485–490.

Çaglar, E., N. Sandalli, S. Twetman, S. Kavaloglu, S. Ergeneli, and S. Selvi. 2005. Effect of yogurt with *Bifidobacterium* DN-173 010 on salivary mutans Streptococci and Lactobacilli in young adults. *Acta Odontologica Scandinavica* 63(6):317–320.

Camelin, I., C. Lacroix, C. Paquin, H. Prevost, R. Cachon, and C. Divies. 1993. Effect of chelatants on gellan gel rheological properties and setting temperature for immobilization of living Bifidobacteria. *Biotechnology Progress* 9(3):291–297.

Caron, C. 1995. Commercial production of baker's yeast and wine yeast. In *Biotechnology*, ed. H.-J. Rehm, and G. Reed, pp. 322–351. Weinheim: VCH Verlag.

Carvalho, A. S., J. Silva, P. Ho, P. Teixeira, F. X. Malcata, and P. Gibbs. 2004. Effects of various sugars added to growth and drying media upon thermotolerance and survival throughout storage of freeze-dried *Lactobacillus delbrueckii* ssp. *bulgaricus*. *Biotechnology Progress* 20(1):248–254.

Champagne, C.P., Fustier, P. 2007. Microencapsulation for the improved delivery of bioactive compounds into foods. *Current Opinion in Biotechnology* 18(2):184–190.

Champagne, C. P., C. Gaudy, D. Poncelet, and R. J. Neufeld. 1992. *Lactococcus lactis* release from calcium alginate beads. *Applied and Environmental Microbiology* 58(5):1429–1434.

Chan, E. S. and Z. Zhang. 2002. Encapsulation of probiotic bacteria *Lactobacillus acidophilus* by direct compression. *Food and Bioproducts Processing: Transactions of the Institution of Chemical Engineers, Part C* 80(2):78–82.

Chan, E. S. and Z. Zhang. 2005. Bioencapsulation by compression coating of probiotic bacteria for their protection in an acidic medium. *Process Biochemistry* 40(10):3346–3351.

Chandramouli, V., K. Kailasapathy, P. Peiris, and M. Jones. 2004. An improved method of microencapsulation and its evaluation to protect *Lactobacillus* spp. in simulated gastric conditions. *Journal of Microbiological Methods* 56(1):27–35.

Charteris, W. P., P. M. Kelly, L. Morelli, and J. K. Collins. 1998. Development and application of an *in vitro* methodology to determine the transit tolerance of potentially probiotic *Lactobacillus* and *Bifidobacterium* species in the upper human gastrointestinal tract. *Journal of Applied Microbiology* 84(5):759–768.

Chavarri, F. J., M. De Paz, and M. Nuñez. 1988. Cryoprotective agents for frozen concentrated starters from non-bitter *Streptococcus lactis* strains. *Biotechnology Letters* 10(1):11–16.

Chen, L. Y., G. E. Remondetto, and M. Subirade. 2006. Food protein-based materials as nutraceutical delivery systems. *Trends in Food Science and Technology* 17:272–283.

Chen, M. J., K. N. Chen, and Y. T. Kuo. 2007. Optimal thermotolerance of *Bifidobacterium bifidum* in gellan-alginate microparticles. *Biotechnology and Bioengineering* 98(2):411–419.

Chen, C. C., C. H. Chiu, T. Y. Lin, H. N. Shi, and W. A. Walker. 2009a. Effect of probiotics *Lactobacillus acidophilus* on *Citrobacter rodentium* colitis: The role of dendritic cells. *Pediatric Research* 65(2):169–175.

Chen, X., J. Fruehauf, J. D. Goldsmith, et al. 2009b. *Saccharomyces boulardii* inhibits EGF receptor signaling and intestinal tumor growth in Apc(min) mice. *Gastroenterology* 137(3):914–923.

Chen, Y. S., Y. L. Lin, R. L. Jan, H. H. Chen, and J. Y. Wang. 2010. Randomized placebo-controlled trial of lactobacillus on asthmatic children with allergic rhinitis. *Pediatric Pulmonology* 45(11):1111–1120.

Cho, Y. H., Shim, H. K., and Park, J. 2003. Encapsulation of fish oil by an enzymatic gelation process using transglutaminase cross-linked proteins. *Journal of Food Science* 68:2717–2723.

Clark, P. A. and J. H. Martin. 1994. Selection of Bifidobacteria for use as dietary adjuncts in cultured dairy foods: III—Tolerance to simulated bile concentrations of human small intestines. *Cultured Dairy Products Journal* 29(3):18–21.

Conrad, P. B., D. P. Miller, P. R. Cielenski, and J. J. de Pablo. 2000. Stabilization and preservation of *Lactobacillus acidophilus* in saccharide matrices. *Cryobiology* 41(1):17–24.

Corcoran, B. M., R. P. Ross, G. F. Fitzgerald, and C. Stanton. 2004. Comparative survival of probiotic lactobacilli spray-dried in the presence of prebiotic substances. *Journal of Applied Microbiology* 96(5):1024–1039.

Corcoran, B., Stanton, C., Fitzgerald, G. and Ross, R. 2005. Survival of probiotic lactobacilli in acidic environments is enhanced in the presence of metabolizable sugars. *Applied and Environmental Microbiology.* 71(6):3060.

Corrêa, N. B. O., L. A. Péret Filho, F. J. Penna, F. M. L. S. Lima, and J. R. Nicoli. 2005. A randomized formula controlled trial of *Bifidobacterium lactis* and *Streptococcus thermophilus* for prevention of antibiotic-associated diarrhea in infants. *Journal of Clinical Gastroenterology* 39(5):385–389.

Coulibaly, I., A. Y. Amenan, G. Lognay, M. L. Fauconnier, and P. Thonart. 2009. Survival of freeze-dried *Leuconostoc mesenteroides* and *Lactobacillus plantarum* related to their cellular fatty acids composition during storage. *Applied Biochemistry and Biotechnology* 157(1):70–84.

Craig, E. A., B. D. Gambill, and R. J. Nelson. 1993. Heat shock proteins: Molecular chaperones of protein biogenesis. *Microbiological Reviews* 57(2):402–414.

Crawford, D. R. and K. J. A. Davies. 1994. Adaptive response and oxidative stress. *Environmental Health Perspectives* 102:25–28.

Cremonini, F., S. Di Caro, M. Covino, et al. 2002. Effect of different probiotic preparations on anti-*Helicobacter pylori* therapy-related side effects: A parallel group, triple blind, placebo-controlled study. *American Journal of Gastroenterology* 97(11):2744–2749.

Crittenden, R., R. Weerakkody, L. Sanguansri, and M. Augustin. 2006. Synbiotic microcapsules that enhance microbial viability during nonrefrigerated storage and gastrointestinal transit. *Applied and Environmental Microbiology* 72(3):2280–2282.

Crowe, L. M., D. S. Reid, and J. H. Crowe. 1996. Is trehalose special for preserving dry biomaterials? *Biophysical Journal* 71(4):2087–2093.

Crowe, J. H., J. F. Carpenter, and L. M. Crowe. 1998. The role of vitrification in anhydrobiosis. *Annual Review of Physiology* 60:73–103.

Cruchet, S., M. C. Obregon, G. Salazar, E. Diaz, and M. Gotteland. 2003. Effect of the ingestion of a dietary product containing *Lactobacillus johnsonii* La1 on *Helicobacter pylori* colonization in children. *Nutrition* 19(9):716–721.

Cukrowska, B., A. Ceregra, I. Rosiak, et al. 2008. The influence of probiotic *Lactobacillus casei* and *paracasei* strains on clinical status of atopic eczema in children with food allergy on cow's milk proteins. *Pediatria Wspolczesna* 10(2):67–70.

Cukrowska, B., A. Ceregra, E. Klewicka, K. Ślizewska, I. Motyl, and Z. Libudzisz. 2010. Probiotic *Lactobacillus casei* and *Lactobacillus paracasei* strains in treatment of food allergy in children. *Przeglad Pediatryczny* 40(1):21–25.

Day, L., M. Xu, P. Hoobin, I. Burgar, and M. A. Augustin. 2007. Characterisation of fish oil emulsions stabilised by sodium caseinate. *Food Chemistry* 105(2):469–479.

De Angelis, M. and M. Gobbetti. 2004. Environmental stress responses in *Lactobacillus*: A review. *Proteomics* 4(1):106–122.

de Vrese, M., P. Winkler, P. Rautenberg, et al. 2005. Effect of *Lactobacillus gasseri* PA 16/8, *Bifidobacterium longum* SP 07/3, *B. bifidum* MF 20/5 on common cold episodes: A double blind, randomized, controlled trial. *Clinical Nutrition* 24(4):481–491.

Desai, K. G. H. and H. J. Park. 2005a. Recent developments in microencapsulation of food ingredients. *Drying Technology* 23:1361–1394.

Desai, K. G. H. and H. J. Park. 2005b. Encapsulation of vitamin C in tripolyphosphate cross-linked chitosan microspheres by spray drying. *Journal of Microencapsulation* 22(2):179–192.

Desai, K. G. H., C. Liu, and H. J. Park. 2005. Characteristics of vitamin C immobilized particles and sodium alginate beads containing immobilized particles. *Journal of Microencapsulation* 22(4):363–376.

Desmond, C., C. Stanton, G. F. Fitzgerald, K. Collins, and R. P. Ross. 2001. Environmental adaptation of pro-biotic lactobacilli towards improvement of performance during spray drying. *International Dairy Journal* 11(10):801–808.

Desmond, C., R. P. Ross, E. O'Callaghan, G. Fitzgerald, and C. Stanton. 2002. Improved survival of *Lactobacillus paracasei* NFBC 338 in spray-dried powders containing gum acacia. *Journal of Applied Microbiology* 93(6):1003–1011.

Dimantov, A., M. Greenberg, E. Kesselman, and E. Shimoni. 2004. Study of high amylose corn starch as food grade enteric coating in a microcapsule model system. *Innovative Food Science and Emerging Technologies* 5(1):93–100.

Ding, W. K. and N. P. Shah. 2009a. An improved method of microencapsulation of probiotic bacteria for their stability in acidic and bile conditions during storage. *Journal of Food Science* 74(2):M53–M61.

Ding, W. K. and N. P. Shah. 2009b. Effect of various encapsulating materials on the stability of probiotic bac-teria. *Journal of Food Science* 74(2):M100–M107.

Doleyres, Y., I. Fliss, and C. Lacroix. 2002a. Quantitative determination of the spatial distribution of pure- and mixed-strain immobilized cells in gel beads by immunofluorescence. *Applied Microbiology and Biotechnology* 59(2–3):297–302.

Doleyres, Y., I. Fliss, and C. Lacroix. 2004. Continuous production of mixed lactic starters containing probiot-ics using immobilized cell technology. *Biotechnology Progress* 20(1):145–150.

Duman, D. G., S. Bor, Ö Özütemiz, et al. 2005. Efficacy and safety of *Saccharomyces boulardii* in prevention of antibiotic-associated diarrhoea due to *Helicobacter pylori* eradication. *European Journal of Gastroenterology and Hepatology* 17(12):1357–1361.

Dziezak, J. D. 1988. Microencapsulation and encapsulated ingredients. *Food Technology* 42(4):136–151.

Eikmeier, H. and H. J. Rehm. 1987. Stability of calcium alginate during citric acid production of immobilized *Aspergillus niger*. *Applied Microbiology and Biotechnology* 26(2):105–111.

FAO/WHO. 2001. *Evaluation of Health and Nutritional Properties of Powder Milk and Live Lactic Acid Bacteria*. Rome/Geneva: FAO/WHO.

Fávaro-Trindade, C. S. and C. R. F. Grosso. 2002. Microencapsulation of *L. acidophilus* (La-05) and *B. lactis* (Bb-12) and evaluation of their survival at the pH values of the stomach and in bile. *Journal of Microencapsulation* 19(4):485–494.

Fonseca, F., C. Béal, and G. Corrieu. 2000. Method of quantifying the loss of acidification activity of lactic acid starters during freezing and frozen storage. *Journal of Dairy Research* 67(1):83–90.

Forrest, S. A., R. Y. Yada, and D. Rousseau. 2005. Interactions of vitamin D_3 with bovine β-lactoglobulin A and β-casein. *Journal of Agricultural and Food Chemistry* 53(20):8003–8009.

Forsythe, P., M. D. Inman, and J. Bienenstock. 2007. Oral treatment with live *Lactobacillus reuteri* inhibits the allergic airway response in mice. *American Journal of Respiratory and Critical Care Medicine* 175(6):561–569.

Fowler, A. and M. Toner. 2005. Cryo-injury and biopreservation. *Annals of the New York Academy of Sciences* 1066:119–135.

Fozo, E. M., J. K. Kajfasz, and R. G. Quivey. 2004. Low pH-induced membrane fatty acid alterations in oral bacteria. *FEMS Microbiology Letters* 238(2):291–295.

Franks, F. 1995. Protein destabilization at low-temperatures. *Advances in Protein Chemistry* 46:105–139.

Fuller, R. 1989. Probiotics in man and animals. *Journal of Applied Bacteriology* 66(5):365–378.

Fuller, R. 1991. Probiotics in human medicine. *Gut* 32(4):439–442.

Fuller, R. 1992. *Probiotic the Scientific Basis*. 1st edn. London: Chapman & Hall, 398 pp.

Furrie, E., S. Macfarlane, A. Kennedy, et al. 2005. Synbiotic therapy (*Bifidobacterium longum*/ Synergy 1) initiates resolution of inflammation in patients with active ulcerative colitis: A randomised controlled pilot trial. *Gut* 54(2):242–249.

Gaón, D., C. Garmendia, N. O. Murrielo, et al. 2002. Effect of *Lactobacillus* strains (*L. casei* and *L. acidophillus* strains cerela) on bacterial overgrowth-related chronic diarrhea. *Medicina* 62(2):159–163.

Gaón, D., H. Garcia, L. Winter, et al. 2003. Effect of *Lactobacillus* strains and *Saccharomyces boulardii* on persistent diarrhea in children. *Medicina* 63(4):293–298.

Gardiner, G. E., E. O'Sullivan, J. Kelly, et al. 2000. Comparative survival rates of human-derived probiotic *Lactobacillus paracasei* and *L. salivarius* strains during heat treatment and spray drying. *Applied and Environmental Microbiology* 66(6):2605–2612.

Gåserød, O., A. Sannes, and G. Skjåk-Bræk. 1999. Microcapsules of alginate-chitosan. II. A study of capsule stability and permeability. *Biomaterials* 20(8):773–783.

Gawronska, A., P. Dziechciarz, A. Horvath, and H. Szajewska. 2007. A randomized double-blind placebo-controlled trial of *Lactobacillus* GG for abdominal pain disorders in children. *Alimentary Pharmacology and Therapeutics* 25(2):177–184.

Gbassi, G. K., T. Vandamme, S. Ennahar, and E. Marchioni. 2009. Microencapsulation of *Lactobacillus plantarum* spp in an alginate matrix coated with whey proteins. *International Journal of Food Microbiology* 129(1):103–105.

Gibbs, B. F., S. Kermasha, I. Alli, and C. N. Mulligan. 1999. Encapsulation in the food industry: A review. *International Journal of Food Sciences and Nutrition* 50(3):213–224.

Gill, H. S., Q. Shu, H. Lin, K. J. Rutherfurd, and M. L. Cross. 2001. Protection against translocating *Salmonella typltimurium* infection in mice by feeding the immuno-enhancing probiotic *Lactobacillus rhamnosus* strain HN001. *Medical Microbiology and Immunology* 190(3):97–104.

Girgis, H., J. Smith, J. Luchansky, and T. Klaenhammer. 2003. Stress adaptations of lactic acid bacteria. In *Microbial Stress Adaptation and Food Safety*, ed. A. E. Yousef, and V. K. Juneja, pp. 159–212. Boca Raton, FL: CRC Press.

Goderska, K. and Z. Czarnecki. 2008. Influence of microencapsulation and spray drying on the viability of *Lactobacillus* and *Bifidobacterium* strains. *Polish Journal of Microbiology* 57(2):135–140.

Goldberg, I. and L. Eschar. 1977. Stability of lactic acid bacteria to freezing as related to their fatty acid composition. *Applied and Environmental Microbiology* 33(3):489–496.

Goñi, I., L. García-Diz, E. Mañas, and F. Saura-Calixto. 1996. Analysis of resistant starch: A method for foods and food products. *Food Chemistry* 56(4):445–449.

González-Sánchez, F., A. Azaola, G. F. Gutiérrez-López, and H. Hernández-Sánchez. 2010. Viability of microencapsulated *Bifidobacterium animalis* ssp. *lactis* BB12 in kefir during refrigerated storage. *International Journal of Dairy Technology* 63(3):431–436.

Gotteland, M., L. Poliak, S. Cruchet, and O. Brunser. 2005. Effect of regular ingestion of *Saccharomyces boulardii* plus inulin or *Lactobacillus acidophilus* LB in children colonized by *Helicobacter pylori*. *Acta Paediatrica, International Journal of Paediatrics* 94(12):1747–1751.

Gotteland, M., M. Andrews, M. Toledo, et al. 2008. Modulation of *Helicobacter pylori* colonization with cranberry juice and *Lactobacillus johnsonii* La1 in children. *Nutrition* 24(5):421–426.

Gottesman, S., S. Wickner, and M. R. Maurizi. 1997. Protein quality control: Triage by chaperones and proteases. *Genes and Development* 11(7):815–823.

Gouesbet, G., G. Jan, and P. Boyaval. 2001. *Lactobacillus delbrueckii* ssp. *bulgaricus* thermotolerance. *Lait* 81(1–2):301–309.

Gouesbet, G., G. Jan, and P. Boyaval. 2002. Two-dimensional electrophoresis study of *Lactobacillus delbrueckii* subsp. *bulgaricus* thermotolerance. *Applied and Environmental Microbiology* 68(3):1055–1063.

Gouin, S. 2004. Microencapsulation: Industrial appraisal of existing technologies and trends. *Trends in Food Science and Technology* 15(7–8):330–347.

Groboillot, A. F., C. P. Champagne, G. D. Darling, D. Poncelet, and R. J. Neufeld. 1993. Membrane formation by interfacial cross-linking of chitosan for microencapsulation of *Lactococcus lactis*. *Biotechnology and Bioengineering* 42(10):1157–1163.

Guérin, D., J. C. Vuillemard, and M. Subirade. 2003. Protection of bifidobacteria encapsulated in polysaccharide-protein gel beads against gastric juice and bile. *Journal of Food Protection* 66(11): 2076–2084.

Gunning, A. P., A. R. Kirby, V. J. Morris, B. Wells, and B. E. Brooker. 1995. Imaging bacterial polysaccharides by AFM. *Polymer Bulletin* 34(5–6):615–619.

Guo, M. R., P. F. Fox, A. Flynn, and P. S. Kindstedt. 1995. Susceptibility of beta-lactoglobulin and sodium caseinate to proteolysis by pepsin and trypsin. *Journal of Dairy Science* 78(11):2336–2344.

Guslandi, M., G. Mezzi, M. Sorghi, and P. A. Testoni. 2000. *Saccharomyces boulardii* in maintenance treatment of Crohn's disease. *Digestive Diseases and Sciences* 45(7):1462–1464.

Guslandi, M., P. Giollo, and P. A. Testoni. 2003. A pilot trial of *Saccharomyces boulardii* in ulcerative colitis. *European Journal of Gastroenterology and Hepatology* 15(6):697–698.

Guyonnet, D., O. Chassany, P. Ducrotte, et al. 2007. Effect of a fermented milk containing *Bifidobacterium animalis* DN-173 010 on the health-related quality of life and symptoms in irritable bowel syndrome in adults in primary care: A multicentre, randomized, double-blind, controlled trial. *Alimentary Pharmacology and Therapeutics* 26(3):475–486.

Halliwell, B., S. Chirico, M. A. Crawford, K. S. Bjerve, and K. F. Gey. 1993. Lipid peroxidation: Its mechanism, measurement, and significance. *American Journal of Clinical Nutrition* 57(5):715S–725S.

Havenaar, R. and J. H. J. Huis In't Veld. 1992. Probiotics: A general view. In *The Lactic Acid Bacteria in Health and Disease,* Volume 1, ed. B. J. B. Wood, pp. 151–170. Amsterdam: Elsevier.

Hecker, M., W. Schumann, and U. Völker. 1996. Heat-shock and general stress response in *Bacillus subtilis*. *Molecular Microbiology* 19(3):417–428.

Heidebach, T., P. Först, and U. Kulozik. 2009a. Microencapsulation of probiotic cells by means of rennet-gelation of milk proteins. *Food Hydrocolloids* 23(7):1670–1677.

Heidebach, T., P. Först, and U. Kulozik. 2009b. Transglutaminase-induced caseinate gelation for the microencapsulation of probiotic cells. *International Dairy Journal* 19(2):77–84.

Heidebach, T., P. Forst, and U. Kulozik. 2010. Influence of casein-based microencapsulation on freeze-drying and storage of probiotic cells. *Journal of Food Engineering* 98(3):309–316.

Hendrick, J. P. and F. U. Hartl. 1993. Molecular chaperone functions of heat-shock proteins. *Annual Review of Biochemistry* 62:349–384.

Hogan, S. A., B. F. McNamee, E. D. O'Riordan, and M. O'Sullivan. 2001. Microencapsulating properties of sodium caseinate. *Journal of Agricultural and Food Chemistry* 49(4):1934–1938.

Homayouni, A., A. Azizi, M. R. Ehsani, M. S. Yarmand, and S. H. Razavi. 2008. Effect of microencapsulation and resistant starch on the probiotic survival and sensory properties of synbiotic ice cream. *Food Chemistry* 111(1):50–55.

Hou, R. C. W., M. Y. Lin, M. M. C. Wang, and J. T. C. Tzen. 2003. Increase of viability of entrapped cells of *Lactobacillus delbrueckii* ssp. *bulgaricus* in artificial sesame oil emulsions. *Journal of Dairy Science* 86(2):424–428.

Hoyos, A. B. 1999. Reduced incidence of necrotizing enterocolitis associated with enteral administration of *Lactobacillus acidophilus* and *Bifidobacterium infantis* to neonates in an intensive care unit. *International Journal of Infectious Diseases* 3(4):197–202.

Hsiao, H. C., W. C. Lian, and C. C. Chou. 2004. Effect of packaging conditions and temperature on viability of microencapsulated bifidobacteria during storage. *Journal of the Science of Food and Agriculture* 84(2):134–139.

Hubálek, Z. 2003. Protectants used in the cryopreservation of microorganisms. *Cryobiology* 46(3):205–229.

Hurduc, V., D. Plesca, D. Dragomir, M. Sajin, and Y. Vandenplas. 2009. A randomized, open trial evaluating the effect of *Saccharomyces boulardii* on the eradication rate of *Helicobacter pylori* infection in children. *Acta Paediatrica, International Journal of Paediatrics* 98(1):127–131.

Hutkins, R. W., W. L. Ellefson, and E. R. Kashket. 1987. Betaine transport imparts osmotolerance on a strain of *Lactobacillus acidophilus*. *Applied and Environmental Microbiology* 53:2275–2281.

Hyndman, C. L., A. F. Groboillot, D. Poncelet, C. P. Champagne, and R. J. Neufeld. 1993. Microencapsulation of *Lactococcus lactis* within cross-linked gelatin membranes. *Journal of Chemical Technology and Biotechnology* 56(3):259–263.

Inoue, R., A. Nishio, Y. Fukushima, and K. Ushida. 2007. Oral treatment with probiotic *Lactobacillus johnsonii* NCC533 (La1) for a specific part of the weaning period prevents the development of atopic dermatitis induced after maturation in model mice, NC/Nga. *British Journal of Dermatology* 156(3):499–509.

Irvine, S. L., R. Hummelen, S. Hekmat, C. W. N. Looman, J. D. F. Habbema, and G. Reid. 2010. Probiotic yogurt consumption is associated with an increase of CD4 count among people living with HIV/AIDS. *Journal of Clinical Gastroenterology* 44(9):e201–e205.

Iyer, C. and K. Kailasapathy. 2005. Effect of co-encapsulation of probiotics with prebiotics on increasing the viability of encapsulated bacteria under *in vitro* acidic and bile salt conditions and in yogurt. *Journal of Food Science* 70(1):M18–M23.

Jagannath, A., P. S. Raju, and A. S. Bawa. 2010. Comparative evaluation of bacterial cellulose (nata) as a cryo-protectant and carrier support during the freeze drying process of probiotic lactic acid bacteria. *Lebensmittel-Wissenschaft und-Technologie—Food Science and Technology* 43(8):1197–1203.

Jin, X., K. Grigas, C. Chen, A. Panda, and M. L. Matheny. 1985. Method and composition for producing stable bacteria and bacterial formulations. US Patent 5,733,774.

Johnson-Henry, K. C., D. J. Mitchell, Y. Avitzur, E. Galindo-Mata, N. L. Jones, and P. M. Sherman. 2004. Probiotics reduce bacterial colonization and gastric inflammation in *H. pylori*-infected mice. *Digestive Diseases and Sciences* 49(7–8):1095–1102.

Kabir, A. M. A., Y. Aiba, A. Takagi, S. Kamiya, T. Miwa, and Y. Koga. 1997. Prevention of *Helicobacter pylori* infection by lactobacilli in a gnotobiotic murine model. *Gut* 41(1):49–55.

Kailasapathy, K. 2002. Microencapsulation of probiotic bacteria: Technology and potential applications. *Current Issues in Intestinal Microbiology* 3(2):39–48.

Kailasapathy, K. and B. S. Sureeta. 2004. Effect of storage on shelf life and viability of freeze-dried and micro-encapsulated *Lactobacillus acidophilus* and *Bifidobacterium infantis* cultures. *Australian Journal of Dairy Technology* 59(3):204–208.

Kalliomäki, M., S. Salminen, H. Arvilommi, P. Kero, P. Koskinen, and E. Isolauri. 2001. Probiotics in primary prevention of atopic disease: A randomised placebo-controlled trial. *Lancet* 357(9262):1076–1079.

Kalliomäki, M., S. Salminen, T. Poussa, H. Arvilommi, and E. Isolauri. 2003. Probiotics and prevention of atopic disease: 4-year follow-up of a randomised placebo-controlled trial. *Lancet* 361(9372):1869–1871.

Kanamori, Y., M. Sugiyama, K. Hashizume, N. Yuki, M. Morotomi, and R. Tanaka. 2004. Experience of long-term synbiotic therapy in seven short bowel patients with refractory enterocolitis. *Journal of Pediatric Surgery* 39(11):1686–1692.

Kanazawa, H., M. Nagino, S. Kamiya, et al. 2005. Synbiotics reduce postoperative infectious complications: A randomized controlled trial in biliary cancer patients undergoing hepatectomy. *Langenbeck's Archives of Surgery* 390(2):104–113.

Karimi, K., M. D. Inman, J. Bienenstock, and P. Forsythe. 2009. *Lactobacillus reuteri*-induced regulatory T cells protect against an allergic airway response in mice. *American Journal of Respiratory and Critical Care Medicine* 179(3):186–193.

Kato, I., K. Endo-Tanaka, and T. Yokokura. 1998. Suppressive effects of the oral administration of *Lactobacillus casei* on type ii collagen-induced arthritis in DBA/1 mice. *Life Sciences* 63(8):635–644.

Kets, E. P. W. and J. A. M. De Bont. 1994. Protective effect of betaine on survival of *Lactobacillus plantarum* subjected to drying. *FEMS Microbiology Letters* 116(3):251–256.

Kets, E. P. W., P. J. M. Teunissen, and J. A. M. DeBont. 1996. Effect of compatible solutes on survival of lactic acid bacteria subjected to drying. *Applied and Environmental Microbiology* 62(1):259–261.

Kilara, A. and M. N. Vaghela. 2004. Whey proteins. In *Proteins in Food Processing*, ed. R. Y. Yada, pp. 72–99. Cambridge: Woodhead Publishing.

Kim, Y. D., C. V. Morr, and T. W. Schenz. 1996. Microencapsulation properties of gum arabic and several food proteins: Liquid orange oil emulsion particles. *Journal of Agricultural and Food Chemistry* 44(5):1308–1313.

Kim, W. S., L. Perl, J. H. Park, J. E. Tandianus, and N. W. Dunn. 2001. Assessment of stress response of the probiotic *Lactobacillus acidophilus*. *Current Microbiology* 43(5):346–350.

Kim, C. J., S. A. Jun, N. K. Lee, et al. 2006. Encapsulation of *Bacillus polyfermenticus* SCD with alginate-methylcellulose and evaluation of survival in artificial conditions of large intestine. *Journal of Microbiology and Biotechnology* 16(3):443–449.

Kim, S. J., S. Y. Cho, S. H. Kim, et al. 2008. Effect of microencapsulation on viability and other characteristics in *Lactobacillus acidophilus* ATCC 43121. *Lebensmittel-Wissenschaft und-Technologie—Food Science and Technology* 41(3):493–500.

Kimoto, H., S. Ohmomo, and T. Okamoto. 2002. Enhancement of bile tolerance in lactococci by Tween 80. *Journal of Applied Microbiology* 92(1):41–46.

King, A. H. 1995. Encapsulation of food ingredients: A review of available technology, focussing on hydrocolloids. In *Encapsulation and Controlled Release of Food Ingredients*, ACS Symposium Series 590, ed. S. J. Risch, and G. A. Reineccius, pp. 26–39. Washington, DC: American Chemical Society.

King, V. A. E. and J. T. Su. 1994. Dehydration of *Lactobacillus acidophilus*. *Process Biochemistry* 28(1):47–52.

Knorr, D. 1998. Technology aspects related to microorganisms in functional foods. *Trends in Food Science and Technology* 9(8–9):295–306.

Kobayashi, H., T. Suzuki, N. Kinoshita, and T. Unemoto. 1984. Amplification of the *Streptococcus faecalis* pro-ton-translocating ATPase by a decrease in cytoplasmic pH. *Journal of Bacteriology* 158(3):1157–1160.

Kobayashi, H., T. Suzuki, and T. Unemoto. 1986. Streptococcal cytoplasmic pH is regulated by changes in amount and activity of a proton-translocating ATPase. *Journal of Biological Chemistry* 261(2):627–630.

Koebnick, C., I. Wagner, P. Leitzmann, U. Stern, and H. J. F. Zunft. 2003. Probiotic beverage containing *Lactobacillus casei* Shirota improves gastrointestinal symptoms in patients with chronic constipation. *Canadian Journal of Gastroenterology* 17(11):655–659.

Kotowska, M., P. Albrecht, and H. Szajewska. 2005. *Saccharomyces boulardii* in the prevention of antibiotic-associated diarrhoea in children: A randomized double-blind placebo-controlled trial. *Alimentary Pharmacology and Therapeutics* 21(5):583–590.

Krasaekoopt, W., B. Bhandari, and H. Deeth. 2003. Evaluation of encapsulation techniques of probiotics for yoghurt. *International Dairy Journal* 13(1):3–13.

Kukkonen, K., E. Savilahti, T. Haahtela, et al. 2008. Long-term safety and impact on infection rates of postnatal probiotic and prebiotic (synbiotic) treatment: Randomized, double-blind, placebo-controlled trial. *Pediatrics* 122(1):8–12.

Kumar, M., A. Kumar, R. Nagpal, et al. 2010. Cancer-preventing attributes of probiotics: An update. *International Journal of Food Sciences and Nutrition* 61(5):473–496.

Kurugöl, Z. and G. Koturoglu. 2005. Effects of *Saccharomyces boulardii* in children with acute diarrhoea. *Acta Paediatrica, International Journal of Paediatrics* 94(1):44–47.

Lahtinen, S. J., A. C. Ouwehand, S. J. Salminen, P. Forssell, and P. Myllärinen. 2007. Effect of starch- and lipid-based encapsulation on the culturability of two *Bifidobacterium longum* strains. *Letters in Applied Microbiology* 44(5):500–505.

Latha, M. S., A. V. Lal, T. V. Kumary, R. Sreekumar, and A. Jayakrishnan. 2000. Progesterone release from glutaraldehyde cross-linked casein microspheres: *In vitro* studies and *in vivo* response in rabbits. *Contraception* 61(5):329–334.

Lee, B. H. 1996. Bacteria-based processes and products. In *Fundamentals of Food Biotechnology*, ed. B. H. Lee, pp. 219–290. New York, NY: Wiley Interscience.

Lee, D. W., S. J. Hwang, J. B. Park, and H. J. Park. 2003. Preparation and release characteristics of polymer-coated and blended alginate microspheres. *Journal of Microencapsulation* 20(2):179–192.

Leslie, S. B., E. Israeli, B. Lighthart, J. H. Crowe, and L. M. Crowe. 1995. Trehalose and sucrose protect both membranes and proteins in intact bacteria during drying. *Applied and Environmental Microbiology* 61(10):3592–3597.

Leyer, G. J., S. Li, M. E. Mubasher, C. Reifer, and A. C. Ouwehand. 2009. Probiotic effects on cold and influenza-like symptom incidence and duration in children. *Pediatrics* 124(2):e172–e179.

Li, J., M. M. O. Eleya, and S. Gunasekaran. 2006. Gelation of whey protein and xanthan mixture: Effect of heating rate on rheological properties. *Food Hydrocolloids* 20(5):678–686.

Li, X. Y., X. G. Chen, D. S. Cha, H. J. Park, and C. S. Liu. 2009. Microencapsulation of a probiotic bacteria with alginate-gelatin and its properties. *Journal of Microencapsulation* 26(4):315–324.

Lian, W. C., H. C. Hsiao, and C. C. Chou. 2002. Survival of bifidobacteria after spray-drying. *International Journal of Food Microbiology* 74(1–2):79–86.

Lian, W. C., H. C. Hsiao, and C. C. Chou. 2003. Viability of microencapsulated bifidobacteria in simulated gastric juice and bile solution. *International Journal of Food Microbiology* 86(3):293–301.

Lin, H. C., B. H. Su, A. C. Chen, et al. 2005. Oral probiotics reduce the incidence and severity of necrotizing enterocolitis in very low birth weight infants. *Pediatrics* 115(1):1–4.

Linders, L. J. M., G. I. W. De Jong, G. Meerdink, and K. Van't Riet. 1997a. Carbohydrates and the dehydration inactivation of *Lactobacillus plantarum*: The role of moisture distribution and water activity. *Journal of Food Engineering* 31(2):237–250.

Linders, L. J. M., W. F. Wolkers, F. A. Hoekstra, and K. Van't Riet. 1997b. Effect of added carbohydrates on membrane phase behavior and survival of dried *Lactobacillus plantarum*. *Cryobiology* 35(1):31–40.

Linders, L. J. M., G. Meerdink, and K. Van't Riet. 1997c. Effect of growth parameters on the residual activity of *Lactobacillus plantarum* after drying. *Journal of Applied Microbiology* 82(6):683–688.

Lindquist, S. and E. A. Craig. 1988. The heat-shock proteins. *Annual Review of Genetics* 22:631–677.

Liserre, A. M., M. I. Ré, and B. D. G. M. Franco. 2007. Microencapsulation of *Bifidobacterium animalis* subsp. *lactis* in modified alginate-chitosan beads and evaluation of survival in simulated gastrointestinal conditions. *Food Biotechnology* 21(1):1–16.

Livney, Y. D. 2010. Milk proteins as vehicles for bioactives. *Current Opinion in Colloid & Interface Science* 15(1–2):73–83.

Lolkema, J. S., B. Poolman, and W. N. Konings. 1995. Role of scalar protons in metabolic energy generation in lactic acid bacteria. *Journal of Bioenergetics and Biomembranes* 27(4):467–473.

Lucey, J. A., T. van Vliet, K. Grolle, T. Geurts, and P. Walstra. 1997. Properties of acid casein gels made by acidification with glucono-delta-lactone. 2. Syneresis, permeability and microstructural properties. *International Dairy Journal* 7(6–7):389–397.

Madene, A., M. Jacquot, J. Scher, and S. Desobry. 2006. Flavour encapsulation and controlled release—A review. *International Journal of Food Science and Technology* 41(1):1–21.

Madsen, K. L., J. S. Doyle, L. D. Jewell, M. M. Tavernini, and R. N. Fedorak. 1999. *Lactobacillus* species prevents colitis in interleukin 10 gene-deficient mice. *Gastroenterology* 116(5):1107–1114.

Makino, S., S. Ikegami, A. Kume, H. Horiuchi, H. Sasaki, and N. Orii. 2010. Reducing the risk of infection in the elderly by dietary intake of yoghurt fermented with *Lactobacillus delbrueckii* ssp. *bulgaricus* OLL1073R-1. *British Journal of Nutrition* 104(7):998–1006.

Maltais, A., G. E. Remondetto, R. Gonzalez, and M. Subirade. 2005. Formation of soy protein isolate cold-set gels: Protein and salt effects. *Journal of Food Science* 70(1):C67–C73.

Mandal, S., A. K. Puniya, and K. Singh. 2006. Effect of alginate concentrations on survival of microencapsulated *Lactobacillus casei* NCDC-298. *International Dairy Journal* 16(10):1190–1195.

Mansour-Ghanaei, F., N. Dehbashi, K. Yazdanparast, and A. Shafaghi. 2003. Efficacy of *Saccharomyces boulardii* with antibiotics in acute amoebiasis. *World Journal of Gastroenterology* 9(8):1832–1833.

Marquis, R. E., G. R. Bender, D. R. Murray, and A. Wong. 1987. Arginine deiminase system and bacterial adaptation to acid environments. *Applied and Environmental Microbiology* 53(1):198–200.

MartyTeysset, C., J. S. Lolkema, P. Schmitt, C. Divies, and W. N. Konings. 1996. The citrate metabolic pathway in *Leuconostoc mesenteroides*: Expression, amino acid synthesis, and alpha-ketocarboxylate transport. *Journal of Bacteriology* 178(21):6209–6215.

Mazur, P. 1977. Role of intracellular freezing in death of cells cooled at supraoptimal rates. *Cryobiology* 14(3):251–272.

McCarthy, J., L. O'Mahony, L. O'Callaghan, et al. 2003. Double blind, placebo controlled trial of two probiotic strains in interleukin 10 knockout mice and mechanistic link with cytokine balance. *Gut* 52(7): 975–980.

McLean, N. W. and I. J. Rosenstein. 2000. Characterisation and selection of a *Lactobacillus* species to re-colonise the vagina of women with recurrent bacterial vaginosis. *Journal of Medical Microbiology* 49(6):543–552.

McMaster, L. D., S. A. Kokott, and P. Slatter. 2005. Micro-encapsulation of *Bifidobacterium lactis* for incorporation into soft foods. *World Journal of Microbiology & Biotechnology* 21(5):723–728.

Meng, X. C., C. Stanton, G. F. Fitzgerald, C. Daly, and R. P. Ross. 2008. Anhydrobiotics: The challenges of drying probiotic cultures. *Food Chemistry* 106(4):1406–1416.

Metchnikoff, E. 1907. *The Prolongation of Life*. New York, NY: Putman.

Miao, S., S. Mills, C. Stanton, G. F. Fitzgerald, Y. Roos, and R. P. Ross. 2008. Effect of disaccharides on survival during storage of freeze dried probiotics. *Dairy Science and Technology* 88(1):19–30.

Miles, M. J., V. J. Morris, and V. Carroll. 1984. Carob gum-κ-carrageenan mixed gels: Mechanical properties and x-ray fiber diffraction studies. *Macromolecules* 17(11):2443–2445.

Mille, Y., J. P. Obert, L. Beney, and P. Gervais. 2004. New drying process for lactic bacteria based on their dehydration behavior in liquid medium. *Biotechnology and Bioengineering* 88(1):71–76.

Miranda, G. and J. P. Pelissier. 1983. Kinetic studies of *in vivo* digestion of bovine unheated skim-milk proteins in the rat stomach. *Journal of Dairy Research* 50(1):27–36.

Mokarram, R. R., S. A. Mortazavi, M. B. H. Najafi, and F. Shahidi. 2009. The influence of multi stage alginate coating on survivability of potential probiotic bacteria in simulated gastric and intestinal juice. *Food Research International* 42(8):1040–1045.

Molenaar, D., A. Hagting, H. Alkema, A. J. M. Driessen, and W. N. Konings. 1993. Characteristics and osmoregulatory roles of uptake systems for proline and glycine betaine in *Lactococcus lactis*. *Journal of Bacteriology* 175(17):5438–5444.

Montalto, M., N. Maggiano, R. Ricci, et al. 2004. *Lactobacillus acidophilus* protects tight junctions from aspirin damage in HT-29 cells. *Digestion* 69(4):225–228.

Morgan, C. A., N. Herman, P. A. White, and G. Vesey. 2006. Preservation of micro-organisms by drying; A review. *Journal of Microbiological Methods* 66(2):183–193.

Mortazavian, A. M., M. R. Ehsani, A. Azizi, S. H. Razavi, S. M. Mousavi, and J. A. Reinheimer. 2008. Effect of microencapsulation of probiotic bacteria with calcium alginate on cell stability during the refrigerated storage period in the Iranian yogurt drink (doogh). *Milchwissenschaft* 63(3):262–265.

Mukai, T., T. Asasaka, E. Sato, K. Mori, M. Matsumoto, and H. Ohori. 2002. Inhibition of binding of *Helicobacter pylori* to the glycolipid receptors by probiotic *Lactobacillus reuteri*. *FEMS Immunology and Medical Microbiology* 32(2):105–110.

Muthukumarasamy, P. and R. A. Holley. 2006. Microbiological and sensory quality of dry fermented sausages containing alginate-microencapsulated *Lactobacillus reuteri*. *International Journal of Food Microbiology* 111(2):164–169.

Muthukumarasamy, P. and R. A. Holley. 2007. Survival of Escherichia coli O157:H7 in dry fermented sausages containing micro-encapsulated probiotic lactic acid bacteria. *Food Microbiology* 24(1):82–88.

Muthukumarasamy, P., P. Allan-Wojtas, and R. A. Holley. 2006. Stability of *Lactobacillus reuteri* in different types of microcapsules. *Journal of Food Science* 71(1):M20–M24.

Nag, A., Han, K. and Singh, H. 2011. Microencapsulation of probiotic bacteria using pH-induced gelation of sodium caseinate and gellan gum. *International Dairy Journal* 21(4):247–253.

Nag, A. and Das, D. 2011. Delivering probiotic bacteria in sheld stable foods. *Food and Beverage Asia* October/November 2011:26–28.

Nannen, N. L. and R. W. Hutkins. 1991. Proton-translocating adenosine-triphosphatase activity in lactic-acid bacteria. *Journal of Dairy Science* 74(3):747–751.

Nase, L., K. Hatakka, E. Savilahti, et al. 2001. Effect of long-term consumption of a probiotic bacterium, *Lactobacillus rhamnosus* GG, in milk on dental caries and caries risk in children. *Caries Research* 35(6):412–420.

Niedzielin, K., H. Kordecki, and B. Birkenfeld. 2001. A controlled, double-blind, randomized study on the efficacy of *Lactobacillus plantarum* 299 V in patients with irritable bowel syndrome. *European Journal of Gastroenterology and Hepatology* 13(10):1143–1147.

Nobaek, S., M. L. Johansson, G. Molin, S. Ahrné, and B. Jeppsson. 2000. Alteration of intestinal microflora is associated with reduction in abdominal bloating and pain in patients with irritable bowel syndrome. *American Journal of Gastroenterology* 95(5):1231–1238.

Norton, S. and C. Lacroix. 1990. Gellan gum gel as entrapment matrix for high temperature fermentation processes: A rheological study. *Biotechnology Techniques* 4(5):351–356.

Oliveira, A. C., T. S. Moretti, C. Boschini, J. C. C. Baliero, O. Freitas, and C. S. Favaro-Trindade. 2007. Stability of microencapsulated B. *lactis* (BI 01) and L. *acidophilus* (LAC 4) by complex coacervation followed by spray drying. *Journal of Microencapsulation* 24(7):685–693.

O'Mahony, L., J. McCarthy, P. Kelly, et al. 2005. *Lactobacillus* and *Bifidobacterium* in irritable bowel syndrome: Symptom responses and relationship to cytokine profiles. *Gastroenterology* 128(3):541–551.

O'Riordan, K., D. Andrews, K. Buckle, and P. Conway. 2001. Evaluation of microencapsulation of a *Bifidobacterium* strain with starch as an approach to prolonging viability during storage. *Journal of Applied Microbiology* 91(6):1059–1066.

Orndorff, G. R. and A. P. MacKenzie. 1973. The function of the suspending medium during the freeze-drying preservation of *Escherichia coli*. *Cryobiology* 10(6):475–487.

Özer, B., Y. S. Uzun, and H. A. Kirmaci. 2008. Effect of microencapsulation on viability of *Lactobacillus acidophilus* la-5 and *Bifidobacterium bifidum* bb-12 during kasar cheese ripening. *International Journal of Dairy Technology* 61(3):237–244.

Özer, B. and H. Avni Kirmaci. 2009. Development of proteolysis in white-brined cheese: Role of microencapsulated *Lactobacillus acidophilus* LA-5 and *Bifidobacterium bifidum* BB-12 used as adjunct cultures. *Milchwissenschaft* 64(3):295–299.

Özer, B., H. A. Kirmaci, E. Senel, M. Atamer, and A. Hayaloglu. 2009. Improving the viability of *Bifidobacterium bifidum* BB-12 and *Lactobacillus acidophilus* LA-5 in white-brined cheese by microencapsulation. *International Dairy Journal* 19(1):22–29.

Peran, L., D. Camuesco, M. Comalada, et al. 2005. Preventative effects of a probiotic, *Lactobacillus salivarius* ssp. *salivarius*, in the TNBS model of rat colitis. *World Journal of Gastroenterology* 11(33):5185–5192.

Peran, L., D. Camuesco, M. Comalada, et al. 2006. *Lactobacillus fermentum*, a probiotic capable to release glutathione, prevents colonic inflammation in the TNBS model of rat colitis. *International Journal of Colorectal Disease* 21(8):737–746.

Peran, L., S. Sierra, M. Comalada, et al. 2007. A comparative study of the preventative effects exerted by two probiotics, *Lactobacillus reuteri* and *Lactobacillus fermentum*, in the trinitrobenzenesulfonic acid model of rat colitis. *British Journal of Nutrition* 97(1):96–103.

Phuapradit, P., W. Varavithya, K. Vathanophas, et al. 1999. Reduction of rotavirus infection in children receiving bifidobacteria-supplemented formula. *Journal of the Medical Association of Thailand* 82(Suppl. 1):S43–S48.

Picot, A. and C. Lacroix. 2003. Production of multiphase water-insoluble microcapsules for cell microencapsulation using an emulsification/spray-drying technology. *Journal of Food Science* 68(9):2693–2700.

Picot, A. and C. Lacroix. 2004. Encapsulation of bifidobacteria in whey protein-based microcapsules and survival in simulated gastrointestinal conditions and in yoghurt. *International Dairy Journal* 14(6):505–515.

Pollock, T. J. 1993. Gellan-related polysaccharides and the genus *Sphingomonas*. *Journal of General Microbiology* 139(8):1939–1945.

Poolman, B. and Glaasker, E. 1998. Regulation of compatible solute accumulation in bacteria. *Molecular Microbiology* 29(2):397–407.

Prasad, J., P. McJarrow, and P. Gopal. 2003. Heat and osmotic stress responses of probiotic *Lactobacillus rhamnosus* HN001 (DR20) in relation to viability after drying. *Applied and Environmental Microbiology* 69(2):917–925.

Prevost, H. and C. Divies. 1992. Cream fermentation by a mixed culture of Lactococci entrapped in two-layer calcium alginate gel beads. *Biotechnology Letters* 14(7):583–588.

Puccio, G., C. Cajozzo, F. Meli, F. Rochat, D. Grathwohl, and P. Steenhout. 2007. Clinical evaluation of a new starter formula for infants containing live *Bifidobacterium longum* BL999 and prebiotics. *Nutrition* 23(1):1–8.

Raharjo, S. and J. N. Sofos. 1993. Methodology for measuring malonaldehyde as a product of lipid peroxidation in muscle tissues: A review. *Meat Science* 35(2):145–169.

Ramos, A., B. Poolman, H. Santos, J. S. Lolkema, and W. N. Konings. 1994. Uniport of anionic citrate and proton consumption in citrate metabolism generates a proton motive force in *Leuconostoc oenos*. *Journal of Bacteriology* 176(16):4899–4905.

Rao, A. V., N. Shiwnarain, and I. Maharaj. 1989. Survival of microencapsulated *Bifidobacterium pseudolongum* in simulated gastric and intestinal juices. *Canadian Institute of Food Science and Technology Journal* 22(4):345–349.

Rautava, S., H. Arvilommi, and E. Isolauri. 2006. Specific probiotics in enhancing maturation of IgA responses in formula-fed infants. *Pediatric Research* 60(2):221–224.

Reddy, I. M., N. K. D. Kella, and J. E. Kinsella. 1988. Structural and conformational basis of the resistance of β-lactoglobulin to peptic and chymotryptic digestion. *Journal of Agricultural and Food Chemistry* 36(4):737–741.

Reid, G., D. Beuerman, C. Heinemann, and A. W. Bruce. 2001. Probiotic Lactobacillus dose required to restore and maintain a normal vaginal flora. *FEMS Immunology and Medical Microbiology* 32(1):37–41.

Reid, A. A., C. P. Champagne, N. Gardner, P. Fustier, and J. C. Vuillemard. 2007. Survival in food systems of *Lactobacillus rhamnosus* R011 microentrapped in whey protein gel particles. *Journal of Food Science* 72(1):M031–037.

Rokka, S. and P. Rantamäki. 2010. Protecting probiotic bacteria by microencapsulation: Challenges for industrial applications. *European Food Research and Technology* 231(1):1–12.

Rosenfeldt, V., K. F. Michaelsen, M. Jakobsen, et al. 2002. Effect of probiotic *Lactobacillus* strains in young children hospitalized with acute diarrhea. *Pediatric Infectious Disease Journal* 21(5):411–416.

Rosenfeldt, V., E. Benfeldt, N. H. Valerius, A. Pærregaard, and K. F. Michaelsen. 2004. Effect of probiotics on gastrointestinal symptoms and small intestinal permeability in children with atopic dermatitis. *Journal of Pediatrics* 145(5):612–616.

Ross, G. R., C. Gusils, and S. N. Gonzalez. 2008. Microencapsulation of probiotic strains for swine feeding. *Biological & Pharmaceutical Bulletin* 31(11):2121–2125.

Ruas-Madiedo, P., J. Hugenholtz, and P. Zoon. 2002. An overview of the functionality of exopolysaccharides produced by lactic acid bacteria. *International Dairy Journal* 12(2–3):163–171.

Rudolph, A. S. and J. H. Crowe. 1985. Membrane stabilization during freezing: The role of two natural cryoprotectants, trehalose and proline. *Cryobiology* 22(4):367–377.

Saarela, M., I. Virkajarvi, H. L. Alakomi, et al. 2005. Influence of fermentation time, cryoprotectant and neutralization of cell concentrate on freeze-drying survival, storage stability, and acid and bile exposure of *Bifidobacterium animalis* ssp *lactis* cells produced without milk-based ingredients. *Journal of Applied Microbiology* 99(6):1330–1339.

Sabikhi, L., R. Babu, D. K. Thompkinson, and S. Kapila. 2010. Resistance of microencapsulated *Lactobacillus acidophilus* LA1 to processing treatments and simulated gut conditions. *Food and Bioprocess Technology* 3(4):586–593.

Saggioro, A. 2004. Probiotics in the treatment of irritable bowel syndrome. *Journal of Clinical Gastroenterology* 38(6 Suppl.):S104–S106.

Sanderson, G. R. 1990. Gellan gum. In *Food Gels*, ed. P. Harris, pp. 201–233. New York, NY: Elsevier.

Sandoval-Castilla, O., C. Lobato-Calleros, H. S. García-Galindo, J. Alvarez-Ramírez, and E. J. Vernon-Carter. 2010. Textural properties of alginate-pectin beads and survivability of entrapped *Lb. casei* in simulated gastrointestinal conditions and in yoghurt. *Food Research International* 43(1):111–117.

Sandra, S., E. A. Decker, and D. J. McClements. 2008. Effect of interfacial protein cross-linking on the *in vitro* digestibility of emulsified corn oil by pancreatic lipase. *Journal of Agricultural and Food Chemistry* 56(16):7488–7494.

Santivarangkna, C., U. Kulozik, and P. Foerst. 2007. Alternative drying processes for the industrial preservation of lactic acid starter cultures. *Biotechnology Progress* 23(2):302–315.

Sarker, S. A., S. Sultana, G. J. Fuchs, et al. 2005. *Lactobacillus paracasei* strain ST11 has no effect on rotavirus but ameliorates the outcome of nonrotavirus diarrhea in children from Bangladesh. *Pediatrics* 116(2):e221–e228.

Schmidt, G., C. Hertel, and W. P. Hammes. 1999. Molecular characterisation of the dnaK operon of *Lactobacillus sakei* LTH681. *Systematic and Applied Microbiology* 22(3):321–328.

Schultz, M., C. Veltkamp, L. A. Dieleman, et al. 2002. *Lactobacillus plantarum* 299V in the treatment and prevention of spontaneous colitis in interleukin-10-deficient mice. *Inflammatory Bowel Diseases* 8(2):71–80.

Selmer-Olsen, E., T. Sorhaug, S. E. Birkeland, and R. Pehrson. 1999. Survival of *Lactobacillus helveticus* entrapped in Ca-alginate in relation to water content, storage and rehydration. *Journal of Industrial Microbiology & Biotechnology* 23(2):79–85.

Semo, E., E. Kesselman, D. Danino, and Y. D. Livney. 2007. Casein micelle as a natural nano-capsular vehicle for nutraceuticals. *Food Hydrocolloids* 21(5–6):936–942.

Sengül, N., B. Aslím, G. Uçar, et al. 2006. Effects of exopolysaccharide-producing probiotic strains on experimental colitis in rats. *Diseases of the Colon and Rectum* 49(2):250–258.

Shah, N. P. and R. R. Ravula. 2000. Microencapsulation of probiotic bacteria and their survival in frozen fermented dairy desserts. *Australian Journal of Dairy Technology* 55(3):139–144.

Sheil, B., J. McCarthy, L. O'Mahony, et al. 2004. Is the mucosal route of administration essential for probiotic function? Subcutaneous administration is associated with attenuation of murine colitis and arthritis. *Gut* 53(5):694–700.

Sheu, T. Y. and R. T. Marshall. 1993. Microentrapment of lactobacilli in calcium alginate gels. *Journal of Food Science* 58(3):557–561.

Shima, M., Y. Morita, M. Yamashita, and S. Adachi. 2006. Protection of *Lactobacillus acidophilus* from the low pH of a model gastric juice by incorporation in a W/O/W emulsion. *Food Hydrocolloids* 20(8):1164–1169.

Siaterlis, A., G. Deepika, and D. Charalampopoulos. 2009. Effect of culture medium and cryoprotectants on the growth and survival of probiotic lactobacilli during freeze drying. *Letters in Applied Microbiology* 48(3):295–301.

Silva, J., A. S. Carvalho, R. Ferreira, et al. 2005. Effect of the pH of growth on the survival of *Lactobacillus delbrueckii* subsp. *bulgaricus* to stress conditions during spray-drying. *Journal of Applied Microbiology* 98(3):775–782.

Simpson, P. J., C. Stanton, G. F. Fitzgerald, and R. P. Ross. 2005. Intrinsic tolerance of *Bifidobacterium* species to heat and oxygen and survival following spray drying and storage. *Journal of Applied Microbiology* 99(3):493–501.

Siró, I., E. Kápolna, B. Kápolna, and A. Lugasi. 2008. Functional food. Product development, marketing and consumer acceptance—A review. *Appetite* 51(3):456–467.

Smeds, A., P. Varmanen, and A. Palva. 1998. Molecular characterization of a stress-inducible gene from *Lactobacillus helveticus*. *Journal of Bacteriology* 180(23):6148–6153.

Smidsrod, O. and G. Skjak-Braek. 1990. Alginate as immobilization matrix for cells. *Trends in Biotechnology* 8(3):71–78.

Soltan Dallal, M. M., M. H. Yazdi, Z. M. Hassan, et al. 2010. Effect of oral administration of *Lactobacillus acidophilus* on the immune responses and survival of BALB/c mice bearing human breast cancer. *Tehran University Medical Journal* 67(11):753–758.

Song, S. H., Y. H. Cho, and J. Park. 2003. Microencapsulation of *Lactobacillus casei* YIT 9018 using a microporous glass membrane emulsification system. *Journal of Food Science* 68(1):195–200.

Stentz, R., C. Loizel, C. Malleret, and M. Zagorec. 2000. Development of genetic tools for *Lactobacillus sakei*: Disruption of the β-galactosidase gene and use of lacZ as a reporter gene to study regulation of the putative copper ATPase, AtkB. *Applied and Environmental Microbiology* 66(10):4272–4278.

Strasser, S., M. Neureiter, M. Geppl, R. Braun, and H. Danner. 2009. Influence of lyophilization, fluidized bed drying, addition of protectants, and storage on the viability of lactic acid bacteria. *Journal of Applied Microbiology* 107(1):167–177.

Sultana, K., G. Godward, N. Reynolds, R. Arumugaswamy, P. Peiris, and K. Kailasapathy. 2000. Encapsulation of probiotic bacteria with alginate-starch and evaluation of survival in simulated gastrointestinal conditions and in yoghurt. *International Journal of Food Microbiology* 62(1–2):47–55.

Sun, W. Q. and A. C. Leopold. 1997. Cytoplasmic vitrification and survival of anhydrobiotic organisms. *Comparative Biochemistry and Physiology—A Physiology* 117(3):327–333.

Sun, W. Q. and P. Davidson. 1998. Protein inactivation in amorphous sucrose and trehalose matrices: Effects of phase separation and crystallization. *Biochimica et Biophysica Acta (BBA)—General Subjects* 1425(1):235–244.

Sun, W. R. and M. W. Griffiths. 2000. Survival of Bifidobacteria in yogurt and simulated gastric juice following immobilization in gellan-xanthan beads. *International Journal of Food Microbiology* 61(1):17–25.

Sýkora, J., K. Valecková, J. Amlerová, et al. 2005. Effects of a specially designed fermented milk product containing probiotic *Lactobacillus casei* DN-114 001 and the eradication of *H. pylori* in children: A prospective randomized double-blind study. *Journal of Clinical Gastroenterology* 39(8):692–698.

Szajewska, H., M. Kotowska, J. Z. Mrukowicz, M. Armánska, and W. Mikolajczyk. 2001. Efficacy of *Lactobacillus* GG in prevention of nosocomial diarrhea in infants. *Journal of Pediatrics* 138(3):361–365.

Tanaka, A., Y. Fukushima, J. Benyacoub, S. Blum, and H. Matsuda. 2008. Prophylactic effect of oral administration of *Lactobacillus johnsonii* NCC533 (La1) during the weaning period on atopic dermatitis in NC/NgaTnd mice. *European Journal of Dermatology* 18(2):136–140.

Tannock, G. W., K. Munro, H. J. M. Harmsen, G. W. Welling, J. Smart, and P. K. Gopal. 2000. Analysis of the fecal microflora of human subjects consuming a probiotic product containing *Lactobacillus rhamnosus* DR20. *Applied and Environmental Microbiology* 66(6):2578–2588.

Teixeira, P., H. Castro, and R. Kirby. 1996. Evidence of membrane lipid oxidation of spray-dried *Lactobacillus bulgaricus* during storage. *Letters in Applied Microbiology* 22(1):34–38.

Thammavongs, B., D. Corroler, J. M. Panoff, Y. Auffray, and P. Boutibonnes. 1996. Physiological response of *Enterococcus faecalis* JH2-2 to cold shock: Growth at low temperatures and freezing/thawing challenge. *Letters in Applied Microbiology* 23(6):398–402.

Thantsha, M. S., T. E. Cloete, F. S. Moolman, and P. W. Labuschagne. 2009. Supercritical carbon dioxide interpolymer complexes improve survival of B. longum Bb-46 in simulated gastrointestinal fluids. *International Journal of Food Microbiology* 129(1):88–92.

Tuomola, E. M., A. C. Ouwehand, and S. J. Salminen. 1999. The effect of probiotic bacteria on the adhesion of pathogens to human intestinal mucus. *FEMS Immunology and Medical Microbiology* 26(2):137–142.

Tursi, A., G. Brandimarte, G. M. Giorgetti, and M. E. Modeo. 2004. Effect of *Lactobacillus casei* supplementation on the effectiveness and tolerability of a new second-line 10-day quadruple therapy after failure of a first attempt to cure *Helicobacter pylori* infection. *Medical Science Monitor* 10(12):CR662–CR666.

Urbancsek, H., T. Kazar, I. Mezes, and K. Neumann. 2001. Results of a double-blind, randomized study to evaluate the efficacy and safety of Antibiophilus® in patients with radiation-induced diarrhoea. *European Journal of Gastroenterology and Hepatology* 13(4):391–396.

Urbanska, A. M., J. Bhathena, and S. Prakash. 2007. Live encapsulated *Lactobacillus acidophilus* cells in yogurt for therapeutic oral delivery: Preparation and *in vitro* analysis of alginate-chitosan microcapsules. *Canadian Journal of Physiology and Pharmacology* 85(9):884–893.

Ushiyama, A., K. Tanaka, Y. Aiba, et al. 2003. *Lactobacillus gasseri* OLL2716 as a probiotic in clarithromycin-resistant *Helicobacter pylori* infection. *Journal of Gastroenterology and Hepatology* 18(8):986–991.

Van de Guchte, M., P. Serror, C. Chervaux, T. Smokvina, S. D. Ehrlich, and E. Maguin. 2002. Stress responses in lactic acid bacteria. *Antonie van Leeuwenhoek, International Journal of General and Molecular Microbiology* 82(1–4):187–216.

Vanderhoof, J. A., D. B. Whitney, D. L. Antonson, T. L. Hanner, J. V. Lupo, and R. J. Young. 1999. *Lactobacillus* GG in the prevention of antibiotic-associated diarrhea in children. *Journal of Pediatrics* 135(5):564–568.

Verdú, E. F., P. Bercík, G. E. Bergonzelli, et al. 2004. *Lactobacillus paracasei* normalizes muscle hypercontractility in a murine model of postinfective gut dysfunction. *Gastroenterology* 127(3):826–837.

Villarruel, G., D. M. Rubio, F. Lopez, et al. 2007. Saccharomyces boulardii in acute childhood diarrhoea: A randomized, placebo-controlled study. *Acta Paediatrica, International Journal of Paediatrics* 96(4):538–541.

Walker, D. C., H. S. Girgis, and T. R. Klaenhammer. 1999. The groESL chaperone operon of *Lactobacillus johnsonii*. *Applied and Environmental Microbiology* 65(7):3033–3041.

Wang, M. F., H. C. Lin, Y. Y. Wang, and C. H. Hsu. 2004. Treatment of perennial allergic rhinitis with lactic acid bacteria. *Pediatric Allergy and Immunology* 15(2):152–158.

Weissbrodt, J. and B. Kunz. 2007. Influence of hydrocolloid interactions on their encapsulation properties using spray-drying. *Minerva Biotecnologica* 19(1):27–32.

Whorwell, P. J., L. Altringer, J. Morel, et al. 2006. Efficacy of an encapsulated probiotic *Bifidobacterium infantis* 35624 in women with irritable bowel syndrome. *American Journal of Gastroenterology* 101(7):1581–1590.

Wildt, S., L. K. Munck, L. Vinter-Jensen, et al. 2006. Probiotic treatment of collagenous colitis: A randomized, double-blind, placebo-controlled trial with *Lactobacillus acidophilus* and *Bifidobacterium animalis* subsp. *lactis*. *Inflammatory Bowel Diseases* 12(5):395–401.

Wolff, E., B. Delisle, G. Corrieu, and H. Gibert. 1990. Freeze-drying of Streptococcus thermophilus: A comparison between the vacuum and the atmospheric method. *Cryobiology* 27(5):569–575.

Xiao, S. D., D. Z. Zhang, H. Lu, et al. 2003. Multicenter, randomized, controlled trial of heat-killed *Lactobacillus acidophilus* LB in patients with chronic diarrhea. *Advances in Therapy* 20(5):253–260.

Yadav, H., S. Jain, and P. R. Sinha. 2007. Antidiabetic effect of probiotic dahi containing *Lactobacillus acidophilus* and *Lactobacillus casei* in high fructose fed rats. *Nutrition* 23(1):62–68.

Yao, A. A., I. Coulibaly, G. Lognay, M. L. Fauconnier, and P. Thonart. 2008. Impact of polyunsaturated fatty acid degradation on survival and acidification activity of freeze-dried *Weissella paramesenteroides* LC11 during storage. *Applied Microbiology and Biotechnology* 79(6):1045–1052.

Yoshida, Y., T. Seki, H. Matsunaka, et al. 2010. Clinical effects of probiotic *Bifidobacterium breve* supplementation in adult patients with atopic dermatitis. *Yonago Acta Medica* 53(2):37–45.

Zárate, G., V. Santos, and M. E. Nader-Macias. 2007. Protective effect of vaginal *Lactobacillus paracasei* CRL 1289 against urogenital infection produced by *Staphylococcus aureus* in a mouse animal model. *Infectious Diseases in Obstetrics and Gynecology* 2007: 1–6, Article ID 48358. doi: 10.1155/2007/48358.

Zink, R., C. Walker, G. Schmidt, M. Elli, D. Pridmore, and R. Reniero. 2000. Impact of multiple stress factors on the survival of dairy lactobacilli. *Sciences des Aliments* 20(1):119–126.

Zocco, M. A., L. Z. Dal Verme, F. Cremonini, et al. 2006. Efficacy of *Lactobacillus* GG in maintaining remission of ulcerative colitis. *Alimentary Pharmacology and Therapeutics* 23(11):1567–1574.

18 Application of Radio Frequency for Military Group Ration Food Package

K. Luechapattanaporn, Y. Wang, J. Wang, J. Tang, L.M. Hallberg, and C.P. Dunne

CONTENTS

18.1 INTRODUCTION

At present, conventional retort heating is generally used to sterilize commercially packaged food. With this method, the heat transfer in solid and semisolid foods is governed by slow conduction heating resulting in severe overheating at the periphery of the container. Dielectric heating, including microwave and radio frequency (RF) heating, offers the potential for quickly heating solid and semisolid foods. Dielectric heating generates heat volumetrically throughout a food product rather than relying on the heat conduction. Thus, dielectric heating can potentially result in less quality (color, texture) degradation of sterilized food.

RF and microwave heating is used extensively in food industries, mainly for drying food ingredients, thawing, and postbaking of biscuits (Tang et al., 2005). The use of dielectric heating at high temperatures for sterilization is still in an early stage of development. According to Electromagnetic Compatibility (EMC) regulations, industrial, scientific, and medical bands for RF heating are standardized at 13.56, 27.12, and 40.68 MHz, respectively. There are two bands standardized for use in microwave application in the United States, that is, 915 and 2450 MHz. The high wavelength in free space, 11 m at 27.12 MHz compared to only 12 cm at 2450 MHz for microwave heating (Rowley, 2001), allowed RF energy to have deeper penetration into the heated food than microwave power.

Thermal processing based on RF is, therefore, suitable for large food tray such as 6-lb capacity military ration polymeric tray.

Scrambled eggs are one of the most popular breakfast entrées in the United States and shelf-stable scrambled eggs are of great interest to the U.S. Army. Due to the heat sensitivity of proteins, fats, and carotenoids in fresh eggs, elements of quality such as color, flavor, and texture are degraded by traditional retort methods at high temperature and pressure. Conductive heat transfer is the dominant thermal mechanism of solid foods in conventional retort heating, and relies on thermally induced vibration between molecules. This is often slower than convective heat transfer in liquid foods. Sterilization value (F_0) and cook value (C_{100}) are commonly used to describe the effect of heat on food in terms of microbiological safety and quality, respectively. Due to the differences in the z values between F_0 and C_{100}, the rate of nutrient destruction is less temperature dependent than that of microbial inactivation. Food heated at higher temperatures requires shorter time to obtain the designated sterilization value (i.e., $F_0 = 4.0$) with smaller cook values. High-temperature-short-time (HTST) processing is preferred to produce safe food while maintaining food quality. However, HTST processes for semisolid and solid food are difficult to achieve with conventional retort heating because of the slow conductive heat transfer within the foods.

Rapid and relatively uniform heating in solid and semisolid food can be achieved by RF heat because RF energy is dissipated through the products based on rapid reversal of individual molecule polarization rather than conductive heating from the surface to the center of the food as found in conventional retorting. RF heating has the potential to improve food quality and reduce surface overheating (Rowley, 2001; Wang et al., 2003b).

A common problem reported frequently in hard-cooked whole eggs and in scrambled eggs is greenish-black discoloration (Tinkler and Soar, 1920; Baker et al., 1967; Gravani, 1969; Wesley et al., 1982; Song and Cunningham, 1985; Cotterill, 1995). In boiled whole eggs, discoloration often occurs at the interface between the yolk and the albumen. This is caused by ferrous sulfide (FeS), a product of the reaction between iron (Fe) from the yolk and hydrogen sulfide (H_2S) from the albumen. The discoloration can extend through the whole yolk if the center of the yolk is overheated. Green color is not observed in egg yolks that were heated and cooled rapidly. After heating, egg yolks become slightly more alkaline, which is a favorable condition for the formation of ferrous sulfide. The amount of discoloration area seemed to be dependent on the heating time (Tinkler and Soar, 1920; Gravani, 1969). Carbon dioxide was also observed to be released rapidly from the albumen during heating, resulting in an increase in pH (Gravani, 1969). However, discoloration may disappear during storage because ferrous sulfide is easily oxidized (Baker et al., 1967). Similar discoloration can be observed in scrambled eggs for the same reason as in the whole eggs (Wesley et al., 1982). Greenish-black discoloration can be prevented by one of the two common methods: (1) chelating the iron to prevent the formation of green color from ferrous sulfide and (2) lowering the pH to create an acidic condition that is unfavorable for ferrous sulfide formation (Cotterill, 1995). Adding chelating agents such as salts of ethylenediaminetetraacetic acid (EDTA) can prevent discoloration in egg products. For example, adding 0.015% disodium ethylenediaminetetraacetic acid (Na_2EDTA) prevented the green-gray color development effectively in retorted liquid whole eggs (Song and Cunningham, 1985). Citric acid is commonly used to lower the pH to about 6.8 (Cotterill, 1995). Citric acid (0.17%) has been shown to prevent the green-gray discoloration in cooked liquid whole eggs; however, there was a significant change of flavor when compared to the control (Gossett and Baker, 1981).

Another major problem in the texture of scrambled eggs is an undesirable change of three-dimensional gel structure (O'Brien et al., 1982) caused by syneresis. Applications of heat denature native egg proteins from helical conformation to long-chain protein molecules (Golding, 1963). At their isoelectric point, proteins aggregate when heated and form a course network with large pores, low gel strength, and minimal water binding. A more uniform gel matrix with high gel strength and better water binding is formed at a pH greater than the isoelectric point (Woodward and Cotterill, 1986). Attractive and repulsive forces within these molecules form a three-dimensional network which increases gel rigidity (Ferry, 1948; Golding, 1963). The addition of modified tapioca starch, sodium carboxymethylcellulose (CMC), and xanthan gum can increase water-holding capacity of frozen omelets (O'Brien et al., 1982). Syneresis of scrambled eggs stored on a steam table can be prevented by the addition of 0.25% each of modified corn starch and hydroxypropylcellulose (Wesley et al., 1982).

There is a current need for fresh-cook-like shelf-stable egg products for military combat rations. A variety of egg products have been introduced by conventional retort heating, but color, flavor, and texture have been degraded by processing. Novel thermal processes that can shorten the heating time and produce better-tasting shelf-stable products are being investigated for combat ration development. RF heating has a potential of rapid heating, but egg formulations for RF heating will need to be optimized to achieve certain lethality level and maintain food quality.

Preliminary research on RF-sterilized scrambled eggs resulted in greenish-black discoloration and undesirable syneresis after processing and storage. The objective of this study was to determine the effects of ingredients, packaging, and pre-fill-cook methods on scrambled egg quality to select an acceptable combination for RF sterilization. Since there was no prior experimental information on the effect of high temperature (121°C) on the quality of egg products, preliminary results on retort-heated eggs were included for complete understanding of heating effect on the egg quality.

18.2   MATERIALS AND METHODS

Our ultimate goal was to develop an acceptable scrambled egg formulation suitable for RF processing of the product in 6-lb capacity combat group-ration polymeric trays. Our current 27 MHz pilot-scale RF sterilization system allows processing of only one 6-lb capacity tray at a time. A prescreening study was thus conducted using a conventional pilot-scale retort (Design RDSW3; Lee Metal Products Co., Philipsburg, PA) to evaluate the influence of citric acid and water-holding substances (e.g., gums and starches) on sterilized-scrambled egg quality. The larger capacity of the conventional retort allowed us to evaluate the influence of high temperatures on egg quality of different formulations with the number of units required of each variable for statistical significance. RF heating of a 6-lb capacity polymeric tray generally requires about 30 min process time to provide a sterilization value (F_0) of ~6 min, about 1/3 of the time needed to achieve the same F_0 when using conventional retort methods (Wang et al., 2003b). For the prescreening study, we chose small capacity polymeric trays (7-oz, $100 \times 140 \times 25$ mm with 3 mm thick wall: Rexam™ Union, MO) and aluminum cans (8-Z short can: 211×300), with processing times about 30 and 50 min, respectively. The results from this prescreening study, thus, represent a conservative estimation of the effect of RF processing on egg quality. RF tests with the selected formation following the prescreening study served to confirm the results of the selection of formulations.

18.3   PREPARATION OF SCRAMBLED EGGS

The prescreening of scrambled eggs formulation using a retort is done. Scrambled eggs in this study were prepared from frozen pasteurized liquid whole eggs which came with 0.15% citric acid from the manufacturer (Michael Foods Egg Products Co., MN). Citric acid was added to prevent discoloration. The amounts of eggs, modified potato starch: a mixture of one-half PenPlus 40™ and one-half PenBind 100™ (Penford Food Ingredients, Co., Englewood, CO), and citric acid were varied in four formulations as shown in Table 18.1. Additional ingredients were 20% water, 2.98% vegetable oil, and 0.59% salt (%wb). The mixture was scrambled on a stainless-steel griddle at 135°C with no additional oil added on the surface until a cohesive structure was established but was not brown. The maximum amount of citric acid should not be greater than 0.17% due to the undesirable sour taste at that level (Gossett and Baker, 1981). The pH of sterilized-scrambled eggs should be in the range of 6.8–7.1 to prevent discoloration (Ziegler et al., 1971; Wesley et al., 1982). Both small-capacity polymeric trays and aluminum cans were filled immediately after precooking with 200 g

TABLE 18.1

Ingredients Used in Different Formulations in the Prescreening Study

	Ingredients (%wb)		
Formulation	Liquid Eggs	Starch	Citric Acid
1	75.28	1	0.15
2	75.43	1	0.11
3	76.28	0	0.15
4	76.43	0	0.11

of either 15% precooked-scrambled eggs and 85% liquid egg mixture to try to simulate the scramble effect, yet have a pumpable fill, or 100% precooked-scrambled eggs. An RTD (resistance temperature detector) thermocouple was placed in the geometric center of the containers, secured, and used to monitor the temperature of the product during heating. The packaged scrambled eggs were heated to reach the desired sterilization value (F_0) of ~4.0 min.

Formulation 1 with 100% precooking was selected for further study. Different amounts and types of water-holding substances such as 0.5–1.0% modified waxy corn starch (PenCling® 570, Penford Food Ingredients, Co., Englewood, CO), 0.5–0.75% carrageenan type J (Genu®, CP Kelco Inc., San Diego, CA), 0.2–0.25% high-acyl gellan gum (Kelcogel®LT100, CP Kelco Inc., San Diego, CA), 0.1–0.25% xanthan gum (Keltrol® RD, CP Kelco Inc., San Diego, CA), and 0.05–0.1% guar gum (Sigma Aldrich, Inc., St Louis, MO) were used to reduce syneresis.

18.4 QUALITY MEASUREMENT

After storage for 1 week at 4°C, elements of quality in the processed scrambled eggs were measured. The samples in the original containers were equilibrated to 20°C overnight before measurement.

pH measurement. A pH meter (Accumet Portable pH meter AP5, Fisher Scientific, Houston, TX) was used to measure the pH of the liquid from syneresis. The pH of scrambled eggs was measured by a flat-surface pH electrode (Corning Flat Surface Combination, Nova Analytics Co., MA).

Amount of syneresis. The amount of liquid from syneresis in the product was collected and weighed. The data are presented as the percent of egg weight:

$$\%\text{Syneresis} = \frac{\text{syneresis (g)}}{\text{sample (g)}} \times 100 \qquad (18.1)$$

Color measurement. CIELAB color scales were used to quantify the color of scrambled eggs in terms of the degree of lightness (L*), ranging from zero for black and 100 for perfectly white, the degree of redness or greenness (+/–a*), and the degree of yellowness or blueness (+/–b*) (Giese, 2003). Color parameters (L*, a*, b*) were measured using a Minolta colorimeter (Minolta Spectrophotometer CM-2002; Minolta Camera Co. Ltd., Japan). The measurements were conducted in triplicate.

Texture measurement. Texture profile analysis (TPA) was used to imitate the action of the jaw by compressing a bite-size piece of food two times (Bourne 2002). Scrambled eggs were cut into cylinders with a diameter of 2.5 cm and a thickness of 1 cm using a stainless-steel tube and a wire cutter. In a double compression test, the samples were pressed to 50% of their original height (Woodward and Cotterill, 1986) by a flat cylindrical aluminum probe at a cross-head speed of 1 mm/s, then allowed to rebound for 12 s and compressed again, using a TA.XT2 Texture Analyzer

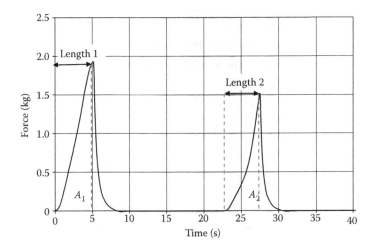

FIGURE 18.1   A typical instrumental texture profile analysis curve for scrambled eggs.

(Texture Technologies Corp., Scarsdale, NY/Stable Micro Systems, Godalming, Surrey, UK) equipped with a 5-kg load cell. The results are reported as the means of duplicate tests. Hardness, springiness, and cohesiveness were computed from a TPA curve and were defined as follows (Bourne, 2002):

- *Hardness:* the maximum height of the force peak on the first compression cycle (g)
- *Springiness:* the distance the sample was compressed during the second compression to the peak force (length 2 in Figure 18.1) divided by the initial sample height (length 1 in Figure 18.1)
- *Cohesiveness:* the ratio of the positive force areas under the first and second compressions (A_2/A_1 in Figure 18.1)

Statistical analysis was performed using Statistical Analysis System software (SAS version 8.1, SAS Institute Inc., Cary, NC). An analysis of variance (ANOVA) method was used to analyze data in color and texture measurements. Differences were considered significant when p values were <0.05. When the ANOVA method showed one or more significant differences, the least significant difference (LSD) method was used to separate treatment means.

18.5   PROCESSING SCRAMBLED EGGS WITH RF HEATING

Based on the results obtained from chemical and physical measurements in the prescreening studies, we selected the best formulation for further studies (Table 18.2). RF heating tests were conducted to ensure that the selected formulation can be processed in the 6-lb capacity polymeric trays to yield an acceptable product.

One of the most important parameters related to this form of dielectric heating, which includes microwave (100–30,000 MHz) and RF (10–100 MHz) processing, is the dielectric property of the food products. Dielectric properties govern how foods react to alternating electric field, at a molecular level, to generate heat. At microwave and higher frequencies, dipolar relaxation (dipolar molecules align within electric field) of water molecules often dominates in dielectric heating. Relaxation effects of water molecules are usually less important at low frequencies (Wang, 2002). Below 200 MHz, the gross ionic conductivity (σ) plays a significant role in dissipating electromagnetic fields, and the loss factor of a material (an ability to dissipate energy in an applied electric field) is directly related to its conductivity (Equation 18.2) (Wang, 2002).

TABLE 18.2

Ingredients of the Selected Formulation for RF Sterilization

Ingredients	Amount (%)
Liquid whole eggs	75.08
Water	20.00
Vegetable oil	2.98
Salt	0.59
Citric acid	0.15
Corn starch	1.00
Xanthan gum	0.10
Guar gum	0.10

$$\sigma = \omega \varepsilon_0 \varepsilon_r'' = 2\pi f \varepsilon_0 \varepsilon_r'' \tag{18.2}$$

where f is the temporal frequency and ω is the radian frequency, which are related by $\omega = 2\pi f$, ε_0 is permittivity related to free space (vacuum); $\varepsilon_0 = 8.854 \times 10^{-12}$ Farads/m, and ε_r'' is the loss factor.

The conductivity of selected formulation was measured. The loss factor (ε_r'') of a material can be expressed in Equation 18.3 (Wang et al., 2003a).

$$\varepsilon_r'' = \varepsilon_d'' + \varepsilon_\sigma'' \tag{18.3}$$

where ε_d'' is relative dipole loss and ε_σ'' is relative ionic loss.

Since ionic conductivity plays an important role below 200 MHz, ionic loss (ε_σ'') can be used to calculate loss factors without considering relative dipole loss (ε_d'') though it is important in microwave frequencies (915 and 2450 MHz).

The power dissipation of dielectric heating in the radio frequency range can be estimated from the food conductivity (Wang, 2002).

$$P_{ave} = \sigma E^2 \tag{18.4}$$

where P_{ave} is the averaged power dissipation per unit volume (W/m^3), σ is the ionic conductivity (S/m), and E is the electric field intensity (V/m).

In order to develop a suitable scrambled egg formulation for RF heating, the electrical conductivity was used as an approximation for averaged power dissipation of the food. The higher the power the less time was needed to achieve the HTST process. Electrical conductivity of the liquid egg mixtures was determined using a conductivity meter (CON-500, Cole-Parmer Instrument Co., Vernon Hills, IL).

Scrambled eggs (2726 g) were prepared based on the selected formulation (Table 18.3) and placed in a tray before heating with a 6-kW pilot-scale RF system developed at Washington State University (Figure 18.2) based on a 27.12-MHz RF generator (COMBI 6-S; Strayfield Fastran, UK) and a water-conditioning system. Detailed information about this RF sterilization system can be found in Luechapattanaporn et al. (2004). The circulating water temperature was controlled by the conditioning system to match the temperature of the heated food during the RF process. This was to reduce localized heating at the interface between the food package and the water in the RF sterilization chamber. For that reason and from preliminary results, the conductivity of the immersion water was adjusted to ~60 µS/cm at 21°C. In previous studies (Wang et al., 2003b), a chemical marker was used to determine hot and cold spots within a package. Based on

TABLE 18.3

Scrambled Egg Quality in 7-oz Capacity Trays and Cans after Storage for 1 Week

Formulation	Mixture	Discolored Area (%)	Syneresis (%)	pH Scrambled Eggs	Syneresis
Freshly cooked		0	0	7.35	—
Trays					
1	a[a]	0	5.58	7.08	6.72
	b[b]	0	1.46	7.46	6.72
2	a	5	5.41	7.32	6.91
	b	0	0.98	7.55	7.25
3	a	5	8.2	7.04	6.75
	b	0	3.22	7.36	6.75
4	a	30	10.53	7.37	6.97
	b	6	6.21	7.17	7.03
Cans					
1	a[a]	0	0	6.91	—
	b[b]	0	0	7.2	—
2	a	0	0	7.17	—
	b	0	0	7.49	—
3	a	0	0	6.95	—
	b	0	0	7.21	—
4	a	0	0	7.17	—
	b	0	0	7.3	—

[a] a = 100% precooked-scrambled eggs filled in the packages.

[b] b = 15% precooked-scrambled eggs with 85% liquid egg mixture in the packages.

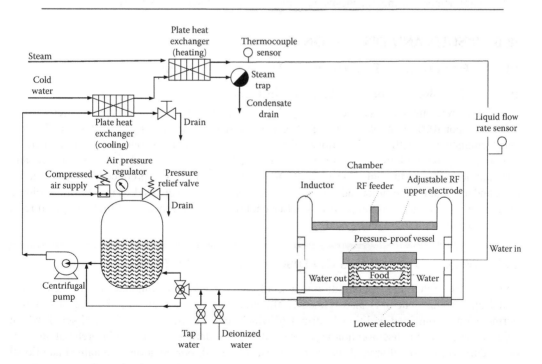

FIGURE 18.2 Simplified schematic diagram of the Washington State University RF sterilization unit with a water-circulating system.

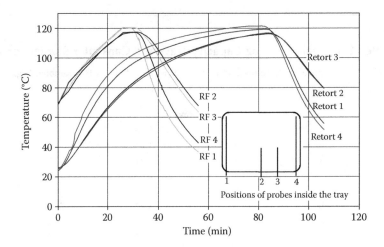

FIGURE 18.3 Time–temperature profile for scrambled eggs thermally processed by RF and retort heating.

this determination, four fiber optic sensors (FISO Technologies, Inc., Quebec, Canada) were inserted into four different locations (Figure 18.3). Thermal processing was conducted based on the temperature profile of the fiber optic probe at the cold spot to reach a sterilization value (F_0) of ~4.0 min.

Scrambled eggs (2726 g) were also processed in a stationary water retort to reach the same F_0 as that of the RF-heated scrambled eggs. A comparison of scrambled egg quality was made between RF- and retort-heated scrambled eggs.

After sterilization, scrambled eggs were measured for pH, color parameters (L*, a*, b*), and texture parameters (hardness, cohesiveness, and springiness) using a TPA test.

18.6   RESULTS AND DISCUSSION

18.6.1   Effect of High Temperature on Scrambled Egg Quality

18.6.1.1   Discoloration of Scrambled Eggs in Trays

Discolored area, amount of syneresis, and pH of scrambled eggs in trays or cans are presented in Table 18.3. For 100% precooked-scrambled eggs processed in 7-oz capacity trays, Table 18.3 shows that formulation 1 (with both additional citric acid and 1% modified potato starch) yielded no discoloration, followed by formulation 2 (without additional citric acid and with starch) and formulation 3 (with additional citric acid but without starch), which both produced 5% of discolored area, and formulation 4 (without additional citric acid or starch) which resulted in 30% of discolored area. There was no undesirable sour taste after cooking and being heated at high temperature in scrambled eggs with 0.15% citric acid.

18.7   EFFECT OF SYNERESIS ON DISCOLORATION IN TRAYS

The results indicated that discoloration is not only influenced by the amount of citric acid in the initial egg mixture but it is also related to the amount of syneresis after thermal processing. Formulation 1 contained additional citric acid which lowered the pH of eggs, and starch which reduced syneresis. No discoloration was observed. In formulation 2, which had starch but no additional citric acid, a small area of discoloration was observed. Formulation 3 contained additional citric acid but no starch, and a greater amount of syneresis was observed. The difference between the pH of scrambled eggs (~7.04) and the syneresis (~6.75) indicated that either the citric acid was

TABLE 18.4

Color and Texture Parameters of Scrambled Eggs in 7-oz Capacity Trays

Formulation	L*	a*	b*	Hardness (g)	Springiness (Ratio)	Cohesiveness (Ratio)
			100% Precooked			
Freshly cooked	84.17 ± 2.04[a]	4.00 ± 0.26[a]	38.76 ± 1.22[a]	N/A[1]	N/A	N/A
1	79.5 ± 0.68[b]	1.94 ± 0.18[b]	31.2 ± 2.48[a]	2378.87 ± 137.39[ab]	0.93 ± 0.02[a]	0.64 ± 0.02[b]
2	74.69 ± 1.80[c]	1.04 ± 0.36[c]	27.66 ± 2.25[c]	2285.19 ± 152.75[b]	0.92 ± 0.01[a]	0.67 ± 0.00[b]
3	79.88 ± 0.99[b]	2.26 ± 0.24[b]	31.80 ± 1.52[b]	3486.74 ± 374.09[a]	0.91 ± 0.00[a]	0.75 ± 0.01[a]
4	69.10 ± 1.91[d]	1.36 ± 0.36[c]	23.08 ± 1.46[d]	3334.73 ± 401.64[ab]	0.90 ± 0.01[a]	0.74 ± 0.01[a]
			15% Precooked			
Freshly cooked	84.17 ± 2.04[a]	4.00 ± 0.26[a]	38.76 ± 1.22[a]	N/A[1]	N/A	N/A
1	81.79 ± 2.07[bc]	1.17 ± 0.07[b]	32.91 ± 1.66[a]	994.89 ± 40.35[a]	0.77 ± 0.01[a]	0.51 ± 0.01[c]
2	81.18 ± 2.19[c]	1.33 ± 0.10[b]	30.21 ± 1.29[b]	984.19 ± 64.49[a]	0.83 ± 0.01[a]	0.52 ± 0.02[c]
3	84.89 ± 0.25[a]	1.09 ± 0.03[b]	27.78 ± 2.42[c]	964.11 ± 100.11[a]	0.78 ± 0.05[a]	0.60 ± 0.02[b]

Note: Values within a column having the same superscript are not significantly different ($p \geq 0.05$, least significant difference test).

[1] Freshly cooked eggs could not be fractioned into portions that allowed repeatable TPA measurements.

dissociated from the eggs to the syneresis or the citric acid was effectively buffered in the eggs resulting in the higher pH of the eggs. Because alkalinity favors the formation of ferrous sulfide (Song and Cunningham, 1985), the discoloration occurred.

Table 18.4 shows that scrambled eggs with added citric acid (formulations 1 and 3) gave a greater degree of lightness (L*), redness (greater a*), and yellowness (greater b*) ($p < 0.05$) than the scrambled eggs without additional citric acid (formulations 2 and 4).

18.8   DISCOLORATION AND SYNERESIS IN CANS

The amount of syneresis was not only affected by the presence of starch but also by different packaging. There was no syneresis and no discoloration observed among all of the formulations of scrambled eggs packaged in cans, even though the pH was as high as 7.5. This might be attributed to the citric acid remaining in the processed-scrambled eggs without syneresis. At high temperatures, a high pressure of ~30 psi was used in the thermal process to prevent the package from bursting. It is possible that the rigid can structure protected the eggs from being compressed under high pressure, which resulted in a smaller amount of syneresis found in the cans. The results indicated that the applied pressure caused syneresis to seep from the scrambled eggs, rather than high temperatures. In addition, the hardness of the eggs packaged in cans was smaller than that in the trays. The protein gel may have been disrupted by reheating during sterilization, resulting in an increase of free water from the protein network, which leads to a rubbery texture (O'Brien et al., 1982).

Scrambled eggs in cans had a more brownish color (smaller L*, greater a*) compared to the same formulations in 7-oz capacity trays. The degree of redness was significantly different between scrambled eggs packaged in cans and trays ($p < 0.05$). Even though the amount of scrambled eggs in both packages was the same, the geometric differences in the packaging resulted in a longer heating time for canned scrambled eggs (57 min) to reach the same sterilization value as the 7-oz capacity trays (30 min).

18.9 EFFECT OF COOKING METHOD ON DISCOLORATION

The cooking method affected the discoloration of scrambled eggs in 7-oz capacity trays. After 1 week of storage, there was a greater area of discoloration observed in trays filled with 100% precooked-scrambled eggs without additional citric acid (Table 18.3), than in trays filled with 15% precooked-scrambled eggs. The difference was attributed to multiple causes, including but not limited to the following two: (1) the stainless-steel griddle used to cook the scrambled eggs resulted in an increase in the percentage of iron in the scrambled eggs (Park and Brittin, 1997), metal ions contributed to the formation of the greenish-black discoloration (Cotterill, 1995) and (2) trays filled with 15% precooked-scrambled eggs yielded less syneresis than trays filled with 100% precooked-scrambled eggs (Table 18.3).

18.10 EFFECT OF FORMULATION AND PROCESS ON SYNERESIS AND TEXTURE OF SCRAMBLED EGGS

Syneresis in eggs was affected by the amount and type of water-holding substances included in the formulation, the cooking method, and the packaging. Adding modified potato starch increased scrambled egg water-holding capacity and reduced the syneresis. In this study, modified potato starch (1%) reduced the amount of syneresis from 10.53% to 5.58% in a tray filled with 100% precooked-scrambled eggs (Table 18.3). The texture profile for a gel is described by hardness, springiness, and cohesiveness. Generally, hardness is correlated to the rupture strength of the egg sample, while springiness (sometimes referred to as elasticity) can be used to represent rubberiness, and cohesiveness is the degree of difficulty to break down a sample (Sanderson, 1990).

The texture parameters of scrambled eggs in 7-oz capacity trays and cans are presented in Tables 18.4 and 18.5. Trays and cans filled with 100% precooked-scrambled eggs without starch (formulations 3 and 4) had greater hardness and cohesiveness than eggs with starch (formulations 1 and 2) ($p < 0.05$), but there was no significant difference in hardness among trays filled with 15% precooked-scrambled eggs.

TABLE 18.5

Color and Texture Parameters of Scrambled Eggs in Cans

Formulation	L*	a*	b*	Hardness (g)	Springiness (Ratio)	Cohesiveness (Ratio)
			100% Precooked			
Freshly cooked	84.17 ± 2.04[a]	4.00 ± 0.26[a]	38.76 ± 1.22[a]	N/A[1]	N/A	N/A
1	77.84 ± 0.88[b]	3.77 ± 0.22[b]	32.28 ± 0.99[b]	1748.75 ± 124.21[c]	0.89 ± 0.01[a]	0.69 ± 0.02[b]
2	74.98 ± 1.28[c]	3.92 ± 0.24[b]	31.02 ± 2.27[b]	1557.73 ± 7.54[c]	0.92 ± 0.05[a]	0.70 ± 0.03[b]
3	74.81 ± 0.81[c]	5.02 ± 0.4[a]	33.37 ± 1.38[b]	2351.47 ± 35.25[a]	1.11 ± 0.00[a]	0.79 ± 0.02[a]
4	77.65 ± 0.18[b]	3.82 ± 0.06[b]	31.63 ± 1.15[b]	2018.11 ± 43.43[b]	1.31 ± 0.32[a]	0.81 ± 0.00[a]
			15% Precooked			
Freshly cooked	84.17 ± 2.04[a]	4.00 ± 0.26[a]	38.76 ± 1.22[a]	N/A[1]	N/A	N/A
1	79.85 ± 2.18[b]	2.46 ± 0.18[c]	29.56 ± 2.49[b]	1007.36 ± 35.90[a]	0.89 ± 0.03[a]	0.49 ± 0.07[a]
2	80.36 ± 0.39[b]	2.89 ± 0.35[b]	30.81 ± 1.33[b]	873.77 ± 8.98[b]	0.85 ± 0.01[a]	0.44 ± 0.01[a]
3	81.23 ± 1.16[b]	2.68 ± 0.06[bc]	32.2 ± 0.74[b]	721.47 ± 39.69[c]	0.88 ± 0.04[a]	0.54 ± 0.01[a]

Note: Values within a column having the same superscript are not significantly different ($p \geq 0.05$, least significant difference test).

[1] Freshly cooked eggs could not be fractioned into portions that allowed repeatable TPA measurements.

TABLE 18.6

Scrambled Egg Quality in 7-oz Capacity Trays with Different Water-Holding Substances after Storage for 1 Week

Type of Water-Holding Substances	Amount (%)	Syneresis (%)	pH		Appearance
			Scrambled Eggs	Syneresis	
Carrageenan type J	0.5–0.75	0	6.90–6.93	—	Exhibit gelatinous syneresis
High-acyl gellan gum	0.2–0.25	0	6.85–6.91	—	Exhibit gelatinous syneresis
Xanthan gum	0.15	5.67	6.97	6.74	Exhibit viscous syneresis after storage

Different types and amounts of water-holding substances were studied to reduce the amount of syneresis after sterilization. The pH, amount of syneresis, and appearance for different types of water-holding substances are presented in Table 18.6. After precooking, there was no gelatinous syneresis observed in scrambled eggs with water-holding substances. However, after sterilization, there was undesirable gelatinous syneresis observed in scrambled eggs prepared with carrageenan gum and high-acyl gellan gum. Even though high-acyl gellan gum forms a gel at temperatures ranging between 70°C and 80°C (Huang et al., 2004), gelatinous syneresis was observed in this study after temperature variation from 121°C to 80°C. Generally, gels are thermally induced three-dimensional polymer networks. The syneresis occurs when the gel is subjected to extreme temperature variations. Combinations of starch and hydrocolloids are usually used to modify texture and reduce syneresis (Sanderson, 1990).

In this study, nongelling hydrocolloids such as xanthan gum and guar gum were used to reduce syneresis. An undesirable viscous syneresis liquid was observed in sterilized-scrambled eggs with 0.15% xanthan gum. The combinations of different modified starch and hydrocolloid were tested. The selected formulation of scrambled eggs for RF sterilization is presented in Table 18.2.

18.11 VERIFICATION OF THE SELECTED FORMULATION WITH RF STERILIZATION

Based on previous results, the addition of citric acid to reach the total amount of 0.15% (wb) was found to be effective in preventing greenish-black discoloration. Sterilized-scrambled eggs with 15% precooked and 85% liquid egg mixture gave a cake-like texture which was found to be undesirable for scrambled eggs. Filling the 6-lb tray with 100% precooked-scrambled eggs was selected as a presterilization method for RF processing.

The conductivity of the selected formulation for the liquid egg mixture was 10.82 mS/cm at 19°C. The loss factor was calculated by Equation 18.2 to be 720 at 27 MHz which is in the optimum RF heating range (~400–900 at 20°C). A time–temperature profile for whey protein gel with a loss factor of 835 at 20°C (Wang et al., 2003a) showed that the heat-up time required for the least heated part to reach the target temperature of 121°C was 30 min as compared to 90 min in a retort (Wang et al., 2003b).

Temperature changes at four different positions within the scrambled eggs (6-lb capacity polymeric tray) during an RF process are shown in Figure 18.3. The RF heat-up time of scrambled eggs to reach 121°C was ~25 min compared to ~70 min for retort heating. There was no greenish-black discoloration and no syneresis observed after RF sterilization. Hardness of RF-heated scrambled eggs as determined by a TPA test was half of that of scrambled eggs prepared by formulation 1 (from 2378 to 928 g).

TABLE 18.7

Color and Texture Parameters of RF-Sterilized Scrambled Eggs

Type of Process	L*	a*	b*	Hardness (g)	Springiness (Ratio)	Cohesiveness (Ratio)
Freshly scrambled eggs	85.92 ± 0.08[a]	2.45 ± 0.16[b]	33.79 ± 1.05[a]	N/A[1]	N/A	N/A
RF-heated scrambled eggs	83.46 ± 2.78[a]	0.95 ± 0.32[c]	28.10 ± 1.29[b]	928.78 ± 90.59[a]	0.82 ± 0.08[a]	0.45 ± 0.02[a]
Retort-heated scrambled eggs	74.12 ± 2.42[b]	6.52 ± 0.72[a]	29.11 ± 1.32[b]	782.40 ± 13.73[a]	0.88 ± 0.05[a]	0.50 ± 0.03[a]

Note: Values within a column having the same superscript are not significantly different ($p \geq 0.05$, least significant difference test).

[1] Freshly cooked eggs could not be fractioned into portions that allowed repeatable TPA measurements.

The comparison of RF- and retort-heated scrambled eggs (Table 18.7) showed significant differences in the degree of lightness and redness. Retort heating produced the darker scrambled eggs. Fresh-cook-like shelf-stable egg products are preferred for military combat rations. There was no significant difference in texture parameters between the two processes. Perhaps subtle texture differences would be detected by sensory mouth feel evaluation.

Even though RF heating has been used extensively in food industries for postbaking of biscuits, drying food ingredients, and thawing meats and fish, the use of RF at high temperatures for sterilization is still in an early stage of development (Tang et al., 2005). Further studies on the design of industrial systems as well as economic studies are needed before this technology can be adopted by the food industry. RF sterilization processing for low-acid food requires FDA approval for application in the United States.

18.12   CONCLUSIONS

Discoloration of sterilized-scrambled eggs can be prevented with the addition of citric acid (0.15%wb) and a combination of different water-holding substances. The color of scrambled eggs heated by RF energy at 27.12 MHz was less degraded (greater L* and smaller a*) than that of retort-heated products. The results from this study can be used for developing sterilized-scrambled eggs as a shelf-stable product for both military and civilian uses. There is a potential to produce heat-sensitive and high-value foods using RF energy not otherwise available.

ACKNOWLEDGMENTS

The authors acknowledge the financial support from the Defense Logistics Agency project CORANET and Washington State University IMPACT Center. They thank Dr. Romeo Toledo of the University of Georgia and Jason Mathews of Michael Foods Egg Products Company for their technical advice.

REFERENCES

Baker, R. C., Darfler, J., Lifshitz, A. 1967. Factors affecting the discoloration of hard-cooked egg yolks. *Poultry Science.* 46, 664–672.

Bourne, M. C. 2002. *Food Texture and Viscosity: Concept and Measurement.* (2nd ed., pp. 182–186). Academic Press, China.

Cotterill, O. J. 1995. Freezing egg products. In *Egg Science and Technology*, ed. W. J. Stadelman and O. J. Cotterill (pp. 265–288). Food Product Press, New York.

Ferry, J. 1948. Protein gels. *Advances in Protein Chemistry*. 4(1), 1–78.

Giese, J. 2003. Color measurement in foods. *Food Technology*. 57(12), 48, 49, 54.

Golding, S. H. 1963. *The effect of rate of heating, final internal temperature, and sugar level on protein gel formation*. [M.S. thesis]. Ithaca, NY: Cornell University. 60 p.

Gossett, P. W, Baker, R. C. 1981. Prevention of the green-gray discoloration in cooked liquid whole eggs. *Journal of Food Science*. 46, 328–331.

Gravani, R. B. 1969. *The formation and prevention of a greenish black discoloration in cooked liquid eggs*. [MSc thesis]. Ithaca, NY: Cornell University. 60 p.

Huang, Y., Singh, P. P, Tang, J., Swanson, B. G. 2004. Gelling temperatures of high acyl gellan as affected by monovalent and divalent cations with dynamic rheological analyses. *Carbohydrate Polymer*. 56, 27–33.

Luechapattanaporn, K., Wang, Y., Wang, J., Tang, J., Hallberg, L. M. 2004. Microbial safety in radio frequency processing of packaged foods. *Journal of Food Science*. 69(7), M201–M206.

O'Brien, S. W., Baker, R. C, Hood, L. F, Liboff, M. 1982. Water-holding capacity and textural acceptability of precooked, frozen, whole-egg omelets. *Journal of Food Science*. 47, 412–417.

Park, J., Brittin, H. C. 1997. Increased iron content of food due to stainless steel cookware. *Journal of American Dietetic Association*. 97(6), 659–661.

Rowley A. T. 2001. Radio frequency heating. In *Thermal Technologies in Food Processing*, ed. P. Richardson (pp. 163–177). Woodhead Publishing, England.

Sanderson, G. R. 1990. Gellan gum. In *Food Gels*, ed. P. Harries (pp. 201–232). Elsevier Science, New York.

Song, I. S., Cunningham, F. E. 1985. Prevention of discoloration in retorted whole egg. *Journal of Food Science*. 50, 841–842.

Tang, J., Wang, Y., Chan, T. V. C. T. 2005. Radio frequency heating in food processing. In *Novel Food Processing Technologies*, eds. G. Barbosa-Cánovas, M. Tapia, and M. P. Cano (pp. 501–524). Marcel Dekker, Boca Raton, Florida.

Tinkler, C. K., Soar, M. C. 1920. The formation of ferrous sulphide in eggs during cooking. *Biochemical Journal*. 14, 114–119.

Wang, Y. 2002. Dielectric properties of foods relevant to RF and microwave pasteurization and sterilization. In *Radio frequency (RF) heating of food*. [DPhil dissertation]. Pullman, Washington: Washington State University. p. 17–45, 62–106.

Wang, Y., Wig. T. D., Tang, J., Hallberg, L. M. 2003a. Dielectric properties of foods relevant to RF and microwave pasteurization and sterilization. *Journal of Food Engineering*. 52, 257–268.

Wang, Y., Wing, T. D., Tang, J., Hallberg, L. M. 2003b. Sterilization of foodstuffs using radio frequency heating. *Journal of Food Science*. 68(2), 539–544.

Wesley, R. D., Rousselle, J. R., Schwan, D. R., Stadelman, W. J. 1982. Improvement in quality of scrambled egg products served from steam table display. *Poultry Science*. 61, 457–462.

Woodward, S. A., Cotterill, O. J. 1986. Texture and microstructure of heat-formed egg white gels. *Journal of Food Science*. 51(2), 333–339.

Ziegler, H. F. Jr., Seeley, R. D., Holland, R. L. 1971. Frozen egg mixture. US Patent. 3,565,638. February 23.

19 Interaction between Food Components and the Innovation Pipeline

Alistair Carr

CONTENTS

19.1 INTRODUCTION

When approaching the subject of interactions of components for a specific functional food, it is imperative that the overall objective for looking at interactions is clearly understood. For this chapter, it is assumed that the overall objective of all functional food innovation is to successfully commercialize a functional food product. In the product development process, there will be many hurdles and decision points and it will not be possible to maximize all options. When faced with such decisions, the developer will need to know which targets are "must haves" and which are "nice to have." To this end, the chapter is structured around the interactions that are key to successfully commercializing functional food innovation.

19.2 WHAT MAKES A FUNCTIONAL FOOD SUCCESSFUL?

The successful launch and subsequent commercial sustainability of new functional foods in the marketplace are largely dependent on perceived-added value of the food. Generally a food which claims some form of health benefit sells at a higher price than foods that do not make such claims. The higher price is in part a necessity due to the inclusion of more costly functional ingredients, and partially due to the need to derive a greater margin to offset the cost of the typically longer development process and thus higher risk that the functional food developer undertakes.

To make functional food claims, a product must comply with the appropriate jurisdictional regulations. For an example of the impact of regulations (in the U.S. setting) on functional food development, the reader can refer to an article by Uzzan et al. (2007). In all cases, the aspect of the food that enables it to be labeled functional must be present at the time of consumption when the product is eaten according to the recommended instructions within the claimed shelf life. Thus, it is important that manufacturers understand how the functional aspect of their food is affected during production, storage, preparation, and consumption.

For many commonplace nutrients, such as vitamins and fats, there is much literature on the impact of ingredient interactions during processing and storage. Most undergraduate food chemistry textbooks describe the mechanisms underpinning degradation of major nutritional components during food manufacture and the importance of considering their degradation kinetics when conducting shelf life studies. Common textbook examples considered include vitamin losses through heat processes, rancidity development, and loss of protein value through Maillard-type reactions.

Curiously however, despite the importance placed on such analyses in undergraduate courses, this most basic step is often not considered in the innovation pipeline for functional foods and ingredients until quite late in the development process.

19.3 WHEN SHOULD AN INNOVATOR IN THE FUNCTIONAL FOOD SPACE CONSIDER PROCESSING?

The focus of functional food innovation has tended to focus on the bio-prospecting for new ingredients and the research that is necessary to find new physiological benefits from compounds or structures and then determine such factors as their dose response, efficacy, and toxicity. Analysis of patent literature suggests that in many cases it is only once the functional side of a compound is established that a researcher/developer then asks the question: "How should the functional compound be delivered to a consumer?" The reason for the relatively late consideration of how exactly a compound might be used in a food is in large part due to where the fundamental bio-prospecting research is conducted: predominantly in pharmaceutical companies and in the biochemistry and associated medical science departments of universities. It is often not until the bioactive functional compound or its use is protected through patent applications that the actual vehicle for commercialization (a food product) is considered.

19.3.1 EVOLUTION OF LACTOFERRIN AS A FUNCTIONAL FOOD INGREDIENT

An interesting example illustrating innovation in the functional food space is the evolution of lactoferrin as a functional food ingredient. This example illustrates how understanding the interactions of a bioactive compound can lead to reduced ingredient manufacturing costs and increased ingredient and product flexibility and use.

A reasonable metric for monitoring the development of commercially useful innovation is by tracking granted patents. For a patent application to proceed to grant, it must not only pass examination for novelty, utility, and obviousness but the granted patent itself represents a significant monetary investment and research investment. For the purpose of this example, I have only considered granted patents in the United States. The data are therefore more likely to approximate the true number of innovations as picking patents from one country avoids artificial inflation of numbers via duplicate family members from other jurisdictions. The data in Figure 19.1 shows the accumulative count of granted U.S. lactoferrin patents as a function of the first patent application filing (i.e., the earliest priority date) associated with each granted patent. The granted patents are linked with the earliest priority date as this is the closest link to the start date of the product development pipeline. The actual concept behind each innovation and the investment decision to initiate and proceed with development would, however, have occurred at least some months and possibly some years earlier. Aside from business and market drivers, the lag between concept and the priority filing would depend on the experiments necessary to prove that the applicants were in full possession of the claimed invention.

The apparent tailing off of patents, post 2005, is likely to be an artifact due to the long lag time between the first patent application filing and the examination and granting of a patent. For a patent

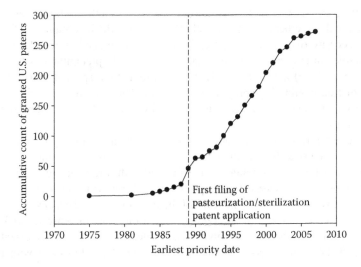

FIGURE 19.1 The accumulative count of granted U.S. lactoferrin patents as a function of the earliest priority date associated with each granted patent.

that has a non-U.S. priority application, national phase entry does not occur until 30 months after filing following which there is a period of several years before examination.

At the time of writing, there have been 273 granted U.S. patents focused on some aspect of commercial opportunities concerned with lactoferrin: from isolation through to specific medical uses (Figure 19.2). In each case, the patent represents a significant research investment.

Aside from perhaps the patents covering analytical techniques and "other," all of the other patented innovations, if commercialized, will require some form of pasteurization or more likely, due to the target consumer typically having a compromised immune system, sterilization before the end product, which may be a functional food or pharmaceutical product, is consumed.

Apart from manufacturing a safe product for the target consumer, the issue of shelf life is key to the financial success of a food product: with a longer shelf life the product is able to be more readily distributed without the need for complicated transportation; additionally, managing stock levels is more important with a short shelf life product due to the increased risk of wastage if product is not sold by the due date. In the case of functional foods, wastage generally results in higher financial losses than nonfunctional foods as functional ingredients are typically more expensive. According to Starling (2008), lactoferrin has sold between 250 and 500 euros per kilogram.

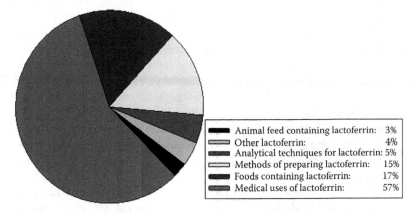

Animal feed containing lactoferrin:	3%
Other lactoferrin:	4%
Analytical techniques for lactoferrin:	5%
Methods of preparing lactoferrin:	15%
Foods containing lactoferrin:	17%
Medical uses of lactoferrin:	57%

FIGURE 19.2 A breakdown of granted lactoferrin patents on the basis of their main inventive IPC code.

Therefore, the success of each of these innovations hinges on the ability to pasteurize or sterilize either the functional ingredient or alternatively the product which contains the functional ingredient. It is this necessity that presents a potential problem to manufacturing lactoferrin-containing products as lactoferrin is known to be heat labile. Lactoferrin precipitates at 65°C/15 min at very low concentrations (0.5%) and in the early days of production, spray drying was not possible as precipitate formation would clog spray-drying nozzles. Thus, the first lactoferrin to be manufactured could only be produced as a sterile ingredient by sterile filtration followed by freeze drying (Dosako et al., 1992).

For the manufacturer, this meant that a product could be made by dry blending to make a powdered product that needs to be rehydrated by the consumer, by sterilizing the food followed by aseptic addition of lactoferrin, or manufacture of a food with sufficient overage addition of lactoferrin to account for processing losses. These options either limit the format of the functional food and thus acceptability to consumers or, in the case of the third option, add cost by increasing the content of an expensive raw ingredient. The preceding limitations thus increase the risk to any product development investment. The key to solving the issues surrounding pasteurization and sterilization has largely been in understanding the interaction of the bioactive with the surrounding environment.

A patent application was filed in 1989 (Dosako et al., 1992) reporting that the heat stability of lactoferrin was dependent on ionic strength. Additionally, Dosako and coworkers claimed that the addition of a desalting operation to an ionic strength of $<10^{-3}$ after isolation (lactoferrin is eluted from ion exchange columns with saline solution) would enable the lactoferrin to be heat treated and to be spray dried.

This innovation created greater flexibility to lactoferrin manufacturing but did not provide a solution for formulators as typical food systems have ionic strengths approaching physiological saline.

The next breakthrough was the work by Tomita et al. (1994) who claimed a novel process for stabilizing lactoferrin against heat denaturation, irrespective of ionic strength, by manipulating the pH of the food system to between 2 and 6. It was this work that first allowed the mixing of ingredients prior to heat treatment and thus offered flexibility in both product processing and format.

The innovations developed after this date (approximately 200 granted U.S. patents) require either access to the claimed technology or a noninfringing work around if the vehicle for commercialization was a functional food and the market of interest was a jurisdiction where the patent was current. Continuing product development and associated clinical trials in the absence of addressing the issue of manufacturing a safe food runs the risk of being prevented, by patents, from commercializing the functional food and hence not generating a return on the development investment.

Since the work by Tomita et al. (1994), there have been several patent applications focused on the manipulation of ingredient interactions to improve lactoferrin heat stability that are yet to be examined or have not been filed in the United States. Horigome et al. (2010) have developed an ingredient-based system to impart thermal stability to lactoferrin over the pH range of 6–9. They reported that the heat stability of lactoferrin, as determined by measuring both the iron-binding capacity and denaturation via SDS-PAGE, is markedly improved by addition of a nucleic acid with a molecular weight in the range of 60–1200 kDa to lactoferrin. From Figure 19.3, very small increases in the nucleic acid content of a formulation can have significant impact on the ability of lactoferrin to retain its iron-binding capability during heat processing. An additional finding by this group (refer Figure 19.4) was that small additions of some metals (copper, zinc, and iron) have a synergistic interaction with the lactoferrin/nucleic acid composition leading to further improvements in heat stability. It is worth noting that Horigome and coworkers did not find any advantage when copper was added in the absence of the nucleic acid.

Other ingredient-based solutions to the problem of heat processing of lactoferrin have been reported by Noriko et al. (2004, 2010). These solutions were not part of the data set reported in Figures 19.1 and 19.2 as patent protection for these innovations was only applied for in Japan.

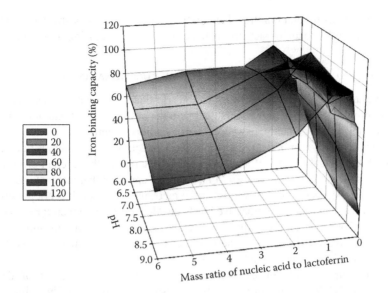

FIGURE 19.3 Contour plot showing the impact of nucleic acid addition and pH manipulation on the iron-binding capacity of lactoferrin that has been heated to 80°C for 5 min. (Adapted from data by Horigome, A. et al. 2010. Substance and composition both capable of imparting heat resistance. US 2010/0310673A1.)

The work of Noriko et al. claims that addition of one of the following ingredients will improve the stability of lactoferrin around neutral pH: soybean polysaccharides, xanthan gum, locust bean gum, carrageenan, sucrose fatty acid ester, a glycerine fatty acid ester, casein sodium, lecithin, pectin, and carboxymethyl cellulose.

In 2008, Fonterra found a pure processing solution that eliminated the dependence on heat treatment for pasteurization and sterilization through the application of high-pressure processing (US20080317823 and US20080166466). In doing so, they also removed the constraint of complex

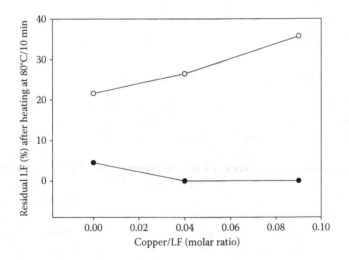

FIGURE 19.4 Impact of copper addition to lactoferrin solutions containing nucleic acid at a weight ratio of 0.1 (○) and 0 (●) on the residual lactoferrin content after heat treatment at 80°C/10 min. (Adapted from data by Horigome, A. et al. 2010. Substance and composition both capable of imparting heat resistance. US 2010/0310673A1.)

ingredient formulations inherent in the other solutions discussed previously. A further advantage of HPP is that if it is applied to an in-pack product, the risk of postprocessing contamination is reduced.

19.3.2 WHAT DO WE MEAN BY NUTRIENT LOSS IN FUNCTIONAL FOODS?

So far we have seen through the example of lactoferrin that ingredient interactions play an important part in stabilizing bioactive ingredients that form the basis of a functional food. However, when we talk about stability what exactly do we mean? For traditional nutrients such as vitamins, we typically use terms such as "vitamin degradation" or "loss of activity" as if there is but one mechanism for deriving physiological benefit. With the increased interest in the interaction of nutrients with physiology over the last 30 years, however, it has become apparent that many nutrients interact on a number of different levels often via several distinct mechanisms. Thus, it is not possible to measure one property and then claim that a bioactive has been "denatured" and therefore of no nutritionally functional value. Conversely, it is equally incorrect to suggest that because formulation and processing has resulted in the maximizing of one functional property, the other benefits the bioactive is known to have will also be maximized.

Returning to our example of lactoferrin, the graphical representation of data tabled by Wakabayashi et al. (2006), shown in Figure 19.5, illustrates the impact of both ingredient interaction, via pH, and thermal processing on three functional properties: iron-binding, antigenicity, and antibacterial properties. In general, these data are in agreement with the method of heat treatment patent of Tomita et al. (1994), that is, irrespective of the heat treatment given, it is more desirable to thermal process lactoferrin under acidic conditions. However, Wakabayashi's group has measured the potency of several lactoferrin targets and we see from Figure 19.5 that it is not possible to maximize all of these properties. For example, increasing the severity of thermal processing from 90°C/5 min to 100°C/min at pH 3 will actually improve the antibacterial properties of lactoferrin relative to the native state whereas for antigenicity and iron binding a significant decrease is observed.

Maximizing the efficacy of the bioactive ingredient for the specific claimed benefit in a functional food does not in itself correlate with a successful product. To be successful, there must be sufficient numbers of customers who want to consume the food product on an ongoing basis for a profitable price. The term "profitable" may not necessarily mean that the individual product makes a profit per se, as is the case for loss-leader-type pricing, but generally the entire business for a company will be better off due to the food's continued sale. For functional foods, the efficacy of the constituent bioactive ingredient is not the sole determining motivation for consumer purchase.

19.3.3 BIOACTIVE INTERACTIONS AND ORGANOLEPTIC PROPERTIES

Like all food products, continued sales are related to the degree to which customers will put up with a product's deficiencies for a perceived benefit. In the general case, food purchasing motivation is the balance between price, organoleptic satisfaction, satisfaction of psychological needs and wants, and satisfaction of perceived health needs and wants. While the satisfaction of health needs and wants is clearly important for functional foods, its optimization at the expense of the other factors may result in an overall decrease in desire to purchase. There have been numerous studies investigating the success factors for the acceptance of functional foods, and sensory has been highlighted as a key factor. For a summary of these studies, the reader is referred to a paper by Verbeke (2006).

The sensory characteristics of a food product may stem from ingredient interactions during the manufacture of the bioactive ingredient, during the manufacture of the food product, throughout the shelf life of the product, or simply through the formulation. It is possible to mitigate sensory issues at each of these stages, but ideally an ingredient solution is preferable as it offers greater flexibility to the food product manufacturer. Ingredient solutions may be either primary (at the point of manufacture) or secondary (manufacturing a new ingredient from the primary bioactive ingredient).

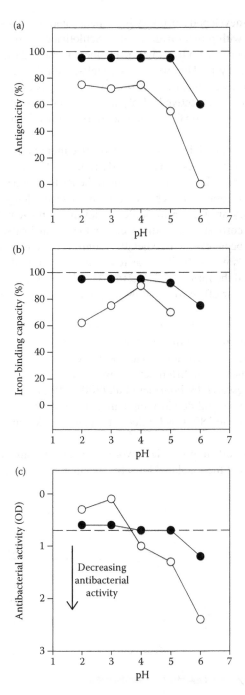

FIGURE 19.5 Impact of heat treatment at 90°C/5 min (●) and 100°C/5 min (○) of lactoferrin over a pH range of 2–6 on antigenicity (a), iron-binding capacity (b), and antibacterial activity (c). All properties were measured at neutral pH. Dashed line in all graphs represents the property of a nonheated lactoferrin solution. (Adapted from data by Wakabayashi, H.; Yamauchi, K.; Takase, M. 2006. *International Dairy Journal*, 16, 1241–1251.)

Schlothauer et al. (2006) developed a primary ingredient solution to solve the issue of bitterness that is commonly associated with protein hydrolysates. Schlothauer's group identified the exact bioactive peptides of interest in a protein hydrolysate and then monitored the release of these peptides as a function of overall hydrolysis. This work was coupled with the sensory analysis of hydrolysate samples and enabled the researchers to discover a unique processing window (see Figure 19.5) allowing the manufacture of a bioactive hydrolysate without the usual concomitant bitterness. This ingredient could be used directly by food manufacturers without the need for further masking technologies (Figure 19.6).

However, it is not always possible to modify a bioactive ingredient at the point of manufacture to achieve improved flavor and in these cases it is desirable to find a secondary ingredient solution wherein the bioactive is combined with other ingredients to produce a new ingredient that has improved attributes. An example of such a case is the omega-3 long-chain polyunsaturated fatty acids which although they are known to be beneficial in the prevention of a variety of diseases, including hypertension, coronary heart disease, rheumatoid arthritis, and Crohn's disease, their consumption has largely been restricted to health recommendations to eat more fish. Attempts have been made to fortify foods with fish oils, so as to avoid the need for drastic changes in diet, but the concentration in foods and the format of the fortified foods has been limited by the inherent "fishy" flavor and the propensity for off-flavors that develop through processing and storage as a result of lipid oxidation.

Common primary ingredient oil solutions such as steam deodorizing techniques to remove undesirable volatiles can be used to minimize undesirable flavors. However, unlike conventional food oils, fish oils contain bioactive fatty acids that have more double bonds and thus are more reactive. Recognition of such compositional differences between standard and bioactive ingredients is important in process design. Research by Fournier et al. (2006, 2007) (refer Figure 19.7) has shown that the use of the standard French oil deodorizing temperature of 220°C results in a significant loss of the bioactive fatty acids (up to 38% loss for docosahexaenoic acid) and suggests modifying process temperatures to 180°C.

While deodorizing fish oils improve the flavor on the day of manufacture, the key to enabling a greater uptake of fish oils or their isolated bioactive compounds such as omega-3 PUFAs in the diet

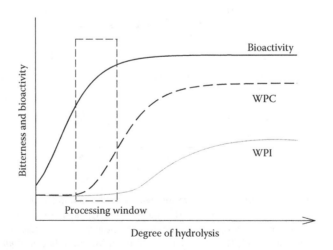

FIGURE 19.6 A schematic plot of ACE-I peptide release relative to bitterness development for whey protein concentrate and whey protein isolate as a function of the degree of hydrolysis. The dashed rectangle denotes a processing window of opportunity where maximum ACE-I peptides are released with minimal bitterness development. (Adapted from Schlothauer, R. et al. 2006. Bioactive whey protein hydrolysate. US7148034.)

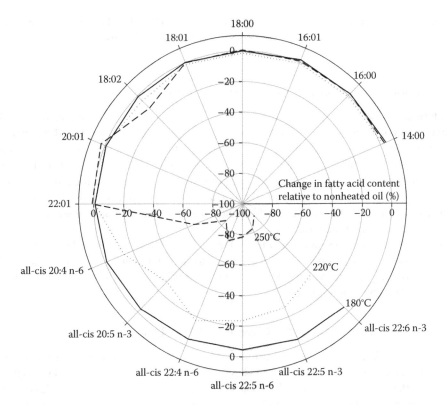

FIGURE 19.7 Effect of deodorizing temperature on fatty acid loss in fish oil. (Drawn from data by Fournier, V. et al. 2006. *European Journal of Lipid Science and Technology*, 108(1), 33–42.)

is to develop an ingredient that also reduces the rate of off-flavors formed during downstream processing by the food formulator and over the intended shelf life of the formulated product.

The main approaches to the shelf life oxidation problem have been through addition of antioxidants to the oil itself (Sims and Fioriti, 1976) and microencapsulation technologies (Drusch and Mannino, 2009; Kralovec et al., 2012). The addition of antioxidants to oil as a sole solution to oxidation limits the ease with which formulators can utilize the ingredient: process lines will require some form of dispersion during which surface area of the oil increases and thus the potential for exposure to oxygen is increased. The risk of oxygen exposure is considerably greater in baked goods, compared to beverages, as there is the additional complication of direct exposure of oils to air. Encapsulation enables multiple ingredient formats from pre-made emulsions to spray-dried powders, which in turn facilitate the usage of the bioactive oils. Encapsulation as the secondary ingredient solution of choice has undergone considerable development over the last couple of decades from relatively simple emulsions using single-component emulsifiers to emulsions that involve multiple components and complex processing (Drusch and Mannino, 2009).

The opportunity to protect expensive bioactive oil does not end with ingredient/emulsion manufacture. A number of workers have reported that the composition of the continuous phase has a potentially significant role to play. Faraji et al. (2004) found that 5% fish oil emulsions stabilized by 1.0% WPI at pH 7.0 washed to remove nonabsorbed protein oxidized at a higher rate than unwashed emulsions with the lipid hydroperoxides levels after 12 days storage at 20°C of approximately 7.5 and 0.1 μmol/mL, respectively. Through addition of protein at levels of 0.05% to washed emulsions, Faraji and coworkers established that oxidation could be significantly reduced and the effect varied with the type of protein: whey protein addition was less effective than casein and soy protein. The mechanism of antioxidant action was shown to be related to the ability to chelate iron and in the case of soy and whey proteins also act as free radical scavengers through their sulfhydryl groups.

19.3.4 FOOD COMPONENT INTERACTIONS AND BIOAVAILABILITY

When formulating a functional food, the impact of ingredient interactions on the bioavailability of the functional compound must be considered. Jeanes et al. (2004) demonstrated that consumption of tocopherol in a capsule format had little or no impact on plasma tocopherol levels unless they were consumed with fat-containing food. Similar results have been reported by Leonard et al. (2004) comparing ingestion of 400 IU of vitamin E as a capsule with a breakfast cereal fortified with a fat emulsion containing only 30 IU of vitamin E. Consumers of the fortified cereal, and therefore concomitantly fat, had a sixfold higher vitamin E absorption despite the level ingested being an order of magnitude lower.

The implication of such synergistic interactions between bioactives and other ingredients during digestion is that there is the opportunity for reduced formulation costs through reduction in the mass of the bioactive ingredient while still maintaining a sufficient benefit to the consumer to fulfill health claim-labeling requirements.

19.3.5 INTERACTIONS OF BIOACTIVE COMPONENTS THAT LEAD TO TOXICITY

One of the main determinants of a consumer's propensity to buy a functional food is trust in the brand and company manufacturing the food. While that trust can be diminished through publicity of evidence that a product does not deliver a stated health claim, a much greater loss of consumer trust is brought about by publicity of sickness, disease, or death that is directly attributable to consumption of a company's product. The impact of the latter is exemplified by the fall from grace of Sanlu Group from their position as one of China's leading manufacturers of infant formula to bankruptcy following melamine adulteration of infant formula that resulted in 1253 cases of illness and two deaths (Chen et al., 2010).

To avoid not delivering a stated health claim, manufacturers should carry out appropriate due diligence, including adequate clinical trials, quality control, shelf life testing, and implementation of good manufacturing practice. Likewise, food poisoning via bacteria or foreign matter contamination can be avoided by utilizing tools such as modern risk management programs, good manufacturing practices, hazard analysis, and critical control point implementation. With all foods, there is a further way in which foods can result in harm to the consumer—formation of toxic compounds either during manufacturing or on storage. These interactions are generally understood for traditional foods: a history of manufacture and consumption has resulted in a knowledge of potential interactions that may cause harm to consumers. With functional foods, however, components not normally associated with each other are often brought together and so the interactions that result may be somewhat more difficult to predict. An interesting example is the formation of biogenic amines in cold-smoked sausage fortified with a prebiotic and/or a probiotic organism (*Lactobacillus sakei*) by Garmiene et al. (2006). In this work, they showed that the concentration, type of biogenic (putrescine, tyramine, and histamine), and the pattern of formation depended on the fortifying component(s). After storage for 35 days, the total biogenic amine concentration was 120.5, 15.97, and 65.21 mg/kg for sausage fortified with prebiotic, probiotic, and both prebiotic and probiotic addition, respectively.

The impact of the formation of toxic by-products will depend on the target consumer. Returning to the example of fish oil, the impact of oxidation on enriched foods can be more than the development of undesirable flavors. Lipid oxidation products are known to be toxic via a range of pathways, including destruction of cellular membranes and mutagenic and carcinogenic effects (Kubow, 1992; Helbock et al., 1993). The effects of oxidation products are of particular importance in infant formulae, which are frequently fortified with long-chain PUFAs, as neonates and some new-born infants are unable to synthesize these developmental essential fatty acids themselves. A recent study by Kleiber et al. (2010) while recognizing potential confounding variables in their study (other lipid-derived peroxides and ascorbic acid) suggests that exposure to H_2O_2 in total parenteral nutritional formulations has consequences for lipid and glucose metabolism later in life.

In addition to the issue of potentially toxic degradation products being formed, there is a concomitant change in the fatty acid profile of the functional food. Not only might the change in individual fatty acid concentrations render health claims associated with a product invalid and the degradation products themselves be potentially toxic to the consumer but the change in the fatty acid profile per se may also be a hazard for the consumer. In a study of lipid oxidation products of enteral formulations, Rufian-Henares et al. (2005) reported an increase in the ratio of omega 6 to omega 3 fatty acids from 6:1 to 6.7, 7.1, and 7.9 at 4°C, 20°C, and 30°C, respectively, after a storage period of 4 weeks. They concluded that on long-term storage, the resulting changes to the fatty acid profile, and of the change to the omega 6 to omega 3 ratio in particular, of the enteral formulations studied would render them more inflammatory and result in increased high-inflammatory stress in patients.

19.4 CONCLUSIONS

This chapter presented some of the key elements that must be considered to ensure the commercial success of a functional food ingredient. There is a strong argument that a developer of functional ingredients, and particularly of new functional ingredients, must consider the format of the food that will finally deliver the ingredient early in the development process irrespective of whether the developer intends to manufacture the functional food per se or merely operate as an ingredient supplier. Failure to understand how a functional ingredient will interact with other components under the environmental conditions encountered during processing and on storage puts at risk the investment that has already been spent through the possibility of a technological hurdle to commercialization. A technological hurdle found after ingredient development will delay the period until the investment is recouped, and in the event that a third party controlling access to a necessary solution may result in reduced margins, restricted food formats, and thus markets or in the worst case, complete restriction from commercializing the ingredient in a food.

The chapter also highlights the importance of getting the basics of process optimization, formulation, and shelf life studies right. To this end, the developer must choose appropriate analytical techniques to measure the bioactive quality that is being claimed for the food. We have seen for instance that a simplistic approach, such as establishing if "denaturation" in the normal sense has occurred, may be of little value in determining the impact on the efficacy of the functional ingredient.

While food safety is an important component for all food manufacturing, it requires a higher degree of consideration in the functional food space as functional foods often contain unusual ingredients or ingredients that are in higher concentrations than are naturally present in their "nonfunctional" counterparts. Thus, there is the possibility of new or unforeseen interactions that may change the composition of the food in a multitude of ways from a mere decrease in the concentration of the bioactive component to the formation of toxic compounds or creation of an imbalance of the nutritional value of the food to the extent that harm is caused to the consumer. Developers should especially be cognizant of functional foods in the medical food space wherein the consumer may be particularly at risk.

With the increasing consumer demand for healthy foods, food technologists can expect to be engaged in functional food development during their careers. To be successful in developing safe, nutritious, organoleptically acceptable products that deliver on claimed health benefits over the expected shelf life, the food technologist will need to consider the interplay of processing and formulation and their combined impact on food component interactions. This is not a trivial exercise and will require input across a range of disciplines.

REFERENCES

Chen, Q.; Zhang, Q.; Huang, S.; Xiao, L. 2010. Evolution mechanism study for food safety emergency—Based on life-cycle theory. *Industrial Engineering and Engineering Management 2010 IEEE 17th International Conference Proceedings.* October 29–31, 2010, pp. 1053–1057.

Dosako, S.; Shinooka, R.; Tanaka, M. 1992. Method for thermally treating lactoferrin. US5116953.

Drusch, S. and Mannino, S. 2009. Patent-based review on industrial approaches for the microencapsulation of oils rich in polyunsaturated fatty acids. *Trends in Food Science and Technology*, 20, 237–244.

Faraji, H.; McClements, D.J.; Decker, E.A. 2004. Role of continuous phase protein on the oxidative stability of fish oil-in-water emulsions. *Journal of Agricultural and Food Chemistry*, 52, 4558–4564.

Fournier, V.; Destaillats, F.; Juanédal, P.; Dionisi, F.; Lambelet, P.; Sébédio, J.; Berdeaux, O. 2006. Thermal degradation of long-chain polyunsaturated fatty acids during deodorization of fish oil. *European Journal of Lipid Science and Technology*, 108(1), 33–42.

Fournier, V.; Destaillats, F.; Hug, B.; Golay, P.-A.; Joffre, F.; Juanéda, P.; Sémon, E. et al. 2007. Quantification of eicosapentaenoic and docosahexaenoic acid geometrical isomers formed during fish oil deodorization by gas–liquid chromatography. *Journal of Chromatography A*, 1154(1–2), 353–359.

Garmiene, G.; Šarkinas, A.; Šalaševičienė, A.; Baltušnikienė, A.; Zaborskienė, G. 2006. Biogenic amines in cool smoked sausages with biological additives. *Veterinarija Ir Zootechnika. T*, 33(55), 31–35.

Helbock, H.J.; Motchnik, P.A.; Ames, B.N. 1993. Toxic hydroperoxides in intravenous lipid emulsions used in preterm infants. *Pediatrics*, 91(1), 83–87.

Horigome, A.; Murata, M.; Yamauchi, K.; Takase, M.; Takeda, Y.; Hashimoto, J.; Kojima, I. 2010. Substance and composition both capable of imparting heat resistance. US 2010/0310673A1.

Jeanes, Y.M.; Hall, W.L.; Ellard, S.; Lee E.; Lodge, J.K. 2004. The absorption of vitamin E is influenced by the amount of fat in a meal and the food matrix. *British Journal of Nutrition*, 92, 575–579.

Kleiber, N.; Chessex, P.; Rouleau, T.; Nuyt, A.-M.; Perreault, M.; Lavoie, J.-C. 2010. Neonatal exposure to oxidants induces later in life a metabolic response associated to a phenotype of energy deficiency in an animal model of total parenteral nutrition. *Pediatric Research*, 68(3), 188–192.

Kralovec, J.A.; Zhang, S.; Zhang, W.; Barrow, C.J. 2012. A review of the progress in enzymatic concentration and microencapsulation of omega-3 rich oil from fish and microbial sources. *Food Chemistry*, 131(2), 639–644.

Kubow, S. 1992. Routes of formation and toxic consequences of lipid oxidation products in foods. *Free Radical Biology & Medicine*, 12, 63–81.

Leonard, S.W.; Good, C.K.; Gugger, E.T.; Traber, M.G. 2004. Vitamin E bioavailability from fortified breakfast cereal is greater than that from encapsulated supplements. *American Journal of Clinical Nutrition*, 79(1), 86–92.

Noriko, U; Yuji, K; Miyako, T.; Takeshi, K.; Kaoru, S.; Toshimitsu, Y. 2004. *Lactoferrin Composition.* JP2004352669A2.

Noriko, U; Yuji, K; Miyako, T.; Takeshi, K.; Kaoru, S.; Toshimitsu, Y. 2010. *Lactoferrin Composition.* JP2010180219A2.

Rufian-Henares, J.A.; Guerra-Hernandez, E.; Garcia-Villanova, B. 2005. Evolution of fatty acid profile and lipid oxidation during enteral formula storage. *Journal of Parenteral and Enteral Nutrition*, 29(3), 204–211.

Schlothauer, R.; Schollum, L.; Reid, J.; Harvey, S.; Carr, A.; Fanshawe, R. 2006. Bioactive whey protein hydrolysate. US7148034.

Sims, R.J.; Fioriti. J.A. 1976. Methional, its dimer or trimer or a combination of these, is added to polyunsaturated oils in small but effective amounts to stabilize the oils against oxidative rancidity. US3957837.

Starling, S. 2008. *Eastern Markets Provide Fresh Lactoferrin Hope.* Downloaded August 18, 2011 from http://www.nutraingredients.com/Industry/Eastern-markets-provide-fresh-lactoferrin-hope.

Tomita, M.; Tamura, Y.; Miyakawa, H.; Saito, H.; Abe, H.; Nagao, E. 1994. Method for heat treatment of lactoferrin without losing physiological without losing physiological activities thereof. US5340924.

Uzzan, M.; Nechrebeki, J.; Labuza T.P. 2007. Thermal and storage stability of nutraceuticals in a milk beverage dietary supplement. *Journal of Food Science*, 72(3), E109–E114.

Verbeke, W. 2006. Functional foods: Consumer willingness to compromise on taste for health? *Food Quality and Preference,* 17(1–2), 126–131.

Wakabayashi, H.; Yamauchi, K.; Takase, M. 2006. Lactoferrin research, technology and applications. *International Dairy Journal*, 16, 1241–1251.

20 Innovation in Technology Development with Reference to Enzymatic Extraction of Flavonoids

Munish Puri and Madan Lal Verma

CONTENTS

20.1 INTRODUCTION

Bioactive compounds such as vitamin C, carotene (β-carotene), flavonoids, limonoids, essential oil, acridone alkaloids, fibers, minerals, vitamin B, and other related nutrients such as thiamine, riboflavin, nicotinic acid/niacin, pantothenic acid, pyridoxine, folic acid, and so on are present in citrus fruits (Benavente-Garcia et al., 1997; Hamdan et al., 2011). Of all the flavonoids, flavanone glycosides (polymethoxy flavones) present in citrus have a constructive influence on human health. In addition, these compounds seek scientific attention because of their physiological and pharmacological benefits. Flavonoids are a large group of phenolic bioactives that are found in a range of plant-derived foods, mainly in citrus peel, skin of grapes, and epidermis of tea leaves (Denny and Buttriss, 2007). Flavonoids have a unique structure based on three phenyl rings, A, B, and C, as shown in Figure 20.1 where ring B may bind to position 3 at fused ring C to form isoflavonone (Bohm, 2006). Variations in substitution pattern to ring C in the structure of these compounds result in the major flavonoid classes: flavonols (found in onions, e.g., quercetin), flavones (found in parsley/celery, e.g., apigenin), flavanones (found abundantly in citrus fruits, e.g., naringin and hesperitin), isoflavones (leguminous plants such as soybean, e.g., genestein), flavanols (found in tea/apple/apricot, e.g., catechins), and anthocynadins (found in blackcurrants/blueberries, e.g., cyanidins). The biological effects of flavonoids depend on their chemical structure. The position of hydroxyl groups (OH) and other features are important for antioxidant and free-radical-scavenging effects (Hosseinimehr, 2010; Martins et al., 2011).

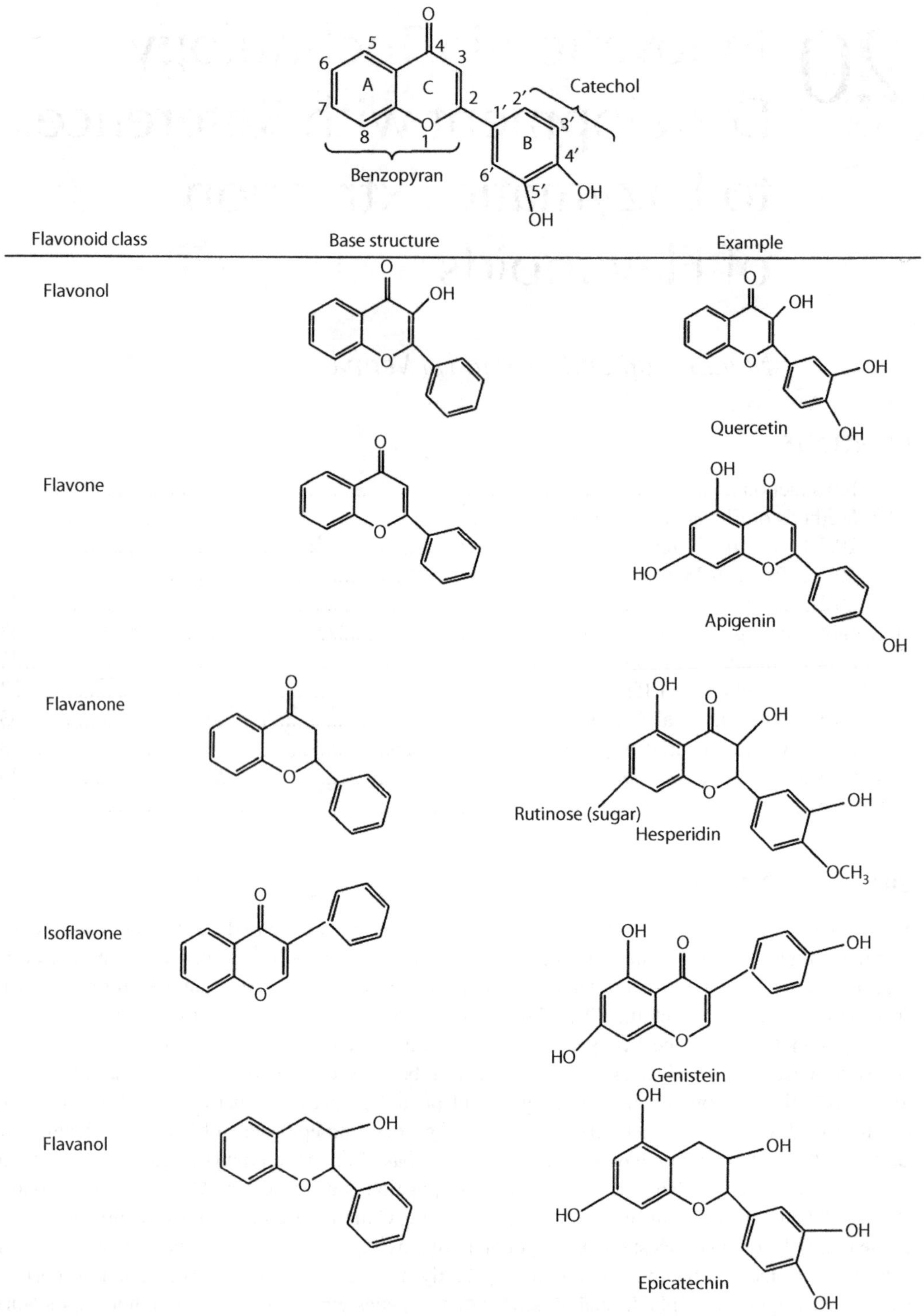

FIGURE 20.1 Structure of flavonoids, its classes, and main examples. (Reproduced from Hosseinimehr, SJ. *Drug Discovery Today* 2010, 15:907–918.)

Flavonoids are of immense interest owing to their observed biological effects *in vitro* such as free-radical scavenging, modulation of enzyme activity, inhibition of cellular proliferation, potential utility as an antibiotic, antiallergic, antiulcer, and anti-inflammatory agent (Havsteen, 2002; Li et al., 2006a; Özçelik et al., 2008; Yoshida et al., 2010; Hamdan et al., 2011). Sources for high flavonoid content are explored because these have beneficial properties for human health. In addition, an efficient method for extraction of flavonoids from fruit, vegetables, plants, and agricultural waste is required to achieve high bioactive yield. Thus, citrus peel because of its high flavonoid content could be exploited for its extraction by both pharmaceutical and food industries (Londoño-Londoño et al., 2010). However, a suitable technology development is the need of the hour.

The methods of flavonoid extraction are attracting the attention of researchers to provide more quantities so that the same can be used as natural food supplements to enhance the quality of life. An effective extraction procedure to obtain the flavonoids from the citrus peel has been described recently (Wang and Weller, 2006). This chapter focuses on the methods of extraction of flavonoids and their potential biotechnological application.

20.2   METHODS OF FLAVONOID EXTRACTION

Interest in citrus plant-derived bioactives has led to an increased need for ideal extraction methods, which could obtain maximum yields in a shorter duration. Several methods like solvent extraction (Manthey and Grohmann, 1996; Jeong et al., 2004; Anagnostopoulou et al., 2006; Li et al., 2006a; Zia-ur-Rehman, 2006), hot water extraction (Xu et al., 2007), alkaline extraction (Curto et al., 1992; Bocco et al., 1998), resin-based extraction (Calvarano et al., 1996; Kim et al., 2007), electron beam- and γ-irradiation-based extractions (Kim et al., 2008), supercritical fluid extraction (Giannuzzo et al., 2003), and enzyme-assisted extraction (Li et al., 2006b; Puri et al., 2011b) have been reported in the literature for the extraction of flavonoids from citrus peel. A few of these innovative approaches are discussed below.

20.2.1   Chemical Methods

Many of the industries, particularly the pharmaceutical and food industries, use solvents for the extraction of bioactive compounds from citrus materials. Chemical methods use organic solvents, such as hexane, methanol, ethanol, petroleum ether, benzene, toluene, ethyal acetate, isopropanaol, acetone, and so on, to extract flavonoids from plant materials. The extraction carried out by diffusion transfers from the solids to the surrounding solvents is known as leaching. The operating temperature and time of extraction are specific to the nature of the plant materials.

Five citrus peels (Yen Ben lemon, Meyer lemon, grapefruit, mandarin, and orange) were used for the extraction of phenolic substances with ethanol. The highest amount of polyphenolics (162 mg per 100 g fresh peel) were obtained when grapefruit peel was extracted with 72% ethanol at 80°C, followed by Yen Ben lemon (118 mg), orange (74 mg), and Meyer lemon (60 mg). Recovery increased with the increase in ethanol concentration of up to 85% ethanol (Li et al., 2006a).

A finger lime (*Citrus australasica*) fruit is one of the five native citrus species endemic to Australia, which grow mainly in the rainforests of Queensland and New South Wales. An extract was prepared from the peel with dichloromethane for the extraction of limonene. The peel was covered again with dichloromethane (SDS, Atrasol, 900 mL) and left at room temperature for 12 h. The combined extracts were dried over magnesium sulfate and concentrated in a column at atmospheric pressure to extract new terpenyl compounds (Delort and Jaquier, 2009).

Dried peel powder of *Citrus decumana* was extracted by the maceration process using solvents of increasing polarity (Sood et al., 2009). Maceration was first carried out with hexane followed by chloroform, ethyl acetate, and methanol, respectively. The powdered material was extracted with each solvent three times at room temperature over a period of 24 h. The material was kept for 24 h between each successive solvent for proper drying. The extracts were filtered and concentrated under vacuum on a rotary evaporator at 40°C and stored in a refrigerator for further analysis.

Naringin isolation from the albedo of Khao Taeng-gwa peel was carried by methanol extraction followed by its crystallization in water. Direct water extraction from the peel was followed and each experiment was repeated three times using methanol extract. The process with highest naringin yield was used for the isolation of naringin from the albedo and flavedo portions of peel from the other Khao Nam Pheung (KN) and Tong Dee (TD) cultivars. Powdered KT cultivar of pomelo peel was macerated in large-scale naringin isolation in methanol for 3 days (Sudto et al., 2009). The extracted slurry with methanol was dried with a rotary evaporator under reduced pressure at 45°C. Water was added to the dry methanolic extract. Dichloromethane was added after stirring at 70°C for 2 h, and the mixture was left for 4 days at 25°C. The naringin crystals formed in the aqueous layer were filtered and harvested (Sudto et al., 2009).

In another study, dry powder (1 g) of plant tissues was homogenized in dimethyl sulfoxide:methanol (1:1, v/v) in an ultraturrax blender (Bermejo et al., 2011). The supernatant after centrifugation (12,000 rpm, 15 min, 4°C) was filtered (0.45 μm) and analyzed by HPLC-diode array detection (DAD) and HPLC-mass spectrometry (MS) for the presence of flavonoids using a reverse-phase column (C18). A gradient mobile phase consisting of acetonitrile (solvent A) and 0.6% acetic acid (solvent B) was used at a flow rate of 1 mL/min. Compounds were indentified on the basis of comparison of their retention times and UV-visible and mass spectrum data with corresponding standards (Weber et al., 2006; Mata Bilbao et al., 2007).

Techniques such as organic solvent extraction require several hours or even days to obtain plant/flavonoid extracts. Also, a large volume of solvent is spent for the extraction of flavonoids. Generally, solvent needs to be evaporated which adds extra cost and loss of quality of the product. Often, these methods may either cause the degradation of the targeted compounds because of high temperature and long extraction times, or pose health-related risks because of the unawareness of safety criterion followed during irradiation. Innovative methods for flavonoid extraction are described in the following section in order to overcome the aforementioned limitations.

20.2.2 PHYSICAL METHODS

Supercritical fluid extraction has been documented as an effective method for preparing bioactive products from plant materials (Modey et al., 1996). The combined liquid-like solvating capabilities and gas-like transport properties of supercritical fluids make them particularly suitable for the extraction of diffusion-controlled matrices such as plant tissues. Moreover, the solvent strength of supercritical fluid can be manipulated by changing pressure (P) and/or temperature (T); therefore, it may achieve a remarkably high selectivity. This tunable solvation power of supercritical fluid is particularly useful for the extraction of complex samples such as plant materials (Reverchon and De Marco, 2006).

High-pressure flavonoid extraction from *Citrus sulcata* was performed. The dried *Citrus sulcata* peel and edible fruit powder (1 g) was mixed with 50 mL of 40% ethanol and extracted for 30 min at 100 atmospheres. The extracted solution was collected, filtered through a 0.4 μm membrane, and concentrated by freeze-drying after depressurization; the collected extract was stored at −20°C in the refrigerator (Wang et al., 2011).

Recently, microwave-assisted extraction (MAE) has received great attention mainly because of considerable saving in processing time, solvent consumption, and energy (Spigno and Faveri, 2009). A laboratory-scale MAE apparatus operated at atmospheric pressure with microwave frequency of 2450 MHz was used for extraction purpose. The process parameters such as microwave power 10–800 W, temperature 1–120°C, and time 1–999 s were linearly adjusted. The extracts were filtered through nylon filter (0.45 μm) and analyzed for free phenolic acid content by HPLC. The yields were better when compared with the traditional methods. MAE showed many advantages, such as shorter time, less solvent requirement, higher extraction rate, saving of energy, and better products with lower cost. The performance of the method was confirmed by different antioxidant assay systems. The results were promising and demonstrated the practical feasibility of MAE to substitute the traditional time-consuming techniques for efficient extraction of phenolic compounds from citrus mandarin peels (Hayat et al., 2009).

Ultrasonic-assisted extraction (UAE) has proven to significantly decrease extraction time and increase extraction yields in many vegetable materials. The cavitation process causes the swelling of cells or the breakdown of cell walls during sonication which allow high diffusion rates across the cell wall or a simple washing out of the cell contents (Vinatoru, 2001). Better recovery of cell contents can be obtained along with solvent, temperature, and pressure by optimizing the ultrasound application factors, including frequency, sonication power and time, as well as ultrasonic wave distribution (Londoño-Londoño et al., 2010; Wang and Weller, 2006). Optimization of UAE has been described recently to extract hesperidin from Penggan (*Citrus reticulata*) peel (Ma et al., 2008a), and phenolic acids and flavanone glycosides from Satsuma mandarin (*Citrus unshiu* Marc.) peel (Ma et al., 2009). Workers further refined their process for extracting hesperidin from *Citrus reticulate* peel by increasing the frequency to 60 kHz for 60 min at 40°C in the presence of methanol (Ma et al., 2008c). The highest yield was obtained with dry material in 30 min versus wet material. Dry material has more porosity and the solvent diffusion rate resulted in higher yield (Khan et al., 2010).

The citrus peels from three species, Tahiti lime (*Citrus latifolia*), sweet orange (*Citrus sinensis*), and oneco tangerine (*Citrus reticulata*), were obtained for the extraction of hesperidin and other related citrus flavonoids such as naringin. The extraction was carried out in ultrasonic cleaning bath, operating at 60 kHz (Ma et al., 2008c). A factorial design (2^2) was used to optimize the extraction process from tangerine peel by identifying the effect of two active factors in improving yield percentage and total phenolic compounds. The effect of water content in the citrus peel material (0% and 75%), extraction time (30 and 90 min), and peel/water ratio (g/mL) were studied. The hesperidin extraction was accomplished by successive acid/base precipitations from flavonoid fraction. The hesperetin was obtained by atmospheric pressure acid-catalyzed hydrolysis of hesperidin and used as a model to establish the differences between glycoside and aglycone. Structural identification of glycoside and aglycone was made by HPLC/MS comparing fragmentation profile with reference standards (Grohmann et al., 2000).

20.2.3 ENZYME ASSISTED

Enzymes have been used safely in a wide variety of foods for centuries. The biodiversity of enzymes is providing the pharmaceutical/food industry with a wide range of functionalities. The application of enzymes for complete extraction of flavonoids without the use of solvents could be an attractive proposal. Enzymes have been used in particular for the pretreatment of plant material before conventional methods for extraction. Various enzymes such as cellulases, pectinases, rhamnosidases, and their combinations are often required to disrupt the structural integrity of the plant cell wall, thereby enhancing the extraction of bioactives from plants (Mamma et al., 2008; Puri et al., 2012). These enzymes act on cell wall components, hydrolyze them, and increase the permeability of the cell wall, thus resulting in higher extraction yields of bioactives. Enzymes can be derived from bacteria, fungi, animal organs, or vegetable/fruit extracts. It is important to understand the catalytic property and mode of action, optimum operational conditions, and which enzyme or enzyme combination is appropriate for the plant material selected in order to use enzymes most effectively for extraction applications.

The application of enzymes in the extraction of oil from oil seeds such as sunflower, corn, coconut, olives, avocado, and so on is reported in the literature (Li et al., 2006b). Various enzyme combinations are used to loosen the structural integrity of botanical material thereby enhancing the extraction of the desired flavor and color components. Recently, enzymes have been used for the extraction of flavonoids from plant materials, as a pretreatment of the raw material before subjecting the plant material to hydro distillation/solvent extraction. A deep knowledge of enzymes, their mode of action, conditions for optimum activity, and selection of the right type of enzymes are essential to use them effectively for extraction. Although the hydrolases enzymes such as lipases, proteases (i.e., chymotrypsin, subtilisin, thermolysin, and papain), and esterases use water as a substrate for the reaction, they are also able to accept other nucleophiles such as alcohols, amines, thio-esters, and oximes (Sowbhagya and Chitra, 2010).

Advantages of enzyme pretreatment are the reduction in extraction time, minimal usage of solvents, and a product with increased yield and quality. A limitation of this method is the cost of the enzymes which could be overcome by balancing the concentration of enzyme preparations and tailor-made enzyme preparations for specific reactions (Sowbhagya and Chitra, 2010; Puri et al., 2011a). Crude enzyme preparations can be used in some commercial applications to reduce the cost of the enzyme preparation. The increased yield of value-added products (volatile oils) obtained by the enzyme pretreatment can balance the increased cost of using enzymes. Knowledge of the cell wall composition of the raw material to be treated helps in the selection of the enzyme and the concentration to be used.

Use of citrozyme CEO (Switzerland) containing hemicelluloytic, pectolytic activity with high polygalactouranase activity for pretreatment of citrus peel to recover oil has been reported elsewhere (Coll et al., 1995). Enzyme treatment reduced emulsion viscosity and assisted in breaking down of the emulsion to recover oil from the aqueous phase. Optimization of the oil recovery process (enzyme addition time, use of a buffer tank, and closed system and optimum enzyme dosage) resulted in advantages such as increase in yield of essential oil, reduction in freshwater consumption, and wastewater production, wastewater being more easily biodegradable, increased centrifuge capacities, improved dewaxing of citrus oils, and had no influence on oil quality.

Citrus bergamia peel is an underutilized by-product of the essential oil and juice-processing industry. As with other citrus peels, it still contains exploitable components, such as pectins and flavonoids. Commercial glycoside hydrolases, specifically a combination of pectolytic and cellulolytic enzymes, solubilized a high percentage of the raw material. The flavonoid profile of the peel consisted of characteristic citrus species flavanone rutinosides and neohesperosides derived from naringenin, eriodictyol, and hesperetin. In addition, a number of minor flavanone and flavone glycosides, not found in orange and lemon peels, were identified (Mandalari et al., 2006). The majority of flavonoids were extracted in the two 70% v/v ethanol extractions. Processing this material clearly has economic potential leading to low environmental impact.

Hydrolysis of grapefruit peel waste was done with cellulase and pectinase enzymes. This study tested different loadings of commercial cellulase and pectinase enzymes and pH levels to hydrolyze grapefruit peel waste to produce flavonoids and sugars. The lowest loadings of pectinase and cellulase per gram of dry matter were reported to yield maximum glucose. Cellulose, pectin, and hemicellulose in grapefruit peel waste were hydrolyzed by pectinase and cellulase enzymes to monomer sugars, which can then be used by microorganisms to produce ethanol and other fermentation products (Wilkins et al., 2007).

The hydrolysis of flavonoids (naringin) from kinnow peel (2%, w/v) was followed by incubating purified recombinant α-L-rhamnosidase (6.5 U) at 50°C for 1 h. α-L-Rhamnosidase (EC 3.2.1.40) catalyzes the cleavage of terminal rhamnoside groups from naringin to prunin and rhamnose was investigated (Puri et al., 2011b). The samples were analyzed for naringin hydrolysis through HPLC. The compound identification was done through matching of retention time between the standard solution and the sample (Puri et al., 2010, 2011b). We have recently demonstrated the feasibility of enzyme-assisted extraction of stevioside from *Stevia rebaudiana* Bertoni, which gives better yield as compared with conventional solvent method of extraction (Puri et al., 2011a).

The enzymatic extraction of flavonoids may be limited at present because of the following factors: (i) procurement of enzymes is expensive for processing large volumes of raw material and (ii) inability of the available enzyme preparations to completely hydrolyze plant cell wall thus limiting the availability of bioactives. However, enzyme-based extraction provides an opportunity that can enhance the quality of flavonoids.

20.3 BIOTECHNOLOGICAL APPLICATION

It is anticipated that increased availability of citrus bioactives as a result of optimizing extraction procedure will lead to the use of flavonoids as food supplements in benefiting human health.

20.3.1 ANTIOXIDANT PROPERTIES

Flavonoids show antioxidant property by scavenging reactive oxygen species (Rice-Evans et al., 1997; Sood et al., 2009) and reactive nitrogen species (Pannala et al., 1997; Brown et al., 1998), in a structure-dependent manner. Antioxidant properties are attributed by virtue of the number and arrangement of their phenolic hydroxyl groups attached to ring structures. Their ability to act as antioxidants by donating an electron to an oxidant critically depends on the reduction potential of their radicals (Jovanovic et al., 1998) and their accessibility of the radical. Flavonoids are ideal scavengers of peroxyl radicals because of their favorable reduction potential relative to alkyl peroxyl radicals. Thus, these bioactive molecules have served as effective inhibitors of lipid peroxidation. The major structural characteristics responsible for their reducing properties are a catechol (3′,4′-dihydroxy) structure in the B ring; an unsaturated 2,3 double bond and a 3-hydroxyl group in the C ring.

Many *in vitro* studies have demonstrated the potent peroxyl radical scavenging abilities of flavonoids in inhibiting lipid peroxidation and oxidation of low-density lipoproteins (LDL) (Castelluccio et al., 1995). There have been a few studies on the ability of flavonoids and phenolic acids to scavenge reactive nitrogen species. Nitrous oxide (NO) is such a species produced by the action of nitric oxide synthase in endothelial cells and neurones. iNOS is also induced and further NO synthesis activated at sites of inflammation. Concomitant production of nitric oxide and superoxide radical at such sites of chronic inflammation induces the production of peroxynitrite. Peroxynitrite is a toxic oxidizing and nitrating species which is produced by rapid interaction of superoxide radical and nitric oxide (Beckman et al., 1994). Nitrated proteins are immunogenic and nitration can alter their function and stability, thus interfering with cell signaling pathways, cytoskeletal structures and repair mechanisms, and nitrosation of tyrosine has been suggested to be responsible for the onset of apoptotosis. Thus the ability to inhibit peroxynitrite-dependent nitration of proteins has a potentially significant contributory role in inhibiting damage to biomolecules mediated by reactive nitrogen species. Flavonoids are ideal candidates for this role.

The activity of flavonoids to inhibit peroxynitrite-dependent nitration of tyrosine is structure dependent. Thus, catechol-containing phenolics inhibit by scavenging peroxynitrite through electron donation whereas monohydroxycinnamates and flavonoids with monophenolic B rings intercept the reaction between tyrosine and peroxynitrite via the anticipated mechanism of competitive nitration. Several flavonoids and phenolic compounds are powerful inhibitors of nitrous acid-dependent nitration and DNA deamination *in vitro* (Oldreive et al., 1998). Thus, flavonoids from plant materials might provide a gastro-protective effect under conditions in which high levels of reactive nitrogen species are produced. Flavonoids and phenolic compounds with hydroxyl groups can also interact with transition metal ions to form chelates. These chelates might be stable, or redox cycling might take place leading to the reduction of iron or copper to a more pro-oxidant form and the oxidized quinone.

20.3.2 ANTIDIABETIC EFFECTS

Flavonoids, especially quercetin, have been reported to possess antidiabetic activity. Vessal et al. (2003) reported that quercetin brings about the regeneration of pancreatic islets and probably increases insulin release in streptozotocin-induced diabetic rats. Quercetin also, in another study, stimulated insulin release and enhanced Ca^{2+} uptake from isolated islets cell which suggest a place for flavonoids in noninsulin-dependent diabetes (Hif and Howell, 1984; Hif and Howell, 1985). The citrus bioflavonoids hesperidin and naringin both play crucial roles in controlling the progression of hyperglycemia. This may be done partly by increasing hepatic glycolysis and glycogen concentration and/or by lowering hepatic gluconeogenesis (June et al., 2004).

20.3.3 ANTIMICROBIAL ACTIVITY

Flavonoids have been used extensively since centuries for the treatment of various diseases. Propolis has high flavonoid (galangin) content. This has been attributed to its healing properties because of its antimicrobial activity of flavonoid content. It has been reported to possess inhibitory actions against *Aspergillus tamarii*, *Aspergillus flavus*, *Cladosporium sphaerospermum*, *Pencillium digitatum*, and *Penicillium italicum* (Cushnie and Lamb, 2005). Flavonoid (5,7,4'-trihydroxy-8-methyl-6-(3-methyl-[2-butenyl])-2S-flavonone) isolated from shrub *Eysenhardtia texana* and flavonoid 7-hydroxy-3',4'-(methylenedioxy) flavan from *Termanalia bellerica* possess antifungal activity against *Candida albicans*, whereas 6,7,4'-trihydroxy-3',5'-dimethoxyflavone and 5,5'-dihydroxy-8,2',4'-trimethoxyflavone are effective against *Aspergillus flavus* (Cushnie and Lamb, 2005). Nobiletin and langeritin isolated from peelings of tangerine orange showed fungistatic action toward *Deuterophoma tracheiphila* while hesperidin stimulates fungal growth slightly (Tapas et al., 2008). Quercetin and naringenin are reported to be inhibitors of *Bacillus subtilis*, *Candida albicans*, *Escherichia coli*, *Staphylococcus nervous*, *Staphylococcus epidermis*, and *Saccharomyces cerevisiae* (Taleb-Contini et al., 2003).

Flavonoids (morin-3-*O*-lyxoside, morin-3-*O*-arabinoside, quercetin, and quercetin-3-*O*-arabinoside) isolated from *Psidium guajava* leaves possess bacteriostatic action against foodborne pathogenic bacteria, including *Bacillus stearothermophilus*, *Brochothrix thermosphacta*, *Escherichia coli*, *Listeria monocytogenes*, *Pseudomonas fluorescens*, *Salmonella enteric*, *Staphyloccus aureus*, and *Vibrio cholera* (Narayana et al., 2001; Rattanachaikunsopon and Phumkhachorn, 2010; Table 20.1).

TABLE 20.1
Antimicrobial Activities of Flavonoids

Activity	Organism	Flavonoid
Antibacterial activity	*Staphylococcus aureus*	Quercetin, baicalin, hesperitin, fisetin, naringin + rutin, naringin + hespertin, *iso*-liquiritigenin
	Staphylococcus albus	Fisetin
	Streptococcus pyrogenes	Apigenin
	Streptococcus viridians	Apigenin
	Streptococcus jaccalis	Chrysin
	Streptococcus baris	Chrysin
	Streptococcus pneumonia	Chrysin
	Pseudomonas aeruginosa	Rutin, naringin, baicalin, hydroxyethylrutosine
	Escherichia coli	Quercetin
	Bacillus subtilis	Quercetin
	Bacillus anthracis	Rutin
	Proteus vulgaris	Datisetin
	Clostridium perfingens	Hydroxyethylrutoside
Antiviral activity	*Rabies virus*	Quercetin, quercetrin, rutin
	Para influenza virus	Quercetin, rutin
	Herpes simplex virus	Galangin, quercetin, kaempferol, apigenin
	Respiratory synctial virus	Quercetin, naringin
	Immunodeficiency virus Auzesky virus	Apigenin
	Auzesky virus	Quercetin, quercetrin, morin, apigenin
	Polio virus	Quercetin
	Mengo virus	Quercetin
	Pseudorabies virus	Quercetin

Flavonones having sugar moiety showed antimicrobial activity, whereas none of the flavonols and flavonolignans showed inhibitory activity on microorganisms. Quercetin has been reported to completely inhibit growth of *Staphylococcus aureus* (Tapas et al., 2008).

20.3.4 OTHER POTENTIAL APPLICATIONS OF FLAVONOIDS

Citrus flavonoids are particularly promising in alleviating obesity and associated illnesses, since a large body of research in humans and animals has shown hypolipidemic and/or antidiabetic effects of citrus fruits and juices (Gorinstein et al., 2004), as well as purified flavonoids (Mulvihill et al., 2009). The human hepatoma *HepG2* cell line has been used extensively to examine the molecular mechanisms of citrus flavonoid action *in vivo* and to establish that citrus flavonoids act through multiple pathways to reduce hepatic lipid secretion, and that the effects are consistent with physiological responses to these compounds in humans and animals (Kurowska et al., 2004). Citrus flavonoids regulated the transcription of the LDL receptor gene in HepG2 cells, and the DNA binding site for the transcription factor, sterol regulatory element binding protein, was necessary for the regulation (Morin et al., 2008). Citrus flavonoid action on inhibition of apolipoprotein B secretion was specifically demonstrated in primary liver cells (Dobrzyn and Ntambi, 2005). Two structural classes of citrus flavonoids reduce stearoyl-CoA desaturase (SCD1) mRNA concentrations in a dose-dependent manner in rat primary hepatocytes (Nichols et al., 2011). Citrus flavonoids have been shown to decrease plasma lipid levels, improve glucose tolerance, and attenuate obesity (Nichols et al., 2011). Citrus flavonoids repress the mRNA for SCD1, a key enzyme in lipid synthesis and obesity control, in rat primary hepatocytes. Repression of this enzyme reduces hyperlipidemia and adiposity.

20.4 CONCLUSION AND FUTURE DIRECTIONS

Citrus flavonoids have received much attention over the past years. A variety of potential beneficial effects of flavonoids have been elucidated and validated. The study of flavonoids is complex in the current scenario, because of the heterogeneity of different molecular structures and limited data on its bioavailability. Therefore, there is requirement of a simple and economically valuable method for the extraction of citrus flavonoids. Chemical and physical extraction methods were employed in flavonoid extraction. Enzyme-assisted extraction keeping the limitation of chemical-based extraction methods in mind, is a sustainable alternative that will benefit the industry immensely. Future investigations will concern scale-up of the process to further enhance flavonoid yield.

REFERENCES

Anagnostopoulou, MA; Kefalas, P; Papageorgiou, VP; Assimopoulou AN; Boskou, D. Radical scavenging activity of various extracts and fractions of sweet orange peel (*Citrus sinensis*). *Food Chemistry* 2006, 94:19–25.

Beckman, J; Chen, S; Ischiropoulos, H; Cow, J. Oxidative chemistry of peroxynitrite. *Methods in Enzymology* 1994, 233:229–240.

Benavente-Garcia, O; Castillo, J; Marin, FR; Ortuno, A; Del Rio, JA. Uses and properties of citrus flavonoids. *Journal of Agricultural and Food Chemistry* 1997, 45:4505–4515.

Bermejo, A; Llosa, MJ; Cano, A. Analysis of bioactive compounds in seven citrus cultivars. *Food Science and Technology International* 2011, 17:55.

Bocco, A; Cuvelier, ME; Richard, H; Berset, C. Antioxidant activity and phenolic composition of citrus peel and seed extracts. *Journal of Agricultural and Food Chemistry* 1998, 46:2123–2129.

Bohm, BA. *Introduction to Flavonoids* 2006, Vol. 2, Harwood Academic Publishers, New York, USA.

Brown, JE; Khodr, H; Hider, RC; Rice-Evans, CA. Structural dependence of flavonoid interactions with Cu^{2+} ions: implications for their antioxidant properties. *Biochemical Journal* 1998, 330:1173–1178.

Calvarano, M; Postorino, E; Gionfriddo, F; Calvarano, I; Bovalo, F. Naringin extraction from exhausted bergamot peels. *Perfumer and Flavorist* 1996, 21:1–4.

Castelluccio, C; Paganga, G; Melikian, N; Bolwell, GP; Pridman, J; Sampson, J; Rice-Evans, CA. Antioxidant potential of intermediates in phenylpropanoid metabolism in higher plants. *FEBS Letter* 1995, 368:88–192.

Coll, L; Saura, D; Ruiz, MP; Canovas, JA. Viscometric control in the enzymatic extraction of citrus peel oils. *Food Control* 1995, 6:143–146.

Curto, RL; Tripodo, MM; Leuzzi, U; Giuffrè, D; Vaccarino, C. Flavonoids recovery and SCP production from orange peel. *Bioresource Technology* 1992, 42:83–87.

Cushnie, TPT; Lamb, AJ. Antimicrobial activity of flavonoids. *International Journal of Antimicrobial Agents* 2005, 26:343–356.

Denny, AR; Buttriss, JL. Plant Foods and Health: Focus on Plant Bioactives. EuroFIR Synthesis Report No. 4. EuroFIR Project Management Office/British Nutrition Foundation, London. 2007.

Delort, E; Jaquier, A. Novel terpenyl esters from Australian finger lime (*Citrus australasica*) peel extract. *Flavour and Fragrance Journal* 2009, 24:123–132.

Dobrzyn, A; Ntambi, JM. Stearoyl-CoA desaturase as a new drug target for obesity treatment. *Obesity Reviews* 2005, 6:169–174.

Giannuzzo, AN; Boggetti, HJ; Nazareno, MA; Mishima, HT. Supercritical fluid extraction of naringin from the peel of Citrus paradise. *Phytochemical Analysis* 2003, 14:221–223.

Gorinstein, S; Caspi, A; Libman, I; Katrich, E; Lerner, HT; Trakhtenberg, S. Preventive effects of diets supplemented with sweetie fruits in hypercholesterolemic patients suffering from coronary artery disease. *Preventive Medicine* 2004, 38:841–847.

Grohmann, K; Manthey, JA; Cameron, RG. Acid-catalyzed hydrolysis of hesperidin at elevated temperatures, *Carbohydrate Research* 2000, 328:141–146.

Hamdan, D; El-Readi, MZ; Tahrani, A; Herrmann, F; Kaufmann, D; Farrag, N; El-Shazly, A; Wink, M. Chemical composition and biological activity of citrus *jambhiri Lush. Food Chemistry* 2011, 127:394–403.

Havsteen, BH. The biochemistry and medicinal significance of the flavonoids. *Pharmacology and Therapeutics* 2002, 96:67–202.

Hayat, K; Sarfraz, H; Shabbar, A; Umar, F; Baomiao, D; Shuqin, X; Chengsheng, J; Xiaoming, Z; Wenshui, X. Optimized microwave-assisted extraction of phenolic acids from citrus mandarin peels and evaluation of antioxidant activity *in vitro. Separation and Purification Technology* 2009, 70:63–70.

Hif, CS; Howell, SL. Effects of epicatechin on rat islets of langerhans. *Diabetes* 1984, 33:291–296.

Hif, CS; Howell, SL. Effects of flavonoids on insulin secretion and Ca^{+2} handling in rat islets of langerhans. *Journal of Endocrinology* 1985, 107:1–8.

Hosseinimehr, SJ. Flavonoids and genomic instability induced by ionizing radiation. *Drug Discovery Today* 2010, 15:907–918.

Jeong, SM; Kim, SY; Kim, DR; Jo, SC; Nam, KC; Ahn, DU; Lee, SC. Effect of heat treatment on the antioxidant activity of extracts from citrus peels. *Journal of Agricultural and Food Chemistry* 2004, 52:3389–3393.

Jovanovic, S; Steenken, S; Simic, MG; Hara, Y. In: *Flavonoids in Health and Disease.* (Rice-Evans, C and Packer, L., eds) Marcel Dekker, New York, 1998, pp. 137–161.

June, UJ; Lee, MK; Jeong, KS; Choi, MS. The hypoglycaemic effects of hesperidin and naringin are partly mediated by hepatic glucose-regulating enzymes in C57BL/KsJ-db/db mice. *The Journal of Nutrition* 2004, 134:2499–24503.

Khan, MK; Vian, MA; Sylvie, A; Tixier, F; Dangles, O; Chemat, F. Ultrasound-assisted extraction of polyphenols (flavanone glycosides) from orange (*Citrus sinensis* L.) peel. *Food Chemistry* 2010, 119:851–858.

Kim, JW; Lee, BC; Lee, JH; Nam, KC; Lee, SC. Effect of electron-beam irradiation on the antioxidant activity of extracts from *Citrus unshiu* pomaces. *Radiation Physics and Chemistry* 2008, 77:87–91.

Kim, MR; Kim, WC; Lee, DY; Kim, CW. Recovery of narirutin by adsorption on a non-ionic polar resin from a water-extract of *Citrus unshiu* peels. *Journal of Food Engineering* 2007, 78:27–32.

Kurowska, EM; Manthey, JA; Casaschi, A; Theriault, AG. Modulation of HepG2 cell net apolipoprotein B secretion by the citrus polymethoxyflavone, tangeretin. *Lipids* 2004, 39:143–151.

Li, BB; Smith, B; Hossain, MM. Extraction of phenolics from citrus peels: I. Solvent extraction method. *Separation and Purification Technology* 2006a, 48:182–188.

Li BB; Smith, B; Hossain, MM. Extraction of phenolics from citrus peels: II. Enzyme-assisted extraction method. *Separation and Purification Technology* 2006b, 48:189–196.

Londoño-Londoño, J; Lima, VRD; Lara, O; Gil, A; Pasa, TBC; Arango, GJ; Pineda, JRR. Clean recovery of antioxidant flavonoids from citrus peel: Optimizing an aqueous ultrasound-assisted extraction method. *Food Chemistry* 2010, 119:81–87.

Ma, Y; Chen, J; Liu, D; Ye, X. Effect of ultrasonic treatment on the total phenolic and antioxidant activity of extracts from citrus peel. *Journal of Food Science* 2008c, 73:115–120.

Ma, Y; Chen, J; Liu, D; Ye, X. Simultaneous extraction of phenolic compounds of citrus peel extracts: Effect of ultrasound. *Ultrasonics Sonochemistry* 2009, 16:57–62.

Ma, Y; Ye, X; Fang, Z; Chen, J; Xu, G; Liu, D. Phenolic compounds and antioxidant activity of extracts from ultrasonic treatment of Satsuma mandarin (*Citrus unshiu* Marc.) peels. *Journal of Agriculture and Food Chemistry* 2008b, 56:5682–5690.

Ma, Y; Ye, X; Hao, Y; Xu, G; Xu, G; Liu, D. Ultrasound-assisted extraction of hesperidin from Penggan (*Citrus reticulata*) peel. *Ultrasonics Sonochemistry* 2008a, 15:227–232.

Mamma, D; Kourtoglou, E; Christakopolulos, P. Fungal multienzyme production on industrial by-products of the citrus-processing industry. *Bioresource Technology* 2008, 99:2373–2383.

Mandalari, G; Bennett, RN; Bisignano, G; Saija, A; Dugo, G; Locurto, RB; Faulds, CB, Waldron, KW. Characterization of flavonoids and pectins from bergamot (*Citrus bergamia* risso) peel, a major byproduct of essential oil extraction. *Journal of Agricultural and Food Chemistry* 2006, 54:197–203.

Manthey, JA; Grohmann, K. Concentrations of hesperidin and other orange peel flavonoids in citrus processing byproducts. *Journal of Agricultural and Food Chemistry* 1996, 44:811–814.

Martins, S; Mussatto, SI; Teixeira, J.A. Bioactive phenolic compounds; production and extraction by solid substrate fermentation. *Biotechnology Advances* 2011, 29:365–373.

Mata Bilbao, ML; Andrés-Lacueva, C; Jauregui, O; Lamuela-Raventós, RM. Determination of flavonoids in a citrus fruit extract by LC-DAD and LC-MS. *Food Chemistry* 2007, 101:1742–1747.

Modey, WK; Mulholland, DA; Raynor, MW. Analytical supercritical fluid extraction of natural products. *Phytochemical Analysis* 1996, 7:1–15.

Morin, B; Nichols, LA; Zalasky, KM; Davis, JW; Manthey, JA; Holland, LJ. The citrus flavonoids hesperetin and nobiletin differentially regulate low density lipoprotein receptor gene transcription in HepG2 liver cells. *The Journal of Nutrition* 2008, 138:274–1281.

Mulvihill, EE; Allister, EM; Sutherland, BG; Telford, DE; Sawyez, CG; Edwards, JY; Markle, JM; Hegele, RA; Huff, MW. Naringenin prevents dyslipidemia, apolipoprotein B overproduction, and hyperinsulinemia in LDL receptor null mice with diet-induced insulin resistance. *Diabetes* 2009, 58:2198–2210.

Narayana, KR; Reddy, SR; Chaluvadi, MR; Krishna, DR. Bioflavonoids classification, pharmacological, biochemical effects and therapeutic potential. *Indian Journal of Pharmacology* 2001, 33:2–16.

Nichols, LA; Jackson, DE; Manthey, JA; Shukla, SD; Holland, LJ. Citrus flavonoids repress the mRNA for stearoyl-CoA desaturase, a key enzyme in lipid synthesis and obesity control, in rat primary hepatocytes. *Lipids in Health and Disease* 2011, 10:36–40.

Oldreive, C; Zhao, K; Paganga, G; Halliwell, B; Rice-Evans, C. Inhibition of nitrous oxide acid-dependent tyrosine nitration and DNA base deamination by flavonoids and other phenolic compounds. *Chemical Research in Toxicology* 1998, 11:1574–1579.

Özçelik, B; Deliorman Orhan, D; Özgen, S; Ergun, F. Antimicrobial activity of flavonoids against extended-spectrum-lactamase (ESβL)-producing *Klebsiella pneumonia*. *Tropical Journal of Pharmaceutical Research* 2008, 7:1151–1157.

Pannala, AS; Rice-Evans, CA; Halliwell, B; Singh, S. Inhibition of peroxynitrite-mediated tyrosine nitration by catechin polyphenols. *Biochemical and Biophysical Research Communications* 1997, 232:164–168.

Puri, M; Kaur, A; Schwarz, WH; Singh, S; Kennedy, JF. Molecular characterization and enzymatic hydrolysis of naringin extracted from kinnow peel waste. *International Journal of Biological Macromolecules* 2011b, 48:58–62.

Puri, M; Sharma, D; Tiwary, AK. Downstream processing of stevioside and its potential applications. *Biotechnology Advances* 2011a, 29:781–791.

Puri, M; Sharma, D; Barrow, CJ. Enzyme assisted extraction of bioactives from plants. *Trends in Biotechnology* 2012, 30:37–44.

Puri, M; Kaur, A; Singh, RS; Schwarz, WH. One step purification and immobilization of His-tagged rhamnosidase for naringin hydrolysis. Process. *Biochemistry* 2010, 45:451–456.

Rattanachaikunsopon, P; Phumkhachorn, P. Contents and antibacterial activity of flavonoids extracted from leaves of *Psidium guajava*. *Journal of Medicinal Plants Research* 2010, 4:393–396.

Reverchon, E; De Marco, I. Supercritical fluid extraction and fractionation of natural matter. *Journal of Supercritical Fluids* 2006, 38:146–166.

Rice-Evans, C; Miller, NJ; Paganga, G. Antioxidant properties of phenolic compounds. *Trends in Plant Sciences* 1997, 2:1532–1539.

Sood, S; Arora, B; Bansal, S; Muthuraman, A; Gill, N; Arora, R; Bali, M; Sharma, P. Antioxidant, anti-inflammatory and analgesic potential of the *Citrus decumana* L. peel extract. *Inflammopharmacology* 2009, 17:267–274.

Sowbhagya, HB; Chitra, VN. Enzyme-assisted extraction of flavorings and colorants from plant materials. *Critical Reviews in Food Science and Nutrition* 2010, 50:146–161.

Spigno, G; Faveri, DMD. Microwave-assisted extraction of tea phenols: A phenomenological study. *Journal of Food Engineering* 2009, 93:210–217.

Sudto, K; Pornpakakul, S; Wanichwecharungruang, S. An efficient method for the large scale isolation of naringin from pomelo (*Citrus grandis*) peel. *International Journal of Food Science and Technology* 2009, 44:1737–1742.

Taleb-Contini, SH; Salvador, MJ; Watanabe, E; Ito, I; Oleveira, DCRD. Antimicrobial activity of flavonoids and steroids isolated from two *Chromolaena* species. *Revista Brasileira de Ciencias Farmaceuticas* 2003, 39:403–408.

Tapas, AR; Sakarkar, DM; Kakde, RB. Flavonoids as nutraceuticals: A review. *Tropical Journal of Pharmaceutical Research* 2008, 7:1089–1099.

Vessal, M; Hemmati, M; Vasei, M. Antidiabetic effects of quercetin in streptozocin induced diabetic rats. *Comparatrive Biochemistry and Physiology—Part C Toxicology and Pharmacology* 2003, 135:357–364.

Vinatoru, F. An overview of the ultrasonically assisted extraction of bioactive principles from herbs. *Ultrasonics Sonochemistry* 2001, 8:303–313.

Wang AY, Zhou MY, Lin WC 2011, Antioxidative and anti-inflammatory properties of *Citrus sulcata* extracts. *Food Chemistry* 2011, 124:958–963.

Wang, L; Weller, CL. Recent advances in extraction of nutraceuticals from plants. *Trends in Food Science and Technology* 2006, 17:300–312.

Weber, B; Hartmann, B; Stockigt, D; Schreiber, K; Roloff, M; Bertram, HJ; Schmidt, CO. Liquid chromatography/mass spectrometry and liquid chromatography/nuclear magnetic resonance as complementary analytical techniques for unambiguous identification of polymethoxylated flavones in residues from molecular distillation of orange peel oils (*Citrus sinensis*). *Journal of Agricultural and Food Chemistry* 2006, 54:274–278.

Wilkins, MR; Widmer, WW; Grohmann, K; Cameron, RG. Hydrolysis of grapefruit peel waste with cellulase and pectinase enzymes. *Bioresource Technology* 2007, 98:1596–1601.

Xu, G; Ye, X; Chen, J; Liu, D. Effect of heat treatment on the phenolic compounds and antioxidant capacity of citrus peel extract. *Journal of Agricultural and Food Chemistry* 2007, 55:330–335.

Yoshida, H; Takamura, N; Shuto, T; Ogata, K; Tokunaga, J; Kawai, K; Kai, H. The citrus flavonoids hesperetin and naringenin block the lipolytic actions of TNF-α in mouse adipocytes. *Biochemical and Biophysical Research Communications* 2010, 394:728–732.

Zia-ur-Rehman, Citrus peel extract: A natural source of antioxidant. *Food Chemistry* 2006, 99:450–454.

21 Novel Extraction Technology for Antioxidants and Phytochemicals

Rajshri Roy, Kerrie Close, and Dilip Ghosh

CONTENTS

21.1 INTRODUCTION

In addition to primary metabolites, plants produce a broad range of bioactive compounds of secondary metabolites and these phytochemicals have been determined to be beneficial to human health (Pathak, 2011). There are hundreds, if not thousands, of these phytochemicals that have a beneficial effect on the body, effects such as antioxidant activity, boosting the immune system, anti-inflammatory, antiviral, antibacterial, and cellular repair. As a result, the incorporation of these compounds into nutraceutical and functional foods has grown significantly throughout the world as consumers seek to utilize more natural substances to reduce the risk of disease as well as for prevention and treatment (Pathak, 2011). Natural antioxidants are preferred over synthetic antioxidants as they are found to impose side effects (Krishnaiah et al., 2007). This interest in the field of antioxidants in recent years and research efforts have led to a better understanding of the mechanisms involved and in the application areas in both food and nonfood commodities as well as in biological systems and as dietary supplements. Therefore, the extraction and purification of these compounds has become an area of increased focus to enable maximum yield and to preserve the bioactivity and quality.

More traditional extraction methods for recovering and concentrating these compounds from plants are time consuming and require large quantities of solvents which have led to an increased demand for novel extraction methods that are more efficient and have less of an environmental impact (Pathak, 2011). There has been research in laboratories all around the world and efforts are underway for devising better methodologies for the extraction, identification, and application of antioxidants as well as methodology development for their evaluation. Some novel extraction technologies are ultrasonic-assisted extraction (UAE), microwave-assisted extraction (MAE), and supercritical fluid extraction (SFE) and these methodologies have the possibility of reducing the extraction time while increasing the yield and quality of the extracts (Pathak, 2011). These novel techniques have been developed for the extraction of nutraceuticals from plants in order to shorten extraction time, decrease solvent consumption, increase extraction yield, as well as enhancing the quality of the extracts (Wang et al., 2010).

The matrix and operating parameters, extraction time, advantages, limitations, and potential applications are discussed in this chapter, and compared to conventional solid–liquid extraction and Soxhlet extraction.

21.2 OVERVIEW

Extraction of phenolic compounds and antioxidants is an operation in which a constituent of a liquid is Soxhlet extraction to another liquid (solvent). The term solid–liquid extraction is restricted to those situations in which a solid phase is present and includes those operations frequently referred to as leaching, lixiviation, and washing.

Extraction always involves two steps:

1. Contact of the solvent with the solid to be treated so as to transfer the soluble constituent (solute) to the solvent
2. Separation or washing of the solution from the residual solid

These two steps may be conducted in separate equipments or in the same piece of equipment. Liquid always adheres to the solid which must be washed to prevent either the loss of solution if the soluble constituent is the desired material or the contamination loss of the solids if these are the desired material. The complete process also includes the separate recovery of the solute and solvent. This is done by another operation such as evaporation or distillation.

21.3 SOLID–LIQUID EXTRACTION BY SOXHLET APPARATUS

Solid–liquid extraction (leaching) is the process of removing a solute or solutes from a solid by using a liquid solvent. Leaching is widely used in chemical industries where mechanical and thermal methods of separation are not possible or practical. Extraction of sugar from sugar beets and oil from oil-bearing seeds, and production of a concentrated solution of a valuable solid material are typical industrial examples of leaching. The leaching process can be considered in three parts:

1. Diffusion of the solvent through the pores of the solid
2. Dissolution of the solutes by the diffused solvent
3. Soxhlet extraction of the solution from porous solid to the main bulk of the solution

21.3.1 COMMERCIAL APPLICATIONS

Extraction of phenolic compounds from natural sources is the most widely studied application of Soxhlet extraction with several hundreds of published scientific papers. Coffee and tea decaffeination, hops extraction, spices extraction, and flavor and fragrance extraction are the major application of this technology. Soxhlet extraction has unique properties, such as (1) it is a flexible process due to the possibility of continuous modulation of the solvent power/selectivity of the Soxhlet extraction, and (2) it allows the elimination of polluting organic solvents and of the expensive postprocessing of the extracts for solvent elimination. Soxhlet extraction is the traditional extraction technique.

Several compounds have been examined as Soxhlet solvents, for example, hydrocarbons such as hexane, pentane, and butane; nitrous oxide; sulfur hexafluoride; and fluorinated hydrocarbons (Azizah et al., 1999). The base Soxhlet process scheme (extraction plus separation) is relatively cheap and very simple to be scaled up to an industrial scale.

21.3.1.1 Essential Oil

This process has been widely studied. Essential oils are the product of hydrocarbonation and oxygenation of terpenes and sesquiterpenes. This is a combination of extraction and fractional processes. This process can be optimized at mild pressures (from 90 to 100 bar) and temperatures (from 40°C to 50°C) since at these process conditions all the essential oil components are largely soluble in liquid (Brown, 1956; Bennett and Myers, 1983; Diplock, 1998).

21.3.1.2 Seed Oils

The hexane extraction from ground seeds is the traditional way to produce vegetable oil. The process is very efficient, but its major problem is the elimination of hexane after extraction. The Soxhlet extraction of several seed oils has been successfully performed up to the pilot scale to overcome the above technical issues (McCabe et al., 1993, 1956; José et al., 2007).

21.3.2 HIGH-ADDED VALUE COMPOUNDS

A selected list of high-added value compounds (mainly nutraceuticals and pharmaceuticals) is reported in Table 21.1. A large spectrum of compounds, including food additives with nutritional and pharmaceutical properties (nutraceuticals), range from tocopherols to carotenoids to alkaloids to unsaturated fatty acids (Sinnott et al., 1983; Perry, 1984, 1988; Wollgast and Anklam, 2000). Pharmaceutical compounds such as artemisinin (antimalarial drug), hyperforin (antidepressant drug), and sterols can be extracted from various materials. In the following, some relevant cases that have been recently studied are discussed in detail.

21.3.2.1 Nutraceuticals

Carotenoids (e.g., lycopene), a large family of compounds that possess antioxidant and coloring properties, have been widely used for food, cosmetic, and medical applications. Variable yields of lycopene ranging from 53.9% to about 80% to almost 90% were found when compared to organic

TABLE 21.1

High-Added Value Compounds Extracted by Soxhlet Extraction Methods

Raw Material	Botanical Name	Extract
	Plant Origin	
Aloe vera leaves	*Aloe barbadensis* Miller	α-Tocopherol
Anise verbena	*Lippia alba*	Limonene and carvone
Apricot pomace	*Prunus armeniaca*	β-Carotene
Artemisia	*Artemisia annua* L.	Artemisinin
Buriti fruit	*Mauritia flexuosa*	Carotenoids and lipids
Chamomile	*Matricaria recutita*	Flavonoids and terpenoids
Cocoa beans	*Theobroma cacao*	Caffeine, theobromine, methylxanthines, butter
Coneflower	*Echinacea angustifolia*	Alkylamides
Coriander seeds	*Coriandrum sativum*	Tocopherols, flavonoids, and terpenoids
Eucalyptus leaves	*Eucalyptus camaldulensis* var. *brevirostris*	Gallic and ellagic acids
Ginger	*Zingiber officinale* Roscoe	Gingerols and shogaols
Ginkgo	*Ginkgo biloba* L.	Ginkgolides and flavonoids
Green tea	*Cratoxylum prunifolium*	Catechins
Hawthorn	*Crataegus* sp.	Flavonoids and terpenoids
Microalgae	*Spirulina maxima*	Carotenoids, astaxanthin, and fatty acids
	Chlorella vulgaris	
Propolis	*Resina propoli*	Flavonoids, galangin, and caffeic acid phenethyl ester
Red yeast	*Phaffia rhodozyma*	Astaxanthin
Saw Palmetto berries	*Serenoa repens*	Fatty acids and β-sitosterol
Soybean lecithin	*Glycine max*	Phosphatidylcholine
St. John's wort	*Hypericum perforatum* L.	Hyperforin, phloroglucinols, and adhyperforin
Tomato	*Lycopersicon esculentum*	Lycopene and β-carotene
	Animal Origin	
Animal liver		Benzimidazoles
Crustaceans		Astaxanthin
Poultry feed, eggs, and muscle tissue		Nicarbazin
Buffalo milk		Buttermilk, butter, and milk fat globule membrane

solvent extraction, the maximum yield being influenced by the maximum pressure and temperature used. Very recently, selective extraction, fractionation, and encapsulation of all-*trans*-lycopene from tomato by Soxhlet extraction in one step have been successfully commissioned at the industrial level (Wollgast and Anklam, 2000).

The extraction and purification of polar lipids derived from milk fat globule membrane have been developed by combining microwave filtration and Soxhlet extraction (Zitko, 1980). Since milk-derived sphingolipids and phospholipids affect numerous physiological functions, such as growth and development, molecular transport systems, stress response, trafficking, and absorption processes, this technological development could be used to tailoring dietary manipulation of dairy lipid components to improve health wellness.

21.3.2.2 Pharmaceuticals

St. John's wort (*Hypericum perforatum*) extracts is a well-known antidepressant having demonstrated clinical effects (even though not based on large scientific trials). Out of two active compounds, hyperforin has been successfully extracted by Soxhlet extraction from plant particles in the pressure range 90–160 bar at 40°C and 50°C, varying CO_2 flow rate, and operating at various extraction times (Xie et al., 2001). Artemisinin, an antimalarial drug, has been commercially extracted using the Soxhlet extraction method (Zhu et al., 2001). Another study demonstrated the comparison of several technologies of extracting artemisinin based on their extraction efficacies, cost, energy efficiency, and global warming potential, and the Soxhlet extraction method was rated very efficient than others.

21.3.3 Antisolvent Extraction

Some essential compounds such as lecithin (Mukhopadhyay, 2000), propolis (Catchpole, 2004), protein from tobacco (Scrugli et al., 2002), and so on cannot be extracted by conventional technology due to their solubility/polarity problem. The supercritical antisolvent extraction (SAE) consisting of the continuous flow of Soxhlet extraction and of the liquid mixture successfully overcame the above limitations and was commissioned commercially.

21.3.4 Advantages of Soxhlet Extraction

The benefits of Soxhlet extraction and especially the supercritical CO_2 versus conventional techniques which are based on the rapid diffusion of the analytes in the fluid (gas-like diffusion) and the fluid solvation power (liquid-like solvation) have led to the promotion of Soxhlet extraction as an alternative to conventional liquid solvent extractions such as ultrasonic extraction. Table 21.2 demonstrates the most significant advantages of the Soxhlet extraction technique, such as its preconcentration effect, its cleanness and safety, its quantitativeness, its expeditiousness, and its simplicity and selectivity.

21.3.5 Limitations of Soxhlet Extraction

Although Soxhlet extraction has very significant benefits, there are significant limitations that are worth studying in order to know the field of application of the technique. The following are the major drawbacks of the Soxhlet extraction and purification technique.

TABLE 21.2

Advantages of Soxhlet Extraction Technology

Types	Advantages
Preconcentration effect	• Solvent concentration
	• Significant reduction of processing time
	• Efficient solvent changeover
Safety	• Cleaner and less hazardous
	• No fire risk
	• No environmentally hazardous wastes
Quantitative	• Complete isolation of the analyte
	• High recovery rate of the analyte
	• Very high diffusivity
Expeditiousness	• Penetrates faster into solid matrices
	• No concentration is required after extraction
	• Short sample preparation time
Simplicity	• Requires minimum number of steps
	• Short analysis and sample extraction time
	• Negligible analytical errors due to reduced steps and analytical time
Selectivity	• Selective extraction of a wide range of analytes
	• No additional manipulation and leads to direct analysis

21.3.5.1 Dealing with Natural Samples

One of the limitations of this technique is difficulties in dealing with natural samples, as the analytes bind more strongly in natural compounds. The best way to overcome this shortcoming is to add polar modifiers (such as methanol).

21.3.5.2 Frequent Need for Clean-Up

Cleaning up the final products from unwanted matrix components is one of the basic problems of the Soxhlet extraction and purification technique, especially when dealing with fat-soluble analytes. A number of sample clean-up methods, such as selective adsorbents, immunoaffinity, and introduction of binary fluid mixture, have been demonstrated sufficient to recover the trapped compound.

21.4 ULTRASONIC-ASSISTED EXTRACTION

UAE has been widely employed recently for the extraction of desired compounds because of its facilitated mass transfer between immiscible phases through superagitation at low frequency (Yan, 2011). Ultrasound utilizes sound waves which are mechanical vibrations that travel through matter that expand and compress molecules that create bubbles and finally cavity collapse (Pathak, 2011). The optimum-processing parameters that need to be determined are the ratio of water (solvent) to raw material, extraction time, and extraction temperature (Yan, 2011). The benefits of ultrasound are generally attributed to acoustic cavitation phenomenon that is formation, growth, and collapse of microbubbles inside a liquid phase submitted to ultrasonic cavitation (Virot et al., 2010). The mechanical, cavitation, and thermal efficacies can result in disruption of cell walls, particle size reduction, and enhanced mass transfer across cell membranes (Pan et al., 2011). It is a simple, efficient, and inexpensive alternative to conventional techniques as ultrasonic cavitation creates shear forces that break cell walls mechanically and enhance material transfer (Zhang et al., 2011). The mechanical effects induce a greater penetration of the solvent into the cellular material and improve mass transfer and by disrupting the cell walls it can facilitate the release of the contents. It has been shown that plant extracts diffuse across cell walls due to ultrasound which causes cell rupture over a shorter period (Wang et al., 2010). This can be done via either continuous mode and/or pulsed mode (Pan et al., 2011). UAE can enable new commercial extraction opportunities and processes for food and allied industries with the opportunity to provide improved bioavailability of micronutrients and avoid degradation of bioactives, and the potential to achieve simultaneous extraction and encapsulation (Vilkhu et al., 2008).

There are two general designs of ultrasonic-assisted extractors, ultrasonic baths and closed extractors fitted with an ultrasonic horn transducer. In order to obtain efficient and effective UAE, it is necessary to take into account various plant characteristics such as moisture content and particle size as well as the solvent used (Wang et al., 2010).

21.4.1 ADVANTAGES OF ULTRASONIC-ASSISTED EXTRACTION

1. High reproducibility at shorter times.
2. Simplified manipulation.
3. Lowered energy input.
4. Reduced operating temperature that allows the extraction of thermolabile compounds.
5. Lowered solvent consumption.
6. Extraction generally enhanced, high extraction efficiency, increased antioxidant activity of the extracts, improved total polyphenol content.
7. Avoidance of structural changes and degradation of polysaccharides.
8. Upscaling of ultrasonic devices is quite easy and cheaper.
9. Simplification of handling and work-up conditions.
10. Can be used with any solvent which allows for extraction of a wide range of natural compounds.

11. No chemical involvement; can prevent possible chemical degradation of target compounds.
12. Apparatus is cheaper and operation is easier.

21.4.2 COMMERCIAL APPLICATIONS

Uses of power ultrasound are considered as a potential energy assistance that can give significant effects on the rate of various chemicals and/or physical processes (Virot et al., 2010). Ultrasonics is one of the most industrially used methods to enhance mass transfer phenomena (Corrales et al., 2008). It is very challenging to attempt extraction on an industrial scale, and the key issues identified are the nature of the tissue being extracted and the location of the components to be extracted; pretreatment of the tissue; the nature of the component being extracted; the effects of ultrasonic involving superficial tissue disruption; increasing surface mass transfer; intraparticle diffusion; loading of extraction chamber with substrate; increased yield of extracted components; increased rate of extraction, enabling reduction in extraction time; and higher process throughput (Vilkhu et al., 2008). The use of coproducts is a growing topic with the possible use of the total food biomass being considered a key process in achieving profitability as well as sustainability in food industries (Virot et al., 2010).

21.5 MICROWAVE-ASSISTED EXTRACTION

Microwaves are composed of electric and magnetic fields and thus emit electromagnetic radiations that are transmitted as waves and these waves penetrate biomaterials and interact with polar molecules, such as water in the biomaterials, to create heat (Wang et al., 2010; Wang, 2011; Pathak, 2011). MAE is a process that uses microwave energy and solvents to extract desired compounds from various plant materials. Due to the temperature and pressure being highly localized, it can cause selective migration of the desired compounds out of the material at a more rapid rate thus reducing the extraction time and solvent usage; this is being employed more increasingly for the extraction of natural products because it is a cheap and rapid technique (Spigno, 2009; Michel et al., 2011). Microwaves can heat a whole material to penetration depth simultaneously (Wang et al., 2010). It has also been shown to result in similar or better recoveries of extract compared to more conventional techniques and without altering the molecular structure and antioxidant potential of the extracted compounds (Spigno, 2009; Wang et al., 2010).

There are two main types of MAE systems commercially available; the first uses closed extraction vessels under controlled pressure and temperature and the second uses a focused microwave oven at atmospheric pressure (Pathak, 2011). Michel et al. (2011) reported the development of a pressurized solvent-free microwave-assisted extraction (PSFME) technique that respects green chemistry as well as the benefits of being rapid and cheap; it does not need sample preparation and/or the evaporation step. The closed MAE system is performed in a closed vessel unit under high extraction temperature and with the pressure being dependent on the volume and boiling point of the solvents (Pathak, 2011).

Advantages

1. Reduced extraction time
2. Reduced solvent usage
3. Improved extraction yield and higher recoveries
4. Process simplicity and low cost
5. Wider choice of solvents and solvent mixtures

Disadvantages/limitations

1. Compared to SFE, an additional filtration or centrifugation step is necessary to remove the solid residue.

2. The efficiency of microwaves can be very poor when the target compounds or the solvents are nonpolar or they are volatile.
3. It is usually performed at higher temperatures of 110–150°C and this may lead to the denaturation of the thermolabile compounds.

21.5.1 Commercial Applications

MAE can extract nutraceuticals from plant materials faster than conventional methods and a higher extraction yield can be achieved in a shorter time, while reducing solvent consumption (Wang et al., 2010).

21.6 SUPERCRITICAL FLUID EXTRACTION

Supercritical state is achieved when the temperature and pressure of a substance are raised over its critical value with a supercritical fluid having properties of both bases and liquids (Pathak, 2011). Supercritical fluids (SCF) are by definition at a temperature and pressure greater than or equal to the critical temperature and pressure of the fluid. Supercritical carbon dioxide ($scCO_2$) is a supercritical fluid because its critical temperature is taken to a point where it is neither a liquid nor a gas but retains both liquid-like solvent properties and gas-like densities. Supercritical fluids are more efficient to spread out along a surface than a true liquid having lower surface tensions than liquids. At the same time, unlike gas, a supercritical fluid maintains a liquid's ability to dissolve substances that are soluble in the compound. In the case of $scCO_2$, this means oils and other organic contaminants can be removed from a surface even if it has an intricate geometry or includes cracks and crevices.

$scCO_2$ is carbon dioxide (CO_2) that has been heated and pressurized above its critical point, which is the highest temperature and pressure at which the gaseous form of pure carbon dioxide can be compressed into a liquid. CO_2's critical pressure is about 1070 pounds per square inch (psi) and the critical temperature is about 31°C, so supercritical applications using CO_2 typically operate at temperatures between 32°C and 49°C and pressures between 1070 and 3500 psi. The physical properties of $scCO_2$ is somewhere between those of a liquid and a gas.

SFE with carbon dioxide as the supercritical fluid is a very attractive method for extraction as CO_2 is an inert, nonflammable, nonexplosive, inexpensive, odorless, colorless, clean solvent and leaves no solvent residue in the product (Krishnaiah et al., 2007).

Many industries throughout the world have started using the nontoxic, environmentally friendly $scCO_2$ as a solvent, replacing harsher volatile organic solvents, such as chlorinated hydrocarbons and chlorofluorocarbons. Since the 1990s, $scCO_2$ has emerged as an environmentally benign substitute for more conventional solvents used for organic synthesis that enter the atmosphere from sprays and similar products. Dry cleaners, plastics manufacturers, food producers, and various industries involved in the extraction of flavors and fragrances have already been using the "benign" solvent, as a part of their environmentally friendly industrial practices. The $scCO_2$ technology is currently extensively used to remove caffeine selectively and leave the flavor of fresh coffee, for example, in decaffeinated coffee beans. Most big pharmaceutical companies have begun using $scCO_2$ for processing drugs into powder consistently. By simply changing pressure and/or temperature, the unique nature of the supercritical fluids can be achieved for organic synthesis purpose. The factors that are considered most important for good recoveries are optimization of operating conditions such as pressure, percentage of modifier, fluid pressure and temperature, and extraction time (Krishnaiah et al., 2007). The dissolving power of a supercritical fluid solvent depends on its density and this is highly adjustable by changing the pressure and temperature, and the supercritical fluid has a higher diffusion coefficient and lower viscosity and surface tension than a liquid solvent, which in turn leads to more favorable mass transfer (Pathak, 2011).

The $scCO_2$ has been researched for potential applications in many areas of food and agriculture industries. Because CO_2 is GRAS, nonflammable, noncorrosive, inexpensive, and easily recyclable, its application in food manufacturing is considered safe. Since CO_2 has low critical temperature, it helps prevent thermal degradation of food products. Moreover, considering stability, structural conformity, and functional properties (such as antioxidant; Stevenson et al., 2008) of the extracted compounds by this method, Blanch et al. (2007) reported these as stable, effective, and without structural change.

High-pressure carbon dioxide pasteurization has been proposed as an alternative of thermal pasteurization for food (Garcia-Gonzalez et al., 2007). This would be an added advantage of supercritical extraction using pure CO_2.

21.6.1 ADVANTAGES OF SFE

The benefits of SFE and especially the supercritical CO_2 versus conventional techniques which are based on the rapid diffusion of the analytes in the fluid (gas-like diffusion) and the fluid solvation power (liquid-like solvation) have led to the promotion of SFE as an alternative to conventional liquid solvent extractions such as Soxhlet and ultrasonic extractions. Table 21.3 demonstrates the most significant advantages of the SFE technique, such as its preconcentration effect, its cleanness and safety, its quantitativeness, its expeditiousness, and its simplicity and selectivity.

The overall advantages of $scCO_2$ extraction technology are (Rozzi and Singh, 2002):

- Supercritical fluids (including CO_2) have a higher diffusion coefficient and lower viscosity than liquids.
- Negligible surface tension allows them to enhance extraction efficiencies by rapid penetration into matrices.
- Selective extraction by manipulating solubility through varying temperature and pressure.
- No chemical residues.
- CO_2 is GRAS, nonflammable, noncorrosive, inexpensive, and recyclable.

TABLE 21.3
Advantages of scCO₂ Extraction Technology

Types	Advantages
Preconcentration effect	• Solvent concentration
	• Significant reduction of processing time
	• Efficient solvent changeover
Cleanness and safety	• Cleaner and less hazardous
	• No fire risk
	• No environmentally hazardous wastes
Quantitativeness	• Complete isolation of the analyte
	• High recovery rate of the analyte
	• Very high diffusivity
Expeditiousness	• Penetrates faster into solid matrices
	• No concentration is required after extraction
	• Short sample preparation time
Simplicity	• Requires minimum number of steps
	• Short analysis and sample transfer time
	• Negligible analytical errors due to reduced steps and analytical time
Selectivity	• Selective extraction of a wide range of analytes
	• No additional manipulation and leads to direct analysis

21.6.2   LIMITATIONS OF SFE

Although the $scCO_2$ extraction has very significant benefits over the traditional extraction and purification processes (as described above), there are significant limitations that are worth studying in
order to know the field of application of the technique. The following are the major drawbacks of the
$scCO_2$ extraction and purification technique.

21.6.2.1   Extraction of Polar Analytes

Due to the low dielectric constant, CO_2 is not a good choice for extraction of polar and ionic compounds (alcohol phenol ethoxylate), although it is an excellent solvent for nonpolar analytes. This
can be overcome by the addition of co-solvents (Yang et al., 1995).

21.6.2.2   Dealing with Natural Samples

One of the limitations of this technique is difficulties in dealing with natural samples, as the analytes bind more strongly in natural compounds. The best way to overcome this shortcoming is to
add polar modifiers (such as methanol).

21.6.2.3   Frequent Need for Clean-Up

Cleaning up the final products from unwanted matrix components is one of the basic problems of
the $scCO_2$ extraction and purification technique, especially when dealing with fat-soluble analytes.
A number of sample clean-up methods, such as selective adsorbents (Pinchon et al., 1997), immunoaffinity (Neubauer et al., 1998), and introduction of binary fluid mixture have been demonstrated
to be sufficient to recover trapped compounds.

21.6.3   COMMERCIAL APPLICATIONS

The SFE is still under industrial development. Extraction of compounds from natural sources is the
most widely studied application of SCFs with several hundreds of published scientific papers. Coffee
and tea decaffeination, hops extraction, spices extraction, and flavor and fragrance extraction are the
major applications of this technology. SFE has unique properties, such as (1) it is a flexible process due
to the possibility of continuous modulation of the solvent power/selectivity of the SCF and (2) it allows
the elimination of polluting organic solvents and of the expensive postprocessing of the extracts for
solvent elimination. The SFE has immediate advantages over traditional extraction techniques.

Several compounds have been examined as SFE solvents. For example, hydrocarbons such as
hexane, pentane, and butane; nitrous oxide; sulfur hexafluoride; and fluorinated hydrocarbons
(Smith, 1999). The CO_2 is the most popular SFE solvent because it is safe, readily available, and has
a low cost that allows supercritical operations at relatively low pressures and at near-room temperatures. The major serious drawback of SFE is the higher investment costs if compared to traditional
atmospheric pressure extraction techniques. However, the base process scheme (extraction plus
separation) is relatively cheap and very simple to be scaled up to industrial scale. Another downside
is that compressing CO_2 supercritical form is energy intensive.

21.6.3.1   Supercritical Carbon Dioxide Cleaning Technology Review

The $scCO_2$ technology is regarded as the best choice for precision cleaning of various components
and assemblies such as metal bearings, electronic assemblies, optical and laser components, and
computer parts (http://www.pprc.org/pubs/techreviews/co2sum.html). A process change from
aqueous or solvent cleaning to $scCO_2$ cleaning is environmentally advantageous, simply because
of its nonflammable, inert, and non-ozone-depleting nature.

21.6.3.2   Solid Extraction Processing

This is the most studied SCF application for the extraction/elimination of one or more compound
families from a solid natural matrix. Some well-established industrial processes use SFE to produce

hops extracts, decaffeinated coffee, and some food nutritional substances that also offer some aspects of therapeutic protection to the human body (nutraceuticals). However, many other applications are possible.

21.6.3.2.1 Essential Oil

The process mentioned in the earlier section can be optimized at mild pressures (from 90 to 100 bar) and temperatures (from 40°C to 50°C) since at these process conditions all the essential oil components are largely soluble in $scCO_2$ (Akgün et al., 1999; Kim and Hong, 1999; Bravi et al., 2007). Data on the supercritical extraction of essential oils is shown in Table 21.4 that is alphabetically organized by the common name (raw material), the botanical name, and the target component (the extract).

21.6.3.2.2 Seed Oils

The hexane extraction from ground seeds is the traditional way to produce vegetable oil. The process is very efficient, but its major problem is the elimination of hexane after extraction. The SFE of several seed oils has been successfully performed up to the pilot scale to overcome the above technical issues (Table 21.4).

TABLE 21.4
SFE of Oleoresins (OR), Essential (EO), Volatile (VO), and Seed (SO) Oils

Raw Material	Botanical Name	Extract
Anise seeds	*Pimpinella anisum* L.	EO
Basil leaves	*Ocimum basilicum*	EO
Cashew	*Anacardium occidentale*	VO
Celery roots	*Apium graveolens* L.	SO
Chamomile flowers	*Chamomilla recutita* L. R.	EO and OR
Clove bud	*Eugenia caryophyllata*	EO
Coriander seeds	*Coriandrum sativum* L.	SO
Eucalyptus leaves	*Eucalyptus globulus* L.	EO
Fennel seeds	*Foeniculum vulgare* Mill.	SO
Grape seeds	*Vitis vinifera*	SO
Juniper fruits	*Juniperus communis* L.	VO
Lemon balm	*Melissa officinalis*	EO
Lemon eucalyptus	*Eucalyptus citriodora*	EO
Lemongrass leaves	*Cymbopogon citrates*	EO
Marjoram leaves	*Origanum majorana*	EO
Mint leaves	*Mentha spicata insularis*	EO
Oregano	*Origanum vulgare* L.	EO
Palm kernel oil	*Elaeis guineensis*	SO
Pepper, black	*Piper nigrum* L.	EO
Pepper, red	*Capsicum frutescens* L.	OR
Rye bran	*Secale cereal*	Alkylresorcinols
Sage leaves	*Salvia desoleana*	EO
Spiked thyme	*Thymbra spicata*	EO
Thyme	*Zygis sylvestris*	EO

Source: Adapted and modified from Reverchon, E. and De Marco, I. 2006. *J. Supercrit. Fluids*, 38: 146–166.

21.6.3.3 High-Added Value Compounds

A selected list of high-added value compounds (mainly nutraceuticals and pharmaceuticals) is reported in Table 21.5. A large spectrum of compounds, including food additives with nutritional and pharmaceutical properties (nutraceuticals), range from tocopherols to carotenoids to alkaloids to unsaturated fatty acids. Pharmaceutical compounds like artemisinin (antimalarial drug), to hyperforin (antidepressant drug), and to sterols can be extracted from various materials. In the following, some relevant cases that have been recently studied are discussed in detail.

21.6.3.3.1 Nutraceuticals

Successful commercial extraction of carotenoids by SCFs from various sources has been studied (Gomez-Prieto et al., 2003, Sanal et al., 2005; Uquiche et al., 2004; Vasapollo et al., 2004). SFE of

TABLE 21.5

High-Added Value Compounds Extracted by SFE Methods

Raw Material	Botanical Name	Extract
Plant Origin		
Aloe vera leaves	*Aloe barbadensis* Miller	α-Tocopherol
Anise verbena	*Lippia alba*	Limonene and carvone
Apricot pomace	*Prunus armeniaca*	β-Carotene
Artemisia	*Artemisia annua* L.	Artemisinin
Buriti fruit	*Mauritia flexuosa*	Carotenoids and lipids
Chamomile	*Matricaria recutita*	Flavonoids and terpenoids
Cocoa beans	*Theobroma cacao*	Caffeine, theobromine, methylxanthines, and butter
Coneflower	*Echinacea angustifolia*	Alkylamides
Coriander seeds	*Coriandrum sativum*	Tocopherols, flavonoids, and terpenoids
Eucalyptus leaves	*Eucalyptus camaldulensis* var. *Brevirostris*	Gallic and ellagic acids
Ginger	*Zingiber officinale* Roscoe	Gingerols and shogaols
Ginkgo	*Ginkgo biloba* L.	Ginkgolides and flavonoids
Green tea	*Cratoxylum prunifolium*	Catechins
Hawthorn	*Crataegus* sp.	Flavonoids and terpenoids
Microalgae	*Spirulina maxima* *Chlorella vulgaris*	Carotenoids, Astaxanthin, and fatty acids
Propolis	*Resina propoli*	Flavonoids, galangin, and caffeic acid phenethyl ester
Red yeast	*Phaffia rhodozyma*	Astaxanthin
Saw Palmetto berries	*Serenoa repens*	Fatty acids and β-sitosterol
Soybean lecithin	*Glycine max*	Phosphatidylcholine
St. John's wort	*Hypericum perforatum* L.	Hyperforin, phloroglucinols, and adhyperforin
Tomato	*Lycopersicon esculentum*	Lycopene and β-carotene
Animal Origin		
Animal liver		Benzimidazoles
Crustaceans		Astaxanthin
Poultry feed, eggs, and muscle tissue		Nicarbazin
Buffalo milk		Buttermilk, butter, and milk fat globule membrane

Source: Adapted and modified from Reverchon, E. and De Marco, I. 2006. *J. Supercrit. Fluids*, 38: 146–166.

lycopene (from tomato) has been commissioned using pure $scCO_2$ (Gomez-Prieto et al., 2003) and with co-solvents (Vasapollo et al., 2004). Very recently, selective extraction, fractionation, and encapsulation of all-*trans*-lycopene from tomato by $scCO_2$ in one step have been successfully commissioned at the industrial level (Blanch et al., 2007).

Astaxanthin is a xanthophyll and is naturally found in various materials such as red yeast (*Phaffia rhodozyma*) (Lim et al., 2002), microalgae (*Chlorella vulgaris*) (Mendes et al., 2003), and crayfish (crustacean). Up to 97% astaxanthin extraction yield was reported by the $scCO_2$ extraction method with ethanol as the cosolvent, when compared to its initial content in the matrix (Valderrama et al., 2003). The extraction and purification of polar lipids derived from milk fat globule membrane has been developed by combining microfiltration and $scCO_2$ (Astaire et al., 2003). Since milk-derived sphingolipids and phospholipids affect numerous physiological functions, such as growth and development, molecular transport systems, stress response, trafficking, and absorption processes, this technological development could be used to tailoring dietary manipulation of dairy lipid components to improve health wellness.

21.6.3.3.2 Pharmaceuticals

St. John's wort (*Hypericum perforatum*) extract is a well-known antidepressant having demonstrated clinical effects. Out of two active compounds, hyperforin has been successfully extracted by $scCO_2$ from plant particles in the pressure range of 90–160 bar at 40°C and 50°C, varying CO_2 flow rate, and operating at various extraction times (Rompp et al., 2004). Artemisinin, an antimalarial drug, has been commercially extracted using the $scCO_2$ method (Quispe-Condori et al., 2005). Another study demonstrated the comparison of several technologies of extracting artemisinin based on their extraction efficacies, cost, energy efficiency, and global warming potential, and $scCO_2$ method was rated very efficient than others (Lapkin et al., 2006). Very recently, Pharmalink marketed an anti-inflammatory compound (MO-CO2SFE95) from New Zealand green-lipped mussel using $scCO_2$ extraction process based on extensive human trials (McPhee et al., 2007; Treschow et al., 2007).

21.6.3.4 Liquid Extraction Processing

The fractionation of liquid mixtures into two or more fractions is another relevant process in $scCO_2$, based on the different solubilities of the liquids to be separated. Hexane elimination from vegetable oils to recover reusable compounds and fried oil fractionation by $scCO_2$ (Sesti Osséo et al., 2004) are the two most commonly used applications.

21.6.3.5 Antisolvent Extraction

Some essential compounds, such as lecithin (Mukhopadhyay, 2000), propolis (Catchpole, 2004), protein from tobacco, and so on cannot be extracted by conventional technology due to their solubility/polarity problem. The SAE consisting of the continuous flow of $scCO_2$ and of the liquid mixture successfully overcame the above limitations and was commissioned commercially.

21.6.4 Safety Analysis

Since the beginning of the green chemistry movement 10 years ago, the need for alternative solvents for reactions has been one of the major issues scientists/technologists have faced (Clark and Tavener, 2007). The use of alternative solvent is reviewed in terms of manufacturing, distribution, usage, and disposal criteria. Table 21.6 shows the relative advantages and disadvantages of alternative solvents.

CO_2 and water do not require manufacture as such, although energy is required for their respective condensation and purification. From a "food miles" point of view, both water and CO_2 are available worldwide and thus may usually be sourced close to the site of use. It has been

TABLE 21.6

Advantages and Disadvantages of Using Alternative Solvents

Key Solvent	Properties	Separation and Reuse	Health and Safety	Cost of Use	Environmental Impact	Arbitrary Score[a] (/25)
$scCO_2$	Poor solvent for many polar compounds, may be improved with cosolvents or surfactants (1)	Excellent, efficient, and selective (5)	Nontoxic and nonflammable (4)	Energy cost is high, CO_2 is cheap and abundant (3)	Sustainable, no significant end-of-life concern (5)	18
Ionic liquids	Wide range of designer solvents, always polar (4)	Easy to remove, reuse may be a problem if high purity is required (2)	Very limited data available, reported to flammable/ toxic (2)	Expensive, except few (2)	Petrochemical-based are nonsustainable, but sustainable ILs exist, synthesis is energy intensive (3)	13
Fluorous solvents	Limited to nonpolar solutes, best used in biphasic systems (3)	May be distilled and reuse (4)	Bioaccumulative, greenhouse gases (2)	Very expensive (1)	Very resource demanding, nonsustainable (2)	12
Water	Dissolves small quantities of many compounds, generally poor for nonpolar (3)	Purification is energy demanding, limited reuse (3)	Nontoxic, nonflammable, and safe to handle (5)	Very cheap, energy cost high (4)	Sustainable and safe to the environment (4)	19
Solvents based on/ derived from renewables	Wide range (4)	May be distilled (4)	Generally low toxicity (4)	Cost will decrease with greater market volume (4)	Sustainable, volatile organic compounds will cause problem (3)	19

Source: Adapted from Clark, J.H. and Tavener, S.J. 2007. *Organic Process Res. Dev.*, 11: 149–155.
[a] Arbitrary scoring on a scale of 1 (poor) to 5 (very good).

estimated that about 50% of the energy used in chemical processes is consumed in purification and recycled streams. CO_2 is considered excellent in this category. CO_2 is a colorless, noncombustible, and nontoxic gas. Because it is heavier than air, it spreads along the ground. Although it forms a portion of exhaled air, high concentration of CO_2 in respirable air can lead, without any observable signs, to asphyxia. Table 21.7 demonstrates the physical, chemical, and toxicological information about the safety specification of CO_2.

Supercritical CO_2 has little environmental impact, and it may be safely released into the environment simply by venting the reaction. SFE is widely used in the food industry, mainly because of its ability to offer an essentially solvent-free final product and to meet the most rigorous environmental regulations.

TABLE 21.7

Comparison of Physical Properties and Health and Safety Data for Some Representative Solvents

Solvent	Relative Cost[a]	LD50 (Rat) (mg/kg)	Environmental Fate
DCM	1	1600	Photo degradation
Hexane	1	28,700	Photo degradation
Water	[a]	N/A	No change
CO_2	[a]	N/A (asphyxiant)	No change
Bioethanol	1	7060	Rapid biodegradation
Ethyl lactate	2	>2000	Rapid biodegradation

Source: Adapted and modified from Clark, J.H. and Tavener, S.J. 2007. *Organic Process Res. Dev.*, 11: 149–155.

[a] From Aldrich Chemical Co.; water and CO_2 are essentially free resources, but cost of use depends on energy efficiency of purification/condensation processes.

21.6.4.1 Safety Analysis of Compounds Derived from This Technology

Supercritical CO_2 technology is currently successfully applied in several food-processing and manufacturing industries, such as essential oils, vegetable oils, and so on. The new horizon of this application in nutraceutical, cosmetic, and pharmaceutical industries is challenging.

Very few animal/human toxicological studies have been done targeting the safety profile of compounds extracted or fractionated by this technology. The triterpenoids, a group of polar components extracted from bamboo shaving using $scCO_2$, were evaluated for toxicological effect on animals (Zhang et al., 2004). The result demonstrated that no significant toxicological effects were found both in rats and in mice at more than 10,000 mg/kg body weight. However, the objective of this study was primarily the safety issues of triterpenoids, but not the technology itself.

Lyprinol, derived from the green-lipped mussel of New Zealand, is another example of the success story of SFE technology. A good number of animal and human studies were performed to evaluate its efficacy and safety profiles (Gruenwald et al., 2004; Lau, 2004). No safety concerns related to the extraction method were raised in assessing this product. Very recently, Pharmalink patented an anti-inflammatory compound (MO-CO2SFE95) from New Zealand green-lipped mussel using the $scCO_2$ extraction process (McPhee et al., 2007; Treschow et al., 2007).

21.7 CONCLUSION

Nowadays, new natural sources for functional ingredients are being searched by the food industry. The final goal is to develop new products that can provide an additional benefit to human health besides the basic energetic and nutritional requirements. Among the more interesting compounds that can be extracted from natural sources, antioxidants are the most intensely studied because they can have a double functionality, that is, they can be useful as a food preservation method while providing important health benefits for humans.

With the objective of isolating antioxidant compounds from natural sources, several plant varieties have been studied along with different natural sources as algae, microalgae, and food by-products.

At the same time, there is a clear need of developing new extraction processes, environmentally clean, safe, and selective enough to extract natural food ingredients with a high yield.

Thus, the Soxhlet extraction technology has grown in importance, mainly when using natural solvents. It allows obtaining extracts free of toxic residues that can be directly used without any further treatment, and with a composition tuneable by changing the extraction conditions (that, of course, affects the extraction selectivity).

Thanks to this technique, intermediate polar compounds can be isolated with high selectivity, which can be achieved by modifying the extraction temperature. At the same time, the extraction procedures are faster than traditional extraction methods without the use of any organic solvent.

The application of advanced technologies has been demonstrated to offer an extraordinary potential and selectivity for extraction purposes. They are a combination of effective extraction techniques and low-cost raw materials that represent environmental and economical alternatives to conventional extraction methods where large amounts of organic solvents and long extraction times are required. Utilizing novel technologies for extraction will reduce food-processing wastes and facilitate the production of natural valuable products which will guarantee food sustainability and meet consumer demands (Sarkar et al., 2011).

REFERENCES

Akgün, M., Akgün, N.A., and Dinçer, S. 1999. Phase behaviour of essential oil components in supercritical carbon dioxide. *J. Supercrit. Fluids*, 15: 117–125.

Astaire, J., Ward, R., German, J.B., and Jimenez-Flores, R. 2003. Concentration of polar MFGM lipids from buttermilk by microfiltration and supercritical fluid extraction. *J. Dairy Sci.*, 86: 2297–2307.

Azizah, A.H., Ruslawati, N.M., and Swee Tee, T. 1999. Extraction and characterization of antioxidants from cocoa by-products. *Food Chem.*, 64: 199–202.

Bennett, C.O. and Myers, J.E. 1983. *Momentum, Heat and Mass Transfer*, 3rd edn. Chemical Engineering Series, McGraw-Hill, New York.

Blanch, G.P., Castillo, M.L., Caja, M.D., Perez-Mendez, M., and Sanchez-Cortes, S. 2007. Stabilization of all-*trans*-lycopene from tomato by encapsulation using cyclodextrins. *Food Chem.*, 105: 1335–1341.

Bravi, M., Spinoglio, F., Verdone, N. et al. 2007. Improving the extraction of α-tocopherol-enriched oil from grape seeds by supercritical CO_2. Optimisation of the extraction conditions. *J. Food Eng.*, 78: 488–493.

Brown, G.G. 1956. *Unit Operations*, John Wiley & Sons, USA.

Catchpole, O.J., Grey, J.B., Mitchell, K.A., and Lan, J.S. 2004. Supercritical antisolvent fractionation of propolis tincture. *J. Supercrit. Fluids*, 29: 97–106.

Clark, J.H. and Tavener, S.J. 2007. Alternative solvents: Shades of green. *Organic Process Res. Dev.*, 11: 149–155.

Corrales, M., Toepfl, S., Butz, P., Knorr, D., and Tauscher, B. 2008. Extraction of anthocyanins from grape by-products assisted by ultrasonics, high hydrostatic pressure or pulsed electric fields: A comparison. *J. Innovative Food Sci. Emerging Tech.*, 9: 85–91.

Diplock, A.T., Charleux, J.L., Crozier-Willi, G. et al. 1998. Functional food science and defence against reactive oxidative species [review]. *Br. J. Nutr.*, 80: 77–112.

Garcia-Gonzalez, L., Geeraerd, A.H., Spilimbergo, S. et al. 2007. High pressure carbon dioxide inactivation of microorganisms in foods: The past, the present and the future. *Int. J. Food Microbiol.*, 117: 1–28.

Gomez-Prieto, M.S., Caja, M.M., Herraiz, M., and Santa-Maria, G. 2003. Supercritical fluid extraction of all-*trans*-lycopene from tomato. *J. Agric. Food Chem.*, 51: 3–7.

Gruenwald, J., Graubaum, H.J., Hansen, K., and Grube, B. 2004. Efficacy and tolerability of a combination of Lyprinol and high concentrations of EPA and DHA in inflammatory rheumatoid disorders. *Advn. Ther.*, 21: 197–201. http://www.pprc.org/pubs/techreviews/co2sum.html.

José, A.D.C., Garcia-Gonzalez, M., and Guerrero, M.G. 2007. Outdoor cultivation of microalgae for carotenoid production: Current state and perspectives. *Appl. Microbiol. Biotechnol.*, 74: 1163–1174.

Kim, K.H. and Hong, J. 1999. Equilibrium solubilities of spearmint oil components in supercritical carbon dioxide. *Fluid Phase Equil.*, 164: 107–115.

Krishnaiah, D., Sarbatly, R., and Bono, A. 2007. Phytochemical antioxidants for health and medicine—A move towards nature. Biotech. *Mol. Biol. Rev.*, 1: 97–104.

Lapkin, A.A., Plucinski, P.K., and Culter, M. 2006. Comparative assessment of technologies for extraction of artemisinin. *J. Nat. Prod.*, 69: 1653–1664.

Lau, C.S. 2004. Treatment of knee osteoarthritis with Lyprinol, lipid extract of the green-lipped mussel, a double-blind placebo-controlled study. *Prog. Nutr.*, 6: 17–31.

Lim, G-B., Lee, S-Y., Lee, E-K., Haam, S-J., and Kim, W-S. 2002. Separation of astaxanthin from red yeast *Phaffia rhodozyma* by supercritical carbon dioxide extraction. *Biochem. Eng. J.*, 11: 181–187.

McCabe, W.L., Smith, J.C., and Harriott, P. 1993. Unit Operations of Chemical Engineering, 5th ed., McGraw-Hill, New York.

Michel, T., Destandau, E., and Elfakir, C. 2011. Evaluation of a simple and promising method for extraction of antioxidants from sea buckthorn (*Hippophaë rhamnoides* L.) berries: Pressurised solvent-free microwave assisted extraction. *Food Chem.*, 126: 1380–1386.

McPhee, S., Hodges, L.D., Wright, P.F.A. et al. 2007. Anticyclooxygenase effects of lipid extracts from the New Zealand grre-lipped mussel (*Perna canaliculus*). *Comp, Biochem. Physiol.*, Part B, 146: 346–356.

Mendes, R.L., Nobre, B.P., Cardoso, M.T., Pereira, A.P., and Palavra, A.F. 2003. Supercritical carbon dioxide extraction of compounds with pharmaceutical importance from microalgae. *Inorg. Chim. Acta*, 356: 328–334.

Mukhopadhyay, M. 2000. *Natural Extracts Using Supercritical Carbon Dioxide*, CRC Press, Boca Raton, FL.

Neubauer, G., King, A., and Rappsilber, J. et al. 1998. Mass spectrometry and EST-database searching allows characterization of the multi-protein spliceosome complex, *Nat. Genet.*, 20: 46–50.

Pan, Z., Qu, W., Mab, H., Atungulu, G., and McHugh, T. 2011. Continuous and pulsed ultrasound-assisted extractions of antioxidants from pomegranate peel. *J. Ultrasonics Sonochem.*, 18: 1249–1257.

Pathak, Y., 2011 May. *Handbook of Nutraceuticals Volume II: Scale-Up, Processing and Automation*, CRC Press, USA.

Perry, R.H. and D.W. Green. 1988. *Perry's Chemical Engineers' Handbook*, 6th edn, McGraw-Hill, New York.

Pinchon, V., Aulard-Macler, E., Oubihi, H., Hennion, M.C., and Caude, M. 1997. *Chromatographia*, 46: 529.

Quispe-Condori, S., Sanchez, D., Foglio, M.A., Rosa, P., Zetzl, C., Brunner, G., and Meireles, A.A. 2005. Global yield isotherms and kinetic of artemisin extraction from *Artemisia annua* L leaves using supercritical carbon dioxide. *J. Supercrit. Fluids*, 36: 40–48.

Reverchon, E. and De Marco, I. 2006. Supercritical fluid extraction and fractionation of natural matter. *J. Supercrit. Fluids*, 38: 146–166.

Rompp, H., Seger, C., Kaiser, C.S., Haslinger, E., and Schmidt, P.C. 2004. Enrichment of Hyperforin from St. John's Wort (*Hypericum perforatum*) by pilot-scale supercritical carbon dioxide extraction. *Eur. J. Pharm. Sci.*, 21:443–451.

Rozzi, N.L. and Singh, R.K. 2002. Supercritical fluids and the food industry. *Comprehensive Rev. Food Sci. Food Safety*, 1: 33–36.

Sanal, I.S., Bayraktar, E., Mehmetoglu, U., and Calimli, A. 2005. Determination of optimum conditions for SC-(CO_2 + ethanol) extraction of β-carotene from apricot pomace using response surface methodology. *J. Supercrit. Fluids*, 34: 331–338.

Sarkar, A., Das, S., Ghosh, D., and Singh, H. 2011. Green concepts in the food industry. In: *Handbook of Nutraceuticals, Vol II, Scale-Up, Processing and Automation*, ed. Pathak, Y, CRC Press, FL, pp. 455–483.

Scrugli, S., Frongia, M., Muscas, M. et al. 2002. A preliminary study on the application of supercritical antisolvent technique to the fractionation of tobacco extracts. In: *Proceedings of the 8th Meeting on Supercritical Fluids Bordeaux.* eds. M. Besnard and F. Cansell, France, 901.

Sesti Osséo, L., Caputo, G., Gracia, I., and Reverchon, E. 2004. Continuous fractionation of used frying oil by supercritical CO_2. *J. Am. Oil Chem. Soc.*, 81: 879–885.

Smith, R.M. 1999. Supercritical fluids in separation science—the dreams, the reality and the future. *J. Chromatogr. A*, 856: 83–115.

Sinnott, R.K., Coulson, J.M., and Richardson, J.F. 1983. *An Introduction to Chemical Engineering Design*, 1st edn, Pergamon Press, Oxford, UK.

Spigno, G. and De Faveri, D.M. 2009. Microwave-assisted extraction of tea phenols: A phenomenological study. *J. Food Eng.*, 93: 210–217.

Stevenson, D., Inglett, G., Chen, D., Biswas, A., Eller, F., and Evangelista, R. 2008. Phenolic content and antioxidant capacity of supercritical carbon dioxide-treated and air-classified oat bran concentrate microwave-irradiated in water or ethanol at varying temperatures. *Food Chem.*, 108: 23–30.

Treschow, A.P., Hodges, L.D., Wright, P.F.A., Wynne, P.M., Kalafatis, N., and Macrides, T.A. 2007. Novel anti-inflammatory ω-3 PUFAs from the New Zealand grre-lipped mussel (*Perna canaliculus*). *Comp. Biochem. Physiol. Part B*, 147: 645–656.

Uquiche, E., del Valle, J.M., and Ortiz, J. 2004. Supercritical carbon dioxide extraction of red pepper (*Capsicum annuum* L.) oleoresin. *J. Food Eng.*, 65: 55–66.

Valderrama, J.O., Perrut, M., and Majewski, W. 2003. Extraction of astaxantine and phycocyanine from microalgae with supercritical carbon dioxide. *J. Chem. Eng. Data*, 48: 827–830.

Vasapollo, G., Longo, L., Restio, L., and Ciurlia, L. 2004. Innovative supercritical CO_2 extraction of Lycopene from tomato in the presence of vegetable oil as co-solvent. *J. Supercrit. Fluids*, 29: 87–96.

Vilkhu, K., Mawson, R., Simons, L., and Bates, D. 2008. Applications and opportunities for ultrasound assisted extraction in the food industry—A review. *J. Innovative Food Sci. Emerging Technol.*, 9: 161–169.

Virot, M., Tomao, V., Le Bourvellec, C., Renard, C.M.C.G., and Chemat, F. 2010. Towards the industrial production of antioxidants from food processing by-products with ultrasound-assisted extraction. *J. Ultrasonics Sonochem.*, 17: 1066–1074.

Wang, J., Zhang, J., Zhao, B., Wang, X., Wu, Y., and Yao, J. 2010. A comparison study on microwave-assisted extraction of *Potentilla anserina* L. polysaccharides with conventional method: Molecule weight and antioxidant activities evaluation. *J. Carbohydrate Polymers*, 80: 84–93.

Wang L. 2011. Advances in extraction of plant products in nutraceutical processing. In: *Handbook of Nutraceuticals Volume II, Scale-Up, Processing and Automation*, ed. Pathak, Y. CRC Press, Boca Raton, FL, Chapter 2, pp. 15–52.

Wollgast, J. and Anklam, E. 2000. Review on polyphenols in *Theobroma cacao*: Changes in composition during the manufacture of chocolate and methodology for identification and quantification. *Food Res. Int.*, 33: 423–447.

Yan, Y., Yu, C., Chen, J., Li, X., Wang, W., and Li, S. 2011. Ultrasonic-assisted extraction optimized by response surface methodology, chemical composition and antioxidant activity of polysaccharides from *Tremella mesenterica*. *J. Carbohydrate Polymers*, 83: 217–224.

Yang, Y., Garaibeth, A., Hawthorne, S.B., and Miller, D.J. 1995. Combined temperature/modifier effects on supercritical CO_2 extraction efficiencies of polycyclic aromatic hydrocarbons from environmental samples. *Anal. Chem.*, 67: 641–646.

Xie, W., Gao, Z., Pan, W.-P., Hunter, D., Singh, A., and Vaia, R. 2001. Effect of monomers on the basal spacing of sodium montmorillonite and the structures of polymer—Clay nanocomposites. *Chem. Mater.*, 13: 2979.

Zhang, G., He, L., and Hu, M. 2011. Optimized ultrasonic-assisted extraction of flavonoids from *Prunella vulgaris* L. and evaluation of antioxidant activities *in vitro*. *J. Innovative Food Sci. Emerging Technol.*, 12: 18–25.

Zhu, J., Morgan, A.B., Lamelas, F.J., and Wilkie, C.A. 2001. Fire properties of polystyrene-clay nanocomposites. *Chem. Mater.*, 13, 3774.

Zitko, V. 1980. *The Handbook of Environmental Chemistry. Part A. Anthropogenic Compounds*, Springer, Heidelberg, Germany.

Section V

Innovation in Functional Food Ingredients

22 Advances in Milk Protein Ingredients

Thom Huppertz and Hasmukh Patel

CONTENTS

22.1 INTRODUCTION

Over the past two decades, the demand worldwide for dairy products and dairy ingredients has grown significantly and this demand is expected to continue to grow in the future. New nutritional science knowledge has contributed to customer and consumer awareness. Today, consumers are more aware of their health and their nutritional requirements. They are making more informed decisions about the food products they consume, which has created much pressure and competition for food manufacturers and has resulted in a consistently increasing range of functional and nutritional food

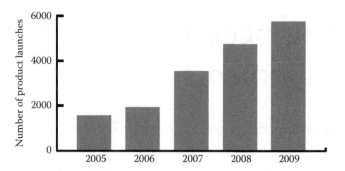

FIGURE 22.1 The number worldwide of new functional food and beverage products introduced between 2005 and 2009. (Adapted from Mintel Group Ltd. 2009. *Global New Products Database*. London: Mintel Group Ltd.)

products being launched every year. According to Mintel Group Ltd (2009), the number of new functional food and beverage products introduced worldwide grew from approximately 1500 in 2005 to approximately 5700 in 2009 (Figure 22.1). Because the market is becoming more and more competitive, food manufacturers are looking for competitively priced food ingredients for their product formulations.

Milk and milk products are excellent sources of nutrition. Milk protein ingredients provide not only nutrition, but also specific technical functionality. They provide unique functional benefits that give formulation flexibility and desired properties in the final products. Milk protein ingredients are natural, trusted food ingredients, and are ideal for unique nutritional and functional applications (Huffman and Harper 1999). Prior to the 1970s, it was difficult to manufacture good quality and reasonably pure protein fractions and dairy ingredients on a commercial scale economically. However, advances in the dairy industry during the 1970s and 1980s in commercially relevant state-of-the-art processing technologies such as ultrafiltration (UF), microfiltration (MF), nanofiltration (NF), and ion exchange (IEX) have meant some radical changes in the commercial processing of dairy ingredients, particularly protein ingredients. With the advent of these technologies, it is now possible to produce, on an industrial scale and with good microbiological quality and in a cost-effective manner, reasonably pure milk protein ingredients, such as whey protein concentrate (WPC), whey protein isolate (WPI), milk protein concentrate (MPC), and isolates of individual proteins, for example, β-lactoglobulin (β-LG), α-lactalbumin (α-LA), lactoferrin (LF), and immunoglobulins (IGs). These ingredients can be tailored for specific functional properties or for specific applications (such as gelling, emulsification, and texture) by manipulating the processing conditions and the processing steps during their manufacture. In addition, many recent clinical studies have proved the nutritional and health-promoting aspects of dairy protein ingredients, which have helped to create much awareness about the nutritional benefits of milk and milk components. In turn, this has boosted the demand for value-added dairy protein ingredients in recent years and has helped these ingredients to fetch premium prices over the standard commodity ingredients, such as skim milk powder (SMP), whole milk powder (WMP), and caseinates. Therefore, converting milk into value-added functional and nutritional ingredients provides more profit, leverages health benefits, and thus provides increased potential for milk.

Recently, detailed studies on specific process-induced interactions of dairy ingredients with other components and their functionality in food systems have helped to design and create tailor-made ingredients with specific functional and/or nutritional quality, many arising from improved knowledge of their impact on structure, texture, flavor, and consumer acceptability of the final product in which the dairy ingredients will be used. Such studies, together with the development of novel, state-of-the art dairy ingredient processing technologies and consumer interest in functional and nutritional products with specific health benefits and sensory properties, are driving the demand for tailor-made, functional, value-added, and nutritional dairy ingredients that are suitable for specific food and beverage applications (Tong 2010).

The recent advances in our knowledge of the effects of processing on the structure of milk proteins and their interactions with other components in food systems, the introduction of manufacturing technologies such as UF, MF, and IEX, and advances in and the adoption of analytical technologies have allowed the commercial development of a range of value-added casein-based ingredients such as MPC and whey-based ingredients such as WPC, WPI, and particular whey protein fractions (β-LG, α-LA, LF, and IGs). Although many dairy-derived ingredients (e.g., milk proteins, complex lipids such as dairy phospholipids, gangliosides, lactose, and complex carbohydrates) are listed in the literature, this chapter deals only with advances in milk powders, caseinates, and the value-added dairy ingredients mentioned above and aims to provide an up-to-date overview of recent advances in dairy protein ingredients, their manufacturing technologies, and their applications.

22.2 MILK POWDERS

22.2.1 INTRODUCTION

In 2009, global production of WMP and SMP, typical compositions of which are shown in Table 22.1, amounted to approximately 3.8 million tons and approximately 3.6 million tons, respectively (IDF 2010). The main reason for manufacturing milk powders is to convert the liquid, perishable milk into a product that can be stored for a substantial period of time without a loss in quality. These milk powders can be transported to nations with dairy industries that cannot fulfill the population demand for dairy products with locally manufactured products. In addition, milk powders are used as functional ingredients in a wide variety of food products, such as clinical and infant nutrition, yogurt, cheese, confectionery, soups and sauces, chocolate, and bakery products. An overview of the functional properties conferred by the main constituents of milk powders, that is, protein, fat, and lactose, in some of their main areas of application is outlined in Table 22.2.

22.2.2 PRODUCTION OF MILK POWDERS

A basic process for the production of milk powder is outlined in Figure 22.2. Similar processes are described by Písecký (1997), Kelly et al. (2003), Westergaard (2004), Baldwin and Pearce (2005), and Walstra et al. (2006). Milk is separated, pasteurized, and, when WMP is produced, standardized to the desired fat content; a solids-not-fat:fat ratio of approximately 2.7 yields a powder containing approximately 26% (m/m) fat. The milk is subsequently preheated. For SMP, depending on typical applications of the final product, three different types of heat treatment, that is, low heat, medium heat, and high heat, yielding different degrees of whey protein denaturation, can be applied. An overview of the different preheating classes is provided in Table 22.3. For WMP, preheating is typically under medium to high heat conditions, that is, 30 s–5 min at 85–95°C. This intense preheating step is aimed at minimizing lipid oxidation in the final product.

TABLE 22.1
Typical Compositions (%, m/m) of Whole Milk Powder and Skim Milk Powder

	Whole Milk Powder	Skim Milk Powder
Fat	25–29	0.5–1.5
Protein	25–28	34–37
Lactose	36–39	48–52
Ash	6–7	7–8
Moisture	2–4	3–5

TABLE 22.2

Functional Properties of Different Constituents of Milk Powders

Constituent	Functional Property	Application
Protein	Water-binding/thickening	Meat products, bakery products, confectionary, soups and sauces, chocolate
	Emulsification	Coffee whiteners, soups, sauces, ice cream, confectionary, meat products
	Foaming/whipping	Ice cream, desserts, whipped toppings
	Gelation	Cheese, yoghurt
	Color/flavor development	Chocolate, confectionary
	Heat stability	Recombined milk, infant and clinical nutrition, soups, and sauces
	Solubility	Recombined milk, infant and clinical nutrition
Fat	Texture/mouthfeel	Cheese, yoghurt, confectionary, chocolate, soups, sauces, coffee whiteners
	Foaming/whipping	Ice cream, desserts, whipped toppings
	Color (whitening)	Confectionary, chocolate, coffee creamers, soups, and sauces
	Flavor	Beverages, ice cream, chocolate
Lactose	Color development	Confectionary, chocolate
	Mouthfeel	Coffee whiteners, confectionary
	Humidity buffering	Bakery products

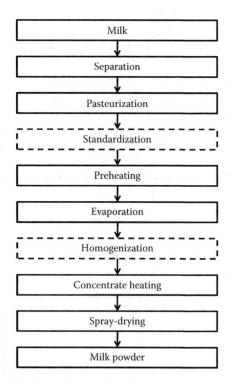

FIGURE 22.2 A basic process for the production of milk powder.

TABLE 22.3

Overview of Different Heat Classes of SMP

Heat Class	WPNI[a]	Typical Preheat Treatment	Potential Applications
Low-heat	>6.0	15–60 s at 70–80°C	Recombined milk, recombined cheese
Medium-heat	1.5–6.0	30–60 s at 90–100°C	Ice cream, confectionary, recombined sweetened condensed milk
High-heat	<1.5	30 s 5 min at 115–125°C	Bakery products, recombined evaporated milk

[a] WPNI = whey protein nitrogen index, expressed as mg undenatured whey protein nitrogen/g powder.

Following preheating, the milk is subsequently concentrated in a falling film evaporator; typical solid contents of the concentrate are 45–50% (m/m) for skim milk, whereas higher solids contents can be achieved for whole milk, because the proportion of protein, the major contributor to viscosity, on a dry matter basis is lower in whole milk than in skim milk (Carr et al. 2003). For SMPs, the maximum achievable degree of concentration decreases with increasing heat class, because denatured whey proteins have a higher voluminosity, and thus contribute more to viscosity, than native whey protein (Snoeren et al. 1982; Carr et al. 2003). For WMP manufacture, the concentrate is subsequently homogenized to stabilize the milk fat globules and thus reduce the level of free, or nonemulsified, fat; homogenization is typically carried out at 60–70°C using a conventional one- or two-stage homogenizer at 5–15 MPa. Subsequently, the concentrate is heated to reduce its viscosity so that it can be atomized readily in the spray drier; in addition, the heating step can inactivate bacteria that may have contaminated the concentrate. The concentrate is usually dried by spray drying, in which it is atomized, using a nozzle or a disk, into droplets of several hundreds of micrometers in diameter, which are subsequently dried. Although roller drying and drum drying are energetically more favorable, and thus cheaper, they yield a flaky powder with, in the case of WMP, a high level of free fat, which is undesirable for most applications, with the exception of milk chocolate manufacture (Liang and Hartel 2004). After spray drying, the moisture content of the powder is generally approximately 8% (m/m) and further drying is required. This is commonly performed in a fluidized bed drier, in which the powder is also agglomerated. In the agglomeration process, porous clusters of powder particles, which have a considerably higher solubility than the individual powder particles, are prepared. The drying of milk, and other products, is described in detail by Písecký (1997), Masters (2002), Refstrup (2003), and Westergaard (2003, 2004).

22.2.3 PHYSICOCHEMICAL PROPERTIES OF MILK POWDERS

22.2.3.1 Milk Powder Composition

Typical compositions of WMP and SMP are outlined in Table 22.1. However, it should be noted that the composition of the surface of WMP particles differs considerably from that of the bulk powder, with fat, lactose, and protein representing 55%, 15%, and 30% of the surface of the particle (Fäldt and Sjöholm 1996). Several processing conditions in the drying process have a direct influence on the moisture content of the final milk powder (Figure 22.3). Concentrate viscosity has a particularly large effect because high viscosity impairs water mobility and high viscosity concentrates produce larger particles on atomization, which retain more water on drying. The moisture content of the powder decreases considerably with increasing outlet temperature. The smaller effects of atomization temperature and atomization intensity are related to the fact that the droplet size at atomization will decrease with temperature and intensity. Preheating intensity increases the concentrate viscosity, thereby increasing the moisture content of the powder.

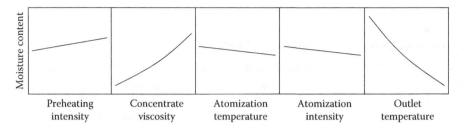

FIGURE 22.3 The approximate influence of processing variables on the moisture content of WMP. (Redrawn with permission from Walstra, P., J. T. M. Wouters, and T. J. Geurts. 2006. *Dairy Science and Technology*, 2nd edn, Boca Raton, FL: CRC Press.)

22.2.3.2 Milk Powder Particles

A milk powder particle generally consists of a continuous mass of lactose and other low molecular mass components in which fat globules, casein micelles, serum proteins, and air vacuoles are embedded (Thomas et al. 2004). Water present in the matrix is bound to both protein and lactose. The lactose is generally present in an amorphous, glassy state because the time and conditions during drying are insufficient for lactose crystallization to be achieved. The vacuoles in the powder particle occur because air is trapped in the particle during the atomization process; nozzle atomization generally yields 0 or 1 air bubbles per droplet, whereas disk atomization yields 10–100 air bubbles per droplet (Walstra et al. 2006). The vacuoles expand further when water vapor enters them during drying. Concentrate viscosity, atomization temperature, and outlet temperature affect the vacuole volume markedly (Figure 22.4). Increasing the concentrate viscosity will reduce the diffusion of air droplets into the atomized droplet and hence will reduce the vacuole volume. Increasing the atomization temperature increases the vacuole volume because it causes a reduction in viscosity. Increasing the outlet temperature does not increase the number of vacuoles, but increases the vacuole volume through expansion of the vacuoles (Walstra et al. 2006).

The average size of the powder particles is generally between 20 and 60 μm, but the size distribution spans from approximately 10 to 200 μm (Thomas et al. 2004). Powder particle size directly affects the solubility of the particles and is influenced by several processing conditions (Figure 22.5). Particle size generally increases with increasing concentrate viscosity but also with increasing vacuole volume. This yields distinct minima for the influence of concentrate viscosity and atomization temperature on particle size; in the absence of vacuole formation, a near-linear increase and a near-linear decrease occur with increasing concentrate viscosity and atomization temperature, respectively (Figure 22.5).

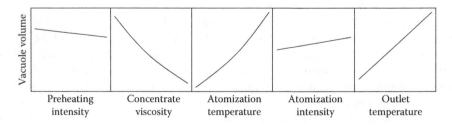

FIGURE 22.4 The approximate influence of some processing variables on the vacuole volume in WMP. (Redrawn with permission from Walstra, P., J. T. M. Wouters, and T. J. Geurts. 2006. *Dairy Science and Technology*, 2nd edn, Boca Raton, FL: CRC Press.)

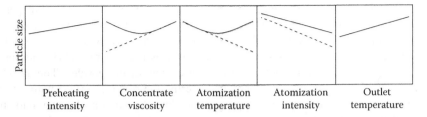

| Preheating intensity | Concentrate viscosity | Atomization temperature | Atomization intensity | Outlet temperature |

FIGURE 22.5 The approximate influence of processing variables on the particle size in WMP. Dashed lines represent the expected influence of processing variables in the absence of vacuole formation. (Redrawn with permission from Walstra, P., J. T. M. Wouters, and T. J. Geurts. 2006. *Dairy Science and Technology*, 2nd edn, Boca Raton, FL: CRC Press.)

22.2.3.3 Free Fat

As mentioned earlier, fat represents approximately 55% of the particle surface material (Fäldt and Sjöholm 1996). The content of free fat, or nonencapsulated fat, that is, the proportion of fat that is readily extractable by solvent, is used as a quality mark for WMPs. Free fat content has considerable effects on the solubility and the flowability of WMP. A detailed review on free fat in milk powders is provided by Vignolles et al. (2007). Free fat that is present on the surface in a layer or in patches is readily extractable, whereas fat that is available in the capillaries and pores takes longer to extract. Emulsified fat present on the surface or in the pores and cracks of the powder particle may also be solvent extractable. Free fat in WMP arises primarily from damage to the milk fat globule membrane (MFGM) during processing and storage of the powder. The main changes in the fat globules during processing occur during evaporation, homogenization, and atomization. Evaporation can disrupt the MFGM as a result of vapor bubble formation (Ye et al. 2004). Homogenization of the concentrate reduces the size of the fat globules, but also changes the composition of the MFGM, from one consisting of a mixture of phospholipids, lipids, and proteins to one consisting predominantly of proteins (Ye et al. 2007). Homogenization pressures that are too low can result in excessive free fat formation. Further disruption of the fat globules can occur during atomization. The free fat content decreases with increasing inlet temperature and decreasing outlet temperature (Vignolles et al. 2007). The free fat content increases significantly when WMP is stored at high temperature and/or humidity, which induces the crystallization of lactose. Growing lactose crystals can damage the fat globules and force them from the lactose matrix to the surface of the particle (Vignolles et al. 2007).

22.2.3.4 Reconstitution Properties

For most applications, milk proteins are reconstituted in an aqueous environment. Full reconstitution, into a suspension of fat globules, casein micelles, and whey proteins in an aqueous serum phase containing lactose and minerals, is crucial in achieving the desired functional properties outlined in Table 22.2. The following stages can be distinguished when milk powder is reconstituted in water or another aqueous medium (Walstra et al. 2006).

1. The powder disperses, that is, the powder particles become fully wetted.
2. The soluble components, for example, lactose and salts, dissolve and the colloidal particles, for example, fat globules and casein micelles, become dispersed in the solution.
3. The physicochemical properties, for example, protein hydration and the mineral balance, equilibrate.

The last stage, in particular, that is, the establishment of protein hydration and the mineral balance of milk, can take a long time if full equilibrium is required. For instance, Anema and Li (2003) showed that full equilibration of the mineral balance when SMP is reconstituted can take >24 h.

The dispersibility of the powder depends primarily on the rate at which water fully penetrates the powder particles. This is dependent on the ability of the powder particle to overcome the surface tension between it and water (Kelly et al. 2003). Because surface fat creates a hydrophobic barrier, the speed of penetration of water into the powder particles is lower for WMP than for SMP and further decreases markedly with increasing free fat content of the powder (Thomas et al. 2004; Walstra et al. 2006). This can be overcome by covering the particle surface with a thin layer of lecithin, which reduces the surface tension considerably. Penetration of water into the powder particle is enhanced with increasing size of the pores and capillaries in the particle.

Insolubility of milk powder relates to the fraction of the powder that does not dissolve under standardized conditions. Insoluble material in milk powder consists largely of aggregated casein micelles and whey proteins, as well as coagulated protein with entrapped fat globules (McKenna et al. 1999; Walstra et al. 2006). As insoluble material forms as a result of heat-induced coagulation during drying, it depends on the time during which the material is at high temperature during drying as well as on the pretreatment of the milk. The influence of various processing variables on the insolubility in milk powders is outlined in Figure 22.6. Outlet temperature has a marked effect probably because most heat-induced coagulation of milk constituents occurs at a moisture content of 10–30% (m/m), that is, during the final stages of drying (Straatsma et al. 1999). The influence of preheating intensity is twofold. On the one hand, increasing preheating intensity will increase viscosity and thereby droplet size during atomization, as a result of which the intensity of heat treatment during drying increases, resulting in the formation of insoluble material. On the other hand, the increase in viscosity as a result of preheating will limit the dry matter content to which the milk can be evaporated, and hence will reduce the solids content of the particles on drying, which would be expected to reduce the development of insolubility, because the stability of milk to heat-induced coagulation decreases markedly with increasing concentration (Walstra et al. 2006). In addition, insolubility also increases markedly when the fraction of casein in the product increases (Kelly et al. 2003). Insolubility in WMP increases further during storage because of sticking and caking, particularly if the product has high moisture content and/or is stored at a relatively high temperature.

22.2.4 Changes in Milk Powders during Storage

During storage, a number of changes that limit the shelf life of the milk powder can occur. The most important are caking of the powder, lipid oxidation, and Maillard reactions, all of which can reduce the functional properties and the desired attributes of milk powders considerably.

22.2.4.1 Caking

Caking of milk powder involves the initial formation of clumps in the powder; eventually the whole product may turn into a solid mass, that is, a cake (Thomas et al. 2004; Walstra et al. 2006). This problem manifests itself primarily when milk powder is stored at a high temperature and/or a high

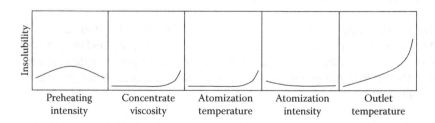

FIGURE 22.6 The approximate influence of processing variables on the insolubility in WMP. (Redrawn with permission from Walstra, P., J. T. M. Wouters, and T. J. Geurts. 2006. *Dairy Science and Technology*, 2nd edn, Boca Raton, FL: CRC Press.)

relative humidity. As the caking of milk powder reduces its flowability, dispersibility, and solubility, it is highly undesirable (Thomas et al. 2004). Milk powders cake as a result of water sorption and the crystallization of lactose; melting and recrystallization of milk fat can also contribute strongly to the caking of WMP (Thomas et al. 2004; Foster et al. 2005). When water vapor condenses on the surface of milk powder particles, very strong interparticle bridges are formed. The water absorbed on the particle surface facilitates molecular diffusion and the crystallization of lactose. Lactose crystallization can result in the formation of solid bridges between powder particles. As the crystallization of lactose results in the release of additional water (amorphous lactose contains more water than crystalline lactose), the problem is further exacerbated and can continue until a solid mass is formed (Thomas et al. 2004). The caking of WMPs can also be induced by fat. Approximately 75% of the fat present on the surface of the milk powder particles is already in liquid form at room temperature, and increasing the temperature further increases the proportion of liquid fat. When the fluidity of the surface fat is sufficiently high, liquid fat bridges may form between particles; on subsequent cooling, they will solidify and will result in caking because of the recrystallization of the milk fat (Foster et al. 2005). Fat-induced caking of WMP particles can be prevented, or at least reduced, by minimizing the amount of free fat in the product and preventing melting of the milk fat during storage at high temperature.

22.2.4.2 Lipid Oxidation

Lipid oxidation is essentially a free-radical chain reaction involving initiation, propagation, and termination stages. Unsaturated fatty acids are oxidized to form odorless, tasteless hydroperoxides, which are unstable and degrade to yield flavorful carbonyls and other compounds, which are perceived as off-flavors. A basic outline of the lipid oxidation reactions is shown in Figure 22.7. The initiation reaction can be promoted by temperature, light, or metal ions; the copper ions present in the natural MFGM are a key catalyst. As oxygen is crucial for the propagation of the reaction, lipid oxidation of WMP has been shown to be far more extensive in WMP that is gas packed with high oxygen content (Van Mil and Jans 1991). The oxygen level in the packages can be reduced through gas flushing, by choosing packaging materials that are impermeable to oxygen, and by using oxygen scavengers (Farkye 2006). Furthermore, free fat should be kept at a minimum, if possible, because it is this proportion of the fat in particular that is readily in contact with the air and thus is most susceptible to lipid oxidation. Lipid oxidation is also affected by moisture content and is less extensive in WMP containing 3.0% moisture than in WMP containing 2.4% moisture (Van Mil and Jans 1991). Walstra et al. (2006) reported that, when the susceptibility of milk powder to lipid oxidation is plotted as a function of moisture content, a distinct minimum is observed at approximately 7% moisture. However, this moisture content is far too high to prevent other undesirable reactions, such as Maillard reactions and the development of insolubility. As a result, the moisture content needs to be optimized so that lipid oxidation, Maillard reactions, and the development of insolubility are minimized; this generally corresponds to a moisture content of approximately 3% (Walstra et al. 2006).

$$
\begin{array}{lll}
\text{Initiation} & RH & \rightarrow R^{\bullet} \\
\text{Propagation} & R^{\bullet} + O_2 & \rightarrow RO_2^{\bullet} \\
& RO_2^{\bullet} + RH & \rightarrow ROOH + R^{\bullet} \\
\text{Termination} & 2\,RO_2^{\bullet} & \rightarrow O_2 + ROOR \\
& RO_2^{\bullet} + R^{\bullet} & \rightarrow ROOR \\
& 2\,R^{\bullet} & \rightarrow RR
\end{array}
$$

FIGURE 22.7 Reaction scheme for lipid oxidation (RH is the unsaturated fatty acid and $R^{\bullet}$ is the radical formed as a result of hydrogen abstraction).

The stability of milk powder to lipid oxidation can also be increased using antioxidants. In addition to antioxidants that can be included as additives, for example, ascorbic acid, sodium ascorbate, ascorbyl palmitate, and butylated hydroxyanisole, some milk constituents have antioxidant capability, which can be exploited in maximizing the oxidative stability of WMP (Farkye 2006). Most notably, the free sulfhydryl group of β-LG has antioxidant activity. It is commonly buried inside the molecule and is thus inaccessible, but heat treatment exposes it and thereby facilitates its use as an antioxidant. Accordingly, for WMPs, the number of exposed sulfhydryl groups increases with increasing preheating intensity (Baldwin and Ackland 1991) and the stability to lipid oxidation increases significantly when the severity of the heat treatment of the milk prior to evaporation is increased (Baldwin et al. 1991; Van Mil and Jans 1991; Stapelfeldt et al. 1997; Farkye 2006).

22.2.4.3 Maillard Reactions

Maillard reactions can occur in milk powders because of the presence of free amino groups, that is, from the lysine residues and the N-termini of the proteins, and the presence of a reducing sugar, that is, lactose. The first step in the Maillard reaction is the reaction of the reactive carbonyl group of the lactose molecule with the nucleophilic amino group, yielding the attachment of the lactose residue to the protein, that is, the lactosylation of the protein. Lactosylation occurs in milk powders even at low temperatures, but the reaction rate is clearly increased when the storage temperature exceeds 20°C (De Block et al. 1998; Guyomarc'h et al. 2000). Moreover, lactosylation in milk powders depends on the moisture content, with powders with lower moisture content showing considerably less lactosylation during storage (De Block et al. 1998; Guyomarc'h et al. 2000). A water activity of approximately 0.5–0.7 appears to be optimal for lactosylation of the protein in milk powder (Troyano et al. 1994). In some cases, lactosylation can even be beneficial to milk protein functionality (Oliver et al. 2006; Oliver 2011). However, further stages in the Maillard reaction can result in the formation of brown pigments, off-flavors, and even carcinogenic compounds, and are thus highly undesirable.

22.3 CASEINS AND CASEINATES

Caseins and caseinates constitute a class of milk protein ingredients that have been produced industrially for nearly a century. Initial applications were primarily as high-quality ingredients in the nonfood sector, for example, in glues, adhesives, plastics, and synthetic fibers. Although some of these application areas still remain today, over the last 50 years or so, caseins and caseinates have also gained importance as an extremely functional class of food ingredient and have become one of the principal functional food proteins. Two different categories of casein can be identified, that is, acid casein and rennet casein. Although there are a wide variety of caseinates, they can be separated into caseinates of monovalent cations, of which sodium caseinate is the predominant form, and caseinates of divalent cations, primarily represented by calcium caseinate. As outlined in Table 22.4, the main constituent of caseins and caseinates is protein, that is, casein, with the remaining constituents being moisture and minerals. They are nearly devoid of fat, lactose, whey protein, and other constituents.

Typical processes for the manufacture of acid casein, rennet casein, and caseinates are given in Figure 22.8. Skim milk is the base material for the production of caseins and caseinates and the first step in the manufacturing process involves destabilization of the casein micelles. For acid casein, this is achieved by lowering the pH sufficiently to induce acid coagulation of the milk. Although lactic acid fermentations are still sometimes used for this purpose, in most cases, a mineral acid such as hydrochloric acid or sulfuric acid is used. Once the desired pH and acid-induced coagulation have been achieved, the coagulum is cooked, commonly to approximately 50–55°C, to enhance whey separation. Subsequently, the whey is removed and the curd is washed several times to remove residual lactose, whey proteins, and minerals. The washed acid casein curd may be dried to obtain acid

TABLE 22.4

Typical Compositions (in %, m/m) of Acid Casein, Sodium Caseinate, Calcium Caseinate, and Rennet Casein

	Acid Casein	Sodium Caseinate	Calcium Caseinate	Rennet Casein
Moisture	8–12	3–5	3–5	8–12
Protein	84–90	90–94	90–94	80–85
Ash	1–2	3.6	3–5	6–9
Lactose	0–1	0–1	0–1	0–1
Fat	0–1	0–1	0–1	0–1
Sodium		1–2		
Calcium			1–2	2–3
pH	4.6–5.2	6.5–7.0	6.5–7.0	7.0–7.5
Solubility in water	0	>98	>95	0

casein. For caseinate production, the acid casein curd is milled and the suspension is subsequently neutralized by the addition of base. The hydroxides of sodium, potassium, calcium, and magnesium are most commonly used for this purpose and yield the caseinates of the respective cations. In addition, ammonia may be used to neutralize acid casein curd to produce ammonium caseinate. The suspension is then heated and dried. The manufacture of rennet casein differs from that of acid casein and caseinates, in that rennet-induced coagulation, rather than acid-induced coagulation, is used. Following rennet-induced coagulation, the coagulum is again cooked, dewheyed, washed, and dried.

On account of the array of functionalities that they possess, caseins and caseinates are used in an extremely wide range of products. The choice of the type of casein is highly application dependent. As outlined in Table 22.4, acid casein and rennet casein are virtually insoluble in water, whereas sodium caseinate and calcium caseinate are highly water soluble. A suspension of sodium caseinate consists of rather small associations of molecules, reaching a size of approximately 20–40 nm. As

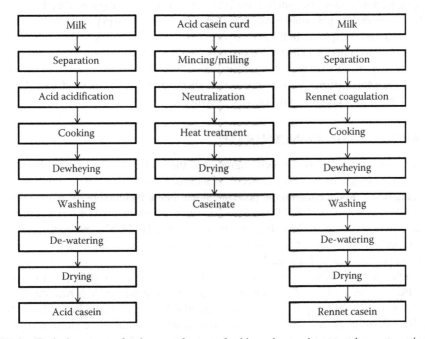

FIGURE 22.8 Typical processes for the manufacture of acid casein, caseinates, and rennet casein.

a result, sodium caseinate suspensions are translucent. Similar properties are seen for other casein-ates of monovalent cations, for example, potassium caseinate and ammonium caseinate. Because of their comparatively low level of particle structure and high degree of flexibility, the caseinates of monovalent cations are excellent emulsifiers and foamers, and also have high heat stability, strong water-binding functionality, and excellent nutritional properties. As a result, these caseinates are widely employed in coffee creamers and other high fat products, cream liqueurs, bakery products, whipped toppings, soups, sauces, ice cream, meat products, and infant and clinical nutrition.

In contrast to the caseinates of monovalent cations, the caseinates of divalent cations, for example, calcium caseinate and magnesium caseinate, form turbid milky-white suspensions in water, contain-ing particles with an average size comparable with that of native casein micelles, that is, several hundred nanometers. The main advantage of using calcium caseinate over sodium caseinate is that, because of the more compact nature of their particles, calcium caseinate suspensions are generally lower in viscosity. As such, calcium caseinates find application predominantly in clinical and infant nutrition and other nutritional products, in which the high viscosity arising from sodium caseinate is of concern. The more aggregated nature of the particles of calcium caseinate also means that its emulsification and foaming properties are poorer than those of sodium caseinate; thus, sodium caseinate is the product of choice when stabilization of oil–water or air–water interfaces is required. Because of their high calcium content, and particularly their high calcium ion activity, calcium caseinates generally have poorer heat stability than sodium caseinates; thus sodium caseinates are also favored when severe heating is to be applied.

Whereas sodium caseinate and calcium caseinate are readily soluble in water, rennet casein and acid casein are virtually insoluble. Although this was not a major concern for some of the initial nonfood applications of acid and rennet caseins, their successful application in many of today's food applications requires the formation of a workable suspension of the caseins. The suspension of acid casein can be achieved by neutralization, through the addition of bases. Therefore, effectively, sodium and calcium caseinate suspensions, for example, are produced, as outlined above. Suspensions prepared in this manner can be used for the applications outlined for the various casein-ates. Advantages of the use of acid casein, rather than sodium caseinate or calcium caseinate, are that the user of the acid casein can control the degree of neutralization and hydration that is required for the specific application. In contrast to acid casein, as rennet casein is already at neutral pH, it cannot be suspended by pH adjustment. For rennet casein, suspension is achieved by the chelation of micellar calcium phosphate. In the primary area of application of rennet casein, that is, processed cheese products and cheese analogs, the suspension of rennet casein is achieved by the addition of so-called melting salts, which are essentially calcium chelators, that is, citrates and (poly)phosphates. By creating such suspensions, the rennet casein is suspended, the fat can be efficiently emulsified in the matrix, and a gelled texture will form on cooling.

22.4   MILK PROTEIN CONCENTRATE

Among the wide variety of milk protein ingredients, the MPCs are a comparatively recent addition that is rapidly gaining wide popularity. MPCs of a range of protein contents, commonly from ~40% to ~85%, are being produced, with the protein content being included in the name of the MPC, for example, MPC42, MPC56, MPC70, and MPC85. Typical compositions of some MPCs are given in Table 22.5, from which it is clear that, compared with SMP, MPCs are enriched in protein and depleted in lactose; the ash, fat, and moisture contents are reasonably constant over the range of protein contents outlined in Table 22.5.

Most high-quality MPCs are prepared using UF of skim milk. A typical process for the produc-tion of MPC is given in Figure 22.9. The first treatment of the skim milk is heat treatment, which is commonly in the low heat region (e.g., 10–20 s at 70–75°C), but should be sufficient to inactivate undesirable microorganisms and enzymes. Subsequently, the milk is concentrated by UF, com-monly using membranes with a pore size of £10 kDa. During the UF step, caseins, whey proteins,

TABLE 22.5

Typical Compositions (in %, m/m) of SMP and Different MPCs

	SMP	MPC42	MPC56	MPC70	MPC80	MPC85
Protein	34.0	42.0	56.0	70.0	80.0	85.0
Fat	0.8	1.0	1.3	1.4	1.8	1.8
Lactose	53.5	45.7	31.2	17.0	5.5	1.2
Ash	7.9	7.8	7.7	7.2	7.4	7.4
Moisture	3.8	3.5	3.8	4.4	4.5	4.6

micellar salts, and residual fat are concentrated in the retentate, whereas lactose, soluble salts, and nonprotein nitrogen are removed with the permeate (Green et al. 1984; Babella 1989; Bastian et al. 1991). For high-protein MPCs, for example, MPC80 and MPC85, UF alone is insufficient to achieve the required protein:solids ratio in the retentate and DF is applied (Singh 2007). The maximum protein content achievable is limited by the presence of residual fat, as well as by the retention of micellar calcium phosphate (Kelly 2011). Once the desired protein:solids ratio has been achieved, the UF retentate is evaporated and spray dried. Because of the considerably higher protein:solids ratio in UF retentate, compared with skim milk, evaporation cannot achieve a solids content for MPCs that is similar to that of SMP. The feed to the spray drier commonly has a solid content of approximately 50% for SMP but of approximately 30% for MPC70, and this will be even lower for MPCs of even higher protein content.

One of the big advantages of MPC over all other milk protein ingredients is that it contains the caseins and whey proteins in their natural ratio and in their native state; that is, the caseins are still

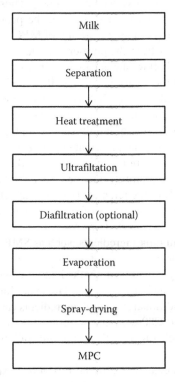

FIGURE 22.9 Typical process for the production of MPC.

in a form that strongly resembles the initial casein micelles in the starting material and the whey proteins are largely undenatured, assuming that the heat load is kept low during processing. As such, MPCs are a popular ingredient for those applications in which the original structure of the milk proteins is desired in terms of functionality, that is, the standardization of cheese milk, the protein fortification of yogurt, ice cream mixes, and clinical and infant nutrition products. Because micellar calcium phosphate is largely retained in the micelles during the UF process, MPCs contain high levels of encapsulated bioavailable calcium, thus further enhancing their popularity for infant and clinical nutrition.

One of the issues for the high-protein MPCs in particular (McKenna 2000; De Castro-Morel and Harper 2002) is that they can suffer from poor solubility, which decreases further on storage, particularly on storage at above ambient temperatures (Mistry and Pulgar 1996a; Mistry 2002; Anema et al. 2006; Fang et al. 2011) and at high moisture content and water activity (Baldwin and Truong 2007). Solubility can often be attained at increased reconstitution temperature (Schuck et al. 1994; McKenna 2000; Mimouni et al. 2009; Fang et al. 2010) or with the application of shear (McKenna 2000); however, in some cases, this is not really feasible; for example, when MPCs are used for the standardization of cheese milk, whey protein denaturation should be avoided and homogenization of the fat globules is undesirable. The poor solubility of high-protein MPCs has been related to excessive protein–protein interactions on the surface of the powder particle (Anema et al. 2006; Havea 2006). The insoluble proteinaceous material has been shown to consist primarily of caseins and involves little or no whey protein (Anema et al. 2006; Havea 2006). In fact, when studying the development of insolubility as a function of storage time, Anema et al. (2006) observed that, even after prolonged storage, approximately 20% of the total protein, equivalent to the proportion of whey protein in MPC, remained soluble. Similar results were recently presented by Mimouni et al. (2010b), who showed that, on the reconstitution of MPC85, lactose, the whey proteins, and the nonmicellar salts, for example, sodium and potassium, dissolved readily into the soluble aqueous phase. In contrast, the caseins, as well as the salts associated with the casein micelles, for example, calcium, magnesium, and phosphate, dissolved only slowly. Thus, it was concluded that the release of casein micelles from the powder particles, and not the penetration of water into the powder particles, was the rate-limiting step in the rehydration of MPC (Mimouni et al. 2010b). Because of the poor release of casein micelles from the powder particles, particularly from the surfaces of the particles, structures resembling hollow shells can remain after the reconstitution of MPC, that is, the constituents disperse from the interior, but a hollow shell of the original particle remains (McKenna 2000; Mimouni et al. 2010a). Babella (1989) reported that the solubility of MPC decreased with an increasing proportion of calcium in the mineral fraction of the product. Based on this report, a process for the production of highly soluble high-protein MPCs has been developed; part of the calcium is removed from the UF retentate and is replaced by monovalent ions, such as sodium, through treatment with a cation exchange resin (Bhaskar et al. 2001; Carr 2002). For MPC60, it has been shown that the solubility and the dispersibility decrease slightly with increasing heat treatment and decreasing pH of the retentate (El-Samragy et al. 1993).

MPCs have been incorporated into a variety of common dairy products, most notably yogurt, ice cream, and particularly cheese. For yogurt, it has been shown that MPCs can be used efficiently as replacements for traditional skim milk ingredients, such as SMP and skim milk concentrate, which are added in many instances to increase the protein content and improve the texture and stability of the product. Replacing these ingredients with MPC had no negative effect on the desired textural properties of the yogurt (Mistry and Hassan 1992; Guzmán-Gonzáles et al. 1999). For ice cream mixes, it has been shown that traditional skim milk ingredients can readily be replaced, on a constant protein basis, with MPC56 or MPC80 without compromising the desired physical properties of the mix (Alvarez et al. 2005), which suggests the suitability of MPC in the production of reduced-carbohydrate ice cream.

Several studies on the rennet coagulation properties of reconstituted MPCs have concluded that particularly high-protein MPCs, for example, MPC80 and MPC90, show poor renneting properties and require the addition of calcium chloride to ensure desirable coagulation properties (Kuo and Harper 2003a; Ferrer et al. 2008; Martin et al. 2010). This is invariably related to excessive removal of soluble calcium during the UF and DF stages applied in the production of the MPCs. The use of MPC for the protein fortification of milk for the production of Gouda cheese not only increased the yield significantly, but also increased the moisture content and thus somewhat impaired the organoleptic properties (Mistry and Pulgar 1996b). MPC was successfully used for the protein fortification of milk for the production of Mozzarella (Harvey 2006; Francolino et al. 2010), Feta (Kuo and Harper 2003b; Harvey 2006), and Cheddar (Harvey 2006) cheeses.

Overall, it can be concluded that MPC is a very suitable ingredient for the protein standardization and fortification of popular dairy products such as cheese, yogurt, and ice cream.

22.5 WHEY PROTEIN INGREDIENTS

22.5.1 WHEY POWDERS

Spray-drying whey into whey powder is still the most common way to process whey in the dairy industry. Three types of whey powder can commonly be distinguished, that is, sweet whey powder, acid whey powder, and demineralized whey powder. The composition of these products is given in Table 22.6. Typically, protein content of whey powder varies from 11% to 15%, whereas lactose content is >60%, but <80%. Fat content is low in all types of whey powder, whereas moisture content typically varies from 3% to 5% (Table 22.6). Ash content shows the strongest variations between the different whey powders; acid whey powder has the lowest ash content, whereas demineralized whey powder has the lowest (Table 22.6). These differences arise as a result of differences in the preparation of the different types of whey. Sweet whey powder is produced from the whey derived from processes which retain (near-)neutral pH of the whey during its preparation, for example, the manufacture of rennet-coagulated cheeses and rennet casein. As such, the ash fraction of sweet whey powder contains the salts that are naturally in the soluble state of milk at neutral pH, that is, most of the monovalent cations and anions, as well as part (i.e., the nonmicellar) di- and trivalent cations and anions. This equates to approximately 30% and 50% of calcium and inorganic phosphate in milk (Walstra et al. 2006). Acid whey powder, in contrast, is produced from whey derived in which acid-induced coagulation of the casein fraction is the mechanism of destabilization of casein and its separation from whey, for example, in the manufacture of acid casein and caseinates, as well as various fermented dairy products, such as quark (Jelen 2009). The addition of production of acid during these processes increases the mineral content of the serum phase of the milk and hence whey. In addition, the reduction in pH leads to an increase in solubility of calcium phosphate, and hence solubilization of micellar calcium phosphate. The combined processes outlined above result in the ash content of acid whey powder being up to 50% higher than that of sweet whey pow-

TABLE 22.6
Composition (in %, m/m) of Sweet, Acid, and Demineralized Whey Powder

	Sweet Whey Powder	Acid Whey Powder	Demineralized Whey Powder
Protein	11–15	11–14	11–15
Lactose	63–75	61–70	70–80
Fat	0–2	0–2	0–2
Ash	8–10	10–13	1–7
Moisture	3–5	3–5	3–5

der. Demineralized whey powder can be prepared from either sweet or acid whey, and has considerably lower ash content than sweet or acid whey powder. This reduction in ash content is achieved through demineralization of the whey by electrodialysis, NF, and/or treatment with IEX resins (Gernigon et al. 2011). Typical levels of demineralization are 30%, 50%, 70%, or 90%, with a demineralization of 90% yielding a powder with an ash content of 1%.

Whey powders are commonly prepared by spray-drying. Typical steps in the preparation of whey powder from liquid whey include a preheating to inactivate residual enzymes and microorganisms, an optional adjustment of pH and demineralization step, followed by clarification and concentration of the whey by reverse osmosis and evaporation to a solids content of typically 58–62%. Subsequently, a precrystallization step is performed, by controlled cooling of the concentrate. This induces crystallization of (part of) the lactose and ensure a low-hygroscopic powder on drying (Písecký 1997; Westergaard 2004).

Whey powder is a relatively-low-cost ingredient which is used in a wide variety of food products. Typical areas of application include the bakery industry, where whey powder is used in crackers, biscuits, and baking mixes. In the dairy industry, whey powders are used in ice cream and desserts, whereas demineralized whey powders are also gaining interest for use in infant formula. Furthermore, whey powders are used in beverage mixes, snacks, flavorings, and animal feed.

22.5.2 Whey Protein Concentrate

WPC is obtained by UF of sweet whey or acid whey. Typically, UF membranes with a molecular weight cut-off of 4–10 kDa are used, so as to retain proteins in the retentate but allow lactose, minerals, and other small constituents to permeate through the membrane. The proportion of protein in dry matter can be increased by increasing the concentration factor in UF. In addition, diafiltration with water can be applied to increase the proportion of proteins in the product further (Morr and Ha 1993; Mulvihill and Ennis 2003; Westergaard 2004; Jelen 2009). The protein content of WPC typically ranges from 35% to 80%, with WPC35, WPC60, WPC75, and WPC80 being the most commonly produced variants. Compositional properties of these WPC properties are given in Table 22.7. Trends displayed in this table highlight that with increasing protein content of the product, fat content also tends to increase, whereas ash and lactose content decrease proportionally.

WPC35 is very similar to SMP in terms of gross composition, and is as such often applied as a cost-effective partial or full skim milk replacer, although it does provide a different protein and mineral composition. Typical applications of WPC35 include dairy beverages, ice cream, and cultured products, such as yoghurt and fresh cheese. WPC35 also finds application in the bakery industry, where it is used in biscuits and crackers, as well as in other fields of application, such as soups, snacks, and nutritional products.

WPC60, WPC75, and WPC80 provide more concentrated sources of highly nutritional protein for protein supplementation for a wide variety of applications. These products provide proteins which are highly soluble, also under acidic conditions, have good emulsifying properties and

TABLE 22.7
Typical Composition (in %, m/m) of WPCs

	WPC35	WPC60	WPC75	WPC80
Protein	34–36	60–62	75–77	80–82
Lactose	48–52	25–30	10–15	4–8
Fat	3–5	3–7	4–8	4–8
Ash	6–8	4–6	4–6	3–4
Moisture	3–5	3–5	3–5	3–5

excellent water-binding, gelling, and thickening properties. As such, these products are widely employed as value-added ingredients for protein fortification. Typical applications include infant formula, clinical nutrition, nutritional bars, beverages, and mixes. In addition, these WPCs are used in processed cheese, yoghurts, desserts, as well as processed meat and fish products.

22.5.3 WHEY PROTEIN ISOLATE

Up until the 1980s, WPC80 was the whey protein ingredient with the highest protein content, but since then, processed for the production of a product with even higher whey protein content, that is, WPI have been developed. WPI typically contains 90–92% protein, a maximum of 1% of fat and lactose, 2–3% ash, and 4–5% moisture. Two main processing sequences can be distinguished for the production of WPI. One involves the use of membrane filtration, whereby the whey is first subjected to MF to reduce the fat content of the whey. Subsequently, the MF permeate is subjected to UF and diafiltration, to achieve the desired proportion of protein in the dry matter of the product (Rowan 1998). Another way to produce WPI is through the use of IEX chromatography. Using this process, the whey proteins are selectively absorbed onto the IEX resin, while the fat, lactose, and minerals are eluted. Subsequently, by increasing ionic strength, the whey proteins are eluted from the IEX resin (Mulvihill and Ennis 2003). Because of the different processing technologies employed, differences in protein and mineral composition are observed between WPI prepared by membrane filtrate and by IEX chromatography. WPI prepared using the latter method generally contains no glycomacropeptide, LF, and peptide fragments, due to the fact that these are not adsorbed by the IEX resin. As a result, levels of α-LA, β-LG, and bovine serum albumin are higher in WPI prepared by IEX than in WPI prepared by membrane filtration (Affertsholt and Nielsen 2007). The mineral composition of the two types of WPI also differs considerably. The minerals in WPI prepared by membrane filtration occur at ratio's similar to those observed in WPC. In contrast, when WPI is prepared by IEX chromatography, the minerals naturally present in the whey are removed. Predominant in this product is the monovalent cation of the mineral used to achieve elution of the proteins from the IEX resin, in most cases this is sodium (Affersholt and Nielsen 2007).

22.5.4 FRACTIONATED WHEY PROTEIN INGREDIENTS

22.5.4.1 α-LA

Since α-LA is the major whey protein in human milk, which is devoid of β-LG, purified α-LA and α-LA-enriched whey protein products are in great demand by the infant formula industry. Rather pure α-LA preparations (>95% protein, of which >90% is α-LA) can be isolated from sweet whey using chromatographic processes (Affersholt and Nielsen 2007). However, the comparable high price for ingredients produced in this manner limits wide-spread use of such products in infant nutrition. More widespread in this area is the use of α-LA-enriched fractions. Most processes for the isolation of α-LA-enriched fractions from whey exploit the low thermal stability of the protein when it is in its, calcium-depleted, apo-form. Holo-α-LA can be converted to apo-α-LA by reducing pH or treatment with a cation exchange resin or calcium-chelating agent. Apo-α-LA denatures and aggregates on heating at approximately 35–55°C. The exact temperature required to induce denaturation depends on pH, ionic strength, and the type of calcium-chelator added. The denatured α-LA can subsequently be separated from the remaining soluble whey proteins using various centrifugation or filtration techniques. The separated apo-α-LA can subsequently be resolubilized in water, neutralized, concentrated, and spray-dried (Pearce 1983, 1987; De Wit and Bronts 1994; Bramaud et al. 1997; Gesan-Guizou et al. 1999). Using aforementioned techniques, α-LA preparation of which >70% of the proteinaceous fraction consists of α-LA can be prepared. Such preparation find wide employ in infant nutrition. In addition, it has been reported that, due to the high water-binding capacity of such fractions, α-LA preparations are more functional in pasta-dough than unfractionated whey protein products.

22.5.4.2 β-LG

β-LG is the most abundant protein in whey. Like α-LA, it can be isolated from milk chromatographically, but the high prices prevent wide-spread application. More economically feasible as β-LG-enriched fraction which are the by-products of the aforementioned procedure for the isolation of α-LA (Pearce 1983, 1987; De Wit and Bronts 1994; Bramaud et al. 1997; Gesan-Guizou et al. 1999). Further removal of other whey proteins, for example, IGs and BSA, can be achieved by membrane filtration, and β-LG preparations containing >80% protein, of which >75% of protein is β-LG, can be prepared. Primary applications for β-LG concentrates are techno-functional, rather than nutritional, since the protein has excellent foaming, emulsification, heat-gelation, water-binding properties, and solubility at low pH. As such, β-LG can be used as an egg white replacer in bakery products, a fat replacer in processed meat products, a source of protein fortification in drinks, and a stabilizer in desserts (De Wit 1998).

22.5.4.3 Lactoferrin

LF has been shown to play an important role in the human cellular immune system response and protect the body against infections. Other reported activities of LF include the primary defense against pathogens, stimulation of the immune system, and regulation of the iron status in the body. As such, its isolation from dairy streams, for subsequent use in infant formula, meat preservation, dietary supplements, pharmaceutical products and cosmetics, and oral hygiene products, has been commercialized. Although LF can be isolated from skim milk as well, it is most commonly isolated from whey by cation exchange chromatography (Paul et al. 1980; Prieels and Peiffer 1986; Martin-Hernandez et al. 1990; Chui and Etzel 1997). The high isoelectric point (approximately 8.7) and thus positive charge at neutral pH of the protein is exploited herein, by using a cationic exchange resin. Using this process, LF preparations with a protein content of 93–96%, of which >95% is LF, can be prepared. Lactoperoxidase, which is also positively charged at neutral pH, is coadsorbed to the cation exchange resin in the isolation of LF. Subsequent separation of the two can be achieved using elution gradients, membrane filtration, or size exclusion chromatography (Prieels and Peiffer 1986; Burling 1989; Chui and Etzel 1997).

22.5.4.4 Immunoglobulins

IGs are commonly present in milk to confer passive immunity to the neonate. As such, IGs are isolated from milk, colostrums, and whey and applied in nutritional and clinical products. Chromatographic technologies, such as IEX chromatography (Bottomly 1989), size exclusion chromatography (Al-Mashikhi and Nakai 1987), metal chelate interaction chromatography (Al-Mashikhi et al. 1988), and affinity-binding chromatography (Chen and Wang 1991; Gani et al. 1992) allow the isolation of preparations of IGs of high purity from whey. Other methods for the isolation of IGs include membrane filtration (Hilpert 1984). Primary applications for isolated IGs are infant formula, clinical nutritional, pharmaceutical products, and animal feed.

22.5.5 WHEY PROTEINS WITH SPECIFIC FUNCTIONALITY

In the last decade, there have been some developments in the preparation of whey protein ingredients with specific technical functionality. Such preparations include microparticulated whey proteins and cold-gelling whey proteins. While they commonly contain the whey proteins in the same ratio's as found in whey powder, WPC and WPI, these products have undergone specific pretreatment to confer specific functionalities to the applications in which they are used.

22.5.5.1 Microparticulated Whey Protein

Microparticulated whey proteins are prepared by a process referred to as microparticulation, which involves the heat treatment of a WPC under high-shear conditions. During this process, the shear breaks up the whey protein aggregates formed by heat treatment, as a result of which fine particles are formed. A variety of microparticulation processes have been reported, including heat treatment under shear (Singer et al. 1988), homogenization of a heated whey protein solution (Paquin et al. 1993), extrusion (Queguiner et al. 1992), and the use of scraped-surface heat exchangers (Spiegel 1999). These microparticulated whey proteins are used primarily as a fat replacer, and have been tested in a wide range of applications, including cheese, yogurt, ice cream, and desserts. Crucial for their successful application is that the microparticulated whey proteins consist of small, smooth, round particles which have the same sensory sensation as emulsion droplets. Whey protein aggregates with sizes ranging from 0.1 to 3 μm were suggested to be optimal for imparting a creamy mouthfeel, whereas larger aggregates may, if they are poorly compressible, suffer from a gritty mouthfeel (Lucca and Tepper 1994).

22.5.5.2   Cold-Gelling Whey Proteins

The term cold gelling "whey proteins" refers to preparations of whey protein, commonly WPCs, which form a stable at ambient temperature on acidification or addition of salts. The advantage that these cold-gelling WPCs offer over traditional WPCs is that no heat treatment is required to induce gelation. Key in the preparation of cold-gelling whey proteins is a heat treatment at relatively low protein concentration (less than 10%), temperature (70–90°C) and ionic strength, and relatively high pH (7–9) (Gao et al. 2006). Advantages of the application of cold-gelling whey proteins have been shown in acidified dairy products, calcium-fortified milk beverages, surimi, and desserts (Keogh 1998; Alting et al. 2003, 2004). Despite such advantages, commercial uptake of cold-gelling WPC has been slow, probably due to the fact that heat treatment and drying needs to be carried out at low concentration and thus involves high production cost.

22.6   CONCLUSIONS AND RECOMMENDATIONS

Extensive research that has been carried out on the biological functions, structures, and physico-chemical and functional characteristics of whey proteins suggests that their structures dictate the physicochemical and functional properties of particular whey proteins As certain functionalities of the milk proteins are linked to their three-dimensional structures and various factors (such as type and source of whey, state and concentration of the whey proteins, pH, ionic environment, and heat treatment) affect the functional properties of whey proteins, it may be possible to identify the processing conditions and parameters to manipulate specific functional properties. The effects of these parameters on the functional properties and how to manipulate them have been researched extensively. We can now obtain tailor-made whey protein ingredients with specific functional properties, selectively isolate particular components of milk, and create value-added milk components that contribute to specific health and nutritional benefits and to the generation of new value-added dairy ingredients with specific functionalities on a commercial scale. All this has ultimately resulted in the development of a variety of new products with specific nutritional and functional benefits and has made more types of food available to the wider population. Consumer trends and the latest scientific research, manufacturing technologies, market opportunities, and food applications for value-added dairy ingredients have provided insights and have helped to create new generations of dairy ingredients that are suitable for applications in specific foods and beverages.

REFERENCES

Affertsholt, T. and M. D. Nielsen. 2007. *The World Market for Whey and Lactose Products*, pp. 2006–2010. Aarhus: 3A Business Consulting.

Al-Mashikhi, S. A. and S. Nakai. 1987. Isolation of bovine immunoglobulins and lactoferrin from whey proteins. *J Dairy Sci* 70:2486–92.

Al-Mashikhi, S. A., E. Li-Chan, and Nakai, S. 1988. Separation of immunoglobulins and lactoferrin from cheese whey by chelating chromatography. *J Dairy Sci* 71:1747–55.

Alting, A. C., R. J. Hamer, C. G. de Kruif, and R. W. Visschers. 2003. Cold-set globular protein gels: Interactions, structure and rheology as a function of protein concentration. *J Agr Food Chem* 51:3150–6.

Alting, A. C., E. T. van der Meulen, J. Hugenholtz, and R. W. Visschers. 2004. Control of texture of cold-set gels through programmed bacterial acidification. *Int Dairy J* 14:323–9.

Alvarez, V. B., C. L. Wolters, Y. Vodovotz, and T. Ji. 2005. Physical properties of ice cream containing milk protein concentrates. *J Dairy Sci* 88:862–71.

Anema, S. G. and Y. Li. 2003. Re-equilibration of the minerals in skim milk during reconstitution. *Milchwissenschaft* 58:174–8.

Anema, S. G., D. N. Pinder, R. J. Hunter, and Y. Hemar. 2006. Effects of storage temperature on the solubility of milk protein concentrate (MPC85). *Food Hydrocolloids* 20:386–93.

Babella, G. 1989. Scientific and practical results with use of ultrafiltration in Hungary. *Bull Int Dairy Fed* 244:7–25.

Baldwin, A. J., and J. D. Ackland. 1991. Effect of preheat treatment and storage on the properties of whole milk powder. Changes in physical and chemical properties. *Neth Milk Dairy J* 45:169–81.

Baldwin, A. J., H. R. Cooper, and K. C. Palmer. 1991. Effect of preheat treatment and storage on the properties of whole milk powder. Changes in sensory properties. *Neth Milk Dairy J* 45:97–116.

Baldwin, A. and D. Pearce. 2005. Milk powder. In *Encapsulated and Powdered Foods*, ed. C. Onwulata, pp. 387–433. Boca Raton, FL: CRC Press.

Baldwin, A. J., and G. N. T. Truong. 2007. Development of insolubility in dehydration of dairy milk powders. *Food Bioprod Process* 85:202–8.

Bastian, E. D., S. K. Collinge, and C. A. Ernstrom. 1991. Ultrafiltration: Partitioning of milk constituents into permeate and retentate. *J Dairy Sci* 74:2423–34.

Bhaskar, G. V., H. Singh, and N. D. Blazey. 2001. Milk protein concentrate products and process. *International Patent Specification* WO01/41578.

Bottomly, R. C. 1989. Isolation of an immunoglobulin rich fraction from whey. *European Patent Application* 0 320152 A2.

Bramaud, C., P. Aimar, and G. Daufin. 1997. Whey protein fractionation: Isoelectric precipitation of α-lactalbumin under gentle heat. *Biotechnol Bioeng* 56:391–7.

Burling, H. 1989. Process for extracting pure fractions of lactoperoxidase and lactoferrin from milk serum. *International Patent Application* WO 89/04608 A1.

Carr, A. J. 2002. Milk protein concentrate products and the uses thereof. *International Patent Application* WO02/196208 A2.

Carr, A. J., C. R. Southward, and L. K. Creamer. 2003. Protein hydration and viscosity of dairy fluids. In *Advanced Dairy Chemistry 1: Proteins*, 3rd edn, eds. P. F. Fox, and P. L. H. McSweeney, pp. 1289–323. New York, NY: Kluwer Academic/Plenum Publishers.

Chen, J.-P. and C.-H. Wang. 1991. Microfiltration affinity purification of lactoferrin and immunoglobulin G from cheese whey. *J Food Sci* 56:701–6, 713.

Chui, C. K. and M. R. Etzel. 1997. Fractionation of lactoferrin and lactoperoxidase from bovine whey using a cation exchange membrane. *J Food Sci* 62:996–1000.

De Block J., M. Merchiers, and R. van Renterghem. 1998. Capillary electrophoresis of the whey protein fraction of milk powders. A possible method for monitoring storage conditions. *Int Dairy J* 8:787–792.

De Castro-Morel, M. and W. J. Harper. 2002. Basic functionality of commercial milk protein concentrates. *Milchwissenschaft* 57:367–70.

De Wit, J. N. 1998. Nutritional and functional characteristics of whey proteins in food products. *J Dairy Sci* 81:597–608.

De Wit, J. N. and Bronts, H. 1994. Process for the recovery of of alpha-lactalbumin and beta-lactoglobulin from a whey product. *European Patent Application* 0 604 864.

El-Samragy, Y. A., C. L. Hansen, and D. J. McMahon. 1993. Production of ultrafiltered skim milk retentate powder. 1. Composition and physical properties. *J Dairy Sci* 76:388–92.

Fäldt, P. and I. Sjöholm. 1996. Characterization of spray-dried whole milk. *Milchwissenschaft* 51:88–92.

Fang, Y., C. Selomulya, S. Ainsworth, M. Palmer, and X. D. Chen. 2011. On quantifying the dissolution behaviour of milk protein concentrate. *Food Hydrocolloids* 25:503–10.

Fang, Y., C. Selomulya, and X. D. Chen. 2010. Characterization of milk protein concentrate solubility using focused beam reflectance measurement. *Dairy Sci Technol* 90:253–70.

Farkye, N. Y. 2006. Significance of milk fat in milk powder. In *Advanced Dairy Chemistry 2: Lipids*, 3rd edn, eds. P. F. Fox, and P. L. H. McSweeney, pp. 451–65. New York, NY: Springer.

Ferrer, M. A., A. R. Hill, and M. Corredig. 2008. Rheological properties of rennet gels containing milk protein concentrates. *J Dairy Sci* 91:959–69.

Foster, K. D., J. E. Bronlund, and A. H. J. Paterson. 2005. The contribution of milk fat towards the caking of dairy powders. *Int Dairy J* 15:85–91.

Francolino, S., F. Locci, R. Ghiglietti, R. Iezzi, and G. Mucchetti. 2010. Use of milk protein concentrate to standardize milk composition in Italian citric Mozzarella making. *Lebensm-Wiss Technol* 43:310–4.

Gani M. M., K. May, and K. Porter. 1992. A process and apparatus for the recovery of immunoglobulins. *European Patent* 0 059 598 A1.

Gao, H., P. Havea, and H. Singh. 2006. Whey products and process. International Patent Application WO/2006/068521.

Gernigon, G., P. Schuck, R. Jeantet, and H. Burling. 2011. Whey processing: Demineralization. In *Encyclopedia of Dairy Sciences*. ed. J. W. Fuquay, P. F. Fox, and P. L. H. McSweeney, 2nd edn , pp. 738–743. San Diego, CA: Academic Press.

Gesan-Guiziou, G., G. Daufin, M. Timmer, D. Allersma, and C. van der Horst. 1999. Process steps for the preparation of purified fractions of α-lactalbumin and β-lactoglobulin from whey protein concentrate. *J Dairy Res* 66:225–36.

Green, M. L., J. K. Scott, M. Anderson, M. C. A. Griffin, and F. A. Glover. 1984. Chemical characterization of milk concentrated by ultrafiltration. *J Dairy Res* 51:267–78.

Guyomarc'h, F., F. Warin, D. D. Muir, and J. Leaver. 2000. Lactosylation of milk proteins during the manufacture and storage of skim milk powders. *Int Dairy J* 10:863–72.

Guzmán-Gonzáles, M., F. Morais, M. Ramos, and L. Amigo. 1999. Influence of skimmed milk concentrate replacement by dry dairy products in a low fat set-type yoghurt model system. I: Use of whey protein concentrates, milk protein concentrates and skimmed milk powder. *J Sci Food Agric* 79:1117–22.

Harvey, J. 2006. Protein fortification of cheese milk using milk protein concentrate—Yield improvement and product quality. *Aust J Dairy Technol* 61:183–5.

Havea, P. 2006. Protein interactions in milk protein concentrate powders. *Int Dairy J* 16:415–22.

Hilpert, H. 1984. Preparation of a milk immunoglobulin concentration from cow's milk. In *Human Milk Banking*. eds. A. F. Williams and J. F. Baums, pp. 17–28. New York: Raven Press.

Huffman, L. M. and W. J. Harper. 1999. Maximizing the value of milk through separation technologies. *J Dairy Sci* 82:2238–44.

IDF. 2010. *The World Dairy Situation*, IDF Bulletin 446. Brussels, Belgium: International Dairy Federation.

Jelen, P. 2009. Dried whey, whey proteins, lactose and lactose derivative products. In *Dairy Powders and Concentrated Products*. ed. A. Y. Tamime. pp. 255–67. Chichester: Blackwell Publishing.

Kelly, P. M. 2011. Milk protein concentrate. In *Encyclopedia of Dairy Sciences*, 2nd edn, ed. J. W. Fuquay, P. F. Fox, and P. L. H. McSweeney, pp. 848–54. San Diego, CA: Academic Press.

Kelly, A. L., J. E. O'Connell, and P. F. Fox. 2003. Manufacture and properties of milk powders. In *Advanced Dairy Chemistry 1: Proteins*, 3rd edn, eds. P. F. Fox, and P. L. H. McSweeney, pp. 1027–61. New York, NY: Kluwer Academic/Plenum Publishers.

Keogh, K. 1998. *The Use of Cold Setting Whey Proteins to Enhance the Gelation Properties of Food*. Fermoy: Moorepark.

Kinsella, J. E. and D. M. Whitehead. 1989. Proteins in whey: Chemical, physical, and functional properties. *Adv Food Nutr Res* 33:343–438.

Kuo, C. J. and W. J. Harper. 2003a. Rennet gel properties of milk protein concentrates. *Milchwissenschaft* 58:181–4.

Kuo, C. J. and W. J. Harper. 2003b. Effect of hydration time of milk protein concentrate on cast Feta cheese and texture. *Milchwissenschaft* 58:283–6.

Liang, B. and R. W. Hartel. 2004. Effects of milk powders in milk chocolate. *J Dairy Sci* 87:20–31.

Lucca, P. A. and Tepper, B. J. 1994. Fat replacers and the functionality of fat in foods. *Trends Food Sci Techn* 5:12–9.

Martin, G. J. O., R. P. W. Williams, and D. E. Dunstan. 2010. Effect of manufacture and reconstitution of milk protein concentrate powder on the size and rennet gelation behaviour of casein micelles. *Int Dairy J* 20:128–31.

Martin-Hernandez, M. C., B. W. Van Markwijk, and H. J. Vreeman.1990. Isolation and properties of lactoperoxidase from milk. *Neth Milk Dairy J* 44:213–31.

Masters, K. 2002. *Spray Drying in Practice*. Charlottenlund: SprayDryConsult International ApS.

McKenna, A. B. 2000. *Effect of Processing and Storage on the Reconstitution Properties of Whole Milk and Ultrafiltered Skim Milk Powders*. PhD diss., Massey Univ., Palmerston North, New Zealand.

McKenna, A. B., R. J. Lloyd, P. A. Munro, and H. Singh. 1999. Microstructure of whole milk powder and of insolubles detected by powder functional testing. *Scanning* 21:305–15.

Mimouni, A., H. C. Deeth, A. K. Whittaker, M. J. Gidley, and B. R. Bhandari. 2009. Rehydration process of milk protein concentrate powder monitored by static light scattering. *Food Hydrocolloids* 23:1958–65.

Mimouni, A., H. C. Deeth, A. K. Whittaker, M. J. Gidley, and B. R. Bhandari. 2010a. Investigation of the microstructure of milk protein concentrate powders during rehydration: Alterations during storage. *J Dairy Sci* 93:463–72.

Mimouni, A., H. C. Deeth, A. K. Whittaker, M. J. Gidley, and B. R. Bhandari. 2010b. Rehydration of high-protein-containing dairy powder: Slow- and fast-dissolving components and storage effects. *Dairy Sci Technol* 90:335–44.

Mintel Group Ltd. 2009. *Global New Products Database*. London: Mintel Group Ltd.

Mistry, V. V. 2002. Manufacture and application of high milk protein powder. *Lait* 82:515–22.

Mistry, V. V. and H. N. Hassan. 1992. Manufacture of nonfat yogurt from a high milk protein powder. *J Dairy Sci* 75:947–57.

Mistry, V. V. and J. B. Pulgar. 1996a. Physical and storage properties of high milk protein powder. *Int Dairy J* 6:195–203.

Mistry, V. V. and J. B. Pulgar. 1996b. Use of high milk protein powder in the manufacture of Gouda cheese. *Int Dairy J* 6:205–15.

Morr, C. V. and E. Y. W. Ha. 1993. Whey protein concentrates and isolates: Processing and functional properties. *Crit Rev Food Sci Nutr* 33:431–76.

Mulvihill D. M. and Ennis, M. P. 2003. Functional milk proteins: Production and utilization. In *Advanced Dairy Chemistry—Volume 1: Proteins*. eds. P. F. Fox and P. L. H. McSweeney. pp. 1175–228. New York: Kluwer Academic/Plenum Publishers.

Oliver, C. M. 2011. Insight into the glycation of milk proteins: An ESI- and MALDI-MS perspective. *Crit Rev Food Sci Nutr* 51:410–31.

Oliver, C. M., L. D. Melton, and R. A. Stanley. 2006. Creating proteins with novel functionality via the Maillard reaction: A review. *Crit Rev Food Sci Nutr* 46:337–50.

Paquin, P., Y. Lebeuf, J. P. Richard, and M. Kalab. 1993. Microparticulation of milk proteins by high pressure homogenization to produce a fat substitute. In *Protein and Fat Globule Modifications by Heat Treatment, Homogenization and Other Technological Means for High Quality Dairy Products*, pp. 389–396. Brussels: International Dairy Federation.

Paul, K. G., P. I. Ohlsson, and A. Hendrikson. 1980. The isolation and some liganding properties of lactoperoxidase. *FEBS Lett* 110:200–4.

Pearce, R. J. 1983. Thermal separation of β-lactoglobulin and α-lactalbumin in bovine Cheddar cheese whey. *Aust J Dairy Technol* 38:144–9.

Pearce, R. J. 1987. Franctionation of whey proteins. *Int Dairy Fed Bul* 212:150–3.

Písecký, J. 1997. *Handbook of Milk Powder Manufacture*. Copenhagen, Denmark: Niro A/S.

Prieels, J. P. and R. Peiffer. 1986. Process for the purification of proteins from a liquid such as milk. UK Patent Application GB2 171 102 A1.

Queguiner, C., E. Dumay, C. Salou-Cavalier, and J-C. Cheftel. 1992. Microparticulation of a whey protein isolate by extrusion cooking at acid pH. *J Food Sci* 57 610–6.

Refstrup, E. 2003. Drying of milk—Drying principles. In *Encyclopedia of Dairy Sciences*, eds. H. Roginski, J. F. Fuquay, and P. F. Fox, pp. 860–71. Amsterdam: Academic Press.

Rowan, C. 1998. The whey ahead. *Food Manuf* 73:19–20.

Schuck, P., M. Piot, S. Méjean, J. Fauquant, C. Brulé, and J. L. Maubois. 1994. Dehydration of an ultra-clean milk and micellar casein enriched milks. *Lait* 74:47–63.

Singer, N. S, S., Yamamoto, and J. Latella. 1988. *Protein product base*. European Patent Application EP250623.

Singh, H. 2007. Interactions of milk proteins during the manufacture of milk powders. *Lait* 87:413–23.

Snoeren, T. H. M., A. J. Damman, and H. J. Klok. 1982. The viscosity of skim-milk concentrates. *Neth Milk Dairy J* 36:305–16.

Spiegel T. (1999). Whey protein aggregation under shear conditions—Effect of lactose and heating temperature on aggregate size and structure. *Int J Food Sci Techn* 34:523–531.

Stapelfeldt, H., B. R. Nielsen, and L. H. Skibsted. 1997. Effect of heat treatment, water activity and storage temperature on the oxidative stability of whole milk powder. *Int Dairy J* 7:331–9.

Straatsma, J., G. Van Houwelingen, A. E. Steenbergen, and P. De Jong. 1999. Spray drying of food products: 2. Prediction of insolubility index. *J Food Eng* 42:73–7.

Thomas, M. E. C., J. Scher, S. Desobry-Banon, and S. Desobry. 2004. Milk powders ageing: Effect on physical and functional properties. *Crit Rev Food Sci Nutr* 44:297–322.

Tong, P. 2010. Dairy Ingredients Symposium press release. U.S. Dairy Export Council. http://www.usdec.org/files/PDFs/Dairy Ingredients Symposium Press Release FINAL.pdf (accessed July 25, 2011).

Troyano, E., A. Olano, and I. Martinez-Castro. 1994. Changes in free monosaccharides during storage of dried milk. *J Agric Food Chem* 42:1543–1545.

Van Mil, P. J. J. M. and A. J. Jans. 1991. Storage stability of whole milk powder: Effects of process and storage conditions on product properties. *Neth Milk Dairy J* 45:145–67.

Vignolles, M.-L., R. Jeantet, C. Lopez, and P. Schuck. 2007. Free fat, surface fat and dairy powders: Interactions between process and product. A review. *Lait* 87:187–236.

Walstra, P., J. T. M. Wouters, and T. J. Geurts. 2006. *Dairy Science and Technology*, 2nd edn, Boca Raton, FL: CRC Press.

Westergaard, V. 2003. Drying of milk—Drying design. In *Encyclopedia of Dairy Sciences*, eds. H. Roginski, J. F. Fuquay, and P. F. Fox, pp. 871–89. Amsterdam: Academic Press.

Westergaard, V. 2004. *Milk Powder Technology: Evaporation and Spray Drying*, 5th edn. Copenhagen, Denmark: Niro A/S.

Ye, A., S. G. Anema, and H. Singh. 2007. Behaviour of homogenized fat globules during the spray drying of whole milk. *Int Dairy J* 17:374–82.

Ye, A., H. Singh, M. W. Taylor, and S. G. Anema. 2004. Interactions of fat globule surface proteins during concentration of whole milk in a pilot-scale multiple-effect evaporator. *J Dairy Res* 71:471–9.

23 Probiotics as Functional Food Ingredients for Augmenting Human Health

Sunita Grover, Ashwani Kumar, A.K. Srivastava, and Virender K. Batish

CONTENTS

Probiotics, particularly those belonging to lactobacilli and bifidobacteria—the two key members of this group, have recently emerged as one of the most powerful microbial agents with multiple health-promoting functions of considerable commercial value and therapeutic potential. The interest in these organisms has grown enormously during the last few years mainly due to the tremendous growth of the market for functional and health foods supplemented with probiotics across the world. The rapid growth and demand for probiotic dairy-based foods is largely attributed to the growing awareness among the consumers about linkage of diet/food with general health, discovery of new probiotics with novel health-promoting physiological functions, and high commercial stakes involved in the probiotic functional dairy food market. It is now well recognized that metabolic inflammatory disorders associated with the malfunctioning of the human gut, such as diarrhea, inflammatory bowel disease (IBD), ulcerative colitis, peptic ulcers, Crohn's disease (CD), constipation along with lactose intolerance, and other chronic lifestyle diseases such as diabetes, rheumatoid arthritis, obesity, colon cancer, hypertension, and allergies can be alleviated through consumption of probiotic cultures directly or their food formulations. Probiotics can be used either as prophylactics or as biotherapeutics as an effective alternative to drug treatment. As compared to many pharmaceutical agents, probiotics are well tolerated by human anatomy and are extremely safe. However, probiotics as a concept is still associated with a large body of unsubstantiated claims, and linking specific health benefits to probiotic functionality is the biggest challenge. Although there is suggestive evidence for each of these functional claims, the exact molecular mechanisms involved therein remain by and large unknown. Hence, to address this issue, genomics-based approaches are currently being explored to identify the relevant molecular properties of probiotics and host cells and their interaction under both *in vitro* and *in vivo* conditions. This information will be extremely valuable for understanding the functionality of the currently available probiotic strains and will also be immensely helpful in the selection of novel probiotics on the basis of their specific molecular functions.

23.1   PROBIOTIC CONCEPT: HISTORICAL PERSPECTIVE

Although the interest in probiotics and probiotic foods, particularly fermented dairy-based products, has grown enormously during the past several years and has been currently the major focus of attention all over the world due to their biotherapeutic potentials, it is not a new concept. Ancient man has been traditionally practicing the same for maintaining health status and well-being since time immemorial without knowing the scientific rationale behind the concept. It figures prominently in Hindu scriptures and even in the Bible. The very first probiotic recorded during prehistoric era was fermented milk. The role of fermented milk in human diet and health was known even in Vedic times. However, the scientific credibility of the concept got a boost with the acceptance of the theory of longevity proposed by Russian scientist Ellie Metchnikoff in 1908 in his book *Prolongation of Life*, wherein he attributed the long life of Bulgarians with the regular consumption of fermented milk such as Bulgarian yoghurt. The probiotic concept gained momentum with the launch of Yakult drink for promoting the health of the Japanese in 1930 by M. Shirota. Finally, it was recognized as the vital health care concept of the twenty-first century because of immense health-promoting physiological functions expressed by probiotics. The probiotic revolution currently witnessed across the world primarily emerged from the shift in the perception of consumers towards their foods not merely as a source of nutrition but beyond that as a medicine to manage their health care needs and protection against diseases. The present-day health-conscious consumers are now looking for safe and cost-effective natural formulations for the management of their routine day-to-day health problems as an alternative to drug therapy due to the exorbitant cost and the undesirable long-term side effects invariably associated with the latter. One such approach that can be quite effective, affordable, and realistic is based on exploring probiotics as functional food ingredients and biotherapeutics through supplementation in foods, particularly dairy-based fermented products which can be extremely beneficial for the target population in their respective countries to address their health problems and well-being.

23.2 DEFINITION AS PER FAO/WHO GUIDELINES

The term "probiotics" was originally derived from the Greek word "pro bios," meaning "for life." An expert panel commissioned by the FAO (Food and Agriculture Organization) and the WHO (World Health Organization) defined probiotics as "live micro-organisms, which, when administered in adequate amounts confer a health benefit on the host." Although this is the most acceptable definition of probiotics used all over the world, several researchers (Lilly and Stilwell, 1965; Fuller, 1989) have given their own definitions with some modifications. However, irrespective of some differences, all definitions agree that probiotic microorganisms must be living and must exert scientifically proven health effects. A probiotic strain must be of human origin, nonpathogenic, technologically suitable for industrial processes, and acid and bile resistant, and must adhere to the gut epithelial tissue, produce antimicrobial substances, modulate immune responses, and influence the metabolic activities of the gut (Dunne et al., 1999).

23.3 PROBIOTIC ATTRIBUTES

Although lactic acid bacteria (LAB), including lactobacilli and bifidobacteria, have been traditionally used as probiotics predominantly since times immemorial, particularly in the preparation of fermented dairy products for therapeutic applications, all the LAB may not be necessarily probiotic. For designating a particular microbial culture as potential probiotic, it must exhibit all the desired probiotic attributes and fulfill the criteria as laid down in the FAO/WHO probiotic guidelines (2002) to qualify for the probiotic status. They must be capable of surviving a passage through the gut, that is, they must have the ability to resist gastric juices, acidic pH and exposure to bile. Simultaneously, they should be able to proliferate and colonize the digestive tract. Finally, they must be safe and effective and maintain their potency during the entire shelf life of the product. Caco2 cell adherence can be used as an effective *in vitro* assay system for evaluating the colonization potential of probiotic strains before conducting clinical studies on human subjects. Apart from these properties, for any microbial culture to be explored as a probiotic candidate, it must be properly identified and characterized.

23.4 IDENTIFICATION AND CHARACTERIZATION OF PROBIOTICS

Since the physiological properties related to probiotic functions are highly strain specific, proper identification and authentication of the probiotic culture at genus, species, and strain level is extremely important to the success of probiotic applications. In this context, both phenotypic and genotypic methods currently in vogue for the identification of all kinds of microbes can also find application in the identification of probiotic organisms. In view of the high stakes involved in exploring the commercial value of probiotics, particularly in the booming functional/health food market, the correct identification of Probiotic cultures has become extremely important in order to rule out the possibility of false claims associated with specific strain and disputes arising out of the mislabeled probiotic preparations.

23.4.1 PHENOTYPIC APPROACHES

Traditionally, probiotic bacteria like any other microorganism can be tentatively identified at the genus and species level by using conventional phenotypic methods based on morphological and biochemical characteristics such as growth at different temperatures, mode of glucose fermentation, lactic acid configuration, fermentation of various carbohydrates, methyl esters of fatty acids (Decallone et al., 1991), and pattern of proteins in the cell wall or entire cell (Gatti et al., 1997). Some of the phenotypic fingerprinting techniques based on phenotypic characteristics include polyacrylamide gel electrophoresis of soluble proteins, fatty acid analysis, bacteriophage typing, as well as sero typing. However, the phenotypic fingerprints obtained are usually less sensitive and changes in the fingerprint may not necessarily mean a different organism, but rather could be attributed to a change in the expression of a particular phenotypic trait. Methods like carbohydrate fermentation and cellular fatty acid methyl ester (FAME) have been widely used to determine the taxonomic relationship of the probiotic lactobacilli and bifidobacteria. However, the conventional methods suffer from lack of reproducibility, type ability, and discriminating power while analyzing the phenotype, since the entire information potential of a genome is never expressed as gene expression is greatly influenced by the environmental conditions (Farber, 1996). Moreover, the plate culturing techniques may not always reveal the true picture of the microbial profile because most of the GIT organisms are difficult to cultivate. All these drawbacks adversely affect the reliability of phenotypic-based methods for culture identification at the genus and species level. Nevertheless, in spite of these drawbacks, phenotypic methods do generate useful data that can be valuable in preliminary identification of probiotic cultures which can be integrated into more advanced techniques currently in vogue for microbial culture identification. Hence, polyphasic approaches combining biochemical, molecular, and morphological data are important for accurate classification of lactic acid bacteria, including probiotics (Klein et al., 1998).

23.4.2 MOLECULAR APPROACHES

Molecular techniques have been found to be quite useful and effective in the characterization of microbial community, composition, enumeration, and monitoring of microbial population and tracking of specific strains of bacteria in the gut microflora. Classification of organisms and evaluation of their evolutionary relatedness by 16S rRNA analysis was first developed by Woese et al. (1987). 16S rRNA has revolutionized the manner in which taxonomists classify and identify bacteria. The 16S rRNA gene has highly variable to highly conserved regions which has allowed meaningful phylogenetic relationships between microbes in natural ecosystems to be discerned. The internal transcribed spacer (ITS) has been explored in the genetic characterization of lactobacilli, bifidobacteria, and LAB. The 16S rRNA gene and the flanking interspacer regions in the microbial genome constitute the most potential molecular markers which are currently used as the "gold standard" for the identification of probiotic at the genus and species level. Since the purported health-benefitting function of probiotics is highly strain specific, identification of these organisms at the strain level is extremely important to substantiate the health claims attributed to a particular strain. Genotypic methods used for strain typing are typically PCR-based methods, for example, randomly amplified polymorphic DNA (RAPD) (Elegado et al., 2004), restriction fragment length polymorphism (RFLP) (Rodas et al., 2005), ribotyping (Yansanjav et al., 2003), pulsed field gel electrophoresis (PFGE) (Sánchez et al., 2004), Rep-PCR, and so on. Gurakan (2004), while exploring ribotyping, used four different restriction enzymes which had different recognition sites in the spacer region. However, no different digestion patterns were observed which showed that sequence variation in the spacer region among *Lactobacillus* strains had not been sufficient for specific identification of *L. plantarum* strains. Therefore, PCR ribotyping was determined as an inefficient method for the identification of *L. plantarum* at the strain level. Nagashima et al. (2003) explored the RFLP and developed new primer–enzyme combinations for terminal restriction fragment length polymorphism (T-RFLP) targeting of the 16S rRNA gene of human fecal DNA. The resulting amplified product was digested with RsaI plus BfaI or with BslI enzymes. Operational taxonomic units (OTUs) were detected with RsaI and BfaI digestion and 14 predominant OTUs were detected with BslI digestion. This new T-RFLP method made it easy to predict what kind of intestinal bacterial group corresponded to each OTU on the basis of the terminal restriction fragment length compared with the conventional T-RFLP. Moreover, it also made possible the identification of the bacterial species that an OTU represents by cloning and sequencing. Coeuret et al. (2004) used PFGE to identify strains to assess the accuracy of labeling with regard to genus and species and found the method to be convenient for identifying probiotic lactobacilli in probiotic food and animal feed. Strain typing has been successfully achieved by PFGE for the *Lactobacillus acidophilus* complex, *L. casei*, *L. delbrueckii*, and its three subspecies (*bulgaricus*, *delbrueckii*, and *lactis*), *L. fermentum*, *L. helveticus*, *L. plantarum*, *L. rhamnosus*, and *L. sakei* (Giraffa and Neviani, 2000). Fluorescent *in situ* hybridization (FISH) has been explored by several investigators in determining the load of viable organisms in the feces and gut. By applying this technique, the number of bacteria in human fecal samples was shown to be approximately 10-fold higher than the number estimated through standard culture techniques, when nonspecific probes to the 16S rRNA for FISH were used (Harmsen et al., 2000). This technique is currently the most advanced technique for enumeration of fecal microbiota in terms of the number of probes available and speed of analysis. Amplification rDNA restriction analysis (ARDRA) has successfully differentiated various species or strains within the *Lactobacillus acidophilus* complex, *L. casei*, *L. delbrueckii*, *L. fermentum*, *L. helveticus*, *L. plantarum*, *L. reuteri*, *L. rhamnosus*, and *L. sakei* (Giraffa and Neviani, 2000; Hozapfel et al., 2001). ARDRA has been used to differentiate a variety of lactobacilli at the species level, including *L. delbrueckii* and its three subspecies (*bulgaricus*, *delbrueckii*, and *lactis*), *L. acidophilus*, and *L. helveticus* (Roy and Sirois, 2001). Amplified fragment length polymorphism (AFLP) has been found to be a very useful fingerprinting technique for bacteria, affording both species resolution and strain differentiation. Species-level discrimination has been shown for the phylogenetically closely related species *L. pentosus*, *L. plantarum*, and *L. pseudoplantarum* using this method (Giraffa and Neviani, 2000). DNA chip/array is also going to be the method of choice for the identification of dairy organisms in the near future because of its high degree of reliability in terms of specificity and sensitivity. The drawbacks associated with the use of the above methods are interlaboratory reproducibility and even in the laboratory with different workers. Hence, the use of housekeeping genes is emerging as an alternative to overcome these hurdles. Since, complete genome sequences of several species of *Lactobacillus* are now available *in silico* studies can provide the basis for establishing sets of housekeeping genes that can accurately predict genome relatedness and improve the accuracy of species identification. In this context, multilocus sequence typing (MLST) has recently been shown to be a powerful technique for bacterial typing. MLST makes use of automated DNA sequencing to characterize the alleles present at different housekeeping gene loci. As it is based on nucleotide sequence, it is highly discriminatory and provides unambiguous results that are directly comparable between laboratories. Recently, a study was carried out by de las Rivas et al. (2006) on the application of MLST system for 16 *L. plantarum* strains that were also characterized by ribotyping and RFLP analysis of the PCR-amplified 16S–23S rDNA intergenic spacer region (ISR). Ribotyping grouped the strains into four groups; however, RFLP analysis of the ISRs showed no differences in the strains analyzed. On the other hand, MLST showed a good discriminatory ability. Naser et al. (2007) used MLST for identification of 201 strains representing 98 species and 17 subspecies. They reported that the housekeeping genes can be used as alternative genomic markers to 16S rRNA gene sequences and have a higher discriminatory power for reliable identification of species of the genus *Lactobacillus*. MLST is a more robust and cost-effective method for ascertaining the genetic structure of large strain collections, particularly when many of the isolates may be isogenic. Since MLST offers accurate and precise identification, easy comparison, and exchange of the results obtained in different laboratories, the future application of this new molecular method could be highly useful for the identification of lactobacillus strains for use in tracking studies in animal as well as human clinical trials besides in probiotic dairy foods.

23.5   STATUS OF PROBIOTIC CULTURES

A number of commercial strains of probiotics mostly of Western gut origin with established health-promoting functions which have been extensively used in different dairy-based functional foods available in the market are listed in Table 23.1 along with their source.

TABLE 23.1
Commercially Available Probiotic Strains

Strain	Source/Producer
L. acidophilus NCFM, also referred to as Howaru Dophilus	Danisco Rhodia, Inc. (Madison, Wisconsin, USA)
L. acidophilus LA-5	Chr. Hansen (Horsholm, Denmark)
L. acidophilus LA-1	
L. paracasei CRL 431	
B. lactis Bb-12	
L. casei Shirota	Yakult (Tokyo, Japan)
B. breve strain Yakult	
L. acidophilus DDS-1	Nebraska Cultures, Inc. (Lincoln, Nebraska, USA)
L. casei DN014001 (Immunitas)	Danone Le Plessis-Robinson (Paris, France)
L. johnsonii La1 (same as Lj1)	Nestlé (Lausanne, Switzerland)
Lactobacillus paracasei St11	
L. fermentum RC-14	Urex Biotech Inc. (London, Ontario, Canada)
L. rhamnosus GR-1	
L. acidophilus R0011	Institut Rosell (Montreal, Canada)
L. rhamnosus R0052	
Bifidobacterium LAFTI®B94	
L. acidophilus LAFTI®L10	
L. casei LAFTI®L26	
L. plantarum 299V	Probi AB (Lund, Sweden)
L. rhamnosus 271	
L. rhamnosus strain GG (under name Gefilus)	Valio Dairy (Helsinki, Finland)
L. reuteri SD2112 (same as MM2)	BioGaia (Raleigh, North Carolina, USA)
L. acidophilus SBT-2062	Snow Brand Milk Products Co., Ltd. (Tokyo, Japan)
B. longum SBT-2928	
L. salivarius UCC118	University College (Cork, Ireland)
B. animalis subsp. *lactis* HN019 (DR10)	Selected from New Zealand Dairy Research Institute and marketed by Danisco as HOWARU Bifido and HOWARU Rhamnosus and by Fonterra as *B. lactis* DR10 and *L. rhamnosus* DR20
L. rhamnosus HN0011 (DR20)	
LGG® EXTRA, a multispecies probiotic combination	Valio (Finland)
Other strains:	
L. rhamnosus Lc705 (DSM, 7061)	
Propinonibacterium freudenreichii subsp *shermanii* JS (DSM, 7067)	
B. animalis subsp. *lactis* BB-12	
B. longum BB536	Morinaga Bifidus Milk Morinaga Milk Industry Co., Ltd. (Zama-City, Japan)
L. rhamnosus LB21	Essum AB (Umeå, Sweden)
Lactococcus lactis L1A	
L. acidophilus LB	Lacteol Laboratory (Houdan, France)

TABLE 23.1   (continued)
Commercially Available Probiotic Strains

Strain	Source/Producer
L. paracasei F19	Arla Dairy (Stockholm, Sweden)
L. crispatus CTV05	Gynelogix (Boulder, Colorado, USA)
L. casei DN114	Danone (Paris, France)
L. delbrueckii subsp. *bulgaricus* 2038	Meiji Milk Products (Tokyo, Japan)
S. boulardii	Biocodex Inc. (Seattle, Washington, USA)
VSL#3—mixture of following eight bacteria	VSL Pharmaceuticals Inc.
Four lactobacilli (*L. acidophilus, L. bulgaricus, L. casei,* and *L. plantarum*), three bifidobacteria (*B. breve, B. infantis,* and *B. longum*) and *S. thermophilus*	
B. infantis 35264	Procter & Gamble (Mason, Ohio, USA)
L. fermentum VRI003 (PCC)	Probiomics (Eveleigh, Australia)
L. paracasei F19	Medipharm (Des Moines, Iowa, USA)
L. paracasei 33	GenMont Biotech (Taiwan)
L. rhamnosus GM	
L. paracasei GMNL	
L. plantarum OM	Bio-Energy Systems, Inc. (Kalispell, Montana, USA)
B. coagulans BC30	Ganeden Biotech Inc. (Cleveland, Ohio, USA)
S. oralis KJ3	Oragenics Inc. (Alachua, Florida, USA)
S. uberis KJ2	
S. rattus JH145	
L. rhamnosus PBO1	Bifodan (Denmark), www.ecovag.com
L. gasseri EB01	
L. VTT E-97800	VTT (Finland)
E. coli M17	BioBalance
E. coli Nissile 1917	Ardeypharm

23.6   SEARCH FOR NOVEL INDIGENOUS PROBIOTIC STRAINS

Although there are already quite a few proven strains of probiotic lactobacilli, bifidobacteria, *Saccharomyces boulardii*, and others with established functional efficacy available commercially as listed above, the list has been expanding steadily over the last few years. Since the novel health-promoting functions of probiotics are highly strain specific and till today there is no report of any universal strain expressing all the desired physiological functions simultaneously, the search for finding novel probiotic strains is a never-ending process and hence should go on unabated to add to the growing list to explore the same for novel product development for specific health applications. The natural habitat of probiotics is the human gut where more than 1000 bacterial species reside as commensals and constitute the gut microbiota. However, the diet plays a key role in the build up of gut microbiota which may vary considerably from person to person and from different geographical locations with different food habits. All the probiotic cultures with established physiological functions commercially available in the world market and used in probiotic foods and formulations have been derived from the human gut of Western/Japanese population. These cultures which are available in limited numbers find it difficult to colonize the native population of other countries with different food habits and hence may not be as effective in combating the gut-related enteric diseases and other chronic disorders prevalent in those countries as in their own native population from where they were derived. Hence, indigenous probiotic cultures with novel physiological properties beneficial to human health isolated from the gut of native population of each country would be a better option to manage inflammatory metabolic disorders as they are likely to be better adapted due to the strong local conditioning effect and have the competitive advantage to stay longer with extended transit in the gut and hence express their desirable functions most optimally. In this context, one of the most crucial issues in this context is the selection of promising strains having strong colonization potential along with better probiotic attributes with novel physiological functions after proper identification and characterization before their application as food supplement in product development for health applications. Realizing the biological significance of the local probiotic strains for possible application in the Indian population, an initiative was taken at the National Dairy Research Institute, Karnal, India with financial support from the Department of Biotechnology, Government of India, for the isolation, identification, and screening of indigenous lactobacilli of Indian gut origin. As a part of this initiative, a collection of more than 100 indigenous probiotic lactobacilli well characterized at the genus, species, and strain level by molecular tools was established in the Molecular Biology Unit at the NDRI. Many of these cultures demonstrated very strong colonization potentials based on their high adherence to *in vitro* epithelial cell culture models such as Caco2 and HT-29. Based on these results, the best colonizing culture was found to be LdCH4 that showed massive adherence capacity towards Caco2 cells followed by *L. plantarum* Lp9 and Lp91 (Batish et al., unpublished data).

23.7 ROLE OF MOLECULAR BIOMARKERS AS AN INDEX OF PROBIOTIC FUNCTIONALITY

With the completion of whole-genome projects related to some proven strains of probiotic lactobacilli and bifidobacteria and the availability of these sequences in the public domain, the locations of various genes encoding probiotic functions, particularly those involved in their survival and colonization in the hostile gut environment along with regulatory elements, have been identified on their genomes. In the light of these advancements, the prospects of exploring these functions as potential probiotic markers have improved considerably. Adhesion is believed to be a very important requirement not only for effective probiotic colonization in the hostile gut environment but also for expressing their putative physiological effects such as immunomodulation (Valeur et al., 2004) and pathogen exclusion (Mack et al., 1999) therein. These biomarkers such as acid and bile tolerance (BSH), surface layer proteins like mucus adhesion-promoting protein (MapA), mucus-binding protein (Mub), collagen-binding protein (CnBP), fibronectin-binding protein (Fbp), elongation factor Tu (EF-Tu), and immunomodulating markers (tumor necrosis factor (TNF-α), interferon-gamma (IFN-γ), transforming growth factor (TGF-β), cyclooxygenase (*Cox*1 and 2), and various cytokines like IL-4, IL-8, IL-10, IL-12, etc.) can play an important role in understanding the functionality of these beneficial microorganisms in the gut. Apart from this, these can be targeted for developing molecular assays for screening and characterization of novel probiotic along with their functional efficacy in animal models before the promising short-listed strains are subjected to clinical trials in human subjects for validation of their specific health claims.

The biomarkers for functional characterization of probiotics can be broadly categorized into two groups, one for general probiotic attributes and the second for more specific health-promoting functions for disease alleviation. Two of our indigenous strains of probiotic lactobacilli were investigated for relative quantification of acid, bile, and surface layer proteins under *in vitro*-simulated gut environmental conditions using RT-qPCR assays. Although both putative probiotic *L. plantarum* isolates investigated in this study were able to survive acid stress under *in vitro* conditions, among the two, Lp91 exhibited relatively greater acid tolerance, as revealed by 4.7-fold upregulation of the *atpD* gene as well as higher log counts at pH 2.5 after 90 min as shown in Figure 23.1 (Duary et al., 2010). Expression of *bsh* gene was similarly upregulated in Lp9, Lp91, and CSCC5276 under different bile concentrations in MRS broth. "*Mub*" gene was highly expressed in media containing mucin (0.01%), bile (1%), pancreatin (1%) (pH 6.5): 13.16 ± 0.45 (Lp9), 6.03 ± 0.24 (Lp91), and

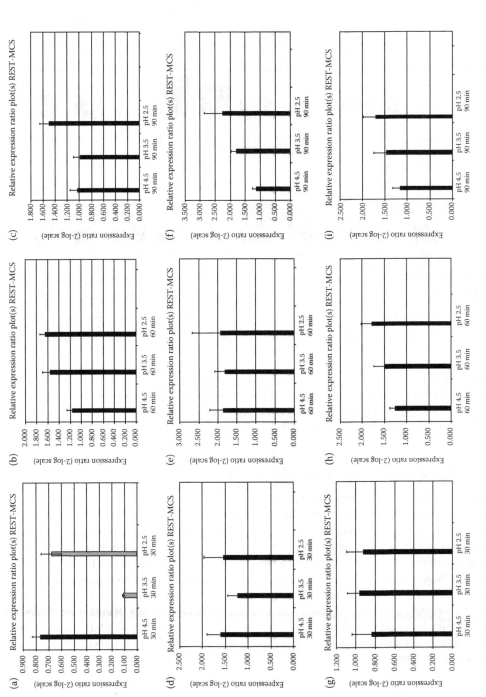

FIGURE 23.1 Expression profile of *apD* gene at different acidic conditions. (a)–(c): Lp9 at pH 4.5, 3.5, and 2.5 after 30, 60, and 90 min, respectively; (d)–(f): Lp91 at pH 4.5, 3.5, and 2.5 after 30, 60, and 90 min, respectively; (g)–(i): CSCC5276 at pH 4.5, 3.5, and 2.5 after 30, 60, and 90 min, respectively. Black bars: significant upregulation of *apD* gene, $p \leq 0.05\%$; gray bars: upregulation of *apD* gene not significant ($p > 0.1$).

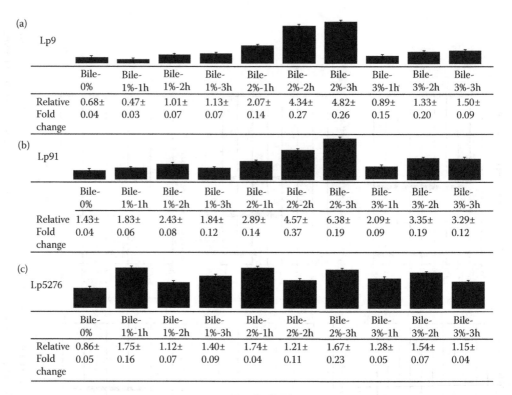

FIGURE 23.2 Expression profile of *Bsh* gene in (a) Lp9, (b) Lp91, and (c) Lp5276 at different bile concentrations.

9.24 ± 0.29 (Lp5276). *MapA* gene was highly expressed in media containing mucin (0.05%), bile (1%), pancreatin (1%) (pH 6.5): 30.92 ± 1.51 (Lp9), 6.24 ± 0.24 (Lp91), and 7.30 ± 0.11 (Lp5276). EF-Tu gene was highly expressed in media containing mucin (0.05%) (pH 7.0): 14.04 ± 1.03 (Lp9), 42.84 ± 5.64 (Lp91), and 12.11 ± 0.84 (Lp5276) as illustrated in Figure 23.2 (Duary et al., 2011).

23.8 COLONIZATION OF PROBIOTICS IN THE GUT

It is generally agreed that in order to permanently establish a bacterial strain in the host intestine, the microorganisms must be able to attach to the intestinal mucosal cells. Even pathogens cannot exert their deleterious effects on the gut unless they adhere to the mucosal epithelial in the gut (Hoepelman and Tuomanen, 1992), and the beneficial action of probiotics has been explored by their purported ability to interfere with the adherence of pathogens to intestinal mucosal cells (Fuller, 1991). Colonization begins as the newborn enters the birth canal with exposure to maternal vaginal and colonic flora (Kohler et al., 2003). Additional stimulation occurs with the introduction of enteric feeding and weaning, and complete colonization occurs with a large variety of organisms by 2 years of age. The effective probiotic colonization in the gut is chiefly mediated by several adhesion factors and surface layer proteins expressed by these organisms in a highly strain-dependent manner as briefly described below.

23.8.1 ADHESION FACTORS

Adhesion to the intestinal mucosa is regarded as a prerequisite for probiotic microorganisms. Adhesion allows the colonization, although transient, of the human intestinal tract and it has been related to many of the health benefits attributed to specific probiotics. Thus, the ability to adhere to

epithelial cells and mucosal surfaces has been suggested to be an important property of many probiotic bacterial strains and combination of probiotics. Several researchers have reported on the roles
of composition, structure, and forces of interaction in bacterial adhesion to intestinal epithelial cells
and mucus. It has been shown that some lactobacilli and bifidobacteria share carbohydrate-binding
specificities with some pathogens wherein this attribute is associated with their pathophysiology.
The adhesion mechanism involves passive forces, electrostatic and hydrophobic interaction, lipoteichoic acids, and specific structures such as polysaccharides and lectins. In general, it is assumed that
probiotic strains are able to inhibit the attachment of pathogenic bacteria by means of steric hin-
drance at enterocyte pathogen receptors. It has been suggested that proteinaceous components are
involved in the adhesion of probiotic strains to intestinal cells. Many specific interactions between
Lactobacilli and host cells seem to be mediated by sortase dependent proteins (SDPs) with a typical
modular structure that includes an N-terminal signal peptide and a–c terminal LPXTG motif. Other
surface proteins can be involved in specific adherence mechanisms.

23.8.2 ROLE OF SURFACE PROTEINS IN ADHERENCE

Apart from adhesion molecules, probiotic cultures, particularly different strains of lactobacillus
species, also express a variety of cell surface proteins such as mannose-specific adhesions (Msa),
mucus-binding protein (Mub), fibronectin-binding protein (FbpA), and surface layer protein A
(slpA). The role of these proteins in the adherence of proven probiotic strains and their colonization
in the gut has been well established by gene knockout mutants by several groups of investigators
(Callanan et al., 2008; Roos and Jonsson, 2002; Bron et al., 2004; Altermann et al., 2004; Pretzer
et al., 2005; Buck et al., 2005; Boekhorst et al., 2006) in *L. plantarum* WCFS1, *L. reuteri* ATCC
53608, *L. gasseri* ATCC 33323, 12 in *L. acidophilus* NCFM, and 9 in *L. johnsonii* NCC533,
L. helveticus DPC4571, *L. acidophilus* NCFM, and *L. salivarius* UCC118.

23.8.3 LIPOTEICHOIC ACIDS

Lipoteichoic acids (LTA) are suggested to provide the main component of the hydrophobicity of the
Lactobacillus cell envelope, although this depends on the D-alanine ester substitutions (Delcour et al.,
1999). The inactivation of *dltD* in the probiotic strain *L. rhamnosus* GG revealed that the D-alanylation
of LTA is not required for short-term adherence to Caco-2 cells (Perea Vélez et al., 2007), while the
dltD mutation increased the biofilm formation capacity of *L. rhamnosus* GG after 72 h of growth on
polystyrene (Lebeer et al., 2007b). The modulation of the LTA structure and charge by mutation can
have a significant impact on the binding and conformational properties of attached cell surface
proteins. The formation of biofilms in the GIT is a more complex process than mere adherence to a
substrate, as was also apparent from *in vitro* simulations of lactobacilli (Lebeer et al., 2007a).

23.8.4 EXOPOLYSACCHARIDE

As for LTA, exopolysaccharides (EPSs) generally play a role in nonspecific interactions of lactobacilli
with abiotic and biotic surfaces by contributing to the cell surface physicochemical properties. EPSs
have also been shown to have an indirect effect on adhesion by shielding other cell surface adhesins.
For example, in *L. johnsonii* NCC533, the deletion of the entire EPS cluster slightly prolonged the gut
persistence of the knockout mutant compared to the persistence of the parental control strains (Denou
et al., 2008). In *L. acidophilus* CRL639, EPSs have also been shown to negatively mediate adhesion
to extracellular matrices (Lorca et al., 2002). Ruas-Madiedo and coworkers found both positive and
negative effects of EPS on the adhesion of probiotics and enteropathogens to human intestinal mucus
(Ruas-Madiedo et al., 2006). EPSs can promote intercellular interactions and the formation of
microcolonies, although this step also depends on many other intrinsic and environmental factors.

23.9 INTERACTION OF PROBIOTICS WITH THE HOST AND THE COMMENSAL GUT FLORA/ORGANISMS

For effective functionality in the gut, probiotic strains have developed a very powerful communication network to have an efficient cross talk with the commensal gut flora, invading pathogens, and the host epithelial cells to exert their physiological functions beneficial to the host health. Given the high number and level of diversity of bacteria that comprise the GIT, it was postulated that the members of this community somehow communicate to coordinate various adaptive processes that include competition and cooperation for nutrients and adhesion sites (Kaper and Sperandio, 2005). Quorum sensing (QS) is a cell-to-cell signaling mechanism through which bacteria produce and/or respond to chemical signals called autoinducers.

23.9.1 COMMUNICATION THROUGH QUORUM SENSING AND SIGNAL TRANSDUCTION

23.9.1.1 Intraspecies Communication

The process of QS operating in bacteria has been extensively investigated in lactic acid bacteria, particularly lactobacilli which fully explore this system to communicate with each other (intrapecies) and with commensal gut micrbiota, the foreign pathogens invading the gut (interspecies) on the one hand and the host's gut mucosal epithelial cells (cross-kingdom signaling) on the other. Lactobacilli are the best example of having a well-knit network of QS, particularly in relation to bacteriocin production. QS has been best studied in lactobacilli in relation to bacteriocin production. As for an intraspecies bacterial communication in Gram-positive bacteria is concerned, it is generally mediated by specific autoinducing signaling peptides that are often posttranslationally modified and exported by dedicated transport systems (Sturme et al., 2007). These signals are sensed by responsive cells via dedicated two-component regulatory systems (2CRSs). *In silico* analysis predicted the presence of five QS signal peptides that include two 2CRSs in *L. plantarum* WCFS1, two in the intestinal species *L. acidophilus* NCFM and *L. johnsonii* NCC533, one in the intestinal species *L. salivarius* UCC118, and the food species *L. delbrueckii* subsp. *bulgaricus* ATCC BAA-365, and none in the intestinal species *L. gasseri* ATCC 33323 (Sturme et al., 2007). The high number of CRSs identified in *L. plantarum* WCFS1 could reflect the ecological flexibility of this species, which can occur on plants, in fermented foods, and in the GIT (Kleerebezem et al., 2003). In comparison, the other lactobacilli described seem to be more restricted to specific environments, possibly resulting in fewer peptide-based QS 2CRSs (Sturme et al., 2007). Nonetheless, an *in vivo* role for these QS systems in the competitive ability of lactobacilli in the GIT remains to be elucidated.

23.9.1.2 Interspecies Communication

Interspecies communication is also very important for the coexistence of two species in a natural ecosystem such as the human gut wherein they can compliment each other and work synergistically or compete with each other by showing antagonism, resulting in predominance of one over the other which can have a significant positive or negative impact on the health and well-being of the host. Surette et al. (1999) described a new family of signal molecules, autoinducer-2 (AI-2), and its cognate synthase LuxS, which are present in both Gram-negative and Gram-positive bacteria. In *Vibrio harveyi*, AI-2, a furanosyl borate diester, is one of the signals that regulate bioluminescence through a complex phosphorelay system (Henke and Bassler, 2004). The binding of AI-2 to the periplasmic receptor LuxP modulates the activity of the inner membrane sensor kinase LuxQ, transducing AI-2 information into the cytoplasm. *V. harveyi* can produce light in response to the AI-2 produced by many other bacterial species. These observations based on the regulation of bioluminescence in *V. harveyi* resulted in the development of a bioassay to detect AI-2 production and led to the suggestion that AI-2 acts as a universal signal molecule that fosters interspecies cell–cell communication

(Bassler et al., 1997). Using the *Vibrio* bioluminescence assay, De Keersmaecker and Vanderleyden (2003) tested the spent culture supernatant of various lactobacilli for the presence of AI-2-type molecules. Strains such as *L. rhamnosus* GG, *L. plantarum* NCIMB8826, *L. johnsonii* VPI1088, and *L. casei* ATCC 393 were shown to produce AI-2-like molecules (De Keersmaecker and Vanderleyden, 2003). The accumulation of two QS signals, cholerae AI-1 (CAI-1) and AI-2 in the gastrointestinal pathogen *Vibrio cholerae*, the accumulation of two QS signals, cholerae AI-1 (CAI-1) and AI-2, represses the expression of virulence factors at high population density. AI-2 functions synergistically with CAI-1 to control virulence gene expression, although CAI-1 is the stronger of the two signals (Higgins et al., 2007). However, apart from bioluminescence in *V. harveyi* and a role in virulence of *V. cholerae*, no obvious phenotype has been associated with the extracellular accumulation of this molecule in most bacteria (Vendeville et al., 2005). The disruption of *luxS in L. reuteri* 100-23 resulted in increased biofilm formation *in vitro* in a bioreactor and on the epithelial surface of the murine fore stomach (Tannock et al., 2005). Whether this was due to disrupted QS control of the biofilm thickness or disturbed metabolism is difficult to discriminate, as the addition of purified AI-2 to the biofilm culture medium could not restore the phenotype to the wild-type level, and the *luxS* mutant showed a reduced ATP level in the exponentially growing cells. Moreover, the ecological performance of the *luxS* mutant, when in competition with *L. reuteri* strain 100-93, was significantly reduced in the highly competitive conditions of the murine cecum but not in the stomach or jejunum (Tannock et al., 2005). In *L. rhamnosus* GG, the disruption of the *luxS* gene resulted in pleiotropic effects on *in vitro* growth, biofilm formation, and *in vivo* persistence in the murine GIT, and these effects were shown to be caused merely by metabolic defects (Lebeer et al., 2007a, 2008).

23.9.1.3 Interkingdom Communication

Recently, it was discovered that bacteria can also exploit QS signals to communicate with the host in a process referred to as cross-kingdom cell-to-cell signaling (Hughes and Sperandio, 2008; Jelcic et al., 2008). This cross-kingdom signaling involves small molecules, such as hormones, that are produced by eukaryotes and hormone-like chemicals that are produced by bacteria. Sperandio and colleagues could show a role for (nor) epinephrine produced by the host, similar to the aromatic signal AI-3 produced by commensal microbiota: both signaling molecules could activate the virulence genes of EHEC mainly by inducing *ler* expression (Sperandio et al., 2003). *Ler* (locus of enterocyte effacement (LEE)-encoded regulator) encodes the principal transcriptional activator of the LEE genes present on a pathogenicity island referred to as LEE of EHEC (Sperandio et al., 2003).

23.9.2 Pattern Recognition Receptors

Many immune responses against the gut microbiota are mediated by pattern recognition receptors (PRRs) such as TLRs that are present on IECs, DCs, and macrophages and intracellular nucleotide-binding oligomerization domain (NOD)-like receptors (NLRs) present in the cytosols of many immune and epithelial cells. These PRRs play a crucial role in the innate immune system and have broad specificities for conserved, invariant, and generally repetitive features of microorganisms, in contrast to the specific antigen receptors of the adaptive immune system (Medzhitov, 2007). The targets of these PRRs are often components of the bacterial cell wall called microbial associated molecular patterns (MAMPs) such as LPS, PG, LTA, and cell wall lipoproteins. For example, triacylated bacterial lipoproteins interact with TLR2, LPS interacts with TLR4, flagellin interacts with TLR5, DNA interacts with TLR9, and muropeptides derived from PG interact with NOD1 or NOD2. These microbial ligands are present in pathogens and nonpathogenic organisms, including lactobacilli. To discriminate between microbes, it seems that the information for the different ligand–PRR interactions is integrated and converged to determine a final response. These signaling events need to be delicately balanced toward tolerance against commensals and reactivity against pathogens, and an imbalance might result in the uncontrolled upregulation of inflammatory responses toward commensal bacteria, as seen in IBD (Medzhitov, 2007).

23.9.2.1 TLR and NLR Signaling

TLRs are transmembrane proteins with an extracellular domain made of leucine-rich repeats involved in ligand recognition and an intracytoplasmic domain containing the highly conserved Toll/IL-1 receptor domain. These Toll/IL-1 receptor domains are homologous to the IL-1 receptor-like intracellular domains and utilize some of the same signaling components involved in response to IL-1, including the cytoplasmic adapter molecule MyD88, the protein kinase IL-1 receptor-associated kinase (IRAK), and the adapter protein TNF receptor-associated factor 6 (TRAF6) as well as Tollip (Toll-interacting protein). Upon stimulation, IRAK is recruited to the TLR through MyD88. IRAK subsequently undergoes phosphorylation and relays the signal downstream by interacting with TRAF6. The cytosolic NLR proteins also have a leucine-rich repeat at the C terminus for ligand recognition, in addition to a Nod domain, and caspase activation and recruitment domains (CARDs) at the N terminus. The TLR and NLR expressions and responsiveness are highly localized and vary extensively with cell type (DCs vs. IECs), location in the body (e.g., spleen vs. mucosa), disease status, and so on. The interaction of these PRRs with their specific ligand induces NF-B signaling and MAPK pathways, with the subsequent secretion of proinflammatory cytokines, chemokines, costimulatory molecules, and antimicrobial peptides (Cario, 2005). NOD and TLR signaling can also modulate each other's pathways.

23.9.2.2 DC-SIGN Signaling

The calcium-dependent C-type lectin DC-SIGN present on DCs is an interesting PRR as it relates to the induction of Treg cells by lactobacilli (Smits et al., 2005). DC-SIGN binds to mannose-containing glycoepitopes, mainly triggering the internalization of microbes for processing and antigen presentation. Certain pathogens also use DC-SIGN as an escape mechanism for immune surveillance and the induction of immunosuppressive effects (Van Kooyk and Geijtenbeek, 2003). It was shown, for instance, that some pathogens trigger DC-SIGN on human DCs to activate the serine and threonine kinase Raf-1, which subsequently leads to the acetylation of the NF-KB subunit p65 but only after the TLR-induced activation of NF-KB, implying cross talk between TLR and DC-SIGN (Gringhuis et al., 2007). The acetylation of p65 both prolonged and increased IL-10 transcription to enhance anti-inflammatory cytokine responses (Gringhuis et al., 2007).

23.10 FUNCTIONALITY OF PROBIOTICS WITH REGARD TO HUMAN HEALTH

Apart from the current application of probiotic bacteria as a general health supplement, an increasing volume of clinical data clearly suggests the effectiveness of probiotics in the treatment of specific diseases. Double-blind placebo-controlled studies have identified potential benefits of ingesting probiotic organisms in patients suffering from lactose intolerance, rota virus diarrhea, IBD/irritable bowel syndrome (IBS), and certain types of allergies. Probiotics are also known to exhibit anticarcinogenic effects by producing antioxidants capable of scavenging free radicals. Probiotics also exert an immunomodulatory role by promoting the endogenous host defense systems, particularly mucosal immunity, by stimulating phagocytosis, macrophages, and other immunological markers such as interleukins, TNFα, natural killer cells, and so on. They are also known to reduce the risk of vaginitis and other sexually transmitted and urinary tract infections by inhibiting the proliferation of pathogens.

Another potential application of probiotic culture is the production of fermented food products enriched with health-promoting substances such as conjugated linoleic acid (CLA). CLA has gained considerable attention in recent years because of several beneficial effects, including anticarcinogenic and antiatherogenic activities, ability to reduce the catabolic effects of immune stimulation, the ability to enhance growth promotion, and the ability to reduce body fat. Of the individual isomers of CLA, *cis*-9,*trans*-11-octadecadienoic acid was implicated as the most biologically active and predominant isomer found in the diet. This arises from the microbial biohydrogenation of dietary linoleic acid to CLA in the rumen.

23.10.1 Hypocholesterolemic Effect

Probiotic lactobacilli and bifidobacterial strains have been explored for the management of hypercholesterolemia, and bile salt hydrolase activity produced by these strains has been attributed to the cholesterol-lowering effect due to direct impact on the host's bile salt metabolism. The use of animal models and human intervention studies to evaluate the effects of probiotics and prebiotics on serum cholesterol levels have been widely used over the years. Milk fermented with lactobacilli was first demonstrated to exhibit hypocholesterolemic effects in humans as early as 1963. Several human studies have shown promising evidence that well-established probiotics possess hypocholesterolemic effects while new strains of probiotics or new type of prebiotics have been evaluated in animal models for their potential hypocholesterolemic effects. Ashar and Chand (2004) reported that serum angiotensin-I converting enzyme (ACE) activity decreased significantly in hypertensive rats when fed milk fermented with *L. delbrueckii* subsp. *bulgaricus, Streptococcus thermophilus*, and *Lactococcus lactis* biovar. *diacetylactis*. The above fermented product when fed to hypertensive humans, decreased systolic as well as diastolic blood pressure and serum cholesterol levels (Ashar and Chand, 2004). In another study, Kapila et al. (2006) reported that feeding of *Lactobacillus casei* subsp. *casei* and its fermented product to rats resulted in reduction in total cholesterol, triglycerides, LDL-cholesterol, and atherogenic index. Increase of serum cholesterol was suppressed to the extent of 22–29% in hyperlipidemic rats fed lyophilized probiotic dahi prepared with *Lactobacillus acidophilus* and *Lactobacillus casei* (Vibha et al., 2007). Chiu et al. (2006) also reported reduced blood and hepatic total cholesterol, triglyceride, and LDL-cholesterol in high-cholesterol-fed hamsters on ingestion of milk fermented with *Lb. paracasei* subsp. *paracasei* NTU 101, *Lb. plantarum* NTU 102, and *Lb. acidophilus* BCRC 17010. Recently, Baroutkoub et al. (2010) reported that consumption of the probiotic yoghurt containing *Lactobacillus acidophilus* and *Bifidobacteria* for 6 weeks resulted in decreased total cholesterol and LDL and increased HDL.

Cardioviva is one of the world's first disease-specific probiotic (cardiovascular diseases) which can be taken as a supplement or added to food products (Micropharma, Montreal, Quebec). Micropharma plans to launch its product as a dietary supplement in Canada and the United States in 2011. Cardioviva is formulated using microencapsulation of bile salt hydrolase (BSH)—active *Lactobacillus reuteri* cardioviva which reaches the GI tract specifically to provide health benefit. Micropharma and Danone have signed a partnership agreement to develop a new marketable dairy product specifically for cardiovascular disease.

Parmalat Canada has also launched Canada's first yoghurt that contains both probiotics and plant sterols, mixing gut health benefits for managing cholesterol levels. The product is marketed under the BioBest Plant Sterols probiotic yoghurt brand.

In a recent study conducted at NDRI by Kumar et al. (2011), two putative indigenous probiotic Bsh$^+$ strains of *L. plantarum* Lp91 and Lp21 (in both free and microencapsulated forms) were able to demonstrate hypocholesterolemic effect after feeding to rats. There was 23.26%, 15.71%, and 15.01% reduction in total cholesterol, 21.09%, 18.77%, and 18.17% reduction in TAG, 38.13%, 23.22%, and 21.42% reduction in LDL-cholesterol after 21 days of dietary treatment, that is, feeding hypercholesterolemic diet (HD) along with Lp91, Cap91, and Lp21, respectively. The corresponding HDL-cholesterol values increased at the rate of 18.94%, 10.30%, and 7.78% in the treated groups as has been recorded in Figure 23.3. The fecal cholic acid levels differed significantly among the various groups ($P < 0.05$). Supplementation of the HD with Bsh-positive *L. plantarum* Lp91 and Lp21 led to considerable increase in the excretion of cholic acid in the feces. After 21 days of feeding, the

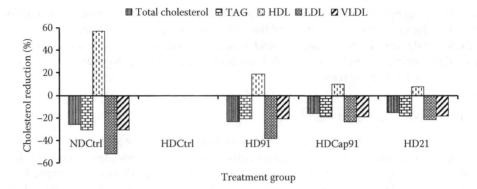

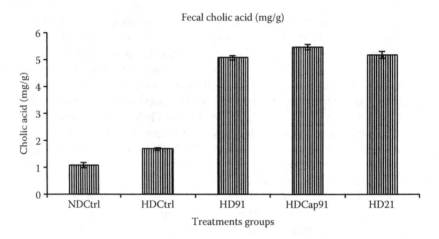

FIGURE 23.3 Percentage decrease in plasma lipids (total cholesterol, TAG, HDL, LDL, and VLDL cholesterol) of dietary treatment groups. NDCtrl, normal diet control; HDCtrl, hypercholesterolemic diet control; HD91, HD containing *Lactobacillus plantarum* Lp91; HDCap91, HD containing microencapsulated *L. plantarum* Lp91; HD21, HD containing *L. plantarum* Lp21.

FIGURE 23.4 Fecal cholic acid concentration for rats fed experimental diets. NDCtrl, normal diet control; HDCtrl, hypercholesterolemic diet control; HD91, HD containing *Lactobacillus plantarum* Lp91; HDCap91, HD containing microencapsulated *L. plantarum* Lp91; HD21, HD containing *L. plantarum* Lp21.

maximum fecal cholic acid excretion (5.489 (SEM 0.09) mmol/g feces) was recorded in the HDCap91 group, whereas in the other probiotic treatment groups HD91 and HD21, the corresponding increase in fecal cholic acid was 5.084 (SEM 0.09) and 5.183 (SEM 0.13) mmol/g, respectively. However, in animals fed on the normal diet, the fecal cholic acid content was found to be 1.084 (SEM 0.09) mmol/g, which was lower than the HDCtrl group (1.703 (SEM 0.04) mmol/g). These results as recorded in Figure 23.4 suggest that *L. plantarum* Lp91 has the potential to be explored as a probiotic biotherapeutic in the management of hypercholesterolemia after validating the safety and efficacy of this strain on dairy-based food formulations prepared with this strain in human subjects through clinical studies.

23.10.2 Diarrhea

Probiotics have preventive as well as curative effect on several types of diarrhea of different etiology. The prevention and therapy of diarrhea have been successfully investigated for numerous dietary probiotic microorganisms. Infectious diarrhea is the most widely investigated area for probiotic use in children, with several meta-analyses published (Van Niel et al., 2002; Huang et al., 2002; Allen et al., 2004). Most of the randomized controlled trials included in these meta-analyses involved children in developed countries in a health care setting. All meta-analyses were challenged by a lack of heterogeneity between studies. However, despite the variability between the probiotics tested, the dose and duration of treatment, the participant groups, and the definitions of diarrhea and the outcome, all reviews concluded that probiotics, coadministered with standard rehydration therapy, decreased the duration of acute diarrhea (E1). A Cochrane review (Allen et al., 2004) comprised 23 studies with a total of 1917 participants (1449 children). The pooled results showed that probiotics reduced the risk of diarrhea by 3 days (relative risk (RR), 0.66; 95% CI, 0.55–0.77; random effects model, 15 studies) and the mean duration of diarrhea by 30.5 h (95% CI, 18.5–42.5 h; random effects model, 12 studies) (E1). None of the studies reported adverse effects. *Lactobacillus rhamnosus* GG (LGG) has been the most investigated probiotic strain for this condition. A meta-analysis of pediatric studies contained a subgroup analysis restricted to LGG therapy, which comprised 10 study arms (Huang et al., 2002). The pooled estimate showed that LGG reduced the duration of diarrhea by 1.2 days (95% CI, −1.6 to −0.8 days; $P < 0.001$) (E1). The Cochrane review (Allen et al., 2004) suggested that LGG may be particularly effective for rotaviral diarrhea (E1). From these meta-analyses (Van Niel et al., 2002; Huang et al., 2002; Allen et al., 2004), it appears that probiotics are more effective if given early in the course of illness and at daily doses of at least 10 billion colony-forming units (CFU). Therefore, there is good evidence to support the use of probiotics in infectious diarrhea of viral etiology, when given early in the illness.

Several probiotics, including *Lactobacillus acidophilus*, *Lactobacillus casei*, LGG, and *S. boulardii*, have been evaluated in treating or preventing AAD, In a meta-analysis on the role of *S. boulardii* in preventing AAD, five randomized controlled trials (1076 participants) were included (Szajewska et al., 2006). The largest of these studies was conducted in 269 children (Kotowska et al., 2005) and concluded that for every 10 patients receiving *S. boulardii* with antibiotics, only fewer will develop diarrhea (E1). The results from the trials studying the role of probiotics in preventing traveler's diarrhea are inconsistent, possibly reflecting the variation in probiotic strains used. However, meta-analysis of 12 studies showed that probiotics decreased the risk of traveler's diarrhea (RR, 0.85; 95% CI, 0.79–0.91; $P < 0.001$) (E1) (McFarland, 2007).

23.10.3 Crohn's Disease and Ulcerative Colitis (Inflammatory Bowel Disease)

A few studies have examined the role of probiotics in inducing or maintaining remission of CD, and in preventing postoperative recurrence. A small pilot study showed that LGG given to four children with active CD led to decreased disease activity scores and improved gut barrier function (E4) (Gupta et al., 2000). A subsequent randomized controlled trial showed that LGG did not maintain remission in children with CD (E2) (Bousvaros et al., 2005). *S. boulardii* has also been evaluated in maintaining remission of CD. Patients with quiescent CD were given aminosalicylic acid alone or with probiotics for 6 months in a blinded fashion (Guslandi et al., 2003), where the relapse rate was found to be substantially lower in patients receiving probiotics (6/16 vs. 1/16; $P = 0.04$) (E2). On the other hand, studies using two different probiotic agents (LGG and *Lactobacillus johnsonii* LA1) have shown that probiotics were not effective in preventing postoperative recurrence of CD (Prantera et al., 2002; Marteau et al., 2006). Probiotics may have roles in both initiating and maintaining remission of UC, with several studies suggesting that probiotics may help to induce remission. The first of these used a synbiotic, combining a probiotic (*Bifidobacterium longum*) and a prebiotic (Synergy 1; Orafti, Tienen, Belgium), for 1 month in 18 adults with active UC (E3) (Furrie et al., 2005). Patients receiving the synbiotic had decreased endoscopic severity scores, clinical activity scores, and decreased levels of key proinflammatory proteins. A second study of 32 adults with acute UC used the high-potency probiotic VSL#3 (Sigma-Tau, Pomezia, Italy), which contains eight separate bacterial strains in large numbers, in an open-label design over 6 weeks (E4) (Bibiloni et al., 2005). Remission or response was seen in 77% of patients following therapy.

23.10.4 PROBIOTICS AND IRRITABLE BOWEL SYNDROME

Clinical studies employing various probiotic agents in adults with IBS have evaluated different outcomes (Quigley and Flourie, 2007). Although some of these studies suggest relief of symptoms such as bloating or flatulence, others show no benefit. For instance, in a study evaluating VSL#3 in a small group of 25 adults with diarrhea predominant IBS, subjects treated with the probiotic had less bloating than those given placebo ($P = 0.046$), but there was no impact on the other symptoms (Kim et al., 2003). Only two published studies have included more than 100 patients. One used a mixture of four probiotics and resulted in improvements in 6 months (Kajander et al., 2005), while the other study assessed an encapsulated form of *Bifidobacterium infantis* 35624 in 362 adults and found that all cardinal symptoms abated, compared with subjects treated with placebo (Whorwell et al., 2006).

23.10.5 PROBIOTICS AND ALLERGIC DISORDERS

Two Scandinavian studies showed that the provision of probiotics alone (LGG) (Kalliomäki et al., 2003) or as synbiotics (Kukkonen et al., 2007) to pregnant mothers and infants after birth reduced the rates of eczema at 2 years of age. Other studies using different probiotics (*L. acidophilus* LAVRI-A152 or *l. reuteri* ATCC 5573053) did not confirm these findings (E2). One of these studies, which involved Western Australian infants at high risk of developing atopic dermatitis receiving probiotics for the first 6 months of life, showed that the rates of atopic dermatitis in treated children were not lower than those in infants who received placebo at 6 and 12 months of age (Taylor et al., 2007). Probiotics may also have a role in treating established atopic dermatitis. A double-blind randomized controlled trial evaluated *L. fermentum* in 53 infants and toddlers with moderate or severe atopic dermatitis (E2) (Weston et al., 2005). The subjects provided with probiotics had reduced severity and extent of dermatitis compared with the controls ($P = 0.03$).

23.11 EFFICACY AND SAFETY OF PROBIOTICS THROUGH CLINICAL TRIALS

As the health benefits of ingesting live bacteria become more evident, foods are now being produced that contain probiotic bacteria. However, the data to support label health claims for probiotic products are often difficult to provide. The experimental evidence to identify probiotic microorganisms and to demonstrate their efficacy in clinical trials is more challenging than for other potential functional foods because the effects are mediated by living microorganisms and may, therefore, be influenced by the status of these microorganisms. A scientific consensus is building to support the claim that the ingestion of certain probiotic bacteria reduces lactose intolerance and can reduce the duration of rotavirus diarrhea. Some probiotic bacteria have "generally accepted as safe" (GRAS) status. Japanese health regulatory officials, using their Foods for Specific Health Use system, have approved human health claims for over 20 probiotic products. This illustrates the considerable discrepancies across countries in the perception of the health effects of probiotics. No single biomarker has been identified that applies to all clinical trials involving probiotics because of the wide variety of diseases and conditions that have been studied. The efficacy of probiotics has been studied for a variety of diseases and metabolic problems, including Crohn's disease (Schultz et al., 2004; Fujimori et al., 2007), IBS (Sen et al., 2002), cholesterol metabolism (Simons et al., 2006), anticancer properties (Russo et al., 2007; Commane et al., 2005), and diverticulitis (White, 2006). However, the degree of success that has been obtained for these conditions/diseases in probiotic feeding trials has not been uniform, and it would be wrong to assume that there exists good evidence to suggest that all of these conditions may be improved with probiotics. In many cases, the GI tract has been the primary target (Gorbach, 2000), but it is becoming evident that other conditions, including allergies, obesity, and urogenital infections, not initially associated with the gut microbiota might also be affected (Ley et al., 2006; Saavedra, 2007). The suggestion that probiotics may be stimulating the immune system has generated a great deal of interest because of the possible consequences to health and metabolism. However, the studies are not often replicated, and therefore, efficacy is hard to establish. Some articles often lack details such as the bacterial strain fed, the numbers of live bacteria consumed, or the timing of the consumption, for example, with or without other foods, which limits their usefulness to prove efficacy. Several studies have reported that the consumption of certain probiotic bacteria resulted in reduced lactose intolerance symptoms in human subjects (de Vrese et al., 2001). Furthermore, a meta-analysis of the treatment of both childhood and rotavirus-associated childhood diarrhea with probiotic bacteria showed a significant reduction in the duration of the diarrhea episode (Huang et al., 2002). These two applications of probiotics appear to be the best documented and have enough reliable data to support a human health claim. The efficacy experiments must be replicated and have an appropriate number of subjects to achieve scientific consensus. The claim of efficacy will be greatly enhanced if a plausible mechanism can be suggested, or demonstrated, that explains the beneficial effect.

23.12 DESIGNING NOVEL PROBIOTIC STRAINS AND FOODS WITH SPECIFIC HEALTH-PROMOTING FUNCTIONS BY GENETIC MANIPULATION

As a result of the rapid advancements in genetic accessibility and protocols for lactobacilli, and availability of the complete genome sequences for common probiotic strains, substantial opportunities and possibilities exist for the development of strains with safe and effective health-promoting effects. The most notable novel recombinant probiotic at present is a derivative of *Lb. johnsonii* La1. La1 is a well-characterized probiotic strain used extensively in the commercial preparation of probiotic foods due to its strong health-related attributes and positive immunomodulatory effects on the host. Milk fermented with this culture produces a racemic mixture of D- and L-lactate in the ratio 60:40. The presence of D-lactate in milk fermented with La1 and the ability of the strain to produce D-lactate after ingestion does not pose any problem to most of the adult population. However it can indeed cause D-acidosis in patients suffering from bowel syndrome and intestinal failure and encephalopathy in new born infants with immature liver. Inactivation of the single-copy D-lactate dehydrogenase (LdhD) gene of La1 resulted in rerouting of pyruvate to many L-lactate with no D-lactate production (Lapierre et al., 1999). This novel strain has the same beneficial properties as the parent probiotic while the absence of D-lactate makes it a safer alternative for specific populations.

Among several other possibilities is the design of recombinant strains with novel properties that confer competitive advantage to their survival. One way to accomplish this strategy is by expressing and secreting colicin V, a narrow host range antibacterial bacteriocin produced by *E. coli* in La1 by replacing the original colicin V leader peptide in colicin with a signal peptide from divergicin A of *Carnobacterium divergens*. This strategy has allowed the expression and secretion of the Gram-negative antimicrobial in probiotic organisms to extend their inhibitory spectrum to Gram-negative enteropathogens too.

The established probiotic lactobacilli can also serve as an attractive candidate for oral vaccination against HIV, tetanus, rota virus, *E. coli*, *Salmonella*, *H. pylori*, and so on in view of their long history of safe use, ease of oral administration, low intrinsic immunogenicity, and extensive industrial handling experience. Recently, a series of expression vectors were constructed that allowed the secretion of human myelin protein by probiotic *L. casei* into the growth medium. This recombinant strain may be useful in oral tolerance induction for intervention in the autoimmune disease, multiple sclerosis.

Currently, the concept of pathophysiology well established in high-risk food pathogens like *Listeria monocytogenes*, *E. coli* 157: H7, *Salmonella enteritidis*, and other species that have evolved strong well-knit adherence systems to survive and colonize in the gut is being explored to mimic the same in proven probiotic strains to improve their colonization potential in the human gut so that their transit period therein is further extended. Attempts are now being made to design novel probiotics by expressing the heterologous genes from the aforesaid pathogens encoding strong adherence properties therein through advanced genetic manipulation techniques (Sleator and Hill, 2008).

23.13   MECHANISM OF ACTION OF PROBIOTICS IN THE GUT

Probiotic bacteria have multiple and diverse influences on the host. Different organisms can influence the intestinal luminal environment, epithelial and mucosal barrier function, and the mucosal immune system. The numerous cell types affected by probiotics involve epithelial cells, dendritic cells, monocytes/macrophages, B cells, and T cells. There are significant differences between probiotic bacterial genera and species. These differences may be due to various mechanisms of action of probiotics. It is crucial that each strain be tested on its own or in products designed for a specific function. Multistrain probiotics seem to be better than single-strain ones, as individual probiotics have different functions and show synergistic effects when administered together (Bengmark, 2005; Meie and Steuerwals, 2005). Molecular research on these probiotics pays attention to these strain-specific properties. Different probiotic strains have been associated with different effects related to their specific capacities to express particular surface molecules or to secrete proteins and metabolites directly interacting with host cells. Several mechanisms such as restoring the normal balance of altered gut microbiota, producing antimicrobial substances (acids, hydrogen

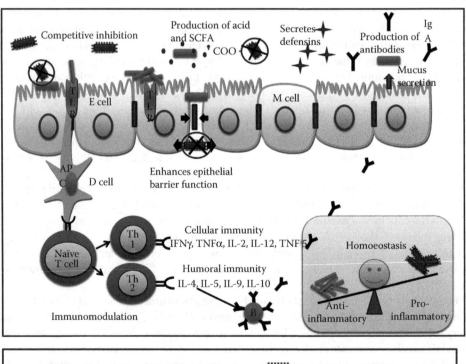

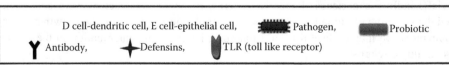

FIGURE 23.5   Possible mechanisms of probiotic action.

peroxide, and bacteriocins and antimicrobial peptides), pathogen exclusion by blocking the receptor sites on the mucosal epithelial cell lining the gut, stimulating mucus secretion, strengthening gut barrier function, competing for adhesion site, stimulating specific and nonspecific immune responses, and so on have been postulated regarding the action of probiotics. However, more in-depth mechanistic studies need to be conducted in appropriate model systems to understand the exact mode of probiotic action at the molecular level. However, some of the scientific evidence-based mechanistics of probiotic functionality having direct impact on human health have been illustrated in Figure 23.5.

23.14 MODULATION OF GUT BY PROBIOTICS

Gut, considered as a superorganism, is the most important organ which is inhabited by 100 trillion bacteria comprising of more than 1000 different species which are responsible for our health and well-being. Any disturbance in the gut flora leads to unhealthy/diseased status. The food we eat modulates the gut flora through immune response and inhibition of pathogens and so on. This is presently an active area of research since several studies have shown the link between gut flora and obesity, diabetes, IBD, and so on. Efforts have been directed to modify the intestinal flora with probiotic bacteria to attenuate IBDs and also prevent relapses in ulcerative colitis, Crohn's disease, and pouchitis. Hence, the modulation of gut flora toward healthy ones can be brought about with the use of probiotics. The modern biotechnological approaches like metagenomics, transcriptomics, proteomics, and metabolomics can throw insight on the mechanism by which probiotics confer gut benefits which will further substantiate the health claims on probiotic dairy products or other foods. Manipulating the gut flora with the use of probiotics will lead to the development of newer designer food-based therapies for the maintenance of health and prevention of diseases. Hence, probiotics are very important for the normal development of the intestine/gut homoeostasis and for defense against infections. The programming of the gut microbiota is of particular interest in infants and the aged population, particularly to control the undesirable population of bacteria. Transcriptomics used to study host response has revealed different cell types and effector molecules, cell receptors, and signaling molecules. Since it is clear that functional health effects are strain specific, different species and strains exhibit diverse and divergent degrees of cell signaling initiation which contributes to health or disease status. Martin et al. (2008) administered probiotic beverages to germ-free mice that had been conventionalized with human baby flora. Using high-density data-generating spectroscopic techniques in combination with multivariate mathematical modeling, it was shown that probiotics resulted in metabolic alterations in a variety of tissues affecting energy, lipid, and amino acid metabolism. Their investigation suggested that probiotics can alter the dynamics of the gut microbiota toward healthy ones. Recently, van Baarlen et al. (2009) analyzed the transcription of genes in the duodenum of healthy humans after probiotic intervention using stationary and log-phase cells as well as dead cells. Stationary-phase cells resulted in the induction of genes such as the NF-kB and JUN transcription factors involved in the establishment of immune tolerance, whereas log-phase cells induced a response targeted toward metabolic function. However, more studies on gene expression analysis at various stages need to be done to demonstrate the potential of probiotic bacteria in the GI tract.

23.15 NEWER APPROACHES FOR STUDYING FUNCTIONALITY OF PROBIOTIC DAIRY PRODUCTS

Newer approaches to study the efficacy of probiotic dairy products for disease management as an adjunct therapy along with drugs include transcriptomics, proteomics, metabolomics, pharmacokinetics, pharmacomimetics, pharmacodynamics, and nutridynamics. However, dairy foods contain a variety of bioactive components in comparison to drugs which have only one specific component and hence can have multiple interactions in consumers consuming these products everyday.

Postgenomic approaches have been exploited to discover the response at the level of the bacterium as well as the host (de Vos et al., 2004; Klaenhammer et al., 2005). Similarly, the nutridynamics approach (de Vos et al., 2006) can be used to study the growth, survival, and persistence of probiotic LAB. Upon ingestion by consumers, probiotics have to face the defense systems of our body, including exposure to gastric juices, bile acids, immunoglobulin A, and other antagonistic compounds. Apart from this, competition with the resident or commensal microbiota is another challenge for the optimal functionality of the probiotic strains.

The advancements in genetic tools have enabled us to understand the functionality of probiotics as well as the complexity of the GI tract. A number of probiotic functional traits such as acid tolerance, bile tolerance, S layer proteins, bacteriocin, and so on in *L. acidophilus* have been confirmed using gene inactivation studies. However, these traits need to be confirmed *in vivo* as different strains exhibit different functions as comparative genomics have shown that all strains are not the same. In a recent study published in *PNAS*, van Baarlen et al. (2010) reported that probiotic strains, viz. *Lactobacillus acidophilus*, *L. casei*, and *L. rhamnosus* each induced differential gene-regulatory networks and pathways in human mucosal biopsies collected during a double-blind placebo-controlled, cross-over probiotic intervention study. Comprehensive analyses revealed that these transcriptional networks regulate major basal mucosal processes and uncovered remarkable similarity to the response profiles obtained for specific bioactive molecules and drugs. The responsiveness of particular individuals consuming probiotics is not only determined by the characteristics of the consumed probiotic strain but also by the host's genetic background, commensal gut flora, diet, as well as lifestyle, thus necessitating the need for personalized probiotics.

23.16 APPLICATION OF PROBIOTICS AS FUNCTIONAL FOOD INGREDIENTS AND BIOTHERAPEUTICS IN PRODUCT DEVELOPMENT: FUNCTIONAL/ HEALTH FOODS

A number of food matrices are being used for the delivery of probiotic bacteria. Among the various foods, dairy products particularly have been the matrix of choice for delivering probiotic organisms (Ross et al., 2002). However, choosing a suitable food system is important in delivering particular species or strains of probiotic cultures. Dairy products, such as milk, yoghurt, dahi, cheese, ice cream, and so on are well suited to promote the positive health image of probiotics. This is because fermented foods and dairy products in particular have already been in constant use by man since times immemorial and the consumers are familiar with the fact that fermented foods contain living microorganisms. Apart from these, dairy products have some inherent properties that can buffer stomach acid and increase the probability of higher survival of probiotic strains in the gut. The interaction of probiotics with either the food matrix or the starter cultures may be even more intensive when probiotics are used as components of starter cultures. Moreover, specific dairy product formulations can influence the functionality of probiotic strains used therein. Hence, it is not always obligatory that by merely adding the selected probiotic strain into the food the same will be replicated in the final product unless it is experimentally proved. In many cases, the efficacy of the probiotic food has yet to be proved in clinical studies involving human subjects although *in vivo* the functionality of many of these dairy-based probiotic foods has been validated in experimental animal models. A few studies have been conducted to determine the effect of varied delivery vehicles such as milk, juice, yoghurt, ice cream, and chocolate (Champagne et al., 2005) on the efficiency of delivery of probiotic bacteria to the GIT. A more recent study in a murine model of colorectal cancer demonstrated an increased positive effect of microencapsulated *L. acidophilus* delivered in yoghurt compared with saline (Urbanska et al., 2009). Azcarate-Peril et al. (2009) have also determined the influence of the delivery matrix effect such as milk on gene expression of the probiotics and reported that optimal conditions of delivery are important to maintain any potential probiotic health attribute in the GI tract.

Due to the wide diversity in food habits, India is enriched with a variety of traditional/ethnic fermented foods which are region specific, produced locally at the domestic level, and constitute an integral part of the Indian diet. One of the most common dairy-based fermented food which invariably figures in the diet of almost the entire ethnic communities inhabiting the country is dahi. Dahi and other dahi-based products such as lassi (butter milk) and srikhand could be the ideal cost-effective candidate of traditional foods for probiotic supplementation. Enrichment of these foods with probiotics can enhance their commercial value considerably. Development of such traditional fermented probiotic foods will add a new dimension for exploring dietary-based probiotic interventions for the management of general health care and specific inflammatory metabolic disorders prevalent in the target population in India. In this context, a lot of R&D work is in progress at the NDRI, Karnal, India and other food processing industries in India to develop probiotic dahi preparations for augmenting human health, well-being, and boosting the immunity.

23.17 EFFECT OF PROCESSING ON THE FATE OF PROBIOTICS IN THE FOODS: VIABILITY AND TECHNOLOGICAL PROPERTIES

The processing parameters used in the production of dairy-based probiotic foods, particularly the fermented products, can have a strong impact on the functionality and technological properties of the probiotic strains used therein. Probiotic viability is the key issue in this regard which must be looked into since many studies have invariably shown low viability of probiotics in market preparations of probiotic foods (Iwana et al., 1993; Shah et al., 1995). The need to monitor the survival of *L. acidophilus* and bifidobacteria in fermented products has often been neglected, with the result that a number of products reach the market containing a few viable bacteria instead of the minimum desired level (10^8 cfu/g in the product) as per FAO/WHO guidelines (Shah et al., 1995). Several factors such as food matrix, starter cultures used in the fermented product, moisture content, oxygen, pH (acidity) preservatives, antimicrobials (acid, hydrogen peroxide) including bacteriocins produced by both the starter cultures and probiotic strain, processing and storage temperature, packaging, and so on, can affect the stability and viability of probiotic bacteria in the product (Ishibashi and Shimamuru, 1993; Iwana et al., 1993). Apart from these, probiotic stability and functionality can also be influenced by the methods of production of the probiotic strains such as fermentation parameters, concentration technology (frozen cultures, freeze-dried, and spray-dried) and preservation methods (lyophilized vs. DVI cultures). Probiotic stability can also be significantly affected by the growth phase of the probiotic strain as the probiotic cells in the logarithmic phase are supposed to be most active as far as their functionality is concerned, although cells in the stationary phase are more stable and can withstand stressed conditions more effectively during the product processing. As per a recent study conducted by Grześkowiak et al. (2011), different sources of the same probiotic strain had demonstrated altered properties which can be influenced by the industrial production of probiotics, processing conditions, as well as food matrix. It was further reported that even small changes in the properties may significantly influence the *in vivo* probiotic functionality, particularly in the human clinical studies. These findings clearly suggest that for ensuring the original properties of probiotic strains and their viability and stability, exactly the same processing protocols and stringent quality control measures should be used during the large-scale production of probiotics to be used as inoculums in product development of uniform quality.

23.18 QUALITY CONTROL OF PROBIOTICS AND PROBIOTICS PREPARATIONS/FOODS

Probiotics are used in both foods and pharmaceuticals or special dietary applications. They have been selected to express strain-specific properties which are of paramount importance for their purported health effects. Such characteristics should be retained throughout food and pharmaceutical processes and storage to be of benefit to the consumer. The most important factor is to retain the strain characteristics and the purity of the preparation. It has been reported especially that dried probiotic preparations may have contaminants. This sets the requirements for hygienic preparation of the products and careful identification of the strains used. All commercial strains should be placed in an international type culture collection for future comparison of the properties and identity. Some probiotic preparations may also mislabel the strains they contain, using old or nonexisting nomenclature. Unlike pharmaceuticals or food chemicals such as additives, the quality criteria for probiotics are largely undefined. This is a key factor for health effects as long-term transfer of probiotic lactic acid bacteria or bifidobacteria in food processing along with the storage may result in changes in their characteristics and health properties. To control these properties, the criteria for assessing such changes should be included in functional foods regulation. The criteria currently used for selecting new probiotics have been suggested as the optimal quality control measure to be used in industrial practice (Tuomola et al., 2001). Since, the specific and novel health claims associated with a specific probiotic or probiotic product are highly strain specific and their functional efficacy, safety, and viability/stability can be significantly influenced during the processing of probiotic foods, there is always a possibility of production of a substandard product of dubious quality. In fact, due to lack of a well-defined regulatory system for managing the overall quality of probiotic functional foods and their strict enforcement, particularly in developing third-world countries including India, a lot of spurious probiotic dairy-based foods have entered the local markets that have put a question mark on the credibility of the health claims associated with such products, resulting in a lot of confusion and mistrust in the minds of the consumers. Hence, in order to ensure the availability of probiotic products of assured quality and safety with consistent efficacy, there is an immediate need for formulating regulatory standards and guidelines and their enforcement in all the countries so that the health benefits of probiotics reach the consumers in letter and spirit.

23.19 REGULATORY ISSUES ON SAFETY AND EFFICACY OF PROBIOTICS AND PROBIOTIC PRODUCTS

As a result of the increasing awareness and belief among the health-conscious consumers towards naturopathy for health care and well-being, the interest in probiotics and probiotic-based functional foods has grown enormously during the last few years and there is a sudden boom in the probiotic foods in the market. Although the optimism associated with the use of probiotic and probiotic foods is undeniable, it is often counterbalanced by the fact that this area has been largely unregulated from a scientific point of view. As a result, quite a few inferior quality products with false health claims have also appeared in the market unscrupulously, thereby creating a lot of confusion in the minds of the consumers. It is, therefore, imperative that these products need to be standardized based on evidence that they produce the desired effects. It is, thus, important to establish a set of uniform guidelines that would ensure product safety, quality and reliability, and a level playing field for all organizations/companies introducing and producing probiotic products. The guidelines should constitute a set of parameters required for a strain/product to be classified as a probiotic. However, as there was no international consensus on the methodology to assess the efficacy and safety of probiotics, the FAO and WHO had initiated the work to compile and evaluate the scientific evidence on the functional and safety aspects of probiotics, and generated "Guidelines for the Evaluation of Probiotics in Food" (FAO/WHO, 2002). The FAO and WHO have established guidelines for probiotics in foods, investigating the levels of scientific evidence needed to make a health claim, and presenting these results to Codex with recommendations on labeling and claims for probiotic foods. Some of the key issues of concern which have been duly addressed and elaborated in these guidelines include a battery of recommended *in vitro* tests as the criteria for designating a culture as probiotic along with its identity at the genus, species, and strain level, followed by assessing the safety, efficacy, and effectiveness *in vivo* using appropriate animal models before validation of purported health claims in clinical studies on human subjects (Phase I, II, and III), proper labeling of the product precisely indicating the identity of the probiotic at the genus, species, and strain level, effective dosage (level of viable cells as cfu/g) during the shelf life and postmarketing surveillance, and the specific health claim made, if any, with scientific evidence-based validation. Although the FAO/WHO guidelines by and large form the basis for formulating probiotic guidelines in most of the developed and developing countries including India, unfortunately, government regulations differ among countries, and hence, the status of probiotics as a component in food is currently not established on an international basis. Hence, there is a need for harmonization of these guidelines to have some uniformity in the product quality, safety, and efficacy effectively at the global level. In this context, it is strongly recommended that in case, any adverse effects are recorded after administration of the probiotic or probiotic food, it must also be properly documented with wide publicity.

23.20 NEGATIVE EFFECTS ON THE HOST-NORMAL AND IMMUNOCOMPROMISED

The side effects of probiotics are rarely reported and generally amount to little more than flatulence or change in bowel habit. A study of long-term consumption of *Bifidobacterium lactis* and *S. thermophilus*-supplemented formula in children aged less than 2 years showed that the product was well tolerated. The use of LGG, which has increased markedly since its introduction in Finland in 1990, has not led to a significant change in the incidence of *Lactobacillus* bacteremia. Complications of treatment with probiotics have been observed in patients who are immunocompromised or in the intensive care setting. *S. cerevisiae* fungemia and *Lactobacillus* bacteremia have been reported in patients with severe underlying illnesses. Cases of infection due to lactobacilli and bifidobacteria are extremely rare and are estimated to represent 0.05–0.4% of cases of infective endocarditis and bacteremia (Gasser, 1994). Increasing consumption of probiotic lactobacilli and bifidobacteria has not led to an increase in such opportunistic infections in consumers. Deaths associated with probiotic infections are also rare, particularly those involving healthy individuals. Despite its ability to cause low-grade infection and endocarditis in immunocompromised individuals, bacteremia due to *Lactobacillus* spp. has a very low mortality rate (Olano et al., 2001). Several studies have found that the correlation between deaths and probiotic infection was low and unconfirmed.

23.21 CONCLUSION

The interest in probiotics and dairy-based probiotic foods has grown enormously during the last few years across the world due to innumerable health-promoting functions. Because of their immense potential directly or indirectly related to human health and well-being, they constitute the key ingredient of the functional/health foods and are currently the major focus of attention not only as bioactive dietary ingredient for boosting overall gut health and immunity but also as potential biotherapeutics in the management of inflammatory metabolic disorders and other chronic diseases. Although almost all the dairy-based foods are excellent carriers of probiotics, traditional fermented dairy products could be the most ideal target for value addition with probiotics for developing into safe, cost–effective, and affordable novel health foods for not only catering to the health care needs of the mass human population, particularly belonging to the low-income and middle-class group especially in developing countries including India, but also for export. Indigenous probiotic strains of lactobacilli and bifidobacteria originating from the gut of the native population are likely to be more effective in the local population to confer their specific health-promoting functions optimally because of better colonization in the gut. Many of the promising indigenous probiotic strains with novel physiological functions have great prospects to be explored either as prophylactics or as biotherapeutics for prevention and cure of specific diseases. However, before the launch of these probiotic cultures as such or in the form of food product in the market for human health applications, the safety and purported health claims associated with such strains need to be critically evaluated in appropriate well-designed animal studies followed by validation in clinical trials on human subjects of the native target population. The mechanistic studies also need to be worked out to understand the exact mode of action of the potential probiotic strains with regard to their functional efficacy against the specific disease. With the recent advancements in molecular biology and genetic engineering techniques and new developments in genomics, proteomics, transcriptomics, and metabolomics along with metagenomics and nutrigenomics, their functional efficacy can be further enhanced by designing novel strains for developing customized/personalized probiotic foods. Probiotics and probiotic foods are going to play a vital role in effective management of human diseases and can help in the creation of a healthy society, particularly in countries like India. Hence, probiotics have a great future ahead to serve mankind.

REFERENCES

Allen, S., J. Okoko, E. Martinez, et al. 2004. Probiotics for treating infectious diarrhoea. Cochrane Database. *Syst. Rev.* (2): CD003048.

Altermann, E., B. L. Buck, R. Cano, and T. R. Klaenhammer. 2004. Identification and phenotypic characterization of the cell division protein CdpA. *Gene* 342: 189–197.

Ashar, M. N. and R. Chand. 2004. Fermented milk containing ACE-inhibitory peptides reduces blood pressure in middle aged hypertensive subjects. *Milchwissenschaft* 59: 363–366.

Azcarate-Peril, M. A., R. Tallon, and T. R. Klaenhammer. 2009. Temporal gene expression and probiotic attributes of *Lactobacillus acidophilus* during growth in milk. *J. Dairy Sci.* 92: 870–886.

Baroutkoub, A., R. Z. Mehdi, R. Beglarian, J. Hassan, S. Zahra, M. S. Mohammad, and E. Mohammad. 2010. Effects of probiotic yoghurt consumption on the serum cholesterol levels in hypercholestromic cases in Shiraz, Southern Iran. *Sci. Res. Essays* 5: 2206–2209.

Bassler, B. L., E. P. Greenberg, and A. M. Stevens. 1997. Cross-species induction of luminescence in the quorum-sensing bacterium. *Vibrio harveyi. J. Bacteriol.* 179: 4043–4045.

Bengmark, S. 2005. Bio-ecology control of the gastrointestinal tract: The role of flora and supplemented probiotics and synbiotics. *Gastroenterol. Clin. North Am.* 34: 13–36.

Bibiloni, R., R. N. Fedorak, G. W. Tannock, et al. 2005. VSL#3 probiotic-mixture induces remission in patients with active ulcerative colitis. *Am. J. Gastroenterol.* 100: 1539–1546.

Boekhorst, J., Q. Helmer, M. Kleerebezem, and R. J. Siezen. 2006. Comparative analysis of proteins with a mucus-binding domain found exclusively in lactic acid bacteria. *Microbiology* 152: 273–280.

Bousvaros, A., S. Guandalini, R. N. Baldassano, et al. 2005. A randomized, double-blind trial of *Lactobacillus* GG versus placebo in addition to standard maintenance therapy for children with Crohn's disease. *Inflamm. Bowel Dis.* 11: 833–839.

Bron, P. A., C. Grangette, A. Mercenier, W. M. de Vos, and M. Kleerebezem. 2004. Identification of *Lactobacillus plantarum* genes that are induced in the gastrointestinal tract of mice. *J. Bacteriol.* 186: 5721–5729.

Bron, P. A., M. Meijer, R. S. Bongers, W. M. de Vos, and M. Kleerebezem. 2007. Dynamics of competitive population abundance of *Lactobacillus plantarum* ivi gene mutants in fecal samples after passage through the gastrointestinal tract of mice. *J. Appl. Microbiol.* 103: 1424–1434.

Buck, B. L., E. Altermann, T. Svingerud, and T. R. Klaenhammer. 2005. Functional analysis of putative adhesion factors in *Lactobacillus acidophilus* NCFM. *Appl. Environ. Microbiol.* 71: 8344–8351.

Callanan, M., P. Kaleta, J. O'Callaghan, O. O'Sullivan, K. Jordan, O. McAuliffe, A. Sangrador-Vegas, L. Slattery, G. F. Fitzgerald, T. Beresford, and R. P. Ross. 2008. Genome sequence of *Lactobacillus helveticus*, an organism distinguished by selective gene loss and insertion sequence element expansion. *J. Bacteriol.* 190: 727–735.

Cario, E. 2005. Bacterial interactions with cells of the intestinal mucosa: Toll-like receptors and NOD2. *Gut* 54: 1182–1193.

Champagne, C. P., N. J. Gardner, and D. Roy. 2005. Challenges in the addition of probiotic cultures to foods. *Crit. Rev. Food Sci. Nutr.* 45: 61–84.

Chiu, C. H., T. Y. Lu, Y. Y. Tseng, and T. M. Pan. 2006. The effects of *Lactobacillus*-fermented milk on lipid metabolism in hamsters fed on high-cholesterol diet. *Appl. Microbiol. Biotechnol.* 71: 238–45.

Coeuret, V., M. Gueguen, and J. P. Vernoux. 2004. Number and strains of lactobacilli in some probiotic products. *Int. J. Food Microbiol.* 97: 147–156.

Commane, D., R. Hughes, C. Shortt, and I. Rowland. 2005. The potential mechanisms involved in the anti-carcinogenic action of probiotics. *Mutat. Res.* 591: 276–289.

De Keersmaecker, S. C. J. and J. Vanderleyden. 2003. Constraints on detection of autoinducer-2 (AI-2) signalling molecules using *Vibrio harveyi* as a reporter. *Microbiology* 149: 1953–1956.

de las Rivas, B., Ángela, Marcobal, and R. Muñoz. 2006. Development of a multilocus sequence typing method for analysis of *Lactobacillus plantarum* strains. *Microbiology* 152: 85–93.

de Vos, W. M., J. J. M. Castenmiller, R. J. Hamer, and R. J. M. Brummer. 2006. Nutridynamics—Studying the dynamics of food components in products and in the consumer. *Curr. Opin. Biotechnol.* 17: 217–225.

de Vos, W. M., P. A. Bron, and M. Kleerebezem. 2004. Post-genomics of lactic acid bacteria and other food-grade bacteria to discover gut functionality. *Curr. Opin. Biotechnol.* 15: 86–93.

de Vrese, M., A. Stegelmann, B. Richter, S. Fenselau, C. Laue, and J. Schrezenmeir. 2001. Probiotics—Compensation for lactase insufficiency. *Am. J. Clin. Nutr.* 73: Suppl 421S–429S.

Decallone, J., M. Delmee, P. Wauthoz, et al. 1991. A rapid procedure for the identification of lactic acid bacteria based on the gas chromatographic analysis of cellular fatty acids. *J. Food Prot.* 54: 217–224.

Delcour, J., T. Ferain, M. Deghorain, E. Palumbo, and P. Hols. 1999. The biosynthesis and functionality of the cell-wall of lactic acid bacteria. *Antonie van Leeuwenhoek* 76: 159–184.

Denou, E., R. D. Pridmore, B. Berger, J. M. Panoff, F. Arigoni, and H. Brussow. 2008. Identification of genes associated with the long gut persistence phenotype of the probiotic *Lactobacillus johnsonii* strain NCC533 using a combination of genomics and transcriptome analysis. *J. Bacteriol.* 190: 3161–3168.

Duary, R .K., V. K. Batish, and S. Grover. 2010. Expression of the atpD gene in probiotic *Lactobacillus plantarum strains* under in vitro acidic conditions by RT-qPCR. *Res. Microbiol.* 161: 399–405.

Duary, R. K., V. K. Batish, and S. Grover. 2011. Relative gene expression of bile salt hydrolase and surface proteins in two putative indigenous *Lactobacillus plantarum* strains under in vitro gut conditions. *Mol. Biol. Rep.* 39: 2541–2552.

Dunne, C., L. Murphy, S. Flynn, et al. 1999. Probiotics: From myth to reality. Demonstration of functionality in animal models of disease and in human clinical trials. *Antonie van Leeuwenhoek* 76: 279–292.

Elegado, F. B., M. A. R. V. Guerra, R. A. Macayan, H. A. Mendoza, and M. B. Lizaran. 2004. Spectrum of bacteriocin activity of *Lactobacillus plantarum* BS and fingerprinting by RAPD-PCR. *Int. J. Food Microbiol.* 95: 11–18.

FAO/WHO. 2002. *Working Group Report on Drafting Guidelines for the Evaluation of Probiotics in Food London*, Ontario, Canada.

Farber, J. M. 1996. An introduction to the hows and whys of molecular typing. *J. Food Prot.* 59: 1091–1101.

Fujimori, S., A. Tatsuguchi, K. Gudis, T. Kishida, K. Mitsui, A. Ehara, T. Kobayashi, Y. Sekita, T. Seo, and C. Sakamoto. 2007. High dose probiotic and prebiotic co-therapy for remission induction of active Crohn's disease. *J. Gastroenterol. Hepatol.* 22: 1199–1204.

Fuller, R. 1991. Probiotics in human medicine. *Gut* 32: 439–442.

Fuller, R. 1989. Probiotics in man and animals. *J. Appl. Bacteriol.* 66: 365–378.

Furrie, E., S. Macfarlane, A. Kennedy, et al. 2005. Synbiotic therapy (*Bifidobacterium longum*/Synergy 1) initiates resolution of inflammation in patients with active ulcerative colitis: A randomized controlled pilot trial. *Gut* 54: 242–249.

Gasser, F. 1994. Safety of lactic acid bacteria and their occurrence in human clinical infections. *Bull Inst Pasteur.* 92: 45–67.

Gatti, M., E. Fornasari, and E. Neviani. 1997. Cell-wall protein profiles of dairy thermophilic lactobacilli. *Lett. Appl. Microbiol.* 25: 345–348.

Giraffa, G. and E. Neviani. 2000. Molecular identification and characterization of food-associated lactobacilli. *Ital. J. Food Sci.* 4: 403–423.

Gorbach, S. L. 2000. Probiotics and gastrointestinal health. *Am. J. Gastroenterol.* 95: Suppl 1: S2–S4.

Gringhuis, S. I., J. den Dunnen, M. Litjens, B. V. Hof, Y. van Kooyk, and T. B. H. Geijtenbeek. 2007. C-type lectin DC-SIGN modulates Toll-like receptor signaling via Raf-1 kinase-dependent acetylation of transcription factor NF-kappa B. *Immunity* 26: 605–616.

Grześkowiak, L., E. Isolauri, S. Salminen, and G. Miguel. 2011. Manufacturing process influences properties of probiotic bacteria. *Br. J. Nutr.* 105: 887–894.

Gupta, P., H. Andrew, B. S. Kirschner, and S. Guandalini. 2000. Is *Lactobacillus* GG helpful in children with Crohn's disease? Results of a preliminary, open-label study. *J. Pediatr. Gastroenterol. Nutr.* 31: 453–457.

Gurakan G. C. 2004 PCR-based typing of *Lactobacillus plantarum* strains. IFT Annual Meeting, July 12–16, Las Vegas, NV.

Guslandi, M, G. Mezzi, M. Sorghi, and P. A. Testoni. 2003. Saccharomyces boulardii in maintenance treatment of Crohn's disease. *Digestive Dis. Sci.* 45: 1462–1464.

Harmsen, H. J. M., G. R. Gibson, P. Elfferich, et al. 2000. Comparison of viable cell counts and fluorescence *in situ* hybridization using specific rRNA-based probes for the quantification of human fecal bacteria. *FEMS Microbiol. Lett.* 183: 125–129.

Henke, J. M. and B. L. Bassler. 2004. Three parallel quorum-sensing systems regulate gene expression in *Vibrio harveyi. J. Bacteriol.* 186: 6902–6914.

Higgins, D. A., M. E. Pomianek, C. M. Kraml, R. K. Taylor, M. F. Semmelhack, and B. L. Bassler. 2007. The major *Vibrio cholerae* auto inducer and its role in virulence factor production. *Nature* 450: 883–886.

Hoepelman, A. I. M and E. I. Tuomanen. 1992. Consequences of microbial attachment: Directing host cell functions with adhesins. *Infect. Immun.* 60: 1729–1733.

Hozapfel, W. H., P. Haberer, R. Geisen, J. Bjorkroth, and U. Schillinger. 2001. Taxonomy and important features of probiotic microorganism in food and nutrition. *Am. J. Clin. Nutr.* 73(S): 365S–373S.

Huang, J. S., A. Bousvaros, J. W. Lee, et al. 2002. Efficacy of probiotic use in acute diarrhea in children: A meta-analysis. *Digestive Dis. Sci.* 47: 2625–2634.

Hughes, D. T., and V. Sperandio. 2008. Inter-kingdom signalling: Communication between bacteria and their hosts. *Nat. Rev. Microbiol.* 6: 111–120.

Ishibashi, N. and S. Shimamura. 1993. Bifidobacteria: Research and Development in Japan. *Food Technol.* 47: 126, 129–130, 132–134.

Iwana, H., H. Masuda, T. Fujisawa, H. Suzuki, and T. Mitsuoka. 1993. Isolation and identification of *Bifidobacterium* spp. in commercial yoghurt sold in Europe. *Bifidobacteria Microflora* 12: 39–45.

Jelcic, I., E. Hufner, H. Schmidt, and C. Hertel. 2008. Repression of the locus of the enterocyte effacement-encoded regulator of gene transcription of *Escherichia coli* O157:H7 by *Lactobacillus reuteri* culture supernatants is LuxS and strain dependent. *Appl. Environ. Microbiol.* 74: 3310–3314.

Kajander, K., K. Hatakka, T. Poussa, et al. 2005. A probiotic mixture alleviates symptoms in irritable bowel syndrome patients: A controlled 6-month intervention. *Aliment Pharmacol. Ther.* 22: 387–394.

Kalliomäki, M., S. Salminen, T. Poussa, et al. 2003. Probiotics and prevention of atopic disease: 4-year follow-up of a randomized placebo-controlled trial. *Lancet* 361: 1869–1871.

Kaper, J. B. and V. Sperandio. 2005. Bacterial cell-to-cell signaling in the gastrointestinal tract. *Infect. Immun.* 73: 3197–3209.

Kapila, S., Vibha, and P. R. Sinha. 2006. Antioxidative and hypocholestrolemic effect of *Lactobacillus casei* ssp *casei. Indian J. Med. Sci.* 59: 361–371.

Kim, H. J., M. Camilleri, S. McKinzie, et al. 2003. A randomized controlled trial of a probiotic, VSL#3, on gut transit and symptoms in diarrhoea-predominant irritable bowel syndrome. *Aliment. Pharmacol. Ther.* 17: 895–904.

Klaenhammer, T. R., R. Barrangou, B. L. Buck, M. A. Azcarate-Peril, and E. Altermann. 2005. Genomic features of lactic acid bacteria effecting bioprocessing and health. *FEMS Microbiol. Rev.* 29: 393–409.

Kleerebezem, M., J. Boekhorst, R. van Kranenburg, D. Molenaar, O. P. Kuipers, R. Leer, R. Tarchini, S. A. Peters, H. M. Sandbrink, M. W. E. J. Fiers, W. Stiekema, R. M. K. Lankhorst, P. A. Bron, S. M. Hoffer, M. N. N. Groot, R. Kerkhoven, M. de Vries, B. Ursing, W. M. de Vos, and R. J. Siezen. 2003. Complete genome sequence of *Lactobacillus plantarum* WCFS1. *Proc. Natl. Acad. Sci. USA* 100: 1990–1995.

Klein, G., A. Pack, C. Bonaparte, and G. Reuter. 1998. Taxonomy and physiology of probiotic lactic acid bacteria. *Int. J. Food Microbiol.* 41: 103–125.

Kohler, H., B. A. McCormick, and A. Walker. 2003. Bacterial-enterocyte crosstalk: Cellular mechanisms in health and diseases. *J. Pediatr. Gastroenterol. Nutr.* 36: 175–185.

Kotowska, M, P. Albrecht, and H. Szajewska. 2005. *Saccharomyces boulardii* in the prevention of antibiotic-associated diarrhoea in children: A randomized double-blind placebo-controlled trial. *Aliment. Pharmacol. Ther.* 21: 583–590.

Kukkonen, K., E. Savilahti, T. Haahtela, et al. 2007. Probiotics and prebiotic galacto-oligosaccharides in the prevention of allergic diseases: A randomized, double blind, placebo-controlled trial. *J. Allergy Clin. Immunol.* 119: 192–198.

Kumar, R., S. Grover, and V. K. Batish 2011. Hypocholesterolemic effect of dietary inclusion of two putative probiotic bile salt hydrolase producing *Lactobacillus plantarum* strains in Sprague–Dawley rats. *Br. J. Nutr.* 105: 561–573.

Lapierre, L., J. E. Jacques-Edouard Germond, A. Ott, M. Delley, and B. Mollet. 1999. D-Lactate dehydrogenase gene (*ldhD*) inactivation and resulting metabolic effects in the *Lactobacillus johnsonii* strains la1 and N312. *Appl. Environ. Microbiol.* 65: 4002–4007.

Lebeer, S., I. J. J. Claes, T. L. A. Verhoeven, C. Shen, I. Lambrichts, J. L. Ceuppens, J. Vanderleyden, and S. C. J. De Keersmaecker. 2008. Impact of luxS and suppressor mutations on the gastrointestinal transit of *Lactobacillus rhamnosus* GG. *Appl. Environ. Microbiol.* 74: 4711–4718.

Lebeer, S., S. C. J. De Keersmaecker, T. L. A. Verhoeven, A. A. Fadda, K. Marchal, and J. Vanderleyden. 2007a. Functional analysis of luxS in the probiotic strain *Lactobacillus rhamnosus* GG reveals a central metabolic role important for growth and biofilm formation. *J. Bacteriol.* 189: 860–871.

Lebeer, S., T. L. A. Verhoeven, M. Perea Vélez, J. Vanderleyden, and S. C. J. De Keersmaecker. 2007b. Impact of environmental and genetic factors on biofilm formation by the probiotic strain *Lactobacillus rhamnosus* GG. *Appl. Environ. Microbiol.* 73: 6768–6775.

Ley, R. E., P. J. Turnbaugh, S. Klein, and J. I. Gordon. 2006. Human gut microbes associated with obesity. *Nature* 444: 1022–1023.

Lilly, D. M. and R. H. Stillwell. 1965. Growth promoting factors produced by probiotics. *Science* 147: 747–748.

Lorca, G., M. I. Torino, G. F. de Valdez, and A. Ljungh. 2002. Lactobacilli express cell surface proteins which mediate binding of immobilized collagen and fibronectin. *FEMS Microbiol. Lett.* 206: 31–37.

Mack, D. R., S. Michail., S. Wei., L. McDougall, and M. A. Hollingsworth. 1999. Probiotics inhibit enteropathogenic *E. coli* adherence *in vitro* by inducing intestinal mucin gene expression. *Am. J. Physiol.* 276: G941–G950.

Marteau, P., M. Lémann, P. Seksik, et al. 2006. Ineffectiveness of *Lactobacillus johnsonii* LA1 for prophylaxis of postoperative recurrence in Crohn's disease: A randomized, double blind, placebo controlled GETAID trial. *Gut* 55: 842–847.

Martin, F. P. J., Y. Wang, and N. Sprenger, N. 2008. Probiotic modulation of symbiotic gut microbial-host metabolic interaction in a humanized microbiome mouse model. *Mol. Syst. Biol.* 4: 157.

McFarland, L. V. 2007. Meta-analysis of probiotics for the prevention of traveler's diarrhea. *Travel. Med. Infect. Dis.* 5: 97–105.

Medzhitov, R. 2007. Recognition of microorganisms and activation of the immune response. *Nature* 449: 819–826.

Meie, R. and M. Steuerwals. 2005. Place of probiotics. *Curr. Opin. Crit. Care* 11: 318–325.

Nagashima, K., T. Hisada., M. Sato, and J. Mochizuki. 2003. Application of new primer-enzyme combinations to terminal restriction fragment length polymorphism profiling of bacterial populations in human feces. *Appl. Environ. Microbiol.* 69: 1251–1262.

Naser, S. M., P. Dawyndt, B. Hoste, et al. 2007. Identification of lactobacilli by pheS and rpoA gene sequence analyses. *Int. J. Syst. Evol. Microbiol.* 57: 2777–2789.

Olano, A., J. Chua, S. Schroeder, A. Minari, M. La Salvia, and H. G. Weissella. 2001. Confusa (Basonym: *Lactobacillus confusus*) bacteremia: A case report. *J. Clin. Microbiol.* 39: 1604–1607.

Perea Vélez, M., T. L. A. Verhoeven, C. Draing, S. Von Aulock, M. Pfitzenmaier, A. Geyer, I. Lambrichts, C. Grangette, B. Pot, J. Vanderleyden, and S. C. J. De Keersmaecker. 2007. Functional analysis of D-alanylation of lipoteichoic acid in the probiotic strain *Lactobacillus rhamnosus* GG. *Appl. Environ. Microbiol.* 73: 3595–3604.

Prantera, C., M. L. Scribano, G. Falasco, et al. 2002. Ineffectiveness of probiotics in preventing recurrence after curative resection for Crohn's disease: A randomized controlled trial with *Lactobacillus* GG. *Gut* 51: 405–409.

Pretzer, G., J. Snel, D. Molenaar, M. Kleerebezem, et al. 2005. Biodiversity based identification and functional characterization of the mannose-specific adhesin of *Lactobacillus plantarum*. *J. Bacteriol.* 187: 6128–6136.

Quigley, E. M. and B. Flourie. 2007. Probiotics and irritable bowel syndrome: A rationale for their use and an assessment of the evidence to date. *Neurogastroenterol. Motility* 19: 166–172.

Rodas, A. M., S. Ferrer, and I. Pardo, I. 2005. Polyphasic study of wine *Lactobacillus* strains: Taxonomic implications. *Int. J. Syst. Evol. Microbiol.* 55: 197–207.

Roos, S. and H. Jonsson. 2002. A high-molecular-mass cell-surface protein from *Lactobacillus reuteri* 1063 adheres to mucus components. *Microbiology* 148: 433–442.

Ross, R. P., G. F. Fitzgerald, J. K. Collins, and C. Stanton. 2002. Cheese delivering biocultures-probiotic cheese. *Aust. J. Dairy Technol.* 57: 71–78.

Roy, D. and S. Sirois. 2001. Molecular differentiation of *Bifidobacterium* species with amplified ribosomal DNA restriction analysis and alignment of short regions of the idh gene. *FEMS Microbiol. Lett.* 191: 17–24.

Ruas-Madiedo, P., M. Gueimonde, A. Margolles, C. G. D. L. Reyes- Gavilan, and S. Salminen. 2006. Exopolysaccharides produced by probiotic strains modify the adhesion of probiotics and enteropathogens to human intestinal mucus. *J. Food Prot.* 69: 2011–2015.

Russo, F., A. Orlando, M. Linsalata, A. Cavallini, and C. Messa. 2007. Effects of *Lactobacillus rhamnosus* GG on the cell growth and polyamine metabolism in HGC-27 human gastric cancer cells. *Nutr. Cancer* 59: 106–114.

Sánchez, I., S. Seseña, and L. L. Palop. 2004. Polyphasic study of the genetic diversity of lactobacilli associated with "Almagro" eggplants spontaneous fermentation, based on combined numerical analysis of randomly amplified polymorphic DNA and pulse-field gel electrophoresis patterns. *J. Appl. Microbiol.* 97: 446–458.

Saavedra, J. M. 2007. Use of probiotics in pediatrics: Rationale, mechanisms of action, and practical aspects. *Nutr. Clin. Practice* 22: 351–365.

Schultz, M., A. Timmer, H. H. Herfarth, R. B. Sartor, J. A. Vanderhoof, and H. C. Rath. 2004. *Lactobacillus* GG in inducing and maintaining remission of Crohn's disease. *BMC Gastroenterol.* 4: 5–8.

Sen, S., M. M. Mullan, T. J. Parker, J. T. Woolner, S. A. Tarry, and J. O. Hunter. 2002. Effect of *Lactobacillus plantarum* 299v on colonic fermentation and symptoms of irritable bowel syndrome. *Digestive Dis. Sci.* 47: 2615–2620.

Shah, N. P., W. E. V. Lankaputhra, M. L. Britz, and W. S. A. Kyle. 1995. Survival of *L. acidophilus* and *Bifidobacterium bifidum* in commercial yogurt during refrigerated storage. *Int. Dairy J.* 5: 515.

Simons, L. A., S. G. Amansec, and P. Conway. 2006. Effect of *Lactobacillus fermentum* on serum lipids in subjects with elevated serum cholesterol. *Nutr. Metab. Cardiovasc. Dis.* 16: 531–535.

Sleator, R D. and C. Hill. 2008. "Bioengineered Bugs"—A patho-biotechnology approach to probiotic research and applications. *Med. Hypotheses* 70(1): 167–169.

Smits, H. H., A. Engering, D. vander Kleij, E. C. de Jong, K. Schipper, T. M. M. van Capel, B. A. J. Zaat, M. Yazdanbakhsh, E. A. Wierenga, Y. van Kooyk, and M. L. Kapsenberg. 2005. Selective probiotic bacteria induce IL-10-producing regulatory T cells *in-vitro* by modulating dendritic cell function through dendritic cell-specific intercellular adhesion molecule 3-grabbing non-integrin. *J. Allergy Clin. Immunol.* 115: 1260–1267.

Sperandio, V., A. G. Torres, B. Jarvis, J. P. Nataro, and J. B. Kaper. 2003. Bacteria-host communication: The language of hormones. *Proc. Natl. Acad. Sci. USA* 100: 8951–8956.

Sturme, M. H. J., C. Francke, R. J. Siezen, W. M. de Vos, and M. Kleerebezem. 2007. Making sense of quorum sensing in lactobacilli: A special focus on *Lactobacillus plantarum* WCFS1. *Microbiology* 153: 3939–3947.

Surette, M. G., M. B. Miller, and B. L. Bassler. 1999. Quorum sensing in *Escherichia coli, Salmonella typhimurium*, and *Vibrio harveyi*: A new family of genes responsible for auto inducer production. *Proc. Natl. Acad. Sci. USA* 96: 1639–1644.

Szajewska, H, M. Ruszcyski, and A. Radzikowski. 2006. Probiotics in the prevention of antibiotic-associated diarrhea in children: A meta-analysis of randomized controlled trials. *J. Pediatr.* 149: 367–372.

Tannock, G. W., S. Ghazally, J. Walter, D. Loach, H. Brooks, G. Cook, M. Surette, C. Simmers, P. Bremer, F. Dal Bello, and C. Hertel. 2005. Ecological behavior of *Lactobacillus reuteri* 100–23 is affected by mutation of the luxS gene. *Appl. Environ. Microbiol.* 71: 8419–8425.

Taylor, A. L., J. A. Dunstan, and S. L. Prescott. 2007. Probiotic supplementation for the first 6 months of life fails to reduce the risk of atopic dermatitis and increases the risk of allergen sensitization in high-risk children. a randomized controlled trial. *J. Allergy Clin. Immunol.* 119(1): 184–191.

Tuomola, E., R. Crittenden, M. Playne, E. Isolauri, and S. Salminen. 2001 Quality assurance criteria for probiotic bacteria. *Am. J. Clin. Nutr.* 73: S393–S398.

Urbanska, A. M., J. Bhathena, C. Martoni, and S. Prakash. 2009. Estimation of the potential antitumor activity of microencapsulated *Lactobacillus acidophilus* yogurt formulation in the attenuation of tumorigenesis in Apc (Min/þ) mice. *Digestive Dis. Sci.* 54: 264–273.

Valeur, N., P. Engel, N. Carbajal, E. Connolly, and K. Ladefoged. 2004. Colonization and immunomodulation by *Lactobacillus reuteri* ATCC 55730 in the human gastrointestinal tract. *Appl. Environ. Microbiol.* 70: 1176–1181.

van Baarlen, P., F. J. Troost, S. van Hemert, C. van der Meer, W. M. de Vos, et al. 2009. Differential NF-kappaB pathways induction by *Lactobacillus plantarum* in the duodenum of healthy humans correlating with immune tolerance. *Proc. Natl. Acad. Sci. USA* 106(7): 2371–2376.

van Baarlen, P., F. Troosta, C. van der Meera, G. Hooivelda, M. Boekschotena, R. J. M. Brummera, and M. Kleerebezem. 2010. Human mucosal *in vivo* transcriptome responses to three lactobacilli indicate how probiotics may modulate human cellular pathways. *Proc. Natl. Acad. Sci. USA* www.pnas.org/cgi/doi/10.1073/pnas.1000079107.

Van Kooyk, Y. and T. B. H. Geijtenbeek. 2003. DC-sign: Escape mechanism for pathogens. *Nat. Rev. Immunol.* 3: 697–709.

Van Niel, C. W, C. Feudtner, M. M. Garrison, and D. A. Christakis. 2002. *Lactobacillus* therapy for acute infectious diarrhea in children: A meta-analysis. *Pediatrics* 109: 678–684.

Vendeville, A., K. Winzer, K. Heurlier, C. M. Tang, and K. R. Hardie. 2005. Making "sense" of metabolism: Autoinducer-2, LuxS and pathogenic bacteria. *Nat. Rev. Microbiol.* 3: 383–396.

Vibha, Sinha, P. R. and H. Yadav. 2007. Antiatherogenic effect of Probiotic dahi in rats feed cholesterol enriched diet. *J. Food Sci. Technol.* 44(2): 127–129.

Weston, S., A. Halbert, P. Richmond, and S. L. Prescott. 2005. Effects of probiotics on atopic dermatitis: A randomized controlled trial. *Archives Dis. Children* 90: 892–897.

White, J. A. 2006. Probiotics and their use in diverticulitis. *J. Clin. Gastroenterol.* 40(7, Suppl 3): S160–2.

Whorwell, P. J., L. Altringer, J. Morel, et al. 2006. Efficacy of an encapsulated probiotic *Bifidobacterium infantis* 35624 in women with irritable bowel syndrome. *Am. J. Gastroenterol.* 101: 1581–1590.

Woese, C. R. 1987. Bacterial evolution. *Microbiol. Rev.* 51: 221–271.

Yansanjav, A., P. Svec, I. Sedlacek, I. Hollerova, and M. Nemec. 2003. Ribotyping of lactobacilli isolated from spoiled beer. *FEMS Microbiol. Lett.* 229, 141–144.

24 Omega-3 Polyunsaturated Fatty Acids

Basic and Contemporary Research Issues

Melinda Phang, Melissa Fry, and Manohar L. Garg

CONTENTS

24.1 INTRODUCTION

The beneficial effects of long-chain omega-3 polyunsaturated fatty acids (LCn-3PUFA) from fish and fish oils in reducing the incidence of cardiovascular disease (CVD) have become a strong clinical focus. Several clinical and epidemiological studies have been conducted to determine the effects of LCn-3PUFA on various biological and physiological indexes. Research on the cardioprotective effects began 30 years ago from the original studies explaining the reduced incidence of CVD in Greenland Eskimos (Dyerberg et al. 1975). The scientific knowledge concerning omega-3 fatty acids (n-3 FA) rapidly expanded and its beneficial effects have now been demonstrated in a wide variety of chronic diseases. Studies have reported that LCn-3PUFA reduces inflammation and the risk of certain cancers and arthritis. Emerging research has also demonstrated the importance of LCn-3PUFA for cognitive and behavioral function, weight management, and skin health. This chapter leads from the early basic research on LCn-3PUFA to the contemporary research of the current and emerging health issues. A brief review of LCn-3PUFA structure and biochemistry will be followed by an extensive review of epidemiological data, animal experiments, and dietary intervention studies.

24.2 OMEGA-3 FATTY ACID STRUCTURE AND BIOCHEMISTRY

The polyunsaturated fatty acids can be divided into two categories, namely the n-3 and the n-6 polyunsaturated (omega-6) fatty acids. This classification is based on the position of the first double bond from the methyl terminal, being located at the third carbon in the n-3PUFA and at the sixth carbon in the n-6PUFA. The n-3PUFA, α-linoleic acid (ALA; 18:3n-3), and the n-6PUFA, linoleic acid (LA; 18:2n-6), are the predominant essential fatty acids that are derived from a variety of animal and plant foods. LA is desaturated and elongated to arachidonic acid (AA; 20:4n-6) while ALA is desaturated and elongated to eicosapentaenoic acid (EPA; 20:5n-3) and docosahexaenoic acid (DHA; 22:6n-3). However, the conversion from ALA to the longer-chain EPA and DHA are modest (<1%), partly due to competition with LA for the rate-limiting enzyme, Δ6 desaturase, to form AA (Gerster 1998). The metabolites derived from EPA or AA are eicosanoids which are further classified into prostaglandins (PGE, PGF), leukotrienes (LTB), or thromboxanes (TxA). These eicosanoids have profound effects on biological responses and are responsible for many of the effects found in inflammatory conditions. In general, eicosanoids derived from AA are proinflammatory and proaggregatory agonists while those derived from EPA are anti-inflammatory and inhibit platelet aggregation (Salmon and Terano 1985). EPA and DHA compete with AA for prostaglandin and leukotriene synthesis at the cyclo-oxygenase (COX) and lipoxygenase (LOX) level to produce eicosanoids of 3-series (PGE_3, PGE_3, TxA_3, and LTB_5) or 2-series (PGE_2, PGE_2, TxA_2, and LTB_4) respectively (Prichard et al. 1995). Eicosanoids derived from AA have opposing effects to those derived from EPA and a dietary imbalance in favor of n-6PUFA may contribute to detrimental effects on health, including CVD (Harris et al. 2009). Therefore, obtaining pre-formed EPA and DHA directly from the diet is important for adequate incorporation into cell membranes and uptake in body tissues (Burdge and Calder 2005). EPA and DHA are found in large quantities in oily fish and marine seafood which indeed are predominantly present in the diet of Greenland Eskimos.

24.3 EPIDEMIOLOGICAL STUDIES

In the 1970s, Dyerberg and Bang conducted a series of prospective studies on Greenland Eskimos (Bang and Dyerberg 1972, 1980; Dyerberg et al. 1975; Bang et al. 1980; Dyerberg and Bang 1980; Dyerberg and Jorgensen 1982) and revealed that the rarity of ischemic heart disease and decreased thrombotic tendency in this population was linked to their consumption of a seafood diet high in LCn-3PUFA. These findings contrasted sharply when compared to the dietary habits of an ethically similar population in Denmark with significantly higher rates of CVD (Dyerberg et al. 1977). The diet of the Danes had a comparable amount of total fat, a higher intake of saturated fat but a much lower intake of LCn-3PUFA, whereas Greenland Eskimos consumed more LCn-3PUFA at the expense of saturated fat (Bang et al. 1980). Greenland Eskimos had lower cholesterol levels due to lower concentrations of LDL and VLDL (Dyerberg et al. 1977) and significantly longer bleeding times than the Danes; the prolonged bleeding time due to decreased platelet aggregation accompanied by a shift from the n-6PUFA to n-3PUFA in platelet fatty acid composition (Dyerberg and Bang 1979). The same phenomenon of lower CVD rates was later reported in other populations consuming a high seafood diet, including populations in Alaska (Newman et al. 1993), Japan (Hamazaki et al. 1988), and China (Yuan et al. 2001). In the Japanese cohort, those that consumed more fish (fisherman) also had a much lower blood pressure as well as the incidence of coronary artery disease (CAD) compared to the Japanese farmers who consumed less fish (Marmot et al. 1975). Observational studies in the Western population reported an inverse relationship between fish consumption and coronary heart disease (CHD) mortality in the Rotterdam (Kromhout et al. 1995) and the Zutphen study (Kromhout et al. 1985) in the Netherlands and the Chicago Western Electric study (Daviglus et al. 1997) in the United States. The Zutphen study reported an inverse dose relation between fish consumption and CHD mortality. Higher fish consumption at baseline with the subsequent 20-year follow-up of CHD mortality was 50% lower in those who consumed more than 30 g of fish per day compared to those who did not consume fish (Kromhout et al. 1985). Similar findings were reported in the Western Electric study with a 30-year follow-up of CHD risk. Fatal myocardial infarction rates were significantly lower in those who ate ≥35 g fish daily than in those who did not (Daviglus et al. 1997). Sudden cardiac death plays a large part in CVD mortality and in most cases is a consequence of cardiac arrhythmia (Huikuri et al. 2001). In the Cardiovascular Health Study, Mozaffarian et al. reported the observational finding that consumption of tuna and broiled or baked fish but not fried fish is associated with lower risk of fatal CHD and arrhythmic death (Mozaffarian et al. 2003). The prevention of fatal arrhythmias by LCn-3PUFA in fish has also been reported in other large cohort studies (Albert et al. 1998; Hu et al. 2002).

In the pathogenesis of cardiovascular events, inflammation plays an important role with the recognition that atherosclerosis is an inflammatory process (Ross 1999). Several epidemiological studies have indicated the beneficial effects of LCn-3PUFA on inflammation and endothelial function. Inverse associations have been found between the intake of LCn-3PUFA and plasma concentrations of biomarkers of inflammation and endothelial activation, including C-reactive protein (CRP), tumor necrosis factor α (TNFα), E-selectin, and intercellular adhesion molecule-1 (ICAM-1) (Lopez-Garcia et al. 2004; Hjerkinn et al. 2005; Zampelas et al. 2005). The association between fish intake and atherosclerosis has also been examined in observational studies and it was reported that serum LCn-3PUFA levels were inversely related to the probability of carotid plaques (Yamada et al. 2000) and significantly less progression of coronary atherosclerosis (Erkkila et al. 2004).

An ecological study was conducted by Zhang et al. (1999) including 36 countries to examine the relation between fish consumption and all causes of mortality, ischemic heart disease (IHD), and stroke. Data were obtained from the Food and Agricultural Organization and the World Health Organization. Significant independent inverse correlations were found between fish consumption and all assessed factors, even after exclusion of countries with the highest amount of fish consumption and lowest all-cause mortality rate. The statistical analyses in the study demonstrated that fish consumption is associated with reduced risk from all-cause, IHD, and stroke mortality at the population level in a diverse number of populations.

24.4 CARDIOVASCULAR DISEASE

Evidences from observational, clinical, animal, and *in vitro* studies have reported the overall cardioprotective role of LCn-3PUFA owing to their antiaggregatory, antiarrhythmic, antihypertensive, and anti-inflammatory effects (Nagakawa et al. 1983; von Schacky and Weber 1985; Knapp et al. 1986; Gaudette and Holub 1990; Kinsella et al. 1990; Axelrod et al. 1994; Prisco et al. 1995; Mori et al. 1997; Wensing et al. 1999; Akiba et al. 2000; Grundt and Nilsen 2008; Harris et al. 2008).

The antiarrhythmic properties of LCn-3PUFA for cardioprotection are suggested by the significant risk reduction of sudden cardiac death associated with LCn-3PUFA intake from fish or fish oil intervention trials. Earlier trials investigated the effects of n-3 FA in the secondary prevention of myocardial infarction (MI). In the Diet and Reinfarction Trial (DART), patients who recovered from MI were randomly allocated dietary advice to reduce the ratio of polyunsaturated to saturated fat, increase fatty fish intake, or increase cereal fiber intake. Patients who were advised to increase their fish to at least two fish meals a week had a 29% decrease in 2 year all-cause mortality compared to those not advised but with no decrease in the rate of nonfatal MI (Burr et al. 1989).

Similar findings were also reported in the GISSI-Prevenzione trial. Recent post-MI patients were randomly assigned to supplements of LCn-3PUFA (1 g/day), vitamin E (300 mg/day), both or none for 3.5 years. Patients receiving treatment of n-3 FA experienced significantly lowered combined risk of mortality, nonfatal myocardial infarction and stroke by 10–15% compared to no LCn-3PUFA. No effect was shown for vitamin E (GISSI 1999).

A meta-analysis including 10 trials reviewed the effects of n-3 FA on cardiovascular events in CHD patients. Daily supplementation with n-3 FA decreased the incidence of all-cause mortality by 16% and decreased the incidence of fatal myocardial infarction by 24%. No significant effects were found for nonfatal myocardial infarction, nonfatal stroke, and angina (Yzebe and Lievre 2004). These studies suggested the antiarrhythmic effects from LCn-3PUFA intake or fatty fish (two per week) may reduce mortality in recent post-MI and CHD patients. However, other studies have also reported unfavorable results. The post-trial follow-up data of the DART trial showed no long-term survival benefit in the post-MI patients. The early reduction in mortality observed in those patients given dietary fish advice over 2 years of the trial was followed by an increased risk (hazard ratio 1.31) over the next 3 years (Ness et al. 2002). Another study also reported that advice to eat two portions of fatty fish per week or 3 g fish oil daily was associated with higher risk of cardiac (hazard ratio = 1.26) and sudden death (hazard ratio = 1.54) in patients with angina over a period of 3–9 years (Burr et al. 2003).

Overall, these studies may suggest an immediate effect of LCn-3PUFA on arrhythmia rather than a slow long-term effect in the regression of other cardiovascular events. However, the conflicting results indicate that the evidence is not conclusive and that more clinical trials are needed.

Elevated blood pressure poses as an independent risk factor for cardiovascular events and indeed the majority of events occur in hypertensive or mildly hypertensive individuals (Stamler et al. 1993). In a U.S. population study, small reductions in blood pressure (BP) of 5 and 10 mmHg were associated with at least 34% and 54% less stroke and at least 21% and 37% less CHD, respectively (Stamler et al. 1993). Several intervention studies have suggested that LCn-3PUFA exerts antihypertensive effects. A meta-analysis of 31 placebo-controlled trials including 1356 subjects reported a dose–response effect of LCn-3PUFA on blood pressure. Minimal BP change was observed with low doses of ≤3 d/day LCn-3PUFA (−1.3/−0.7 mmHg), a significant moderate reduction with 3.3–7 g/day (−2.9/−1.6 mmHg), and a substantial reduction in BP with 15 g/day (−8.1/−5.8 mmHg). Furthermore, the hypotensive effects were only observed in patients with hypertension, atherosclerosis, or hypercholesterolemia (Morris et al. 1993). Other reviews also reported similar findings of a greater BP reduction in hypertensive populations suggesting an increased beneficial effect of LCn-3PUFA in the presence of arterial stiffness (Appel et al. 1993; Geleijnse et al. 2002). In the metaregression analysis including 36 trials, the median dose of 3.7 g/day LCn-3PUFA reduced BP by 2.1/1.6 mmHg in a total of 2114 subjects. Subgroup analyses by subject type revealed larger reduction in BP in hypertensive compared with normotensive subjects (−3.65/−2.51 vs. −1.21/−1.14 mmHg, respectively) (Geleijnse et al. 2002). These studies suggest that relatively high doses of LCn-3PUFA (>3 g/day) can lead to clinically relevant reductions in BP in hypertensive individuals; however, effects of lower doses of LCn-3PUFA and the long-term efficacy on BP are yet to be established.

Apart from the lowering of BP and the regulation of vascular health and dilator function, vasoactive mediators also play an important role in the control of vascular tone for endothelial function. One of the most important mechanisms that underlie the beneficial effects of LCn-3PUFA on endothelial function is through the enzymatic conversion of LCn-3PUFA-derived eicosanoids. Thromboxanes (Tx) and prostaglandins (PG) regulate platelet and endothelial vessel–wall interactions and thus play an important role in the balance between hemostasis and thrombosis which are relevant in the initiation of CHD and stroke. TxA_2 derived from AA is a potent aggregatory substance synthesized via COX pathway while PGI_2 has opposing effects and is synthesized via the LOX pathway in the vascular endothelium. In contrast, the eicosanoids derived from EPA, TxA_3, and PGI_3 have opposing effects and act as a weaker stimulus for platelet aggregation and vasoconstriction. Incorporation of LCn-3PUFA into platelet phospholipids displaces AA from the platelet membranes to compete as a substrate for the COX enzyme and catalyze the biosynthesis of TxA_3, and reduced conversion to TxA_2 (Needleman et al. 1976; Calder 2001; Grundt and Nilsen 2008; Calder 2009) hence lowering the risk of inappropriate thrombus formation and associated vascular diseases. As a result, supplementation with EPA and DHA on platelet function has been extensively studied. EPA and DHA have been reported to reduce aggregation in hypertensive subjects (Mori et al. 1997), diabetic subjects (Tamura et al. 1987; Axelrod et al. 1994), and in healthy controls both *in vitro* and *ex vivo* (Nagakawa et al. 1983; von Schacky and Weber 1985; Gaudette and Holub 1990;

Prisco et al. 1995; Wensing et al. 1999). Studies have reported that LCn-3PUFA supplementation reduces formation of TxA_2 (Srivastava 1985; von Schacky et al. 1985; Scheurlen et al. 1993; Mori et al. 1997), prolongs bleeding time (Sanders et al. 1980; Harris et al. 1981), reduces platelet count (Saga et al. 1994), and is inversely associated with several coagulation factors (Shahar et al. 1993).

24.5 INFLAMMATORY DISEASE

Inflammation is an important component of the early immunologic response; however, when inflammation occurs in an uncontrolled manner, disease may arise. Thus, inappropriate or dysfunctional immune response underlies inflammatory diseases and conditions (Calder 2001). A large body of evidence has suggested that LCn-3PUFA has profound effects on the immune function as they exert a great influence on both cell-mediated and humoral immunity (Kelley et al. 1991). The marked anti-inflammatory effects of LCn-3PUFA might explain the beneficial effect that they have on the various inflammatory conditions characterized by an immune dysregulation. Clinical and experimental trials have suggested that LCn-3PUFA possesses anti-inflammatory effects by several different mechanisms. These include the decreased production of AA-derived eicosanoids, suppressed production of proinflammatory cytokines such as TNFα and CRP, and by modulating adhesion molecule expression (Lopez-Garcia et al. 2004; Zampelas et al. 2005). Indeed, clinical studies have reported that LCn-3PUFA supplementation has beneficial effects on inflammatory bowel disease, psoriasis, and rheumatoid arthritis supporting the anti-inflammatory properties of LCn-3PUFA (Calder 2001). Healthy female subjects (23–33 years) when given 2.4 g LCn-3PUFA/day for 3 months experienced decreased interleukin (IL)-1 beta synthesis by 48%, decreased IL-6 by 30%, and TNFα was reduced by 58% (Meydani et al. 1991). In patients with Crohn's disease (CD) recovering from relapse, those randomly assigned 5.1 g of LCn-3PUFA ethyl esters required a much lower amount of prednisolone necessary to control the disease compared to those on placebo. The investigators concluded that LCn-3PUFA supplementation has an effect on extending the remission of the chronic inflammatory condition, CD (Lorenz-Meyer et al. 1996). When 6 months of LCn-3PUFA (5.2 g) supplementation was given to MS patients, it resulted in significantly decreased production of IL-2 (Gallai et al. 1995), and in patients after abdominal surgery, parental nutrition supplemented with fish oil significantly decreased serum TNFα and IL-6 concentrations compared to those with the n-6PUFA-enriched parental nutrition (Wachtler et al. 1997).

Inflammation also plays an important role in the initiation and progression of atherosclerosis. It has been suggested that inflammation increases the risk of CVD and indeed there is a strong association between systemic inflammation and coronary artery disease (Ross 1999). Studies have reported significant reductions in lymphocyte proliferation after fish oil feeding (Molvig et al. 1991; Thies et al. 2001). Lower levels of ICAM-1 expression on the surface of blood monocytes in healthy male and female subjects (Hughes et al. 1996) and decreased circulating levels of VCAM-1 in elderly subjects (Miles et al. 2001) after an n-3 FA-enriched diet suggest that fish oil decreases cellular adhesion and endothelial activation. In conclusion, these studies show that LCn-3PUFA is potential anti-inflammatory agents providing benefits in chronic inflammatory diseases as well as in systemic inflammation and response to surgery.

24.6 BRAIN AND MENTAL HEALTH

Lipids comprise over 50% of the brain's dry weight and make up important structural components of membrane phospholipids. EPA and DHA are the PUFA that are incorporated into neuronal phospholipids (Yuen et al. 2005). The nervous system, particularly the brain, contains the highest concentration of DHA in the body (Salem et al. 2001). DHA is an important determinant of membrane fluidity, and it facilitates signal transduction, gene expression, ion channel, and the biodynamic activity of neuronal membranes (Sinn and Howe 2008). DHA also stimulates remyelination by stimulating the expression of peroxisomal enzymes, which is essential for plasmalogen synthesis in myelin formation. EPA also plays an important role in brain function via competition with AA for the synthesis of 3-series eicosanoids, which have vasodilatory, anti-inflammatory, and antithrombotic properties.

Since the importance of LCn-3PUFA in brain structure and function became apparent in the 1970s, interest in their functionality has steadily increased (Crawford and Sinclair 1971; Sinclair and Crawford 1972). Studies have revealed that LCn-3PUFA may be beneficial in a number of neurological and psychiatric disorders. Evidence suggests that the diminished LCn-3PUFA concentrations are associated with mood disorders. Many observational and intervention studies have been carried out on the effects of LCn-3PUFA in mental health, including Alzheimer's disease, dementia, depression, Parkinson's disease, and bipolar disorder and developmental disorders, including attention deficit hyperactivity disorder (ADHA).

24.6.1 ALZHEIMER'S DISEASE

Late-onset Alzheimer's disease (AD) is a multifactorial disease that results from the effect of aging and a complex interaction of both environmental and genetic risk factors (Blennow et al. 2006). Due to increased life expectancy in the Western countries, AD is becoming a major public health concern. No effective curative treatments are currently available for AD; therefore, developing novel preventative strategies are of great importance. Many epidemiologic studies have revealed that a reduction in levels or intake of LCn-3PUFA is inversely correlated with an increase in the risk for age-related cognitive decline or forms of dementia such as AD.

Previous studies have shown that an increased dietary consumption or blood levels of DHA appear beneficial in protection against AD and other forms of dementia; however, there are a few studies which suggest that people who carry the Apolipoprotein E (ApoE4) are at a greater risk of developing AD as the genotype limits protection (Rubinsztein et al. 1999). ApoE appears to act as an AD risk factor due to its effects on amyloid-beta (Aβ) metabolism by influencing soluble Aβ clearance and Aβ aggregation. The aggregation of the β-amyloid peptide into toxic Aβ oligomers is widely considered to be the effector in the early stages of AD. Interactions of Aβ oligomers with the synaptic membrane in turn activate proapoptotic signaling pathways. DHA has been shown to limit Aβ production and accumulation and also suppresses several Aβ-induced signal transduction pathways. DHA has been found to be neuroprotective via many mechanisms which include reduced arachidonic acid metabolites, neuroprotective DHA metabolites, and increased factors or downstream trophic signal transduction. DHA appears to reduce Aβ production by several mechanisms, including the induction of increased neuronal expression of an amyloid precursor-sorting protein, SorLa (also called LR11).

Compared to other methods studied to prevent AD such as antioxidants and nonsteroidal antiinflammatory drugs (NSAIDs), LCn-3PUFA is relatively inexpensive and have an excellent safety profile. Based on the findings in the epidemiological studies and research carried out to date, experts suggest that further clinical trials are needed to establish LCn-3PUFA, notably DHA, as a prevention or treatment of age-related cognitive decline, with a focus on the major public health concern, AD. Current clinical trials are being conducted to examine whether the effectiveness of DHA may be increased if it is begun early in life or if taken in conjunction with antioxidants.

24.6.2 DEPRESSION

Epidemiological studies have shown that societies with a diet that includes a large amount of fish, rich in LCn-3PUFA, appear to have a lower prevalence of major depression (Hibbeln 1998; Tanskanen et al. 2001), suggesting a link between LCn-3PUFA and depression. The neuronal cell membrane of the central nervous system contains high concentrations of LCn-3PUFA, and reduction in the LCn-3PUFA level can alter the membrane microstructure which could alter signal transduction and cause immunologic dysregulation, all of which could possibly increase the risk of developing depression (Horrobin and Bennett 1999; Logan 2003). It has been reported that patients with major depressive disorder have lower levels of LCn-3PUFA in serum and red blood cell membranes (Maes et al. 1996; Edwards et al. 1998). This suggests that LCn-3PUFA may have an antidepressant effect. It has been reported that studies using LCn-3PUFA alone has antidepressant effects in patients who suffer from treatment-resistant major depressive disorder, women with postpartum depression, and pregnant women with major depressive disorder and also schizophrenia (Puri et al. 2001, 2002; Su et al. 2001; Chiu et al. 2003; Freeman et al. 2006).

Many studies have been carried out on the association between depression and LCn-3PUFA intake. The first study on the beneficial effect of LCn-3PUFA in reducing symptoms in bipolar disorder was carried out by Stoll et al. in 1999. The results for this study were encouraging as it showed that LCn-3PUFA had a positive outcome in patients with bipolar disorder. LCn-3PUFA does appear to prevent depression but not mania among patients with bipolar disorder (Su et al. 2000; Chiu et al. 2005). Double-blind, placebo-controlled clinical trials have been carried out on the effect of LCn-3PUFA as antidepressants; however, these studies have reported inconsistent results. It is difficult to conclude whether LCn-3PUFA possesses antidepressive effects from the studies which have been carried out due to inadequate sample size, heterogeneity of the patients involved, and the composition and dose of LCn-3PUFA used (Nemets et al. 2002; Peet and Horrobin 2002; Llorente et al. 2003; Marangell et al. 2003; Su et al. 2003; Silvers et al. 2005; Frangou et al. 2006). It has also been found that in juvenile bipolar disorder (JBD), lower intakes of EPA, and DHA may contribute to increased symptoms, as it has been found that red blood cell membrane concentrations of DHA are negatively correlated to depression symptoms (Clayton et al. 2008). Many studies have provided evidence that the higher dosage of EPA does not significantly change the antidepressant efficacy. Due to depression being associated with diabetes mellitus, pregnancy and breast feeding, and heart diseases, LCn-3PUFA is a favorable supplementation which would be beneficial to the physical states of these patients. In order to determine the long-term efficacy of LCn-3PUFA in treating depression, as well as the optimal EPA and DHA composition and dosage, more large-scale, controlled studies are needed.

24.6.3 BIPOLAR DISORDER

Very few studies have examined for supplementation for bipolar disorder. Since the first placebo-controlled study by Stoll et al. on the beneficial effect of LCn-3PUFA in reducing symptoms in bipolar disorder revealed promising results, there has been a broad interest in the use of LCn-3PUFA for the treatment of bipolar disorder. Epidemiological studies have shown that the rates of bipolar disorder in various countries are negatively related to fish and seafood consumption (Hibbeln 2002). LCn-3PUFA may modulate the metabolism of neurotransmitters and are thought to inhibit neuronal signal transduction in a similar way to that of the two effective treatments of bipolar disorder, lithium and valproate (Osher et al. 2005). Previous studies have also supported the hypothesis that LCn-3PUFA alters neuronal membrane fluidity, with MRI results showing that patients with bipolar disorder who took LCn-3PUFA supplements experienced a significant dose-dependent decrease in their brain-water proton transverse (T2) relaxation times (Hirashima et al. 2004). Overall results involving LCn-3PUFA interventions have been conflicting; therefore, further studies to clarify the role, purity, and optimal dosage are required before LCn-3PUFA can be confidently recommended to patients.

24.6.4 PARKINSON'S DISEASE

Parkinson's disease (PD) is one of the most common neurodegenerative disorders. It is characterized primarily by motor symptoms but also includes pathological features such as mood disorders, autonomic system failures, and cognitive deficits. The prevalence of PD increases with age and is considered to be an important cause of chronic disability in the older population. It has become increasingly important for developing therapeutic strategies in order to delay the onset and prevent the progression of PD. Currently, there is no curative treatment for PD but there are pharmacological agents to treat the motor traits of PD such as levodopa (Fahn 2008) and other symptomatic treatments such as dopaminergic agonists (Lees et al. 2009). However, these treatments are unfavorable due to their side effects. Levodopa can cause motor complications, such as dyskinesias, with long-term use. As with other neurodegenerative disorders, LCn-3PUFA as a preventative treatment for PD has been considered.

Recent epidemiological studies and studies carried out in animal models have revealed that low plasma LCn-3PUFA levels may indicate therapeutic strategy for PD. A questionnaire-based study revealed that participants with Mediterranean diets, traditionally composed of vegetable, fruit, and fish, showed a reduced incidence of PD (Gao et al. 2007). This suggests that EPA and DHA are likely to play a role in this positive association. Similar findings have also been revealed in population-based cohort study, where participants were evaluated for the risk of developing PD in relation to a questionnaire-based assessment of dietary intake of FAs. A 6-year follow-up revealed that a high consumption of LCn-3PUFA was related to a reduced risk of PD (de Lau et al. 2005). These studies have provided strong clinical evidence; however, further intervention studies are required to confirm these correlative data.

It has been shown that LCn-3PUFA could be an inexpensive method as a neuroprotective strategy or a disease-modifying option to delay the appearance of symptoms of PD. LCn-3PUFA is also a favorable option as they are readily transferable to the clinical setting and further investigation into LCn-3PUFA and their potential symptomatologic effect as an add-on therapy to levodopa and other dopaminergic agonists need to be carried out.

24.6.5 ATTENTION-DEFICIT HYPERACTIVITY DISORDER

ADHD is a chronic neurobehavioral disorder which affects 3–5% of children globally (Association 2000). Symptoms include inattention, hyperactivity, and impulsivity (Barkley 1997). The exact mechanisms involved in ADHD are not fully understood, and current treatments involved in controlling ADHD symptoms are targeted at modulating dopaminergic and/or noradrenergic systems. These compounds include atomoxetine or methylphenidate (Curatolo et al. 2009). Many studies have indicated significant differences between ADHD and normal children in their fatty acid status. Generally, it appears that children with ADHD tend to have lower LCn-3PUFA, and also an elevated n-6/n-3 PUFA ratio. The first study that revealed a relationship between FA and ADHD was published in 1981 reporting that children with ADHD showed greater thirst compared to controls, which indicated that there were reduced nutritional levels of EFAs in these subjects (Colquhoun and Bunday 1981). This was further supported by several other studies which showed a difference in amounts of PUFA in the blood. A study carried out in 1987 by Mitchell et al. revealed that the serum levels of DHA, dihomogammalinolenic acid (DGLA), and arachidonic acid (AA) were significantly reduced in 44 children with ADHD compared to 45 control children of the same age. Stevens et al. (1995) also reported significantly lower EPA, DHA, and AA levels, as well as total LCn-3PUFA in plasma phospholipids of 53 boys with ADHD compared to 43 controls (Stevens et al. 1995).

It has recently been observed in a specific population that ADHD subjects had significantly higher EPA and DHA levels in both plasma and erythrocytes than healthy age-matched subjects (Spahis et al. 2008). The results were observed on a small sample size; however, it did reveal the importance of taking into account the origin of the population when making comparisons for a particular disorder across countries. Several reasons have been proposed to explain the abnormal EFA status in ADHD subjects such as increased metabolism of PUFAs, lower conversion of EFAs to LC-PUFAs and reduced PUFA intake (Burgess et al. 2000). However, many studies have contradicted these hypotheses, for example, a study which observed increased LCn-3PUFA levels in both plasma phospholipids and erythrocytes in a diagnosed ADHD population revealed no difference in LCn-3PUFA consumption (Antalis et al. 2006; Brookes et al. 2006). Therefore, more studies are needed to provide convincing results to support these hypotheses.

A recent genetic study has identified a significant relationship between the gene which codes for the enzyme involved in the metabolism of LCn-3PUFA, fatty acid desaturase 2 (FADS2), and ADHD. This preliminary finding may have highlighted a potential factor of abnormal LCn-3PUFA status in people with ADHD.

Despite the unknown exact mechanisms involved in the relationship between low EFA and ADHD, the findings of these previous studies have paved the way for further studies into the potential benefits of EFA supplementation to treat ADHD.

Many studies which have been carried out to observe the effects of EFA supplementation in ADHD have very different parameters such as the type and amount of supplement given, the form in which the supplement is given, the duration of the treatment, and also the tests used to evaluate ADHD symptoms. The wide variety of neuropsychological tests used demonstrates the difficulties of defining cognitive and behavioral performance and of identifying specific functions. Also, the diagnosis of ADHD in reported studies has not always been according to DSM-IV criteria and comorbidity existed with behavioral disorders in a number of subjects. These factors may have contributed to heterogeneity within groups.

It can be concluded from the reported studies to date that there is a link between low LC-PUFA and the occurrence of ADHD; however, the beneficial effects of nutritional supplementation have not yet been clearly demonstrated. New and improved studies are needed to observe the beneficial effects of LC-PUFA. Further studies which include placebo-controlled studies with sufficient sample size are required. The inclusion of homogenous populations which include nonmedicated ADHD subjects would also be preferable to determine specific responders' profiles. Studies which include supplements combining both n-3 and n-6 over a prolonged period also need to be conducted (Brookes et al. 2006).

In summary, there are still conflicting indications derived from studies for their possible use of LCn-3PUFA as a supplementary treatment for symptoms. Further clinical studies are needed to investigate the long-term effects of LCn-3PUFA supplementation and also the biological mechanisms for their effects on mental health and brain function.

24.7 WEIGHT MANAGEMENT

The etiology of diabetes, CVD, and inflammatory disease is often associated with obesity. Obesity is a global epidemic throughout the world, affecting developed as well as many developing countries (WHO 2000; Ma et al. 2003). LCn-3PUFA has been shown to suppress appetite, improve blood circulation, increase fat oxidation and energy expenditure, and reduce fat deposition (Buckley and Howe 2010). Several animal studies have suggested that an increased consumption of EPA and DHA can prevent obesity and can reduce body fat in already obese animals. Reduction in body weight in these studies has been associated with alterations in gene expression in tissues that favor increased fat oxidation and reduced fat disposition (Hainault et al. 1993). Some of these studies have shown that reduction in body weight is related to a decrease in food intake and apoptosis of adipocytes (Perez-Matute et al. 2007). Limited human studies also provide evidence that suggests LCn-3PUFA may decrease body fat in humans (Parra et al. 2008). These studies have also revealed that in some cases this reduction may be linked to appetite suppression and increases in fat oxidation and energy expenditure (Buckley and Howe 2009). Carefully designed long-term intervention studies, especially when combined with low-calorie diets and/or increased exercise levels, are required to delineate efficacy and to confirm whether increased LCn-3PUFA is an effective strategy in combating obesity.

24.8 SKIN HEALTH

The first study which identified the benefit of dietary fats in the treatment of skin disease was carried out by Burr and Burr in 1929. It was found that when rats were fed a diet containing no fat, they experienced growth retardation, reproductive failure, and scaling erythema with greater transepidermal water loss. These symptoms were reduced when the diet was supplemented with LA and ALA. Early experiments also revealed that dermatitis could be treated by consumption of these PUFAs (Burr and Burr 1929).

These original investigations have been criticized due to the lack of distinction between supplementation with omega-6 (LA) and omega-3 (ALA) FAs. This differentiation is important due to their roles which we have now found to be distinct.

Linoleic acid and its derivatives play an important role in the structure and function of the permeability barrier for the stratum corneum. ALA derivatives are able to modulate the immune response of the epidermis by activating T lymphocytes, acting on Toll-like receptors (TLRs), and also by activating caspase cascades which influence a number of inflammatory dermatoses, such as psoriasis, acne vulgaris, systemic lupus erythematosus, atopic dermatitis, and skin cancer.

LCn-3PUFA serves as ligands for the peroxisome proliferator-activated receptors (PPARs), an important class of transcription factors in lipid metabolism, insulin sensitization, and sugar homeostasis. They have also been shown to be natural options for treatment of inflammatory skin disease and carcinogenesis of the skin (McCusker and Grant-Kels 2010). DHA and EPA are not major components of the epidermis; this is likely to be due to insufficient dietary intake or greater cellular utilization. It appears that LCn-3PUFA plays an immune-modulating role in the epidermis. EPA appears to reduce T-lymphocyte proliferation, reduce expression of intracellular adhesion molecule-1, and inhibit delayed-type hypersensitivity (Kelley et al. 1991; Hughes et al. 1996). Also, it has been revealed that an enzyme, 15-lipoxygenase, in the epidermis converts PUFAs into anti-inflammatory mediators that lower production of the potent anti-inflammatory and antimicrobial mediator, leukotriene B4, which is formed from the proinflammatory. Increased levels of leukotriene B4 has been discovered in guttate psoriasis lesions (Fogh et al. 1989).

DHA and EPA have been shown to improve psoriasis in hospitalized patients where individuals supplemented with 4 g of EPA daily showed an increased sunburn threshold, reduced p-53 expression, and a reduction in strand breaks in peripheral blood leukocytes (Mayser et al. 1998). LCn-3PUFA has also been a focus for many studies for treatment and prevention of cancer. A 20-year observational study of the Inuit, a population which is known for its large fish consumption, has reported lower rates of both melanoma and nonmelanoma skin cancer (Miller and Gaudette 1996). In the prevention of nonmelanoma skin cancer, DHA and EPA have been of interest to oncologists due to their ability to enhance the effect of chemotherapeutic drugs and also for the protection against bowel cancer (Biondo et al. 2008; Giros et al. 2009). DHA and EPA have been shown to have a proapoptotic effect on colorectal cancer cells by activation of intrinsic and extrinsic caspase cascades. There is strong evidence that DHA and EPA enhance the effectiveness of treatments for many malignancies (Biondo et al. 2008).

24.9 DIETARY DELIVERY OF LCn-3PUFA: TECHNOLOGICAL CHALLENGES

Since LCn-3PUFA has been shown to be essential for brain development and cognitive function as well as for the prevention of CVD, inflammatory diseases, dyslexia, and depression, health authorities all over the world recommend increased consumption of foods containing LCn-3PUFA. However, a large majority of people do not eat seafood on a regular basis because of its cost and availability, and many individuals do not like the flavor/taste/odor of seafood. Functional foods enriched with LCn-3PUFA could play an important role in meeting the dietary recommendations for optimal health. Recent developments in food technology have made possible the enrichment of foods, such as dairy products, bread, eggs, biscuits, lollies, pasta, margarines, and other spreads, with reasonable shelf life but without undesirable fish odor/taste. Microemulsification and nanotechnologies allow fortification of the foods with a relatively large amount of LCn-3PUFA per serve with optimized bioavailability following consumption.

24.10 CONCLUSIONS AND FUTURE RESEARCH DIRECTIONS

It is evident from the information presented in this chapter that there is a need to develop functional foods that can deliver the recommended levels of LCn-3PUFA. It is noteworthy that the total fat content, particularly the level of SFA, must not exceed the dietary guidelines. The fortified food must be convenient, palatable, with no fishy odor/flavor and no fishy eructation following consumption. The food matrix should provide minimum or no resistance for the release of LCn-3PUFA in the gastrointestinal tract to ensure bioavailability. Particular attention needs to be paid to the matrix used for microemulsification, as this may be an important criterion for the bioavailability of LCn-3PUFA. Quantitative data on bioavailability of LCn-3PUFA from the enriched foods are lacking in the literature and warrant investigations. It may also be beneficial to combine LCn-3PUFA with other ingredients in a single food to optimize their health benefits. One such ideal combination may be the synergistic effects of LCn-3PUFA and plant sterols on plasma lipids and the risk for developing CVD. Plant sterols are known to reduce plasma and LDL-cholesterol, while the triglyceride-lowering properties of LCn-3PUFA are well established. The combination of the two may be ideal to achieve overall lipid-lowering effects from a single food and maximum cardioprotection (Micallef and Garg 2008, 2009a,b). Similarly, LCn-3PUFA can be combined with other dietary ingredients, such as carotenoids, in order to maximize the anti-inflammatory effects for the prevention of rheumatoid arthritis, diabetes, asthma, and inflammatory bowel disease. The development of functional foods enriched with larger amounts of LCn-3PUFA and testing for bioavailability, and biological and clinical effects require a concerted team effort, including food technologists, clinical nutritionists, and food manufacturers in close association with regulatory bodies.

REFERENCES

Akiba, S., T. Murata et al. 2000. Involvement of lipoxygenase pathway in docosapentaenoic acid-induced inhibition of platelet aggregation. *Biol Pharm Bull* 23(11): 1293–7.

Albert, C. M., C. H. Hennekens et al. 1998. Fish consumption and risk of sudden cardiac death. *JAMA* 279(1): 23–8.

Antalis, C. J., L. J. Stevens et al. 2006. Omega-3 fatty acid status in attention-deficit/hyperactivity disorder. *Prostaglandins Leukot Essent Fatty Acids* 75(4–5): 299–308.

Appel, L. J., E. R. Miller, 3rd et al. 1993. Does supplementation of diet with 'fish oil' reduce blood pressure? A meta-analysis of controlled clinical trials. *Arch Intern Med* 153(12): 1429–38.

Association, A. P. 2000. *Diagnostic and Statistical Manual of Mental Disorders*. Arlington, VA, American Psychiatric Association.

Axelrod, L., J. Camuso et al. 1994. Effects of a small quantity of omega-3 fatty acids on cardiovascular risk factors in NIDDM. A randomized, prospective, double-blind, controlled study. *Diabetes Care* 17(1): 37–44.

Bang, H. O. and J. Dyerberg 1972. Plasma lipids and lipoproteins in Greenlandic west coast Eskimos. *Acta Med Scand* 192(1–2): 85–94.

Bang, H. O. and J. Dyerberg 1980. The bleeding tendency in Greenland Eskimos. *Dan Med Bull* 27(4): 202–5.

Bang, H. O., J. Dyerberg et al. 1980. The composition of the Eskimo food in north western Greenland. *Am J Clin Nutr* 33(12): 2657–61.

Barkley, R. A. 1997. Behavioral inhibition, sustained attention, and executive functions: Constructing a unifying theory of ADHD. *Psychol Bull* 121(1): 65–94.

Biondo, P. D., D. N. Brindley et al. 2008. The potential for treatment with dietary long-chain polyunsaturated n-3 fatty acids during chemotherapy. *J Nutr Biochem* 19(12): 787–96.

Blennow, K., M. J. de Leon et al. 2006. Alzheimer's disease. *Lancet* 368(9533): 387–403.

Brookes, K. J., W. Chen et al. 2006. Association of fatty acid desaturase genes with attention-deficit/hyperactivity disorder. *Biol Psychiatry* 60(10): 1053–61.

Buckley, J. D. and P. R. Howe 2009. Anti-obesity effects of long-chain omega-3 polyunsaturated fatty acids. *Obes Rev* 10(6): 648–59.

Buckley, J. D. and P. R. C. Howe 2010. Long chain omega-3 polyunsaturated fatty acids may be beneficial for reducing obesity. *Nutrients* 2: 1212–30.

Burdge, G. C. and P. C. Calder. 2005. Conversion of alpha-linolenic acid to longer-chain polyunsaturated fatty acids in human adults. *Reprod Nutr Dev* 45(5): 581–97.

Burgess, J. R., L. Stevens et al. 2000. Long-chain polyunsaturated fatty acids in children with attention-deficit hyperactivity disorder. *Am J Clin Nutr* 71(1 Suppl): 327S–30S.

Burr, G. O. and M. M. Burr 1929. A new deficiency disease produced by the rigid exclusion of fat from the diet. *J Biol Chem* 82: 345–67.

Burr, M. L., P. A. Ashfield-Watt et al. 2003. Lack of benefit of dietary advice to men with angina: Results of a controlled trial. *Eur J Clin Nutr* 57(2): 193–200.

Burr, M. L., A. M. Fehily et al. 1989. Effects of changes in fat, fish, and fibre intakes on death and myocardial reinfarction: Diet and reinfarction trial (DART). *Lancet* 2(8666): 757–61.

Calder, P. C. 2001. Polyunsaturated fatty acids, inflammation, and immunity. *Lipids* 36(9): 1007–24.

Calder, P. C. 2009. Polyunsaturated fatty acids and inflammatory processes: New twist in an old tale. *Biochimie* (91): 791–95.

Chiu, C. C., S. Y. Huang et al. 2003. Omega-3 fatty acids for depression in pregnancy. *Am J Psychiatry* 160(2): 385.

Chiu, C. C., S. Y. Huang et al. 2005. Omega-3 fatty acids are more beneficial in the depressive phase than in the manic phase in patients with bipolar I disorder. *J Clin Psychiatry* 66(12): 1613–4.

Clayton, E. H., T. L. Hanstock et al. 2008. Long-chain omega-3 polyunsaturated fatty acids in the blood of children and adolescents with juvenile bipolar disorder. *Lipids* 43(11): 1031–8.

Colquhoun, I. and S. Bunday 1981. A lack of essential fatty acids as a possible cause of hyperactivity in children. *Med Hypotheses* 7(5): 673–9.

Crawford, M. A. and A. J. Sinclair 1971. Nutritional influences in the evolution of mammalian brain. In: Lipids, malnutrition & the developing brain. *Ciba Found Symp* 267–92.

Curatolo, P., C. Paloscia et al. 2009. The neurobiology of attention deficit/hyperactivity disorder. *Eur J Paediatr Neurol* 13(4): 299–304.

Daviglus, M. L., J. Stamler et al. 1997. Fish consumption and the 30-year risk of fatal myocardial infarction. *N Engl J Med* 336(15): 1046–53.

de Lau, L. M., M. Bornebroek et al. 2005. Dietary fatty acids and risk of Parkinsons disease: Rotterdam study. *Neurology* 12(64): 2040–5.

Dyerberg, J. and H. O. Bang 1979. Haemostatic function and platelet polyunsaturated fatty acids in Eskimos. *Lancet* 2(8140): 433–5.

Dyerberg, J. and H. O. Bang 1980. Proposed method for the prevention of thrombosis. The Eskimo model. *Ugeskr Laeger* 142(25): 1597–600.

Dyerberg, J., H. O. Bang et al. 1975. Fatty acid composition of the plasma lipids in Greenland Eskimos. *Am J Clin Nutr* 28(9): 958–66.

Dyerberg, J., H. O. Bang et al. 1977. Plasma cholesterol concentration in Caucasian Danes and Greenland West-coast Eskimos. *Dan Med Bull* 24(2): 52–5.

Dyerberg, J. and K. A. Jorgensen 1982. Marine oils and thrombogenesis. *Prog Lipid Res* 21(4): 255–69.

Edwards, R., M. Peet et al. 1998. Omega-3 polyunsaturated fatty acid levels in the diet and in red blood cell membranes of depressed patients. *J Affect Disord* 48(2–3): 149–55.

Erkkila, A. T., A. H. Lichtenstein et al. 2004. Fish intake is associated with a reduced progression of coronary artery atherosclerosis in postmenopausal women with coronary artery disease. *Am J Clin Nutr* 80(3): 626–32.

Fahn, S. 2008. The history of dopamine and levodopa in the treatment of Parkinson's disease. *Movement. Disorders* 23: S497–508.

Fogh, K., T. Herlin et al. 1989. Eicosanoids in acute and chronic psoriatic lesions: Leukotriene B4, but not 12-hydroxy-eicosatetraenoic acid, is present in biologically active amounts in acute guttate lesions. *J Invest Dermatol* 92(6): 837–41.

Frangou, S., M. Lewis et al. 2006. Efficacy of ethyl-eicosapentaenoic acid in bipolar depression: Randomised double-blind placebo-controlled study. *Br J Psychiatry* 188: 46–50.

Freeman, M. P., J. R. Hibbeln et al. 2006. Randomized dose-ranging pilot trial of omega-3 fatty acids for postpartum depression. *Acta Psychiatr Scand* 113(1): 31–5.

Gallai, V., P. Sarchielli et al. 1995. Cytokine secretion and eicosanoid production in the peripheral blood mononuclear cells of MS patients undergoing dietary supplementation with n-3 polyunsaturated fatty acids. *J Neuroimmunol* 56(2): 143–53.

Gao, X., H. Chen et al. 2007. Prospective study of dietary pattern and risk of Parkinson disease. *Am J Clin Nutr* 86(5): 1486–94.

Gaudette, D. C. and B. J. Holub 1990. Albumin-bound docosahexaenoic acid and collagen-induced human platelet reactivity. *Lipids* 25(3): 166–9.

Geleijnse, J. M., E. J. Giltay et al. 2002. Blood pressure response to fish oil supplementation: Metaregression analysis of randomized trials. *J Hypertens* 20(8): 1493–9.

Gerster, H. 1998. Can adults adequately convert alpha-linolenic acid (18:3n-3) to eicosapentaenoic acid (20:5n-3) and docosahexaenoic acid (22:6n-3)? *Int J Vitam Nutr Res* 68(3): 159–73.

Giros, A., M. Grzybowski et al. 2009. Regulation of colorectal cancer cell apoptosis by the n-3 polyunsaturated fatty acids docosahexaenoic and eicosapentaenoic. *Cancer Prev Res (Phila)* 2(8): 732–42.

GISSI 1999. Dietary supplementation with n-3 polyunsaturated fatty acids and vitamin E after myocardial infarction: Results of the GISSI-Prevenzione trial. Gruppo Italiano per lo Studio della Sopravvivenza nell'Infarto miocardico. *Lancet* 354(9177): 447–55.

Grundt, H. and D. W. Nilsen 2008. n-3 Fatty acids and cardiovascular disease. *Haematologica* 93(6): 807–12.

Hainault, I., M. Carolotti et al. 1993. Fish oil in a high lard diet prevents obesity, hyperlipemia, and adipocyte insulin resistance in rats. *Ann N Y Acad Sci* 683: 98–101.

Hamazaki, T., M. Urakaze et al. 1988. Comparison of pulse wave velocity of the aorta between inhabitants of fishing and farming villages in Japan. *Atherosclerosis* 73(2–3): 157–60.

Harris, W. S., W. E. Connor et al. 1981. Dietary fish oils, plasma lipids and platelets in man. *Prog Lipid Res* 20: 75–9.

Harris, W. S., M. Miller et al. 2008. Omega-3 fatty acids and coronary heart disease risk: Clinical and mechanistic perspectives. *Atherosclerosis* 197(1): 12–24.

Harris, W. S., D. Mozaffarian et al. 2009. Omega-6 fatty acids and risk for cardiovascular disease: A science advisory from the American Heart Association Nutrition Subcommittee of the Council on Nutrition, Physical Activity, and Metabolism; Council on Cardiovascular Nursing; and Council on Epidemiology and Prevention. *Circulation* 119(6): 902–7.

Hibbeln, J. R. 1998. Fish consumption and major depression. *Lancet* 351(9110): 1213.

Hibbeln, J. R. 2002. Seafood consumption, the DHA content of mothers' milk and prevalence rates of postpartum depression: A cross-national, ecological analysis. *J Affect Disord* 69: 15–29.

Hirashima, F., A. M. Parow et al. 2004. Omega-3 fatty acid treatment and T(2) whole brain relaxation times in bipolar disorder. *Am J Psychiatry* 161(10): 1922–4.

Hjerkinn, E. M., I. Seljeflot et al. 2005. Influence of long-term intervention with dietary counseling, long-chain n-3 fatty acid supplements, or both on circulating markers of endothelial activation in men with long-standing hyperlipidemia. *Am J Clin Nutr* 81(3): 583–9.

Horrobin, D. F. and C. N. Bennett 1999. Depression and bipolar disorder: Relationships to impaired fatty acid and phospholipid metabolism and to diabetes, cardiovascular disease, immunological abnormalities, cancer, ageing and osteoporosis. Possible candidate genes. *Prostaglandins Leukot Essent Fatty Acids* 60(4): 217–34.

Hu, F. B., L. Bronner et al. 2002. Fish and omega-3 fatty acid intake and risk of coronary heart disease in women. *JAMA* 287(14): 1815–21.

Hughes, D. A., A. C. Pinder et al. 1996. Fish oil supplementation inhibits the expression of major histocompatibility complex class II molecules and adhesion molecules on human monocytes. *Am J Clin Nutr* 63(2): 267–72.

Huikuri, H. V., A. Castellanos et al. 2001. Sudden death due to cardiac arrhythmias. *N Engl J Med* 345(20): 1473–82.

Kelley, D. S., L. B. Branch et al. 1991. Dietary alpha-linolenic acid and immunocompetence in humans. *Am J Clin Nutr* 53(1): 40–6.

Kinsella, J. E., B. Lokesh et al. 1990. Dietary n-3 polyunsaturated fatty acids and amelioration of cardiovascular disease: Possible mechanisms. *Am J Clin Nutr* 52(1): 1–28.

Knapp, H. R., I. A. Reilly et al. 1986. In vivo indexes of platelet and vascular function during fish-oil administration in patients with atherosclerosis. *N Engl J Med* 314(15): 937–42.

Kromhout, D., E. B. Bosschieter et al. 1985. The inverse relation between fish consumption and 20-year mortality from coronary heart disease. *N Engl J Med* 312(19): 1205–9.

Kromhout, D., E. J. Feskens et al. 1995. The protective effect of a small amount of fish on coronary heart disease mortality in an elderly population. *Int J Epidemiol* 24(2): 340–5.

Lees, A. J., J. Hardy, T. Revesz. 2009. Parkinson's disease. *Lancet* 373: 2055–2066.

Llorente, A. M., C. L. Jensen et al. 2003. Effect of maternal docosahexaenoic acid supplementation on postpartum depression and information processing. *Am J Obstet Gynecol* 188(5): 1348–53.

Logan, A. C. 2003. Neurobehavioral aspects of omega-3 fatty acids: Possible mechanisms and therapeutic value in major depression. *Altern Med Rev* 8(4): 410–25.

Lopez-Garcia, E., M. B. Schulze et al. 2004. Consumption of (n-3) fatty acids is related to plasma biomarkers of inflammation and endothelial activation in women. *J Nutr* 134(7): 1806–11.

Lorenz-Meyer, H., P. Bauer et al. 1996. Omega-3 fatty acids and low carbohydrate diet for maintenance of remission in Crohn's disease. A randomized controlled multicenter trial. Study Group Members (German Crohn's Disease Study Group). *Scand J Gastroenterol* 31(8): 778–85.

Ma, Y., E. R. Bertone et al. 2003. Association between eating patterns and obesity in a free-living US adult population. *Am J Epidemiol* 158(1): 85–92.

Maes, M., R. Smith et al. 1996. Fatty acid composition in major depression: Decreased omega 3 fractions in cholesteryl esters and increased C20: 4 omega 6/C20:5 omega 3 ratio in cholesteryl esters and phospholipids. *J Affect Disord* 38(1): 35–46.

Marangell, L. B., J. M. Martinez et al. 2003. A double-blind, placebo-controlled study of the omega-3 fatty acid docosahexaenoic acid in the treatment of major depression. *Am J Psychiatry* 160(5): 996–8.

Marmot, M. G., S. L. Syme et al. 1975. Epidemiologic studies of coronary heart disease and stroke in Japanese men living in Japan, Hawaii and California: Prevalence of coronary and hypertensive heart disease and associated risk factors. *Am J Epidemiol* 102(6): 514–25.

Mayser, P., U. Mrowietz et al. 1998. Omega-3 fatty acid-based lipid infusion in patients with chronic plaque psoriasis: Results of a double-blind, randomized, placebo-controlled, multicenter trial. *J Am Acad Dermatol* 38(4): 539–47.

McCusker, M. M. and J. M. Grant-Kels 2010. Healing fats of the skin: The structural and immunologic roles of the omega-6 and omega-3 fatty acids. *Clin Dermatol* 28(4): 440–51.

Meydani, S. N., S. Endres et al. 1991. Oral (n-3) fatty acid supplementation suppresses cytokine production and lymphocyte proliferation: Comparison between young and older women. *J Nutr* 121(4): 547–55.

Micallef, M. A. and M. L. Garg 2008. The lipid-lowering effects of phytosterols and (n-3) polyunsaturated fatty acids are synergistic and complementary in hyperlipidemic men and women. *J Nutr* 138(6): 1086–90.

Micallef, M. A. and M. L. Garg 2009a. Anti-inflammatory and cardioprotective effects of n-3 polyunsaturated fatty acids and plant sterols in hyperlipidemic individuals. *Atherosclerosis* 204(2): 476–82.

Micallef, M. A. and M. L. Garg 2009b. Beyond blood lipids: Phytosterols, statins and omega-3 polyunsaturated fatty acid therapy for hyperlipidemia. *J Nutr Biochem* 20(12): 927–39.

Miles, E. A., F. Thies et al. 2001. Influence of age and dietary fish oil on plasma soluble adhesion molecule concentrations. *Clin Sci (Lond)* 100(1): 91–100.

Miller, A. B. and L. A. Gaudette 1996. Cancers of skin, bone, connective tissues, brain, eye, thyroid and other specified and unspecified sites in Inuit. *Acta Oncol* 35(5): 607–16.

Mitchell, E. A., M. G. Aman et al. 1987. Clinical characteristics and serum essential fatty acid levels in hyperactive children. *Clin Pediatr* 26(8): 406–411.

Molvig, J., F. Pociot et al. 1991. Dietary supplementation with omega-3-polyunsaturated fatty acids decreases mononuclear cell proliferation and interleukin-1 beta content but not monokine secretion in healthy and insulin-dependent diabetic individuals. *Scand J Immunol* 34(4): 399–410.

Mori, T. A., L. J. Beilin et al. 1997. Interactions between dietary fat, fish, and fish oils and their effects on platelet function in men at risk of cardiovascular disease. *Arterioscler Thromb Vasc Biol* 17(2): 279–86.

Morris, M. C., F. Sacks et al. 1993. Does fish oil lower blood pressure? A meta-analysis of controlled trials. *Circulation* 88(2): 523–33.

Mozaffarian, D., R. N. Lemaitre et al. 2003. Cardiac benefits of fish consumption may depend on the type of fish meal consumed: The Cardiovascular Health Study. *Circulation* 107(10): 1372–7.

Nagakawa, Y., H. Orimo et al. 1983. Effect of eicosapentaenoic acid on the platelet aggregation and composition of fatty acid in man. A double blind study. *Atherosclerosis* 47(1): 71–5.

Needleman, P., M. Minkes et al. 1976. Thromboxanes: Selective biosynthesis and distinct biological properties. *Science* 193(4248): 163–5.

Nemets, B., Z. Stahl et al. 2002. Addition of omega-3 fatty acid to maintenance medication treatment for recurrent unipolar depressive disorder. *Am J Psychiatry* 159(3): 477–9.

Ness, A. R., J. Hughes et al. 2002. The long-term effect of dietary advice in men with coronary disease: Follow-up of the Diet and Reinfarction trial (DART). *Eur J Clin Nutr* 56(6): 512–8.

Newman, W. P., J. P. Middaugh et al. 1993. Atherosclerosis in Alaska Natives and non-natives. *Lancet* 341(8852): 1056–7.

Osher, Y., Y. Bersudsky et al. 2005. Omega-3 eicosapentaenoic acid in bipolar depression: Report of a small open-label study. *J Clin Psychiatry* 66(6): 726–9.

Parra, D., A. Ramel et al. 2008. A diet rich in long chain omega-3 fatty acids modulates satiety in overweight and obese volunteers during weight loss. *Appetite* 51(3): 676–80.

Peet, M. and D. F. Horrobin. 2002. A dose-ranging study of the effects of ethyl-eicosapentaenoate in patients with ongoing depression despite apparently adequate treatment with standard drugs. *Arch Gen Psychiatry* 59(10): 913–9.

Perez-Matute, P., N. Perez-Echarri et al. 2007. Eicosapentaenoic acid actions on adiposity and insulin resistance in control and high-fat-fed rats: Role of apoptosis, adiponectin and tumour necrosis factor-alpha. *Br J Nutr* 97(2): 389–98.

Prichard, B. N., C. C. Smith et al. 1995. Fish oils and cardiovascular disease. *BMJ* 310(6983): 819–20.

Prisco, D., M. Filippini et al. 1995. Effect of n-3 fatty acid ethyl ester supplementation on fatty acid composition of the single platelet phospholipids and on platelet functions. *Metabolism* 44(5): 562–9.

Puri, B. K., S. J. Counsell et al. 2001. Eicosapentaenoic acid in treatment-resistant depression associated with symptom remission, structural brain changes and reduced neuronal phospholipid turnover. *Int J Clin Pract* 55(8): 560–3.

Puri, B. K., S. J. Counsell et al. 2002. Eicosapentaenoic acid in treatment-resistant depression. *Arch Gen Psychiatry* 59(1): 91–2.

Ross, R. 1999. Atherosclerosis—An inflammatory disease. *N Engl J Med* 340(2): 115–26.

Rubinsztein, D. C., J. Hon et al. 1999. Apo E genotypes and risk of dementia in Down syndrome. *Am J Med Genet* 88(4): 344–7.

Saga, T., T. Aoyama et al. 1994. Changes in platelet count and mean volume of platelet after administration of icosapentaenoic acid ethyl-ester, and factors that may affect those changes. *Nippon Ronen Igakkai Zasshi* 31(7): 538–47.

Salem, N., Jr., B. Litman et al. 2001. Mechanisms of action of docosahexaenoic acid in the nervous system. *Lipids* 36(9): 945–59.

Salmon, J. A. and T. Terano 1985. Supplementation of the diet with eicosapentaenoic acid: A possible approach to the treatment of thrombosis and inflammation. *Proc Nutr Soc* 44(3): 385–9.

Sanders, T. A., D. J. Naismith et al. 1980. Cod-liver oil, platelet fatty acids, and bleeding time. *Lancet* 1(8179): 1189.

Scheurlen, M., M. Kirchner et al. 1993. Fish oil preparations rich in docosahexaenoic acid modify platelet responsiveness to prostaglandin-endoperoxide/thromboxane A2 receptor agonists. *Biochem Pharmacol* 46(2): 245–9.

Shahar, E., A. R. Folsom et al. 1993. Associations of fish intake and dietary n-3 polyunsaturated fatty acids with a hypocoagulable profile. The Atherosclerosis Risk in Communities (ARIC) Study. *Arterioscler Thromb* 13(8): 1205–12.

Silvers, K. M., C. C. Woolley et al. 2005. Randomised double-blind placebo-controlled trial of fish oil in the treatment of depression. *Prostaglandins Leukot Essent Fatty Acids* 72(3): 211–8.

Sinclair, A. J. and M. A. Crawford 1972. The accumulation of arachidonate and docosahexaenoate in the developing rat brain. *J Neurochem* 19(7): 1753–8.

Sinn, N., P. R. C. Howe 2008. Mental health benefits of omega-3 fatty acids may be mediated by improvements in cerebral vascular function. *Bioscience Hypotheses* 1: 103–8.

Spahis, S., M. Vanasse et al. 2008. Lipid profile, fatty acid composition and pro- and anti-oxidant status in pediatric patients with attention-deficit/hyperactivity disorder. *Prostaglandins Leukot Essent Fatty Acids* 79(1–2): 47–53.

Srivastava, K. C. 1985. Docosahexaenoic acid (C22:6 omega 3) and linoleic acid are anti-aggregatory, and alter arachidonic acid metabolism in human platelets. *Prostaglandins Leukot Med* 17(3): 319–27.

Stamler, J., R. Stamler et al. 1993. Blood pressure, systolic and diastolic, and cardiovascular risks. US population data. *Arch Intern Med* 153(5): 598–615.

Stevens, L. J., S. S. Zentall et al. 1995. Essential fatty acid metabolism in boys with attention-deficit hyperactivity disorder. *Am J Clin Nutr* 62(4): 761–8.

Su, K. P., S. Y. Huang et al. 2003. Omega-3 fatty acids in major depressive disorder. A preliminary double-blind, placebo-controlled trial. *Eur Neuropsychopharmacol* 13(4): 267–71.

Su, K. P., W. W. Shen et al. 2000. Are omega3 fatty acids beneficial in depression but not mania? *Arch Gen Psychiatry* 57(7): 716–7.

Su, K. P., W. W. Shen et al. 2001. Omega-3 fatty acids as a psychotherapeutic agent for a pregnant schizophrenic patient. *Eur Neuropsychopharmacol* 11(4): 295–9.

Tamura, Y., A. Hirai et al. 1987. Anti-thrombotic and anti-atherogenic action of eicosapentaenoic acid. *Jpn Circ J* 51(4): 471–7.

Tanskanen, A., J. R. Hibbeln et al. 2001. Fish consumption and depressive symptoms in the general population in Finland. *Psychiatr Serv* 52(4): 529–31.

Thies, F., G. Nebe-von-Caron et al. 2001. Dietary supplementation with gamma-linolenic acid or fish oil decreases T lymphocyte proliferation in healthy older humans. *J Nutr* 131(7): 1918–27.

von Schacky, C., S. Fischer et al. 1985. Long-term effects of dietary marine omega-3 fatty acids upon plasma and cellular lipids, platelet function, and eicosanoid formation in humans. *J Clin Invest* 76(4): 1626–31.

von Schacky, C. and P. C. Weber 1985. Metabolism and effects on platelet function of the purified eicosapentaenoic and docosahexaenoic acids in humans. *J Clin Invest* 76(6): 2446–50.

Wachtler, P., W. Konig et al. 1997. Influence of a total parenteral nutrition enriched with omega-3 fatty acids on leukotriene synthesis of peripheral leukocytes and systemic cytokine levels in patients with major surgery. *J Trauma* 42(2): 191–8.

Wensing, A. G., R. P. Mensink et al. 1999. Effects of dietary n-3 polyunsaturated fatty acids from plant and marine origin on platelet aggregation in healthy elderly subjects. *Br J Nutr* 82(3): 183–91.

WHO 2000. Obesity: Preventing and managing the global epidemic. Report of a WHO consultation. *World Health Organ Tech Rep Ser* 894: i–xii, 1–253.

Yamada, T., J. P. Strong et al. 2000. Atherosclerosis and omega-3 fatty acids in the populations of a fishing village and a farming village in Japan. *Atherosclerosis* 153(2): 469–81.

Yuan, J. M., R. K. Ross et al. 2001. Fish and shellfish consumption in relation to death from myocardial infarction among men in Shanghai, China. *Am J Epidemiol* 154(9): 809–16.

Yuen, A. W., J. W. Sander et al. 2005. Omega-3 fatty acid supplementation in patients with chronic epilepsy: A randomized trial. *Epilepsy Behav* 7(2): 253–8.

Yzebe, D. and M. Lievre 2004. Fish oils in the care of coronary heart disease patients: A meta-analysis of randomized controlled trials. *Fundam Clin Pharmacol* 18(5): 581–92.

Zampelas, A., D. B. Panagiotakos et al. 2005. Fish consumption among healthy adults is associated with decreased levels of inflammatory markers related to cardiovascular disease: The ATTICA study. *J Am Coll Cardiol* 46(1): 120–4.

Zhang, J., S. Sasaki et al. 1999. Fish consumption and mortality from all causes, ischemic heart disease, and stroke: An ecological study. *Prev Med* 28(5): 520–9.

25 Assessment of Polyphenol-Rich Foods and Beverages on Endothelial (Vascular) Function in Healthy Humans

Mark L. Dreher

CONTENTS

25.1 INTRODUCTION

Although established cardiovascular disease (CVD) risk factors such as dyslipidemia, hypertension, and type 2 diabetes are the primary focus of lifestyle modification, emerging clinical evidence indicates that lifestyle factors such as poor dietary habits, mental stress, inactivity, and excess body weight can also increase endothelial dysfunction in healthy people, which may accelerate early atherosclerosis progression (Marin et al., 2011; USDA and HHS, 2010; Caballero et al., 2008; Hamilton et al., 2007; Ignarro et al., 2007; Mozaffarian et al., 2005; Desideri et al., 2005; Aggoun et al., 2005; Spieker et al., 2002; Ghiadoni et al., 2000; McGill et al., 2000; Duffy et al., 1999; Hashimoto et al., 1998; Clarkson et al., 1996). There is growing clinical evidence that dietary and other lifestyle factors can help to maintain healthy endothelial function (Pase et al., 2011; Marin et al., 2011; Raghuveer, 2010; Heiss et al., 2010; Yeboah et al., 2009; Aggoun et al., 2008; Caballero et al., 2008; Juonala et al., 2008; Mozaffarian et al., 2008; Kato et al., 2006; Mancini, 2004;

Quyyumi, 2003; Teragawa et al., 2001; Anderson et al., 1995; Reddy et al., 1994). The objective of this review is to highlight the growing clinical research on dietary factors, especially polyphenol-rich foods and beverages, to help maintain normal endothelial function and slow down the vascular aging process in healthy adults and children.

25.2 VASCULAR ENDOTHELIUM AND CARDIOVASCULAR HEALTH

The vascular endothelium is recognized as critical for the maintenance and regulation of cardiovascular health (Franzini et al., 2012; Yeboah et al., 2009; Forstermann, 2008; Vita and Keaney, 2002; Singh et al., 2002; Luscher and Barton, 1997). The endothelium is the inner lining of blood vessels (Verma and Anderson, 2000), which helps maintain normal vascular homeostasis by regulating vasomotor tone and smooth muscle cell proliferation and migration (Wilson, 2006; Ross, 1999). The strategic location of the endothelium allows it to sense changes in hemodynamic forces and blood-borne signals and respond by releasing vasoactive substances. Maintenance of an intact monolayer endothelial cell barrier is crucial for normal vascular structure and function and exerts atheroprotective effects *in vivo* through the release of substances that promote anticoagulation, inhibit inflammation and oxidative stress, and induce vasodilatation (Versari et al., 2009; Ashfaq et al., 2008; Verma and Anderson, 2000). Enhanced endothelial function may also improve cerebral blood flow and brain health (Ghosh and Scheepens, 2009; Widlansky et al., 2003; Mombouli and Vanhoutte, 1999).

Endothelial dysfunction is an early pathophysiologic subclinical feature and it appears to be an independent predictor of atherosclerotic disease process involving the initiation and progression of many forms of cardiovascular diseases (Caballero et al., 2008; Groner et al., 2006; Bonetti et al., 2003; Brown and Hu, 2001; Cai and Harrison, 2000; De Vriese et al., 2000; Suwaidi et al., 2000; Drexler and Hornig, 1999; Ruschitzka et al., 1997; Celermajer et al., 1994). The mechanisms by which endothelial vascular dysfunction occurs are complex and incompletely understood, and preventative approaches for endothelial function are evolving but not completely understood. Endothelial dysfunction is a broad term that generally implies diminished production or availability of nitric oxide (NO) and/or an imbalance in the relative contribution of endothelium-derived relaxing and contracting factors (Schini-Kerth et al., 2010; Verma and Anderson, 2000; Joannides et al., 1995). NO is a key endothelium-derived relaxing factor that plays a role in the maintenance of vascular tone and reactivity (Schini-Kerth et al., 2010; Verma and Anderson, 2000). In addition to its vasodilator effect, NO opposes the actions of potent endothelium-derived contracting factors such as angiotensin-II and endothelin-1 (ET-1). NO inhibits platelet and leukocyte activation and maintains the vascular smooth muscle in a nonproliferative state. Oxidative stress, especially related to the excessive production of reactive oxygen species (ROS), is considered an important factor influencing NO half-life (Couillard et al., 2005; Bae et al., 2003; Ceriello, 2002; Ceriello et al., 2002; Bae et al., 2001). Superoxide ion reacts with NO, yielding peroxinitrite, a product that maintains the oxidant properties of ROS but loses NO vasodilatatory capacity. Oxidative stress can uncouple endothelial NO synthetase (eNOS) diverting its activity to the production of free radicals of oxygen instead of NO. Endothelial dysfunction appears mostly as a result of an imbalance between the activity of endogenous prooxidative enzymes such as NADPH oxidase, xanthine oxidase, and antioxidant enzymes such as superoxide dismutase, glutathione peroxidase, or paraoxonase. Certain types of polyphenols such as flavonoids appear to help maintain healthy endothelial function (Heiss et al., 2010; Schini-Kerth et al., 2010; Ghosh and Scheepens, 2009; Karatzi et al., 2009; Forstermann, 2008; Hooper et al., 2008; Nicholson et al., 2008; Schewe et al., 2008; Biesalski, 2007; Santangelo et al., 2007; Hodgson and Croft, 2006; Couillard et al., 2005).

A novel surrogate marker of endothelial dysfunction is the presence of inflammatory endothelial microparticles (EMPs) (Chironi et al., 2009; Jimenez et al., 2005). Microparticles of various cellular origins (platelets, leukocytes, granulocytes, and endothelial cells) are found in the plasma of healthy subjects, and their amount increases under early pathologic conditions beginning in childhood. Given their biochemical composition, nature, and biological effects, EMPs appear to be extensively involved in the initiation of atherosclerosis (Van Wijk et al., 2003). Increases in plasma EMP concentrations, particularly those of endothelial origin, reflect oxidative stress-related cellular injury (Boulanger et al., 2008; Piccin et al., 2007). Elevated EMP concentrations are known to increase endothelial dysfunction in both CVD symptomatic and asymptomatic subjects from childhood to adulthood (Bulut et al., 2009; Schachinger et al., 1999). On the other hand, endothelial progenitor cells (EPCs) may contribute to the maintenance of the endothelium by replacing injured mature endothelial cells (Hristov et al., 2003). The EPC number has been shown to be reduced in patients with cardiovascular disease, diabetes mellitus, and multiple coronary risk factors, which leads to speculation that atherosclerosis is caused by a loss of endothelial-repairing capacity (Roberts et al., 2005; Werner et al., 2005; Hristov et al., 2004). Lifestyle factors such as diet, stress, and excess weight may influence this EMP process (Ignarro et al., 2007).

25.2.1 Noninvasive Measures of Endothelial Dysfunction

Measures of vascular function are becoming increasingly used as clinical measure and outcome marker of CVD risk in various research studies (Chong et al., 2010; Corretti et al., 2002; Kelm, 2002; Celermajer, 1997). Vascular function is generally assessed by noninvasive clinical measurements for enhanced and maintained endothelial activation, and impaired endothelium-dependent vasodilation. The most common noninvasive techniques of measuring endothelium-dependent vasodilatation include flow-mediated dilation (FMD), peripheral arterial tonometry (PAT), and carotid intima–media thickness (CIMT) (Charakida et al., 2010; Fisher et al., 2006; Sattar and Ferns, 2005; Vogel and Benitez, 2000). These techniques generally require specialized technical expertise and equipment for assessment (Grassi et al., 2009). These methods may be useful in detecting subclinical atherosclerosis in children and young adults (Le et al., 2010; Caballero et al., 2008; Mozaffarian et al., 2008). With the ever-increasing prevalence of obesity and metabolic syndrome in children and adults because of sedentary lifestyles and poor nutrition, early detection using these tools seems to be becoming increasingly important in CVD prevention management.

Endothelial function as measured by FMD has been widely used and has proved to be sensitive and accurate in reflecting endothelial function (Yeboah et al., 2007; Patel and Celermajer, 2006; Moens et al., 2005). FMD of the brachial artery is currently the most widely used as a noninvasive method of determining changes in NO-regulated vascular tone and thus endothelial function (Charakida et al., 2010; Yeboah et al., 2009). FMD is designated as an endothelium-dependent process that reflects the relaxation of a conduit artery when exposed to increased flow, for example, after the release of an inflatable cuff. When blood flow increases through a vessel, the vessel dilates. A diminished FMD blood flow response reflects endothelial dysfunction. Impaired brachial FMD response is regarded as a potential early and reversible manifestation of vascular disease and may represent an integrated measure of the impact of various insults to the endothelium. FMD appears to be a potential predictor of incident cardiovascular events in general population-based adults (Yeboah et al., 2009). The addition of FMD to the Framingham Risk Score helps to classify subjects as low, intermediate, and high CVD risk in the Multi-Ethnic Study of Atherosclerosis (MESA), a large prospective cohort study that began in July 2000 to investigate the prevalence, correlates, and progression of subclinical CVD in individuals without known CVD at baseline (Yeboah et al., 2009). Some studies have shown an independent inverse association between brachial FMD and CVD events (Yeboah et al., 2007; Brevetti et al., 2003; Gokce et al., 2002, 2003) but others have not (Frick et al., 2005; Witte et al., 2005; Fathi et al., 2004). The PAT is a rapidly emerging option to the traditional FMD.

CIMT is a frequently used clinical surrogate marker for atherosclerotic disease to assess subclinical vascular dysfunction and prevention measures (Cobble and Bale, 2010). CIMT uses B-mode ultrasound to measure combined thickness of the intimal and medial layers of the carotid artery. CIMT measurement allows health care providers to gain insight into the "lifetime risk" of an individual and investigate potential reasons for premature arterial thickening (i.e., prediabetes,

diabetes, dyslipidemia, obesity, or poor lifestyle). CIMT has been used in a wide range of lifestyle interventions (Bemelmans et al., 2002; Markus et al., 1997). CIMT has several advantages: (1) it can be repeatedly and reproducibly performed with no adverse effects on the patient; (2) it allows for observation of the arterial wall, the actual site of atherosclerotic disease; and (3) it uses equipment readily available and relatively inexpensive. The weakness of CIMT is the lack of standardized protocols and potential inaccurate estimation of the progression or regression of atherosclerosis between measurements. However, the implementation of carotid intima border edge detection software programs can reduce reader variation and improve reproducibility.

25.3 MEAL PATTERNS AND ENDOTHELIAL DYSFUNCTION

The effect of high-saturated fat (SF), high-cholesterol, and high-sodium diets on increasing blood lipoproteins and hypertension and elevating the risk of CVD is widely accepted (USDA and HHS, 2010; Lichtenstein et al., 2006). However, less appreciated is the concept of repeated postprandial hyperglycemia and hypertriglyceridemia effects of meals rich in calories and SF and sodium on subclinical endothelium dysfunction, which can accelerate the early stages of atherosclerotic disease initiation and progression (accelerated vascular aging) in otherwise healthy, relatively CVD-free individuals (Dickinson et al., 2011; Le et al., 2010; Romero-Corral et al., 2010; Tentolouris et al., 2008; Puchau et al., 2009; Groner et al., 2006; Tushuizen et al., 2006; Vogel et al., 1997).

25.3.1 High-Calorie and High-Saturated Fat Meals Patterns

Clinical studies have shown that repeated consumption of meal(s) high in calories and SF by healthy people free of primary CVD risk factors may cause a significant temporary endothelial dysfunction or reduction in FMD response. In the first clinical study, a high-calorie and high-SF meal consumed by healthy adults was followed by a significant, acute decrease in endothelium-dependent vasodilation as measured by FMD response corresponding with increased plasma triglyceride levels (Vogel et al., 1997). In another study with healthy, physically active, lean and insulin-sensitive young males exposed to two consecutive SF-rich fast food meals (breakfast and lunch), the results reported a significant acute impaired FMD and elevation of oxidized low-density lipoprotein (oxLDL) and malondialdehyde (MDA) concentrations, which paralleled a mild increase in glucose and triglycerides (Tushuizen et al., 2006). A study conducted using three high-calorie fast food meals (meal 1: beef burger and French fries; meal 2: vegetarian burger and French fries; and meal 3: vegetarian burger, salad, and yogurt) showed that FMD response was reduced after all meals but the meal 3 diet tended to show a more rapid recovery of FMD response back to baseline (Rudolph et al., 2007). A clinical study comparing the consumption of an SF-rich meal with a monounsaturated fat (MUFA)-rich meal in subjects with type 2 diabetes showed that the SF meal decreased FMD response and the MUFA-rich meal did not impair FMD (Tentolouris et al., 2008). Even low-calorie diets high in SF decreased the FMD response compared to a low-fat weight loss diet (Varady et al., 2011; Phillips et al., 2008). Other studies have shown that the chronic consumption of a Mediterranean diet rich in virgin olive oil can improve endothelial function in both fasting and postprandial states compared to Western diet rich in saturated fat (Marin et al., 2011; Buscemi et al., 2009; Fuentes et al., 2008). Also, diets enriched in nuts such as walnuts and pistachios may improve endothelial health and increase FMD response compared to MUFA-rich or Mediterranean diets (Sari et al., 2010; Cortes et al., 2006; Ros et al., 2004). However, another clinical study in young healthy adults showed that high levels of refined olive, soybean, or palm oil consumption produced similar decreases in FMD response (Rueda-Clausen et al., 2007). These clinical trials tend to demonstrate that high-SF diets promote endothelial dysfunction (reduced FMD response and accelerate vascular aging) and unsaturated fat tend to be neutral or improve FMD response over time; however, more clinical research is needed to better understand the effects of unsaturated fat-rich oils and foods on endothelial function.

The chronic consumption of excessive calories and inactivity may contribute to the prevalence of obesity, which is associated with endothelial dysfunction and the subclinical progression of atherosclerosis in both children and adults (Steinberger and Daniels, 2003; Kimm and Obarzanek, 2002; Srinivasan et al., 1996; Must et al. 1992). Obese children and adolescents tend to have lower FMD and more inelastic carotid arteries than their normal-weight peers (Kapiotis et al., 2006; Pena et al., 2006; Zhu et al., 2005; Woo et al., 2004; Tounian et al., 2001; Celermajer et al., 1992). A cross-sectional study of prepubertal children found an inverse relationship between FMD response and percentage of body fat (Aggoun et al., 2008). Obese children and adolescents also have increased CIMT levels compared to normal-weight children (Le et al., 2010; Urbina et al., 2009). Childhood obesity can advance to adult obesity with progressive increases to higher FMD and CIMT (Gupta et al., 2010; Oren et al., 2003).

Recent research shows that adult weight loss can significantly affect endothelial function as measured by FMD response. In one randomized controlled study, normal-weight healthy subjects with a mean age of 29 years were assigned to gain weight (about 10 lbs) for 8 weeks followed by weight loss for 16 weeks or to maintain weight (Romero-Corral et al., 2010). FMD response remained unchanged for the weight maintainers but decreased significantly for the weight gainers, especially in those with increased visceral fat. However, when the weight gainers shed their excess weight, their FMD response returned to baseline. Also, severely obese adults who lost ≥10% body weight compared to obese individuals who failed to lose weight showed a significant improvement in FMD response with an increase of 30% after weight loss (Bigornia et al., 2010).

25.3.2 HIGH-SODIUM MEALS

Dietary salt reduction has been shown to improve endothelial function as assessed by FMD in a chronic study (Dickinson et al., 2009). However, the mechanisms relating salt and endothelial dysfunction are still not clear. Even the amount of sodium found in commonly eaten meals impairs FMD response in the postprandial phase compared with a low-sodium meal in a group of healthy normotensive adults (Dickinson et al., 2011). The reduction in FMD observed with the high-sodium meal is similar in magnitude to that found in healthy subjects after a high-calorie and high-SF meal (Dickinson et al., 2011; Tentolouris et al., 2008; Vogel et al., 1997). Thus, chronic high consumption of sodium meals may further accelerate endothelial dysfunction in addition to high-calorie and high-SF meals.

25.3.3 LOW ANTIOXIDANT DIETARY PATTERNS

Dietary patterns rich in total antioxidant capacity (TAC) and foods and beverages rich in polyphenols may help to improve endothelial function compared to diets low in these foods (Heiss et al., 2010; Karatzi et al., 2009; Loke et al., 2008; Hodgson and Croft, 2006; Engler et al., 2004; Ros et al., 2004; Steinberg et al., 2003; Hodgson et al., 2002). Dietary TAC has been proposed as a potential marker of diet quality and reduced CVD risk in healthy subjects (Franzini et al., 2012; Puchau et al., 2009). In a randomized, crossover clinical study, healthy subjects with low CVD risk (aged 61 ± 3 years) consuming controlled food patterns based on TAC level (including foods and beverages either high or low in polyphenol content) were assessed for FMD response (Franzini et al., 2012). Subjects consumed diets containing five portions of fruits and vegetables from a list of items with either high TAC (HTAC), including grapes, berries, and oranges, or low TAC (LTAC), including salad, bananas, and apples. The HTAC diets also included red wine, walnuts, dark chocolate, berry ice cream, and the LTAC diets included white wine, white chocolate, or vanilla ice cream. The supply of foods was delivered to subjects at home on a weekly basis. The energy, macronutrient, dietary fiber, and alcohol levels were the same between the HTAC and LTAC diet but the TAC was about four times higher in the HTAC diet compared with the LTAC diet by design. The study reported that HTAC diets resulted in significantly improved FMD response compared to LTAC diets after 2 weeks. Compared to the

LTAC diet response, the mean FMD response was about 60% higher on the HTAC diet and the response was similar for males and females. Also, there were no observed significant differences in body weight, body mass index (BMI), blood pressure, fasting plasma glucose, or lipid profile changes between diets. Conversely, C-reactive protein (hs-CRP) concentrations decreased significantly and α-tocopherol concentrations increased significantly during the HTAC diet compared with the LTAC diet, with no other significant changes in plasma concentrations of TAC. This difference in FMD was observed while controlling for other dietary factors known to have an effect on endothelial function (e.g., dietary fiber, alcohol, and fat). It is important to note that the FMD response decreased with the LTAC diet despite the substantial increase in low polyphenol antioxidant fruit and vegetable intake, whereas HTAC diet with increase in fruit and vegetables with higher polyphenol antioxidant levels resulted in a significant increase in FMD. Similar improvements in FMD have been observed with a Mediterranean-type diet after 2 months (Rallidis et al., 2009). The level of improved FMD response with higher TAC diets was in the range considered to be of prognostic relevance for potentially predicting future cardiovascular events (Gokce et al., 2002).

25.3.4 LOW FRUIT AND VEGETABLE MEAL PATTERNS

Studies have found an inverse relationship between CIMT and intake and plasma levels of antioxidant levels (Franzini et al., 2012; Dwyer et al., 2004; Rissanen et al., 2003; Iribarren et al., 1997). In recent analyses from the Nurses' Health Study and the Health Professionals' follow-up study, fruit was associated with a greater reduction in the risk of CVD than vegetables (Hung et al., 2004). The risk of CVD was decreased by 4% for each additional portion per day of fruit and vegetable intake and by 7% for each additional portion of fruit intake (Dauchet et al., 2006). Survivors from a cohort of 1232 men who participated in the Oslo Diet and Antismoking Study in 1972–1973 were assessed in elderly men (age 70 ± 5 years) with a high risk of CVD for an association between CIMT and dietary intake of vegetables, fruit, and berries (Ellingsen et al., 2008). The CIMT for participants in the highest quartile of dietary intake of fruit and berries was significantly lower than for those in the lowest quartile, giving a mean difference of 0.075 (SE 0.027) mm ($p = 0.033$). In multivariate regression analysis, increased intake of fruit and berries remained inversely associated with CIMT after adjustment for age, cigarette smoking, dietary cholesterol and saturated fat, consumption of milk, cream, and ice cream, and energy intake. The difference of about 350 g of fruit and berries per day between the lowest and highest quartile of intake was associated with a 5.5% adjusted difference in mean CIMT.

Fruit contains a wide range of potentially cardioprotective components, including dietary fiber, vitamins, and a large number of phytochemicals such as carotenoids and polyphenols. Preliminary clinical evidence suggests that polyphenols may, in part, explain the endothelial health benefits of increased fruit intake (Davidson et al., 2009; George et al., 2009; Aviram et al., 2004; Clifton, 2004; Chou et al., 2001; Stein et al., 1999). The potential intake of polyphenols from the minimum recommended five-a-day fruit and vegetables can be as high as 500 mg/day, among the highest of all the phytochemicals (Williamson and Holst, 2008). The exact contribution of polyphenols to endothelial function is not yet fully understood, which depends on the type of fruit and its unique polyphenol make-up.

25.4 POLYPHENOL-RICH FOODS AND VASCULAR ENDOTHELIAL FUNCTION

25.4.1 BACKGROUND

Diet can have a major influence on the risk of CVD (Schini-Kerth et al., 2010). A number of clinical studies indicate that regular intake of certain polyphenol-rich beverages and foods, especially those rich in flavonoids such as certain fruits like grapes, cocoa, and tea, may help maintain normal endothelial function (slow vascular aging) (Pan et al., 2010; Schini-Kerth et al., 2010). These flavonoids are biologically active polyphenolic compounds which may promote healthier NO-mediated endothelium-dependent function and vascular tone (Gonzalez-Gallego et al., 2010). The composition of flavonoids in different plant foods varies greatly. In fruits, there are a number of flavonoids: (1) quercetin, kaempferol, myricetin, and isorhamnetin are common flavonols, with quercetin being the predominant one; (2) proanthocyanidins and their monomer units, catechins (procyanidin) or gallocatechins (prodelphinidins); (3) anthocyanins are glycosides of different anthocyanidins, mainly cyanidin, which are widespread and commonly contribute to the pigmentation of fruits; and (4) citrus fruits differ in their flavonoid profiles from other fruit species, containing flavanones and flavones (hesperidin and naringenin) that are not common in other fruits. The major polyphenolic constituents present in green tea are epicatechin, epigallocatechin, epicatechin-3-gallate, and epigallocatechin-3-gallate (EGCG), whereas black tea contains a small amount of catechins but higher levels of thearubigins and theaflavins, polymerized forms of catechin monomers that are the major components formed during enzymatic oxidation and the fermentation process. Cocoa and soy are rich in flavonols and isoflavones, respectively. Pomegranates contain nonflavonoid polyphenols such as ellagitannins.

Dietary flavonoids vary in their ability to improve endothelial function. A randomized, placebo-controlled, crossover trial in healthy men was conducted to compare the acute effects of the oral administration of 200 mg quercetin, epicatechin, or EGCG on NO, endothelin-1, and oxidative stress after NO production was assessed via the measurement of plasma S-nitrosothiols and plasma and urinary nitrite and nitrate concentrations (Loke et al., 2008). Plasma and urinary concentrations of quercetin, epicatechin, and EGCG were measured to establish the absorption of these flavonoids. Relative to water (control), quercetin and epicatechin resulted in a significant increase in plasma S-nitrosothiols, plasma nitrite, and urinary nitrate concentrations. EGCG did not alter any of the measures of NO production. Quercetin and epicatechin resulted in a significant reduction in plasma endothelin-1 concentration, but only quercetin significantly decreased the urinary endothelin-1 concentration. Significant increases in the circulating concentrations of all the flavonoids were observed after their consumption. Of the dietary flavonoids studied, only quercetin and epicatechin augmented NO status and reduced endothelin-1 concentrations, which reflect improved endothelial function.

25.4.2 TEA

Some 15 clinical studies have shown that both short- and long-term consumption of tea improves endothelial function, as assessed primarily by FMD response (Grassi et al., 2009; Alexopoulos et al., 2008; Tinahones et al., 2008; Jochmann et al., 2007; Lorenz et al., 2007; Widlansky et al., 2007; Hodgson et al., 2006, 2005, 2002; Kim et al., 2006; Reddy et al., 2005; Hirata et al., 2004; Nagaya et al., 2004; Duffy et al., 2001; Serafini et al., 1996) and several reviews summarize the tea studies (Hodgson, 2006; Hodgson and Puddey, 2005). In healthy women, green and black tea significantly increased FMD response in a comparable manner (Jochmann et al., 2007). Similar positive effects on FMD have also been shown for males (Grassi et al., 2009). Both black and green tea have been demonstrated to equally stimulate NO production and vasodilation (Lorenz et al., 2009). The effect was dose dependent, and 800 mg tea flavonoids per day improved FMD significantly more than 100 mg, but the daily consumption of one cup of tea for 1 week can also improve the FMD and coronary flow reserve of healthy volunteers (Grassi et al., 2009; Hirata et al., 2004). Although studies have shown that the addition of milk to tea blunts the FMD response (Lorenz et al., 2007; Serafini et al., 1996), several other studies have demonstrated that the addition of milk does not impair flavonoid or antioxidant bioavailability (Reddy et al., 2005; van het Hof et al., 1998, 1999). The human intervention studies on tea and vascular function were reviewed by Hodgson and Croft (2006) who concluded that, overall, the available clinical studies support the effects of tea flavonoids on improving endothelial function, although the response varies between individuals (Hodgson et al., 2006). The degree of a subject's O-methylation of flavonoids could alter activity, and thus influence any effect on endothelial function. Improvement in FMD following ingestion of tea tends to be higher in individuals with lower gastrointestinal flavonoid O-methylate capacity (Hodgson et al., 2006).

25.4.3 COCOA

Some 15 clinical studies have shown that both short- and long-term consumption of high flavanol cocoa and dark chocolate improves endothelial function, as assessed most of the time by FMD (Westphal and Luley, 2011; Balzer et al., 2008; Faridi et al., 2008; Grassi et al., 2005, 2008; Heiss et al., 2007; Farouque et al., 2006; Hermann et al., 2006; Wang-Polagruto et al., 2006; Schroeter et al., 2006; Heiss et al., 2003, 2005; Vlachopoulos et al., 2005; Engler et al., 2004; Fisher et al., 2003). One clinical study found that the consumption of flavanol-rich cocoa when consumed with a high-fat meal improved acute endothelial dysfunction over low flavanol cocoa (Westphal and Luley, 2011). After the flavanol-poor fat loading, the FMD deteriorated over 4 h but the consumption of flavanol-rich cocoa, in contrast, improved this deterioration in hours 2, 3, and 4 without abolishing it completely. Flavanol-rich cocoa can alleviate the lipemia-induced endothelial dysfunction. Another study showed that solid dark chocolate and liquid cocoa ingestion improved FMD response compared with placebo in overweight subjects but the endothelial function improved significantly more with sugar-free than with regular sweetened cocoa. Further, flavanol-rich cocoa consumption for 4 days induced peripheral vasodilation as tonometry in the finger (PAT) (Fisher et al., 2003). The effect of flavanol-rich cocoa on PAT was significantly more effective in people over 50 years of age after 6 days compared to people under 50 years of age (Fisher and Hollenberg, 2006). Epicatechins in cocoa are primarily responsible for the vascular effects (Schroeter et al., 2006).

Additionally, clinical studies suggest that cocoa flavonoids improve brain blood flow. The ingestion of flavanol-rich cocoa (5 days of 150 mg of cocoa flavanols) increased the BOLD (blood oxygenation level-dependant) signal intensity in response to a cognitive task (Francis et al., 2006). These findings were replicated in another study, which showed an increase in cerebral blood flow velocity in healthy elderly subjects after 2 weeks of intake of flavanol-rich cocoa (900 mg flavonols daily) (Sorond et al., 2008).

25.4.4 RED WINE

Some 11 clinical studies have studied the effects of red wine consumption on short-term and postprandial FMD endothelial function (Hijmering et al., 2007; Boban et al., 2006; Coimbra et al., 2005; Guarda et al., 2005; Zilkens et al., 2005; Karatzi et al., 2004; Whelan et al., 2004; Hashimoto et al., 2001; Cuevas et al., 2000; Agewall et al., 2000; Djousse et al., 1999). The effects of red wine and dealcoholized red wine are reviewed by Karatzi et al. (2009). Although four clinical trials report that red wine improves FMD response (Boban et al., 2006; Whelan et al., 2004; Hashimoto et al., 2001; Cuevas et al., 2000), four studies show neutral FMD effects (Zilkens et al., 2005; Guarda et al., 2005; Agewall et al., 2000; Djousse et al., 1999), and three demonstrated an impaired FMD response (Hijmering et al., 2007; Coimbra et al., 2005; Karatzi et al., 2004). Additionally, four of five trials using dealcoholized red wine have demonstrated improved endothelial function (Boban et al., 2006; Zilkens et al., 2005; Karatzi et al., 2004; Hashimoto et al., 2001; Agewall et al., 2000). Although the clinical studies on red wine FMD response are mixed, this is not surprising since there are many types of wines, diets, and subjects studied. Probably the red wines with higher flavonoid content are more likely to show improved FMD endothelial function and new clinical research is needed to explore the effect of wine flavonoid levels.

25.4.5 FRESH GRAPES

The consumption of a standardized product derived from fresh grapes (GP; freeze-dried preparation of red, green, and blue-black California seeded and seedless table grapes equivalent to 1.25 cups of fresh grapes)* by healthy young subjects resulted in significant improvement in FMD response

---

* Contains 612 μmol of flavans, 43 μmol of anthoncyanins, 3 μmol of flavanols, and 1 μmol of resveratrol.

within 3 h of consumption, when compared with control consumption of a sugar solution (Chaves et al., 2009). When GP was consumed twice daily for 3 weeks, FMD response was further improved and plasma TAC was slightly but significantly increased, with no change in heart rate, hemodynamics, or lipid profiles. Additionally, these researchers evaluated the effect of a high-calorie and high-SF fast food meal and found a 50% reduction in FMD response but the addition of GP to the fast food meal completely prevented a drop in FMD response. This research suggests that a modest intake of fresh grapes may have acute favorable effects on vascular endothelial function in normal healthy people consuming typical Western diets. However, extracts of wine grape and grape seed polyphenols had no impact on increasing FMD response in fasting or postprandial subjects (van Mierlo et al., 2010). Additional clinical research on fresh grapes would be important to confirm these results.

25.4.6 GRAPE JUICE

Some 10 clinical studies have investigated the effects of a grape juice and dealcoholized red wine in healthy to coronary artery disease subjects. Four of the five grape juice clinical studies support improved FMD endothelial function. In the first study, subjects consumed approximately 640 mL of grape juice daily (in addition to their already-established prescription medications), and endothelial performance was assessed with FMD response. Significant improvement in FMD was demonstrated after 14 days of juice intake (Stein et al., 1999). This study was confirmed by Chou et al. (2001). Sixteen healthy adult subjects with hypercholesterolemia (8 men and 8 women; mean age 51.6 ± 8.1 years) without other risk factors consumed 500 mL purple grape juice per day for 14 days (Coimbra et al., 2005). During this time, the FMD significantly increased in the grape juice group (10.1 ± 7.1 before vs. $16.9 \pm 6.7\%$ after) compared to baseline. However, in a clinical study with prehypertensive and stage 1 hypertensive subjects, consuming 7 mL/kg of purple grape juice for 8 weeks did not improve endothelial function as measured by PAT (Dohadwala et al., 2010). In adolescent children with metabolic syndrome, 18 mL/kg grape juice was shown to significantly increase FMD response (Hashemi et al., 2010). Also, five clinical trials using dealcoholized red wine further support improved FMD endothelial function in adults (Boban et al., 2006; Zilkens et al., 2005; Karatzi et al., 2004; Hashimoto et al., 2001; Agewall et al., 2000). As with the grape juice studies, four of the five clinical dealcoholized red wine studies also support improved FMD endothelial function.

25.4.7 POMEGRANATE JUICE

There are only two very exploratory published clinical studies assessing the endothelial health by CIMT and FMD. A randomized, double-blind, parallel trial evaluated the influence of pomegranate juice consumption on anterior and posterior CIMT progression rates in subjects at moderate risk for coronary heart disease (Davidson et al., 2009). Subjects were men (45–74 years old) and women (55–74 years old) with >1 major coronary heart disease risk factor and baseline posterior wall CIMT 0.7–2.0 mm, without significant stenosis. Participants consumed 240 mL/day of pomegranate juice ($n = 146$) or a control beverage ($n = 143$) for up to 18 months. The composite measurement of CIMT showed a significantly smaller value at 12 months in the pomegranate juice group compared to the control group (0.79 vs. 0.81 mm, $p = 0.022$). However, this difference was no longer significant at the end of the 18 month treatment period (0.79 vs. 0.80 mm, $p = 0.168$). A subgroup analysis in Davidson's study revealed that improvement in anterior and/or composite CIMT after 18 months was only found in subjects who had the greatest risk factors (i.e., the top tertiles for baseline triglycerides (TGs), total cholesterol:HDL-cholesterol ratio, TG:HDL-cholesterol ratio, apo-B100, and lowest tertile for HDL-cholesterol). However, results from post hoc exploratory analyses should be interpreted with caution, as these findings will need to be confirmed in future investigations. FMD was not measured in this trial. There is only one published clinical study on pomegranate juice and FMD (Hashemi et al., 2010). In this study, 30 adolescent children with metabolic syndrome consumed 240 mL of pomegranate juice daily, which appeared to slightly improve FMD. More rigorous clinical research on the effect of pomegranate juice on endothelial function is needed before an accurate determination can be made.

25.4.8 SOY ISOFLAVONES

The risks of cardiovascular diseases increase with the decline in estrogen production after menopause in women (Kannel et al., 1976). Dietary intake of compounds with estrogenic properties reduces the incidence of cardiovascular events, according to recent epidemiologic studies (Cassidy et al., 2006; Nagata, 2000). Isoflavone, mainly produced by soybeans, has been suggested to have estrogenic and potentially cardioprotective effects and improved endothelial dysfunction in many experimental studies (Chacko et al., 2007; Chan et al., 2007; Hall et al., 2006; Squadrito et al., 2000). Experimental studies suggest that isoflavone can stimulate the production of NO via estrogen receptor-mediated activation of eNOS (Squadrito et al., 2002). The effect of oral isoflavone consumption on endothelial function in postmenopausal women has been investigated in over 20 studies (Chan et al., 2008; Hall et al., 2006, 2008; Cupisti et al., 2007; Evans et al., 2007; Katz et al., 2007; Hallund et al., 2006; Kreijkamp-Kaspers et al., 2005; Teede et al., 2001, 2003, 2005; Colacurci et al., 2005; Hermansen et al., 2005; Lissin et al., 2004; Cuevas et al., 2003; Howes et al., 2003; Nikander et al., 2003; Steinberg et al. 2003; Squadrito et al., 2003; Hale et al., 2002; Simons et al., 2000). However, the results of these studies were not consistent. In a meta-analysis of all published, double-blind, randomized, placebo-controlled trials on isoflavone intake and FMD response in postmenopausal women, it was determined that isoflavone intake does not improve endothelial function in postmenopausal women with high baseline FMD levels (>5.2%). However, there was significant improvement when the baseline FMD levels were low (<5.2%), although significant heterogeneity was still detected. The baseline FMD profile appears to be an important and potential factor influencing the effect of isoflavones on endothelial function. Additional rigorous studies in women and men are needed to better understand the mechanisms and clinical effects of isoflavones on endothelial function and vascular aging.

25.5 CONCLUSION

Lifestyle risk factors, including poor dietary habits, inactivity, mental stress, and excess body weight, may accelerate CVD progression in otherwise healthy people by promoting endothelial dysfunction. Over the last decade, there have been a growing number of clinical studies on the effects of diet on endothelial function as a potential early indicator of atherosclerosis and arterial damage (vascular aging). The effects of chronic high-calorie, high-SF, and high-sodium meals on repeated postprandial hyperglycemia and hypertriglyceridemia have been shown in several clinical studies to trigger temporary endothelium dysfunction, which may accelerate early stages of vascular aging in otherwise healthy, relatively CVD-free individuals. A number of clinical studies have shown that the TAC content of food patterns and certain polyphenol-rich foods and beverages may increase FMD response (positive effect) compared with foods low in these dietary components. Polyphenol-rich foods with the best clinical evidence are black and green tea, cocoa (high flavanol content), fresh grapes, grape juice, and possibly red wine. However, the clinical evidence for soy isoflavones and pomegranate juice requires more clinical research to confirm their benefits on FMD and/or CIMT. Although there are a number of clinical studies on diet and endothelial function, more clinical trials are needed to better understand the effect of endothelial function on early vascular aging in healthy people, so that authoritative dietary guidance can be developed as appropriate.

REFERENCES

Agewall S., Wright S., Doughty R.N., Whalley G.A., Duxbury M., and Sharpe, N. 2000. Does a glass of red wine improve endothelial function? *Eur Heart J.* 211:74–78.

Aggoun Y., Szezepanski I., and Bonnet D. 2005. Noninvasive assessment of arterial stiffness and risk of atherosclerotic events in children. *Pediatr Res.* 58:173–178.

Aggoun Y., Farpour-Lambert N.J., Marchland L.M., Golay E., Maggie A.B.R., and Begetter M. 2008. Impaired endothelial and smooth muscle functions and arterial stiffness appear before puberty in obese children and are associated with elevated ambulatory blood pressure. *Eur Heart J.* 29, 792–799.

Alexopoulos N., Vlachopoulos C., Aznaouridis K., Baou K., Vasiliadou C., Oietri P., Xaplanteris P., Stefanadi E., and Stefanadis C. 2008. The acute effect of green tea consumption on endothelial function in healthy individuals. *Eur J Cardiovasc Prev Rehabil.* 15(3):300–305.

Anderson T.J., Uehata A., Gerhard M.D., Meredith I.T., Knab S., Delagrange D., Lieberman E.H., Ganz P., Creager M. A., and Yeung A.C. 1995. Close relation of endothelial function in the human coronary and peripheral circulations. *J Am Coll Cardiol.* 265, 1235–1241.

Ashfaq S., Abramson J.L., Jones D.P., Rhodes S.D., Weintraub W.S., Hooper W.C., Vaccarino V., Alexander R.W., Harrison D.G., and Quyyumi A.A. 2008. Endothelial function and amino thiol biomarkers of oxidative stress in health adults. *Hypertension.* 52:80–85.

Aviram M., Rosenblat M., Gaitini D., Nitecki S., Hoffman A., Dornfeld L., Volkova N. et al. 2004. Pomegranate juice consumption for 3 years by patients with carotid stenosis reduces common carotid intima-media thickness, blood pressure and LDL oxidation. *Clin Nutr.* 23:423–433.

Bae J.H., Bassenge E., Kim K.B., Kim Y.N., Kim K.S., Lee H.J., Moon K.C., Lee M.S., Park K.Y., and Schwemmer M. 2001. Postprandial hypertriglyceridemia impairs endothelial function by enhanced oxidant stress. *Atherosclerosis.* 1552:517–523.

Bae J.H., Schwemmer M., Lee I.K., Lee H.J., Park K.R., Kim K.Y., and Bassenge E. 2003. Postprandial hypertriglyceridemia-induced endothelial dysfunction in healthy subjects is independent of lipid oxidation. *Int J Cardiol.* 872:259–267.

Balzer J., Rassaf T., Heiss C., Kleinbongard P., Lauer T., Merx M., Heussen N. et al. 2008. Sustained benefits in vascular function through flavanol-containing cocoa in medicated diabetic patients a double masked, randomized, controlled trial. *J Am Coll Cardiol.* 51:2141–2149.

Bemelmans W.J.E., Lefrandt J.D., Feskens E.J.M., Broer J., Tervaert J.W., May J.F., and Smit A.J. 2002. Change in saturated fat intake is associated with progression of carotid and femoral intima media thickness, and with levels of soluble intercellular adhesion molecule-1. *Atherosclerosis.* 163:113–120.

Biesalski H.K. 2007. Polyphenols and inflammation: Basic interactions. *Curr Opin Clin Nutr Metab Care.* 10:724–728.

Bigornia S.J., Mott M.M., Hess D.T., Apovian C.M., McDonnell M.E., Duess M.A., Kluge M.A., Fiscale A.J., Vita J.A., and Gokce N. 2010. Long-term successful weight loss improves vascular endothelial function in severely obese individuals. *Obesity.* 18(4):754–759.

Boban M., Modum D., Music I., Vukovic J., Brizic I., Salamunic I., Obad A., Palada I., and Dujic Z. 2006. Red wine induced modulation of vascular function: Separating the role of polyphenols, ethanol and urates. *J Cardiovasc Pharmacol.* 47:695–701.

Bonetti P.O., Lerman L.O., and Lerman A. 2003. Endothelial dysfunction: A marker of atherosclerotic risk. *Arterioscler Thromb Vasc Biol.* 23:168–175.

Boulanger C.M., Leroyer A.S., Amabile N., and Tedgui A. 2008. Circulating endothelial microparticles: A new marker of vascular injury. *Ann Cardiol Angeiol.* 57:149–154.

Brevetti G., Silverstro A., Schiano V., and Chiariello M. 2003. Endothelial dysfunction and cardiovascular risk prediction in peripheral arterial disease: Additive value of flow-mediated dilation to ankle-brachial pressure index. *Circulation.* 108(17):2093–2098.

Brown A.A. and Hu F.B. 2001. Dietary modulation of endothelial function: Implications for cardiovascular disease. *Am J Clin Nutr.* 73:673–686.

Bulut D., Tuns H., and Mugge A. 2009. CD31/Annexin V microparticles in healthy offspring of patients with coronary artery disease. *Eur J Clin Invest.* 39:17–22.

Buscemi S., Verga S., Tranchina M.R., Cottone S., and Cerasola G. 2009. Effects of hypocaloric very-low-carbohydrate diet vs mediterranean diet on endothelial function in obese women. *Eur J Clin Invest.* 39(5):339–347.

Caballero A.E., Bousquett-Santos K., Robles-Osorio L., Montagnani V., Soodini G., Porramatikul S., Hamdy O., Nobrega A.C., and Horton E.S. 2008. Overweight latino children and adolescents have marked endothelial dysfunction and subclinical vascular inflammation in association with excess body fat and insulin resistance. *Diabetes Care.* 31:576–582.

Cai H. and Harrison D.G. 2000. Endothelial dysfunction in cardiovascular diseases: The role of oxidant stress. *Circ Res.* 87:840–844.

Cassidy A., Albertazzi P., Nielsen L.I., Hall W., Williamson G., Tetens I., Atkins S. et al. 2006. Critical review of health effects of soyabean phyto-oestrogens in post-menopausal women. *Proc Nutr Soc.* 65:76–92.

Celermajer D.S. 1997. Endothelial dysfunction: Does it matter? Is it reversible? *J Am Coll Cardiol.* 302:325–333.

Celermajer D.S., Sorensen K.E., Gooch V.M., Spiegelhalter D.J., Miller O.I., Sullivan I.D., Lloyd J.K., and Deanfield J.E. 1992. Non-invasive detection of endothelial dysfunction in children and adults at risk of atherosclerosis. *Lancet*. 340:1111–1115.

Celermajer D.S., Sorensen K.E., Spiegelhalter D.J., Georgakopoulos D., Robinson J., and Deanfield J.E. 1994. Aging is associated with endothelial dysfunction in healthy-men years before the age-related decline in women. *J Am Coll Cardiol*. 24:471–476.

Ceriello A. 2002. Nitrotyrosine: New findings as a marker of postprandial oxidative stress. *Int J Clin Pract Suppl*. 129:51–58.

Ceriello A., Taboga C., Tonutti L, Quagliaro L., Piconi L., Da Ros R., and Motz E. 2002. Evidence for an independent and cumulative effect of postprandial hypertriglyceridemia and hyperglycemia on endothelial dysfunction and oxidative stress generation: Effects of short- and long-term simvastatin treatment. *Circulation*. 10610:1211–1218.

Chacko B.K., Chandler R.T., D'Alessandro T.L., Mundhekar A., Khoo N.K., Botting N., Barnes S., and Patel R.P. 2007. Anti-inflammatory effects of isoflavones are dependent on flow and human endothelial cell PPAR gamma. *J Nutr*. 137:351–356.

Chou E.J., Keevil J.G., Aeschlimann S., Wiebe D.A., Folts J.D., and Stein J.H. 2001. Effect of ingestion of purple grape juice on endothelial function in patients with coronary heart disease. *Am J Cardiol*. 88:553–555.

Chan Y.H., Lau K.K., Yiu K.H., Li S.W., Chan H.T., Fing D.Y., Tam S., Lau C.P., and Tse H.F. 2008. Reduction of C-reactive protein with isoflavone supplement reverses endothelial dysfunction in patients with ischaemic stroke. *Eur Heart J*. 29:2800–2807.

Chan Y.H., Lau K.K., Yiu K.H., Li S.W., Chan H.T., Tam S., Shu X.O., Lau C.P., and Tse H.F. 2007. Isoflavone intake in persons at high risk of cardiovascular events: Implications for vascular endothelial function and the carotid atherosclerotic burden. *Am J Clin Nutr*. 86:938–945.

Charakida M., Masi S., Luscher T.F., Kastelein J.J.P., and Deanfield J.E. 2010. Assessment of atherosclerosis: The role of flow-mediated dilatation. *Eur Heart J*. 31:2854–2861.

Chaves A.A., Joshi M.S., Coyle C.M., Brady J.E., Dech S.J., Schanbacher B.L., Baliga R., Basuray A., and Bauer J.A. 2009. Vasoprotective endothelial effects of a standardized grape product in humans. *Vasc Pharm*. 50:20–26.

Chironi G.N., Boulanger C.M., Simon A., Dignat-George F., Freyssinet J.M., and Tedgui A. 2009. Endothelial microparticles in diseases. *Cell Tissue Res*. 335:143–151.

Chong M.F.F., Macdonald R., and Lovegrove J.A. 2010. Fruit polyphenols and CVD risk: A review of human intervention studies. *Br J Nutr*. 104:S28–S39.

Chou E.J., Keevil J.G., Aeschlimann S. et al. 2001. Effect of ingestion of purple grape juice on endothelial function in patients with coronary heart disease. *Am J Cardiol*. 88:553–555.

Clarkson P., Celermajer D.S., Donald A.E., Sampson M., Sorensen K.E., Adams M., Yue D.K., Betteridge D.J., and Deanfield J.E. 1996. Impaired vascular reactivity in insulin-dependent diabetes mellitus is related to disease duration and low density lipoprotein cholesterol levels. *J Am Coll Cardiol*. 28:573–579.

Clifton P.M. 2004. Effect of grape seed extract and quercetin on cardiovascular and endothelial parameters in high risk subjects. *J Biomed Biotechnol*. 2004(5):272–278.

Cobble M. and Bale B. 2010. Carotid intima-media thickness: Knowledge and application to everyday practice. *Postgraduate Med*. 122:1.

Coimbra S.R., Lage S.H.L., Brandizzi L., Yoshida V., and da Luz P.L. 2005. The action of red wine and purple grape juice on vascular reactivity is independent of plasma lipids in hypercholesterolemic patients. *Braz J Med Biol Res*. 38:1339–1347.

Colacurci N., Chiantera A., Fornaro F., de Novellis V., Manzella D., Arciello A., Chiantera V., Improta L., and Paolisso G. 2005. Effects of soy isoflavones on endothelial function in healthy postmenopausal women. *Menopause*. 12:299–307.

Corretti M.C., Anderson T.J., Benjamin E.J., Celermajer D., Charbonneau F., Creager M.A., Deanfield J. et al. 2002. Guidelines for the ultrasound assessment of endothelial-dependent flow-mediated vasodilation of the brachial artery: A report of the international brachial artery reactivity task force. *J Am Coll Cardiol*. 392:257–265.

Cortes B., Nunez I., Cofan M., Gilabert R., Perez-Heras A., Casals E., Deulofeu R., and Ros E. 2006. Acute effects of high-fat meals enriched with walnuts or olive oil on postprandial endothelial function. *J Am Coll Cardiol*. 48(8):1666–1671.

Couillard C., Ruel G., Archer W.R., Pomerleau S., Bergeron J., Couture P., Lamarche B., and Bergeron N. 2005. Circulating levels of oxidative stress markers and endothelial adhesion molecules in men with abdominal obesity. *J Clin Endocrinol. Metab*. 90(12):6454–6459.

Cuevas A., Guasch V., Castillo O., Irribarr V., Mizon C., San Martin A., Strobel P., Perez D., Germain A.M., and Leighton F. 2000. A high fat diet induces and red wine counteracts endothelial dysfunction in human volunteers. *Lipids*. 35:143–148.

Cuevas A.M., Irribarra V.L., Castillo O.A., Yanez M.D., and Germain A.M. 2003. Isolated soy protein improves endothelial function in postmenopausal hypercholesterolemic women. *Eur J Clin Nutr* 57:889–894.

Cupisti A., Ghiadoni L., D'Alessandro C., Kardasz I., Morelli E., Panichi V., Locati D. et al. 2007. Soy protein diet improves endothelial dysfunction in renal transplant patients. *Nephrol Dial Transplant.* 22:229–234.

Dauchet L., Amouyel P., Hercberg S., and Dallongeville J. 2006. Fruit and vegetable consumption and risk of coronary heart disease: A meta-analysis of cohort studies. *J Nutr.* 136:2588–2593.

Davidson M.H., Maki K.C., Dicklin M.R., Feinstein S.B.,Witchger M., Bell M., McGuire D.K., Provost J.C., Liker H., and Aviram M. 2009. Effects of consumption of pomegranate juice on carotid intima–media thickness in men and women at moderate risk for coronary heart disease. *Am J Cardiol.* 104:936–942.

Desideri G., De S.M., Iughetti L., Rosato T., Iezzi M.L., Marinucci M.C., Cofini V. et al. 2005. Early activation of vascular endothelial cells and platelets in obese children. *J Clin Endocrinol Metab.* 90:3145–3152.

De Vriese A.S., Verbeuren T.J., Van de Voorde J., Lameire N.H., and Vanhoutte P.M. 2000. Endothelial dysfunction in diabetes. *Br J Pharmacol.* 130:963–974.

Dickinson K.M., Clifton P.M., and Keogh J.B. 2011. Endothelial function is impaired after a high-salt meal in healthy subjects. *Am J Clin Nutr.* 93(3):500–505.

Dickinson K.M., Keogh J.B., and Clifton P.M. 2009. Effects of a low-salt diet on flow-mediated dilatation in humans. *Am J Clin Nutr.* 89:485–490.

Djousse L., Ellison C., McLennan C., Cupples L.A., Lipinska I., Tofler G.H., Gokce N., and Vita J.A. 1999. Acute effects of a high fat meal with and without red wine on endothelial function in healthy subjects. *Am J Cardiol.* 84:660–664.

Dohadwala M.M., Hamburg N.M., Holbrook M., Kim B.H., Duess M.A., Levit A., Titas M. et al. 2010. Effects of condord grape juice on ambulatory blood pressure in prehypertensive and stage 1 hypertension. *Am J Clin Nutr.* 92(5):1052–1059.

Drexler H. and Hornig B. 1999. Endothelial dysfunction in human disease. *J Mol Cell Cardiol.* 311:51–60.

Duffy S.J., Keaney Jr. J.F., Holbrook M., Gokce N., Swerdloff P.L., Frei B., and Vita J.A. 2001. Short- and long-term black tea consumption reverses endothelial dysfunction in patients with coronary artery disease. *Circulation.* 104:151–156.

Duffy S.J., New G., Harper R.W., and Meredith I.T. 1999. Metabolic vasodilation in the human forearm is preserved in hypercholesterolemia despite impairment of endothelium- dependent and independent vasodilation. *Cardiovasc Res.* 43:721–730.

Dwyer J.H., Paul-Labrador M.J., Fan J., Shircore A.M., Merz C.N.B., and Dwyer K.M. 2004. Progression of carotid intima-media thickness and plasma antioxidants: The los angeles atherosclerosis study. *Arterioscler Thromb Vasc Biol.* 24:313–319.

Ellingsen I., Hjerkinn E.M., Seljeflot I., Arnesen H., and Tonstad S. 2008. Consumption of fruit and berries is inversely associated with carotid atherosclerosis in elderly men. *Br J Nutr.* 99:674–681.

Engler M.B., Engler M.M., Chen C.Y., Malloy M.J, Browne A., Chiu E.Y., Kwak H.K. et al. 2004. Flavonoid-rich dark chocolate improves endothelial function and increases plasma epicatechin concentrations in healthy adults. *J Am Coll Nutr.* 23:197–204.

Evans M., Njike V.Y., Hoxley M., Pearson M., and Katz D.L. 2007. Effect of soy isoflavone protein and soy lecithin on endothelial function in healthy postmenopausal women. *Menopause.* 14:141–149.

Faridi Z., Valentine N.V.Y., Dutta S., Ali A., and Katz D.L. 2008. Acute dark chocolate and cocoa ingestion and endothelial function: A randomized controlled crossover trial. *Am J Clin Nutr.* 88:58–63.

Farouque H.M., Leung M., Hope S.A., Baldi M., Schechter C., Cameron J.D., and Meredith I.T. 2006. Acute and chronic effects of flavanol-rich cocoa on vascular function in subjects with coronary artery disease: A randomized double-blind placebo-controlled study. *Clin Sci.* 111:71–80.

Fathi R., Haluska B., Isbel N., Short L., and Marwick T.H. 2004. The relative importance of vascular structure and function in predicting cardiovascular events. *J Am Coll Cardiol.* 43:616–623.

Fisher N.D.L., Hughes M., Gerhard-Herman M., and Hollenberg N.K. 2003. Flavanol-rich cocoa induces nitric-oxide-dependent vasodilation in healthy humans. *J Hypertens.* 21(12):2281–2286.

Fisher N.D.L., Norman K., and Hollenberg N.K. 2006. Aging and vascular responses to flavanol-rich cocoa. *J Hypertens.* 24:1575–1580.

Flegal K.M., Carroll M.D., and Ogden C.L. 2010. Trends in obesity and extreme obesity among US adults. *JAMA.* 303(3):235–241.

Forstermann U. 2008. Oxidative stress in vascular disease: Cause, defense mechanisms and potential therapies. *Cardiovasc Med.* 5(6):338–349.

Francis S.T., Head K., Morris P.G., and Macdonald I.A. 2006. The effect of flavonol-rich coca on the fMRI response to a cognitive task in healthy young people. *J Cardiovasc Pharmacol.* 2006, 47(Suppl 2):215–220.

Franzini L., Ardigo D., Valtuena S., Pellergrini N., del Rio D., Bianchi M.A., Scazzina F., Piatti P.M., Brighenti F., and Zavaroni I. 2012. Food selection based on high total antioxidant capacity improves endothelial function in a low cardiovascular risk population. *Nutr Metab Cardiovasc Dis*. 22(1):50–57.

Frick M., Suessenbacher A., Alber H.F., Dichtl W., Ulmer H., Pachinger O., and Weidinger F. 2005. Prognostic value of brachial artery endothelial function and wall thickness. *J Am Coll Cardiol*. 46:1006–1010.

Fuentes F., Lopez-Miranda J., Perez-Martinez P., Jimenez Y., Marin C., Gomez P., Fernandez J.M., Caballero J., Delgado-Lista J., and Perez-Jimenez F. 2008. Chronic effect of a high-fat diet enriched with linolenic acid on postprandial endothelial function in healthy men. *Br J Nutr*. 100:159–165.

George T.W., Niwat C., Waroonphan S., Gordon M.H., and Lovegrove J.A. 2009. Effects of chronic and acute consumption of fruit- and vegetable-puree-based drinks on vasodilation, risk factors for CVD and the response as a result of the eNOS G298T polymorphism. *Proc Nutr Soc*. 68(2):148–161.

Ghiadoni L., Donald A.E., Cropley M., Mullen M.J., Oakley G., Taylor M., O'Connor G. et al. 2000. Mental stress induces transient endothelial dysfunction. *Circulation*. 102:2473–2478.

Ghosh D. and Scheepens A. 2009. Vascular action and polyphenols. *Mol Nutr Food Res*. 53(3):322–331.

Gokce N., Keaney J.F. Jr., and Hunter L.M. 2003. Predictive value of noninvasively determined endothelial dysfunction for long term cardiovascular events in patients with peripheral vascular disease. *J Am Coll Cardiol*. 41:1769–1775.

Gokce N., Keaney J.F. Jr, Hunter L.M., Watkins M.T., Menzoian J.O., and Vita J.A. 2002. Risk stratification for postoperative cardiovascular events via noninvasive assessment of endothelial function: A prospective study. *Circulation*. 105:1567–1572.

Gonzalez-Gallego J., Garcıa-Mediavilla M.V., Sonia Sanchez-Campos S., and Tunon M.J. 2010. Fruit polyphenols, immunity and inflammation. *Br J Nutr*. 104:S15–S27.

Grassi D., Desideri G., Croce G., Tiberti S., Aggio A., and Ferri C. 2009. Flavonoids, vascular function and cardiovascular protection. *Curr Pharm Des*. 15:1072–1084.

Grassi D., Desideri G., Necozione S., Lippi C., Casale R., Properzi G., Blumberg J., and Ferri C. 2008. Blood pressure is reduced and insulin sensitivity increased in glucose-intolerant, hypertensive subjects after 15 days of consuming high polyphenol dark chocolate. *J Nutr*. 138:1671–1676.

Grassi D., Mulder T.P., Draijer R., Desideri G., Moluizen H.O., and Ferri C. 2009. Black tea consumption dose-dependently improves flow-mediated dilation in healthy males. *J Hypertens*. 27(4):774–781.

Grassi D., Necozione S., Lippi C., Croce C, Croce G., Valeri L., Pasqualetti P., Blumberg J., and Ferri C. 2005. Cocoa reduces blood pressure and insulin resistance and improves endothelium-dependent vasodilation in hypertensives. *Hypertens*. 46:398–405.

Groner J.A., Joshi M., and Bauer J.A. 2006. Pediatric precursors of adult cardiovascular disease: Noninvasive assessment of early vascular changes in children and adolescents. *Pediatrics*. 1184:1683–1691.

Guarda E., Godoy I., Foncea R., Perez D.D., Romero C., Venegas R., Venegas R., and Leighton F. 2005. Red wine reduces oxidative stress in patients with acute coronary syndrome. *Int J Cardiol*. 104:35–38.

Gupta A.K., Cornelissen G., Greenway F.L., Dhoopati V., Halberg F., and Johnson W.D. 2010. Abnormalities in circadian blood pressure variability and endothelial function: Pragmatic markers for adverse cardiometabolic profiles in asymptomatic obese adults. *Cardiovasc Diabetol*. 9:58.

Hale G., Paul-Labrador M., Dwyer J.H., and Merz C.N. 2002. Isoflavone supplementation and endothelial function in menopausal women. *Clin Endocrinol*. 56:693–701.

Hall W.L., Formanuik N.L., Harnpanich D., Cheung M., Talbot D., Chowienczyk P.J., and Sanders T.A. 2008. A meal enriched with soy isoflavones increases nitric oxide-mediated vasodilation in healthy postmenopausal women. *J Nutr*. 138:1288–1292.

Hall W.L., Vafeiadou K., Hallund J., Bugel S., Reimann M., Koebnick C., Zunft H.J. et al. 2006. Soy-isoflavone-enriched foods and markers of lipid and glucose metabolism in postmenopausal women: Interactions with genotype and equol production. *Am J Clin Nutr*. 83:592–600.

Hallund J., Bugel S., Tholstrup T., Ferrari M., Talbot D., Hall W.L., Raimann M., Williams C., M., and Wiinberg N. 2006. Soya isoflavone-enriched cereal bars affect markers of endothelial function in postmenopausal women. *Br J Nutr*. 95:1120–1126.

Hamilton S.J., Chew G.T., and Watts G.F. 2007. Therapeutic regulation of endothelial dysfunction in type 2 diabetes. *Diabetes Vasc Dis Res*. 4:89–102.

Hashemi M., Kelishadi R., Hashemipour M., Zakeameil A., Khavarian N., Ghatrehsamani S., and Poursafa P. 2010. Acute and long-term effects of grape and pomegranate juice consumption on vascular reactivity in paediatric metabolic syndrome. *Cardiol Young*. 20:73–77.

Hashimoto M., Akishita M., Eto M., Lijima K., Ako J., Yoshizumi M., Akishita M. et al. 1998. The impairment of flow-mediated vasodilatation in obese men with visceral fat accumulation. *Int J Obes Relat Metab Disord*. 225:477–484.

Hashimoto M., Seungbum K., Masato E. et al. 2001. Effect of acute intake of red wine on flow mediated vasodilation of the brachial artery. *Am J Cardiol.* 88:1457–1459.

Heiss C., Dejam A., Kleinbongard P., Schewe T., Sies H., and Kelm M. 2003. Vascular effects of cocoa rich in flavan-3-ols. *JAMA* 290:1030–1031.

Heiss C., Finis D., Kleinbongard P., Hoffmann A., Rassaf T., Kelm M., and Sies H. 2007. Sustained increase in flow-mediated dilation after daily intake of high-flavanol cocoa drink over 1 week. *J Cardiovasc Pharmacol.* 49:74–80.

Heiss C., Kleinbongard P., Dejam A., Perre S., Schroeter H., Sies H., and Kelm M. 2005. Acute consumption of flavanol-rich cocoa and the reversal of endothelial dysfunction in smokers. *J Am Coll Cardiol* 46:1276–1283.

Heiss C., Keen C.L., and Kelm M. 2010. Flavanols and cardiovascular disease prevention. *Eur Heart J.* 31(21):2583–2592.

Hermann F., Spieker L.E., Ruschitzka F., Sudano I., Hermann M., Binggeli C., Luscher T.F., Riesen W., Noll G., and Corti R. 2006. Dark chocolate improves endothelial and platelet function. *Heart.* 92:119–120.

Hermansen K., Hansen B., Jacobsen R., Clausen P., Dalgaard M., Dinesen B., Holst J.J., Pedersen E., and Astrup A. 2005. Effects of soy supplementation on blood lipids and arterial function in hypercholesterol-aemic subjects. *Eur J Clin Nutr.* 59:843–850.

Hijmering M., Lange D., Lorsheyd A., Kraaijenhagen R., and Van de Wiel A. 2007. Bing drinking causes endothelial dysfunction which is not prevented by wine polyphenols: A small trial in healthy volunteers. *J Med.* 65(1):29–35.

Hirata K., Shimada K., Watanabe H., Otsuka R., Tokai K., Yoshiyama M., Homma S., and Yshikawa J. 2004. Black tea increases coronary flow velocity reserve in healthy male subjects. *Am J Cardiol.* 93:1384–1388.

Hodgson J.M. 2006. Effects of tea and tea flavonoids on endothelial function and blood pressure: A brief review. *Clin Exp Pharmacol Physiol.* 33:838–841.

Hodgson J.M., Burke V., and Puddey I.B. 2005. Acute effects of tea on fasting and postprandial vascular function and blood pressure in humans. *J Hypertens.* 23:47–54.

Hodgson J.M. and Croft K.D. 2006. Dietary flavonoids: Effects on endothelial function and blood pressure, a review. *J Sci Food Agric.* 86:2492–2498.

Hodgson J.M. and Puddey I.B. 2005. Dietary flavonoids and cardiovascular disease: Dose the emperor have any clothes? *J Hypertens.* 23:1461–1463.

Hodgson J.M., Puddey I.B., Burke V., and Croft K.D. 2006. Is reversal of endothelial dysfunction by tea related to flavonoid metabolism? *Br J Nutr.* 95:14–17.

Hodgson J.M., Puddey I.B., Burke V., Watts G.F., and Beilin L.J. 2002. Regular ingestion of black tea improves brachial artery vasodilator function. *Clinical Sci.* 102:195–201.

Hooper L., Kroon P.A., Rimm E.B., Cohn J.S., Harvey I., Le Cornu K.A., Ryder J.J., Hall W.L., and Cassidy A. 2008. Flavonoids, flavonoid-rich foods, and cardiovascular risk: Meta-analysis of randomized controlled trials. *Am J Clin Nutr.* 88:38–50.

Howes J.B., Tran D., Brillante D., and Howes L.G. 2003. Effects of dietary supplementation with isoflavones from red clover on ambulatory blood pressure and endothelial function in postmenopausal type 2 diabetes. *Diabetes Obes Metab.* 5:325–332.

Hristov M., Erl W., Linder S., and Weber P.C. 2004. Apoptotic bodies from endothelial cells enhance the number and initiate the differentiation of human endothelial progenitor cells in vitro. *Blood.* 104:2761–2766.

Hristov M., Erl W., and Weber P.C. 2003. Endothelial progenitor cells: Mobilization, differentiation, and homing. *Arterioscler Thromb Vasc Biol.* 23:1185–1189.

Hung H-C., Joshipura K.J., Jiang R., Hu F.B., Hunter D., Smith-Warner S.A., Colditz G.A., Rosner B., Spiegelman D., and Willett W.C. 2004. Fruit and vegetable intake and risk of major chronic disease. *J Natl Cancer Inst.* 96:1577–1584.

Ignarro L.J., Balestrieri M.L., and Napoli C. 2007. Nutrition, physical activity, and cardiovascular disease: An update. *Cardiovasc Res.* 73:326–340.

Iribarren C., Folsom A., Jacobs D.R Jr., Gross M.D., Belcher J.D., and Eckfeldt J.H. 1997. Association of serum vitamin levels, LDL susceptibility to oxidation, and autoantibodies against MDA-LDL with carotid atherosclerosis. *Arterioscler Thromb Vasc Biol.* 17:1171–1177.

Jimenez J.J., Jy W., Mauro L.M., Horstman L.L., Bidot C.J., and Ahn Y.S. 2005. Endothelial microparticles (EMP) as vascular disease markers. *Adv Clin Chem.* 39:131–157.

Joannides R., Haefeli W.E., Linder L., Richard V., Bakkali E.H., Thuillez C., and Luscher T.F. 1995. Nitric oxide is responsible for flow-dependent dilation of human peripheral conduit arteries in vivo. *Circulation.* 91:1314–1319.

Jochmann N., Lorenz M., von Krosigk A., Martus P., Bohm V., Baumann G., Stangl K., and Stangl V. 2007. The efficacy of black tea in ameliorating endothelial function is equivalent to that of green tea. *Br J Nutr.* 99(4):863–868.

Juonala M., Viikari J.S., Ronnemaa T., Marniemi J., Jula A., Loo B.M., and Raitakari O.T. 2008. Associations of dyslipidemias from childhood to adulthood with carotid intima-media thickness, elasticity, and brachial flow-mediated dilatation in adulthood: The cardiovascular risk in young Finns study. *Arterioscler Thromb Vasc Biol.* 28(5):1012–1017.

Le J., Zhang D., Menees S., Chen J., and Raghuveer G. 2010. "Vascular Age" Is advanced in children with atherosclerosis-promoting risk factors. *Circ Cardiovasc Imaging.* 3:8–14.

Lichtenstein A.H., Appel L.J., Brands M., Carnethon M., Daniels S., Franch H.A., Franklin B. 2006. Diet and lifestyle recommendations revision 2006: A scientific statement from the American Heart Association Nutrition Committee. *Circulation.* 1141:82–96.

Lissin L.W., Oka R., Lakshmi S., and Cooke J.P. 2004. Isoflavones improve vascular reactivity in postmenopausal women with hypercholesterolemia. *Vasc Med.* 9:26–30.

Loke W.M., Hodgson J.M., Proudfoot J.M., McKinley A.J., Puddey I.B., and Croft K.D. 2008. Pure dietary flavonoids quercetin and (−)-epicatechin augment nitric oxide products and reduce endothelin-1 acutely in healthy men. *Am J Clin Nutr.* 88:1018–1025.

Lorenz M., Jochmann N., von Krosigk A., Martus P., Baumann G., Stangl K., and Stangl V. 2007. Addition of milk prevents vascular protective effects of tea. *Eur Heart J.* 28:219–223.

Lorenz M., Urban J., Engelhardt U., Baumann G., Stangl K., and Stangl V. 2009. green and black tea are equally potent stimuli of NO production and vasodilation: New insights into tea ingredients involved. *Basic Res Cardiol.* 104(1):100–110.

Luscher T.F. and Barton M. 1997. Biology of the endothelium. *Clin Cardiol.* 20(11 Suppl. 2):3–10.

Kannel W.B., Hjortland M.C., McNamara P.M., and Gordon T. 1976. Menopause and risk of cardiovascular disease: The Framingham Study. *Ann Intern Med.* 85:447–452.

Kapiotis S., Holzer G., Schaller G., Haumer M., Widhalm H., Weghuber D., Jilma B. et al. 2006. A proinflammatory state is detectable in obese children and is accompanied by functional and morphological vascular changes. *Arterioscler Thromb Vasc Biol.* 26:2541–2546.

Karatzi K., Karatzus E., Papamichael C., Lekakis J., and Zampelas A. 2009. Effects of red wine on endothelial function: Postprandial studies vs clinical trials. *Nutr Metab Cardio Dis.* 19:744–750.

Karatzi K., Papamichael C., Aznaourisis K., Karatzis E., Lekakis J., Matsouka C., Boskou G. 2004. Constituents of red wine other than alcohol improve endothelial function in patients with CAD. *Coronary Arter Dis.* 15:485–490.

Kato T., Inoue T., Morooka T., Yoshimoto N., and Node K. 2006. Short-term passive smoking causes endothelial dysfunction via oxidative stress in nonsmokers. *Can J Physiol Pharmacol.* 84:523.

Katz D.L., Evans M.A., Njike V.Y., Hoxley M.L., Nawaz H., Comerford B.P., and Sarrel P.M. 2007. Raloxifene, soy phytoestrogens and endothelial function in postmenopausal women. *Climacteric.* 10:500–507.

Kelm M. 2002. Flow-mediated dilatation in human circulation: Diagnostic and therapeutic aspects. *Am J Physiol Heart Circ Physiol.* 282:H1–H5.

Kim W., Jeong M.H., Cho S.H., Yun J.H., Chae H.J., Ahn Y.K., Cheng X., Kondo T., Murohara T., and Kang J.C. 2006. Effect of green tea consumption on endothelial function and circulating endothelial progenitor cells in chronic smokers. *Circ J.* 70:1052–1057.

Kimm S.Y. and Obarzanek E. 2002. Childhood obesity: A new pandemic of the new millennium. *Pediatrics.* 110:1003–1007.

Kreijkamp-Kaspers S., Kok L., Bots M.L., Grobbee D.E., Lampe J.W., and van der Schouw Y.T. 2005. Randomized controlled trial of the effects of soy protein containing isoflavones on vascular function in postmenopausal women. *Am J Clin Nutr.* 81:189–195.

Mancini G.B. 2004. Vascular structure versus function: Is endothelial dysfunction of independent prognostic importance or not? *J Am Coll Cardiol.* 43:624–628.

Markus R.A., Mack W.J., Azen S.P., and Hodis H.N. 1997. Influence of lifestyle modification on atherosclerotic progression determined by ultrasonographic change in the common carotid intima-media thickness. *Am J Clin Nutr.* 65, 1000–1004.

Marin C., Ramirez R., Delgado-Lista J., Perez-Martinez P., Carracedo J., Garcia-Rios A., Rodriguez F. et al. 2011. Mediterranean diet reduces endothelial damage and improves the regenerative capacity of endothelium. *Am J Clin Nutr.* 93:267–274.

McGill H.C., McMahon A., Henderick E.E., Malcom G.T., Tracy R.E., and Strong J.P. 2000. Origin of atherosclerosis in childhood and adolescence. *Am J Clin Nutr.* 72:1307S–1315S.

Moens A.L., Goovaerts I., Claeys M.J., and Vrints C.J. 2005. Flow-mediated vasodilation: A diagnostic instrument, or an experimental tool? *Chest.* 127:2254–2263.

Mombouli J.V. and Vanhoutte P.M. 1999. Endothelial dysfunction: From physiology to therapy. *J Mol Cell Cardiol.* 311:61–74.

Mozaffarian D., Wilson P.W.F., and Kannel W.B. 2008. Beyond established and novel risk factors: Lifestyle risk factors for cardiovascular disease. *Circulation.* 117:3031–3038.

Must A., Jacques P.F., Dallal G.E., Bajema C.J., and Dietz W.H. 1992. Long-term morbidity and mortality of overweight adolescents. A follow-up of the Harvard Growth Study of 1922 to 1935. *N Engl J Med.* 327:1350–1355.

Nagata C. 2000. Ecological study of the association between soy product intake and mortality from cancer and heart disease in Japan. *Int J Epidemiol.* 29:832–836.

Nagaya N., Yamamoto H., Uematsu M., Itoh T., Nakagawa K., Miyazawa T., Kangawa K., and Miyatake K. 2004. Green tea reverses endothelial dysfunction in healthy smokers. *Heart.* 90:1485–1486.

Nicholson S.K., Tucker G.A., and Brameld J.M. 2008. Effects of dietary polyphenols on gene expression in human vascular endothelial cells. *Proc Nutr Soc.* 67:42–47.

Nikander E., Metsa-Heikkila M., Tiitinen A., and Ylikorkala O. 2003. Evidence of a lack of effect of a phytoestrogen regimen on the levels of C-reactive protein, E-selectin, and nitrate in postmenopausal women. *J Clin Endocrinol Metab.* 88:5180–5185.

Oren A., Vos L.E., Uiterwaal C.S., Gorissen W.H., Grobbee D.E., and Bots M.L. 2003. Change in body mass index from adolescence to young adult and increased CIMT at 28 years: The atherosclerosis in young adult study. *Int J Obes Relat Metab Disorder.* 27(1):1383–1390.

Pan M-H., Lai C-S., and Ho C-T. 2010. Anti-inflammatory activity of natural dietary flavonoids. *Food Function.* 1:161–166.

Pase M.P., Grima N.A., and Sarris J. 2011. The effects of dietary and nutrient interventions on arterial stiffness: A systematic review. *Am J Clin Nutr.* 93(2):446–454.

Patel S. and Celermajer D.S. 2006. Assessment of vascular disease using arterial flow mediated dilatation. *Pharmacol Rep.* 58:3–7.

Pena A.S., Wiltshire E., MacKenzie K., Gent R., Piotto L., Hirte C., and Couper J. 2006. Vascular endothelial and smooth muscle function relates to body mass index and glucose in obese and nonobese children. *J Clin Endocrinol Metab.* 91:4467–4471.

Phillips S.A., Jurva J.W., Syed A.Q., Kulinski J.P., Pleuss J., Hoffmann R.Q., and Gutterman D.D. 2008. Benefit of low-fat over low carbohydrate diet in endothelial health. *Hypertens.* 51(2):376–382.

Piccin A., Murphy W.G., and Smith O.P. 2007. Circulating microparticles: Pathophysiology and clinical implications. *Blood Rev.* 21:157–171.

Puchau B., Zulet M.A., Gonzalez de Echavarri A., Hermsdorff H.H.M., and Martınez J.A. 2009. Dietary total antioxidant capacity: A novel indicator of diet quality in healthy young adults. *J Am Coll Nutr.* 28(6):648–656.

Quyyumi A.A. 2003. Prognostic value of endothelial function. *Am J Cardiol.* 91(12A):19H–24H.

Raghuveer G. 2010. Lifetime cardiovascular risk of childhood obesity. *Am J Clin Nutr.* 91:1514S–1519S.

Rallidis L.S., Lekakis J., Kolomvotsou A., Zampelas A., Vamvakou G., Efstathiou S., Dimitriadis G., Raptis S.A., and Kremastinos D.T. 2009. Close adherence to a Mediterranean diet improves endothelial function in subjects with abdominal obesity. *Am J Clin Nutr.* 90:263–268.

Reddy K.G., Nair R.N., Sheehan H.M., and Hodgson J.M. 1994. Evidence that selective endothelial dysfunction may occur in the absence of angiographic or ultrasound atherosclerosis in patients with risk-factors for atherosclerosis. *J Am Coll Cardiol.* 23:833–843.

Reddy V.C., Sagar G.V., Sreeramulu D., Venu L., and Raghunath M. 2005. Addition of milk does not alter the antioxidant activity of black tea. *Ann Nutr Metab.* 49:189–195.

Rissanen T.H., Voutilainen S., Nyyssonen K., Salonen R., Kaplan G.A., and Salonen J.T.2003. Serum lycopene concentrations and carotid atherosclerosis: The kuopio ischaemic heart disease risk factor study. *Am J Clin Nutr.* 77:133–138.

Roberts N., Jahangiri M., Xu Q. 2005. Progenitor cells in vascular disease. *J Cell Mol Med.* 9:583–591.

Romero-Corral A., Sert-Kuniyoshi F.H., Sierra-Johnson J., Orban M., Gami M., Davison D., Singh P. et al. 2010. Modest visceral fat gain causes endothelial dysfunction in health humans. *J Am Coll Cardio.* 56(8):662–666.

Ros E., Nunez I., Pérez-Heras A., Serra Gilabert R., Casals E., and Deulofeu R. 2004. Walnut diet improves endothelial function in hypercholesterolemic subjects: A randomized crossover trial. *Circulation.* 109:1609–1614.

Ross E. 1999. Atherosclerosis: An inflammatory disease. *N Engl J Med.* 340:115–126.

Rudolph T.K., Ruempler K., Schwedhelm E., Tan-Andresen J., Reederer U., Boger R.H., and Maas R. 2007. Acute effects of various fast-food meals on vascular function and cardiovascular disease risk markers: The Hamburg burger trial. *Am J Clin Nutr*. 86:334–340.

Rueda-Clausen C.F., Silva F.A., Lindarte M.A., Villa-Roel C., Gomez E., Gutierrez R., Cure-Cure C., and Lopez-Jaramillo P. 2007. Olive, soybean and palm oils intake have similar acute detrimental effects over the endothelial function in health young subjects. *Nutr Metab Cardiobasc Dis*. 17(1):50–57.

Ruschitzka F.T., Noll G., and Luscher T.F. 1997. The endothelium in caronary artery disease. *Cardiology*. 88(Suppl. 3):3–19.

Santangelo C., Vari R., Scazzocchio B., Di Benedetto R., Filesi C., and Masella R. 2007. Polyphenols, intracellular signalling and inflammation. *Ann Ist Super Sanita*. 43(4):394–405.

Sari I., Baltaci Y., Bagci C., Davutoglu V., Erel O., Celik H., Ozer O., Aksoy N., and Aksoy M. 2010. Effect of pistachio diet on lipid parameters, endothelial function, inflammation, and oxidative status: A prospective study. *Nutrition*. 26(4):399–404.

Sattar N. Ferns G. 2005. Endothelial dysfunction. In *Cardiovascular Disease: Diet Nutrition and Emerging Risk Factors*, pp. 63–77 (S Stanner, editor). Oxford: Blackwell Science.

Schachinger V., Britten M.B., Elsner M., Walter D.H., Scharrer I., and Zeiher A.M. 1999. A positive family history of premature coronary artery disease is associated with impaired endothelium-dependent coronary blood flow regulation. *Circulation*. 100:1502–1508.

Schewe T., Steffen Y., and Sies H. 2008. How do dietary flavanols improve vascular function? A position paper. *Arch Biochem Biophys*. 476(2):102–106.

Schini-Kerth V.B., Auger C., Kim J-H., Étienne-Selloum N., and Chataigneau T. 2010. Nutritional improvement of the endothelial control of vascular tone by polyphenols: Role of NO and EDHF. *Pflugers Arch—Eur J Physiol*. 459:853–862.

Schroeter H., Heiss C., Balzer J., Kleinbongard P., Keen C.L., Hollenberg N.K., Sies H., Kwik-Uribe C., Schmitz H.H., and Kelm M. 2006. (–)-Epicatechin mediates beneficial effects of flavanol-rich cocoa on vascular function in humans. *Proc Natl Acad Sci*. 103:1024–1029.

Serafini M., Ghiselli A., and Ferro-Luzzi A. 1996. *In vivo* antioxidant effect of green and black tea in man. *Eur J Clin Nutr*. 50:28–32.

Simons L.A., von Konigsmark M., Simons J., and Celermajer D.S. 2000. Phytoestrogens do not influence lipoprotein levels or endothelial function in healthy, postmenopausal women. *Am J Cardiol*. 85:1297–1301.

Singh N., Graves J., Taylor P.D., MacAllister R.J., and Singer D.R. 2002. Effects of a healthy diet and of acute and long-term vitamin C on vascular function in healthy older subjects. *Cardiovasc Res*. 56(1):118–125.

Sorond F.A., Lipsitz L.A., Hollenberg N.K., and Fisher N.D. 2008. Cerebral blood flow response to flavanol-rich cocoa in healthy elderly humans. *Neuropsychiatr Dis Treat*. 4(2):433–440.

Spieker L.E., Hürlimann D., Ruschitzka F., Corti R., Enseleit F., Shaw S., Hayoz D., Deanfield J.E., Luscher T.F., and Noll G. 2002. Mental stress induces prolonged endothelial dysfunction via endothelin-a receptors. *Circulation*. 105:2817–2820.

Squadrito F., Altavilla D., Crisafulli A., Saitta A., Cucinotta D., Morabito N., D'Anna R., Ruggeri Frisina N., and Squadrito G. 2003. Effect of genistein on endothelial function in postmenopausal women: A randomized, double blind, controlled study. *Am J Med*. 114:470–476.

Squadrito F., Altavilla D., Morabito N., Crisafulli A., D'Anna R., Corrado F., Ruggeri P. et al. 2002. The effect of the phytoestrogen genistein on plasma nitric oxide concentrations, endothelin-1levels and endothelium dependent vasodilation in postmenopausal women. *Atherosclerosis*. 163:339–347.

Squadrito F., Altavilla D., Squadrito G., Saitta A., Cucinotta D., Minutoli L., Deodato B. et al. 2000. Genistein supplementation and estrogen replacement therapy improve endothelial dysfunction induced by ovariectomy in rats. *Cardiovasc Res*. 45:454–462.

Srinivasan S.R., Bao W., Wattigney W.A., and Berenson G.S. 1996. Adolescent overweight is associated with adult overweight and related multiple cardiovascular risk factors: The bogalusa heart study. *Metabolism*. 45:235–240.

Stein J.H., Keevil J.G., Wiebe D.A., Aeschlimann S., and Folts J.D. 1999. Purple grape juice improves endothelial function and reduces the susceptibility of LDL cholesterol to oxidation in patients with coronary artery disease. *Circulation*. 10010:1050–1055.

Steinberger J. and Daniels S.R. 2003. Obesity, insulin resistance, diabetes, and cardiovascular risk in children. *Circulation*. 107(10):1448–1453.

Steinberg F.M., Guthrie N.L., Villablanca A.C., Kumar K., and Murray M.J. 2003. Soy protein with isoflavones has favorable effects on endothelial function that are independent of lipid and antioxidant effects in healthy postmenopausal women. *Am J Clin Nutr*. 78:123–130.

Suwaidi J.A., Hamasaki S., Higano S.T., Nishimura R.A., Holmes D.R. Jr., and Lerman A. 2000. Long-term follow-up of patients with mild coronary artery disease and endothelial dysfunction. *Circulation*. 101:948–954.

Teede H.J., Dalais F.S., Kotsopoulos D., McGrath B.P., Malan E., Gan T.E., and Peverill R.E. 2005. Dietary soy containing phytoestrogens does not activate the hemostatic system in postmenopausal women. *J Clin Endocrinol Metab*. 90:1936–1941.

Teede H.J., Dalais F.S., Kotsopoulos D., Liang Y.L., Davis S., and McGrath B.P. 2001. Dietary soy has both beneficial and potentially adverse cardiovascular effects: A placebo-controlled study in men and postmenopausal women. *J Clin Endocrinol Metab*. 86:3053–3060.

Teede H.J., McGrath B.P., DeSilva L., Cehun M., Fassoulakis A., and Nestel P.J. 2003. Isoflavones reduce arterial stiffness: A placebo-controlled study in men and postmenopausal women. *Arterioscler Thromb Vasc Biol*. 23:1066–1071.

Tentolouris N., Arapostathi C., Perrea D., Kyriaki D., Revenas C., and Katsilambros N. 2008. Differential effects of two isoenergetic meals rich in saturated or monounsaturated fat on endothelial function in subjects with type 2 diabetes. *Diabetes Care*. 31:2276–2278.

Teragawa H., Kato M., Kurokawa J., Yamagata T., Yamagata T, Matsuura H., and Chayama K. 2001. Usefulness of flow-mediated dilation of the brachial artery and/or the intima-media thickness of the carotid artery in predicting coronary narrowing in patients suspected of having coronary artery disease. *Am J Cardiol*. 88:1147–1151.

Tinahones F.J., Rubio M.A., Garrido-Sanchez L., Ruiz C., Gordillo E., Cabrerizo L., and Cardona F. 2008. Green tea reduces LDL oxidability and improves vascular function. *J Am Coll Nutr*. 27(2):209–213.

Tounian P., Aggoun Y., Dubern B., Varille V., Guy-Grand B., Sida D., Girardet J.P., and Bonnet D. 2001. Presence of increased stiffness of the common carotid artery and endothelial dysfunction in severely obese children: A prospective study. *Lancet*. 358:1400–1404.

Tushuizen M.E., Nieuwland R., Scheffer P.G.A., Sturka R.J., Heine R.J., and Diamant M. 2006. Two consecutive high-fat meals affect endothelial-dependent vasodilation, oxidative stress and cellular microparticles in healthy men. *J Thromb Haemostasis*, 4:1003–1010.

Urbina E.M., Kimball T.R., McCoy C.E., Khoury P.R., Daniels S.R., and Dolan L.M. 2009. Youth with obesity and obesity-related type 2 diabetes mellitus demonstrate abnormalities in carotid structure and function. *Circulation*. 119:2913–2919.

USDA and HHS. 2010. Report of the Dietary Guidelines Advisory Committee on the Dietary Guidelines for Americans. Part D. Section 3: Fatty Acids and Cholesterol. D-3:1–65.

van het Hof K.H., Kivits G.A., Weststrate J.A., and Tijburg L.B.1998. Bioavailability of catechins from tea: The effect of milk. *Eur J Clin Nutr*. 52:356–359.

van het Hof K.H., Wiseman S.A., Yang C.S., and Tijburg L.B. 1999. Plasma and lipoprotein levels of tea catechins following repeated tea consumption. *Proc Soc Exp Biol Med*. 220:203–209.

van Mierlo L.A., Zock P.L., van der Knaap H.C.M., and Draijer R. 2010. Grape polyphenols do not affect vascular function in healthy men. *J Nutr*. 140:1769–1773.

Van Wijk M.J., VanBavel E., Sturk A., and Nieuwland R. 2003. Microparticles in cardiovascular diseases. *Cardiovasc Res*. 59:277–287.

Varady K.A., Bhutani S., Klempel M.C., and Phillips S.A. 2011. Improvements in vascular health by a low-fat diet, but not a high-fat diet, are mediated by changes in adipocyte biology. *Nutrition J*. 10:10–18.

Verma S. and Anderson T.J. 2000. Fundamentals of endothelial function for the clinical cardiologist. *Circulation*. 105:546–549.

Versari D., Daghini E., Virdis A., Ghiadoni L., and Taddei S. 2009. Endothelial dysfunction as a target for prevention of cardiovascular disease. *Diabetes Care*. 32:S314–S321.

Vita J.A. and Keaney J.F. Jr. 2002. Endothelial function: A barometer for cardiovascular risk? *Circulation*. 106:640–642.

Vlachopoulos C., Aznaouridis K., Alexopoulos N., Economou E., Andreadou I., and Stefanadis C. 2005. Effect of dark chocolate on arterial function in healthy individuals. *Am J Hypertens*. 18:785–791.

Vogel R.A. and Benitez R.M. 2000. Noninvasive assessment of cardiovascular risk: From framingham to the future. *Rev Cardiovasc Med*. 11:34–42.

Vogel R.A., Corretti M.C., and Plotnick G.D. 1997. Effect of a single high-fat meal on endothelial function in healthy subjects. *Am J Cardiol*. 793:350–354.

Wang-Polagruto J.F., Villabianca A.C., Polagruto J.A., Lee L., Holt R.R., Schrader H.R., Ensunsa J.L., Steinberg F.M., Schmitz H.H., and Keen C.L. 2006. Chronic consumption of flavanol-rich cocoa improves endothelial function and decreases vascular cell adhesion molecule in hypercholesterolemic postmenopausal women. *J Cardiovasc Pharmacol*. 47(Suppl. 2):S177–S186.

Werner N., Kosiol S., Schiegl T., Ahlers P., Walenta K., Link A., Bohm M., and Nickenig G. 2005. Circulating endothelial progenitor cells and cardiovascular outcomes. *N Engl J Med*. 353:999–1007.

Westphal S. and Luley C. 2011. Flavanol-rich cocoa ameliorates lipemia-induced endothelial dysfunction. *Heart Vessels*. Ahead of Publication.

Whelan A., Sutherland W., McCormick M., Yeoman D., Jong S., and Williams M. 2004. Effects of white and red wine on endothelial function in subjects with coronary artery disease. *Int Med J*. 34:224–228.

Widlansky M.E., Gokce N., Keaney J.F., and Vita J.A. 2003. The clinical implications of endothelial dysfunction. *J Am Coll Cardiol*. 42:1149–1160.

Widlansky M.E., Hamburg N.M., Anter E., Holbrook M., Elliott J.G., Keaney J.F., and Vita J.A. 2007. Acute EGCG supplementation reverses endothelial dysfunction in patients with coronary artery disease. *J Am Coll Nutr*. 26:95–102.

Wilson A.M. 2006. Are vascular function measurements ready for the clinic? *Eur Heart J*. 27:255–257.

Williamson G. and Holst B. 2008. Dietary reference intake (DRI) value for dietary polyphenols: Are we heading in the right direction? *Br J Nutr*. 99:3, S55–S58.

Witte D.R., Westerink J., de Koning E., Van der Graaf Y., Grobbee D.E., and Bots M.L. 2005. Is the association between flow-mediated dilation and cardiovascular risk limited to low-risk populations? *J Am Coll Cardiol*. 45:1987–1993.

Woo K.S., Chook P., Yu C.W., Sung R.Y., Qiao M., Leung S.S., Lam C.W., Metreweli C., and Celermajer D.S. 2004. Overweight in children is associated with arterial endothelial dysfunction and intima-media thickening. *Int J Obes Relat Metab Disord*. 28:852–857.

Yeboah J., Crouse J.R., Hsu F., Burke G.L., Herrington D.M. 2007. Brachial flow-mediated dilation predicts incident cardiovascular events in older adults: The cardiovascular health study. *Circulation*. 115:2390–2397.

Yeboah J., Folsom A.R., Burke G.L., Johnson C., Polak J.F., Post W., Lima J.A., Crouse J.R., and Herrington D.M. 2009. Predictive value of brachial flow-mediated dilation for incident cardiovascular events in a population-based study the multi-ethnic study of atherosclerosis. *Circulation*. 120:502–509

Zilkens R., Burke V., Hodgson J., Barden A., Beilin L., and Puddey I. 2005. Red wine and beer elevated blood pressure in normotensive men. *Hypertens*. 45:874–879.

Zhu W., Huang X., He J., Li M., and Neubauer H. 2005. Arterial intima-media thickening and endothelial dysfunction in obese Chinese children. *Eur J Pediatr*. 164:337–344.

26 Traditional Understanding, Modern Science, and Usage of Herbal Medicine for Diabetes

Dennis Chang, Srinivas Nammi, and Suzanne Grant

CONTENTS

26.1 INTRODUCTION

Herbal medicine refers to the use of medicinal plants for therapeutic purposes and is one of the main complementary medicine (CM) modalities contributing to human health care throughout the world. The use of herbal medicine predates written history, with a pouch of medicinal herbs found in the personal effects of "Otzi the Iceman" whose body has been frozen for more than 5700 years. Written herbal medicinal history may be dated to around 2500 years ago with records of herbs used by *Shen Nong* in ancient China, documenting around 365 medicines including plants, animals, and mineral products (such as tiger bone, deer antler, and earth dragon). Ayurvedic medicine, the traditional healing system of India, is detailed in several classical texts that date back to around 2000 years ago. Plants for medicine have continued to be used throughout the world in the management of disease, to enhance general health, and to promote longevity.

Modern use of plants for medicine continues as an integral part of the holistic systems of healing in traditional Chinese medicine (TCM) and Ayurvedic medicine. In other Asian countries such as Japan and Korea and in the West, herbal medicine is also widely used as a stand-alone modality or as part of other practices such as naturopathy.

Most manufactured drugs have been developed from medicinal plants (World Health Organisation 2005). Of note, metformin, the current first-line treatment for impaired glucose tolerance (IGT) and type-2 diabetes mellitus (T2DM), is derived from *Galega officinalis* (French lilac). *Galega officinalis* is rich in guanidines which have hypoglycemic effects. Contemporary pharmacology was also founded based on the knowledge of herbal medicine (Burke et al. 2005; McHughes and Timmermann 2005).

In this chapter, herbal medicine for diabetes is discussed in the context of TCM to illustrate the traditional understanding and clinical usage of herbal medicine. Scientific research into chemical properties, mechanisms of action, as well as clinical efficacies of some commonly used herbs for diabetes is overviewed. Safety issues and research strategies associated with herbal medicine are also briefly discussed at the end.

Diabetes is a group of metabolic diseases affecting multiple body systems of the human body as a result of the increased plasma glucose level. It is estimated that 285 million adults between the age of 20 and 79 years worldwide suffer from diabetes, accounting for 6.4% of the world population (International Diabetes Federation 2008). A further 344 million patients have IGT or prediabetes. It is suggested that without intervention, 7.8% of overweight individuals with IGT can develop diabetes within a 3-year period (Diabetes Prevention Program Research Group 2009).

Evidence of the severity of diabetes as a burden on international health is startling. Diabetes was estimated to be the cause of 3.96 million excess deaths among the worldwide adult population in 2010. This is equivalent to 6.8% of global all-ages mortality (Roglic and Unwin 2010). The World Health Organization (WHO) projects that, without urgent intervention, deaths caused by diabetes will increase by more than 50% in the next 10 years (WHO 2008).

Diabetes also carries a huge financial burden. In the United States, the total annual economic cost of diabetes in 2007 was estimated to be $174 billion (American Diabetes Association 2008). The cost of diabetes in Australia was around $3 billion a year according to 2003 figures, with average costs per patient at $5360 plus $5540 in benefits, totaling $10,900 (Colagiuri et al. 2003).

Given the high prevalence and substantial financial burden of diabetes, there is considerable merit in exploring therapeutic approaches that will help manage diabetes and reduce the risk of diabetes in subjects with IGT with minimal or no adverse effects where lifestyle modifications have failed, and pharmaceutical interventions are not warranted or suitable. Herbal medicine may provide safe, cost-effective solutions.

26.2 HERBAL MEDICINE FOR DIABETES: TRADITIONAL MEDICINE PERSPECTIVE

26.2.1 Understanding, Diagnosis, and Patterns of Diabetes in TCM

TCM is a system of healing that originated thousands of years ago. It has evolved into a well-developed, coherent system of medicine that uses several modalities (herbal medicine, acupuncture, qigong, etc.) to treat and prevent illness. Differing from Western medicine diagnosis, which focuses on the "macromolecular" level, TCM emphasizes the whole person, diagnosing through careful examination and identifying patterns of disharmony (Bensoussan and Myers 1996). The aim of treatment is to harmonize imbalances and enhance self-healing.

At the heart of TCM is the selection of treatment for a disease guided specifically by the full range of presenting symptoms and the individualization of a treatment strategy based on those symptoms. Of the many diagnostic tools used in TCM, a commonly used paradigm is the identification of patterns of disharmony (*Bian Zheng*). This diagnostic framework consists of looking, hearing, smelling, asking, and feeling in such a way that extends well beyond what is considered typical in Western medicine. For example, asking may reveal the absence of thirst thereby indicating a *cold* or *damp* condition; asking, looking, and feeling may expose problems with the sinews and tendons and thereby point to a disharmony with the Liver.* Looking at face areas and colors reflect the health of the inner Organs and the eyes reveal the health of *shen* or the spirit. Feeling by palpation along the meridians may also help to guide clinical reasoning and diagnosis. These clinical signs and symptoms are drawn together to identify a pattern of imbalance or disharmony. Any disease may have numerous *patterns of disharmony*, depending on the individual's manifestation of the disease.

A patient with diabetes, for example, may present with symptoms of obesity/overweight, heaviness of the limbs, loose stools, abdominal distension, fatigue, vaginal discharge (or recurrent thrush), a pale tongue, possibly teethmarks, and a distinct coat on the tongue. The pulse may be considered "soggy." These symptoms would be referred to in TCM as *dampness* and *heat* damaging the Spleen. *Damp stagnation* is seen as pathological body fluids clogging the organs and channels, similar to peripheral tissue resistance, due to obesity. The main treatment principle is to tonify the Spleen *qi* and dry *damp* and clear *heat*. Regulating *blood*, which has often been used in modern times for its ability to penetrate congested tissues, may also be valuable in overcoming tissue resistance. Herbs are selected according to the treatment principle.

Diabetes appeared in one of the earliest texts of Chinese herbal medicine, the *Yellow Emperor's Inner Classic* (the *Neijing*) compiled roughly 2000 years ago. The Chinese called diabetes—*xiao ke* meaning "thirst-emaciation." Traditionally, diabetes is divided into three types of *xiao ke* depending on the predominance of three main symptoms: thirst, hunger, and excessive urination, related to the Lung, Spleen, and Kidney, respectively (Choate 1999).

Upper *xiao ke* refers to the lack of body fluids due to Lung *heat* which manifests mainly as excess thirst along with other symptoms of *yin* with additional symptoms such as dry mouth, dry throat, and a dry cough. Middle *xiao ke* refers to the injury of *yin* by Stomach *dryness* which manifests as excessive hunger that may be accompanied by bad breath, burning in the epigastric region, and restlessness. Lower *xiao ke* involves the exhaustion of Kidney *essence* (*jing*) and Kidney *yin* with the main symptom of excessive urination accompanied by symptoms such as lower back pain, weakness at the knees, and malar flush. These patterns rarely present so neatly and often overlap. Treatment is individualized to meet these variations.

In TCM, diabetes is typically considered to be caused by congenital deficiency, inappropriate diet, overwork, and insufficient rest (Lu et al. 1999). Recent theorists in TCM have posited that diabetes has its origins in the following dysfunctions:

- Poor innate constitution, specifically Spleen and Kidney deficiency which leads to the impairment of the transportation and transformation of *fluids* and *yin* deficiency (Li et al. 2006; Liu et al. 2008).
- Inappropriate diet and excessive consumption of sweet, rich, and greasy foods may generate *phlegm* and *damp* which impairs the Spleen and Stomach, damages the Spleen *qi*, and damages the *jing*. This damage leads to the generation of *heat* and *damp* which consumes *yin* and *fluid* (Wu 2004).
- Disorders of the emotions (Wang et al. 1999; Lian 2004; Sun 2005): In TCM when Liver *qi* stagnates, it disturbs the proper ascending and descending of *qi*, leading to *heat* and consumption of both Lung and Kidney *yin* (Li et al. 2006).
- Too much work and insufficient rest can lead to Spleen deficiency which is the source of fluid and excessive sex can consume the Kidney *jing* (Wu 2004; Li et al. 2006). In TCM organ pathology, the pancreas is not mentioned but is functionally included within the "Spleen."

---

* Bodily organs and fluids in TCM do not correspond directly to the Western medicine equivalent. When an organ or fluid is referred in the TCM sense, it is capitalized.

TABLE 26.1

Common Patterns of Disharmony and Associated TCM Signs and Symptoms for Diabetes

TCM Disharmony Pattern	TCM Signs and Symptoms
Qi and *yin* deficiency	Fatigue, lack of strength, thirst, five palm heat (*Wu xin fan re*), polyphagia, polyuria, shortness of breath, reluctance to talk, spontaneous sweating, night sweats, constipation, red tongue with scanty coat or fat tongue, with teethmarks on its edges with a thick coat, bowstring, fine or rapid, forceless pulse
Accompanying *blood stasis*	Stuffiness in the chest, chest pain, numbness in the limbs
Spleen deficiency with *damp*	Stuffiness in the chest, torpid intake, heaviness of limbs, lack of strength, abdominal distension, loose stools, pale red tongue with slimy white coat, soggy pulse
Yin xu with empty-heat	Dry mouth and parched throat, fear of heat, heart vexation, thirst, rapid hungering, tension, agitation and easy to anger, frequent profuse urination, possible constipation, red tongue with scanty and or yellow coat, bowstring, rapid or slippery rapid pulse

In the early stages of diabetes, certain patterns of disharmony dominate (Lian 2004; Wu 2004; Li et al. 2006; Chen et al. 2007; Song 2007) and as the disease progresses, different patterns emerge. The symptoms of patterns of disharmony apparent in the early diabetes are summarized in Table 26.1. Among these, Spleen deficiency with *damp*, and *qi* and *yin* deficiency appear to be dominant patterns and blood stasis was a common accompanying pattern. Recent findings have expanded the symptoms of TCM patterns of disharmony to include a correlation to distinct biochemical markers. For example, Spleen *qi* deficiency with *damp* is characterized by higher levels of insulin, a higher BMI, and higher triglycerides while *qi* and *yin* deficiency is accompanied with lower levels of insulin and higher levels of fasting blood glucose.

26.2.2 TREATMENT PRINCIPLES AND FORMULATIONS IN TCM

As stated earlier, a Chinese medicine practitioner attends to the individual, not the disease. In clinic, there is no absolutely definitive way to treat a disease or a pattern of disharmony. Different herbs and herbal compositions will be used to treat the different patterns of disharmony, and standard formulations are often modified to take into consideration other symptoms such as sleep disturbance or foggy-headedness. Treatment principles and herbs for early-stage diabetes include

- Tonify *qi* and nourish *yin*: Herbal formulae include Jiangtang Bushen Tang (Fan et al. 2004); Danzhi Jiang Tang (Fang 2007); Tang Ping San (Qu 2002); Jianpi Zishen Huo Xue (Tang et al. 2007); and Shengqi Di Huang Tang (Wang 2008). Common *qi* tonics herbs in these formulae include Huang qi (*Astragalus propinquus*), Shao yao (*Paeonia lactiflora*), and Ren shen (*Panax ginseng*). Some of the commonly selected herbs to nourish Kidney *yin*: Shu di huang (processed *Rehmannia glutinosa*), Mai dong (*Ophiopogon japonicas*), Nu zhen zi (*Ligustrum lucidum*), and Han lian cao (*Eclipta prostrata*).
- Strengthen Spleen (and tonify *qi*): Tonifying *qi* and/or strengthening the Spleen was used as the main treatment principle in several clinical trials (Wei et al. 2001; Li et al. 2002; Hao et al. 2004; Luo et al. 2005; Yin 2007). Common *qi* tonics such as Huang qi (*Astragalus propinquus*) were frequently combined with damp draining herbs such as Fu ling (*Wolfiporia extensa*) (Li et al. 2002; Huang 2003).
- Nourish *yin* (and clear empty-heat): Herbal formulae included Ke Tang Ling (Dai 2005), Qimai Jiang Tang (Li et al. 2004), and Liu Wei Di Huang Tang (Zeng et al. 2000). Nourishing *yin* was combined with generating fluids using herbs such as Tian hua fen (*Trichosanthes kirilowii*) (Dai 2005) and Ge gen (*Pueraria lobata*) (Zhou 2001); and clearing heat. In the latter case, herbs such as Huang lian (*Coptis chinensis*) were added along

with Xia ku cao (*Prunella vulgaris*) and Mu dan pi (*Paeonia suffruticosa*) (Zhou 2001; Fan et al. 2004; Yang et al. 2004; Luo et al. 2005).

26.3 MODERN SCIENTIFIC UNDERSTANDING OF HERBAL MEDICINE FOR DIABETES

Numerous herbal medicines have been used for the treatment of type-2 diabetes (T2D) and metabolic disorders (Schoenberg et al. 2004; Lind et al. 2006). Early evidence suggests that herbal medicine interventions could help reduce the risk of mortality-associated diabetes (Yeh et al. 2002, 2003). A meta-analysis of eight trials showed that those people with prediabetes receiving Chinese herbal medicines combined with lifestyle modification were more than twice as likely to have their fasting plasma glucose levels return to normal levels compared to lifestyle modification alone. Those receiving Chinese herbs were less likely to progress to diabetes over the duration of the trial (Grant et al. 2009).

Research on individual herbs helps us understand the chemical properties, pharmacokinetics, pharmacodynamics, and clinical effectiveness of these medicines. Six commonly used herbs for diabetes are discussed below, including bitter melon, fenugreek, ginseng, garlic, prickly pear, and ginger. Their pharmacological effects, associated key evidence, and interactions/contraindications are summarized in Table 26.2.

26.3.1 BITTER MELON

Momordica charantia (bitter melon, bitter gourd, balsam pear, karela) is a tropical vegetable widely cultivated in Asia, Africa, and South America for culinary purpose. The fruit and other parts of the

TABLE 26.2
Summary of Commonly-Used Herbal Medicine Used in Diabetes

Name	Effect	Key Evidence	Interaction/ Contraindication
Bitter melon (*Momordica charantia*)	Hypoglycemic activity	Animal studies: hepatic glucose production, glycogen synthesis; clinical trials: lack of adequate design	Hypoglycemic agents; pregnancy
Fenugreek (*Trigonella foenum*)	Carbohydrate absorption; insulin secretion; lipid lowering; increase HDL	Several clinical trials demonstrated positive effects but lack of quality	Hypoglycemic agents; anticoagulants; MAO inhibitors; pregnancy
Ginseng (*Panax ginseng*)	Hypoglycemic effect, immune stimulant effects; enhance psycho-physiological performance	Animal studies: insulin mimic, alter hepatic glucose metabolism; clinical trials: conflicting results	Hypoglycemic agents; corticosteroids; oral contraceptives; anticoagulants; MAO inhibitors
Garlic (*Allium sativum*)	Increase insulin secretion	Animal studies: insulin secretion; clinical trials failed to show changes in glucose and insulin levels	Anticoagulants; antiplatelet agents
Prickly pear (*Opuntia streptacantha*)	Decrease carbohydrate absorption	Animal studies: hypoglycemic effect; but strong clinical evidence is lacking	Diarrhea, nausea, abdominal fullness
Ginger (*Zingiber officinale*)	Hypoglycemic activity; lipid lowering	Animal studies: reduction of blood glucose; inhibit LDL oxidation; clinical trials: limited RCTs in diabetes	Anticoagulants; antiplatelet agents

plant have been extensively used in folk medicine as a remedy for diabetes and other ailments (Grover and Yadav 2004). The plant contains several biologically active compounds including glycosides such as momordins, momordicosides, and goyaglycosides; saponins such as charantins and charantosides; alkaloids such as momordicin; fixed oils such as stearic acid and elaeostearic acid; triterpenes such as momordicins and cucurbitacins; and proteins such as polypeptide-P and momorcharins (Husain et al. 1994; Xie et al. 1998; Yuan et al. 1999; Murakami et al. 2001; Parkash et al. 2002; Chang et al. 2006). The antidiabetic principles of bitter melon are a mixture of steroidal saponins, insulin-like peptides, alkaloids, and triterpenoids (Ali et al. 1993).

All parts of bitter melon have been widely studied for their glucose and insulin-regulating activities (Grover and Yadav 2004; Leung et al. 2009). Bitter melon extracts and their bioactive compounds have shown to improve glucose tolerance (Chen et al. 2003), suppress postprandial hyperglycemia (Matsuur et al. 2002; Uebanso et al. 2007), and enhance insulin sensitivity (Chen and Li 2005), through pancreatic and extrapancreatic mechanisms, which have been attributed to the regeneration of beta-cells in pancreatic islets (Ahmed et al. 1998; Singh and Gupta 2007), promotion of insulin release (Yibchok-anun et al. 2006; Fernandes et al. 2007), insulin-like activity (Cummings et al. 2004; Yibchok-anun et al. 2006), inhibition of intestinal glucose absorption (Kumar Shetty et al. 2005), upregulation of GLUT4 transporter protein in muscles (Miura et al. 2001; Shih et al. 2009), stimulation of glucose utilization pathways (Rathi et al. 2002), and inhibition of glucose-producing pathways (Shibib et al. 1993). Recent studies have also demonstrated that bitter melon regulates 5′ AMP-activated protein kinase (AMPK) (Cheng et al. 2008) and peroxisome proliferator-activated receptor (PPAR) (Chuang et al. 2006; Shih et al. 2008) pathways and thus is attributed to its mechanisms of action. Bitter melon has also been shown to have protective effects by delaying the progression of diabetic complications in target organs (Srivastava et al. 1987; Ahmed et al. 2004; Kumar et al. 2008).

In an early case study conducted over 11 weeks, the administration of fresh fruit juice and fried fruit of bitter melon to nine T2D patients significantly improved glucose tolerance (Leatherdale et al. 1981). In another case study with 100 patients with T2D, single treatment with fresh bitter melon significantly lowered fasting blood glucose and blood glucose level at 2 h after a glucose meal (Ahmad et al. 1999). In controlled trials, 1-week treatment with methanolic extract of bitter melon in 15 diabetic patients significantly lowered the fasting as well as postprandial blood glucose level (Tongia et al. 2004) whereas a single treatment with an insulin-like compound derived from bitter melon significantly lowered the blood glucose in nine diabetic patients (Baldwa et al. 1977). However, a 4-week randomized controlled trial studied in 50 T2D patients using the dried whole fruit failed to reduce the blood glucose level (John et al. 2003). A recent Cochrane review highlights the gaps and identifies the flaws of previous studies such as small sample size, lack of control, and poor study design and warrants further rigorous studies (Ooi et al. 2010).

26.3.2 Fenugreek

Trigonella foenum-graecum (fenugreek), indigenous to Asian and Mediterranean regions, has been cultivated for thousands of years. Its seeds and leaves are widely used to treat diabetes in Ayurvedic and traditional Chinese medical systems. The seeds are well known for their pungent aromatic properties and often used as a spice to enhance the flavor of food preparations, while the leaves are consumed widely in India as a leafy vegetable (Max 1992). Fenugreek seeds contain nearly 50% fiber, comprising around 30% of soluble fiber and 20% of mucilaginous insoluble fiber. The seeds also contain trigonelline—an alkaloid; trigoneosides, glycoside D, and trigofaenoside A—saponins; diosgenin and yamogenin—sapogenins; galactomannan—a polysacharride; and 4-hydroxy isoleucine—an amino acid (Ali et al. 1995).

Numerous studies have shown the antidiabetic and hypoglycemic activity of fenugreek seed extracts in diabetic mice (Ajabnoor and Tilmisany 1988; Zia et al. 2001), rats (Riyad et al. 1988; Khosla et al. 1995), rabbits (Satyanarayana et al. 2003), and dogs (Ribes et al. 1986). The subfractions of fenugreek seeds containing the fiber, saponins, and proteins showed significant antidiabetic and antiglycosuric effect along with reduction in high plasma glucagon and somatostatin in alloxan-diabetic dogs (Ribes et al. 1986). Earlier studies on the active compounds have shown the hypoglycemic activity of trigonelline (Mishkinsky et al. 1967). However, opinion varies regarding the active compounds and their mechanisms of action (Ali et al. 1995) in isolating galactomannan from fenugreek seeds, which has shown lowering of postprandial glucose levels in rats through delayed gastric emptying and reduced intestinal glucose absorption (Madar et al. 1988). 4-Hydroxyisoleucine, extracted and purified from fenugreek seeds, has shown to increase insulin secretion through a direct action on pancreatic beta-cells (Sauvaire et al. 1998; Broca et al. 1999). Further studies in rats have demonstrated improved peripheral glucose utilization by fenugreek which is attributable to increased glycolytic enzymes activities and reduced activities of gluconeogenic enzymes (Gupta et al. 1999; Raju et al. 2001).

In several small human trials, fenugreek seeds have been shown to lower fasting blood glucose levels. In a double-blind placebo-controlled trial with 25 patients, fenugreek seeds have shown an improved fasting blood glucose and oral glucose tolerance without significant difference between the groups and increased insulin sensitivity (Gupta et al. 2001). In another small crossover trial over 15 days in 10 patients with T2D, fenugreek seed supplementation improved peripheral glucose utilization (Raghuram et al. 1996). In another study in 15 patients, treatment with fenugreek for 10 days improved fasting blood glucose levels (Sharma et al. 1990). The studies conducted to date have been small and methodologically weak. Additional studies of fenugreek are warranted in this area before firm conclusions can be drawn.

26.3.3 Ginseng

Panax ginseng (ginseng) has been widely used for the management of diabetes for thousands of years in many Asian countries. Its root is used medicinally, although active compounds are also present in many other parts of the plant. The major active compounds of ginseng are triterpene glycosides or saponins, commonly referred to as ginsenosides, and more than 40 different ginsenosides have been identified (Liu and Xiao 1992; Baek et al. 1996; Attele et al. 1999). Based on their structural differences, ginsenosides are classified into three major subtypes: the protopanaxadiol group (Rb1, Rb2, Rb3, Rc, Rd, Rg3, Rh2), the protopanaxatriol group (Re, Rf, Rg1, Rg2, Rh1), and the oleanolic acid group (R0) (Tachikawa et al. 1999; Liu et al. 2011). Studies on the metabolism of ginsenosides indicate that they undergo biotransformation by intestinal bacteria through deglycosylation and esterification (Hasegawa et al. 1996).

The vast amount of literature on the chemistry and pharmacology of ginseng exemplifies the renewed interest on ginseng among scientific community. Data from various *in vitro*, *in vivo*, and clinical studies have demonstrated the antidiabetic activity of ginseng and its bioactive compounds (Xie et al. 2005). Multiple studies have demonstrated that ginseng increases insulin release from pancreatic beta-cells (Waki et al. 1982; Rotshteyn and Zito 2004). Ginseng has also shown to improve insulin-stimulated glucose disposal, which is attributed to its ability to increase glycolysis and increase GLUT2 transporter activity (Attele et al. 2002).

Data from randomized-controlled trials of ginseng shows conflicting results. In a double-blind placebo-controlled study for 8 weeks, the efficacy of ginseng (100 or 200 mg) was examined in T2D patients ($n = 36$) (Sotaniemi et al. 1995). Compared with the placebo group, the 200 mg dose of ginseng reduced fasting blood glucose and body weight. In another 12-week double-blind randomized-controlled trial, 19 T2D patients received the ginseng preparation or placebo (2 g/meal = 6 g/day) as an adjunct to their usual antidiabetic therapy (Vuksan et al. 2008). A significant 8–11% decrease in glucose on the oral glucose tolerance test and 33% decrease in plasma insulin was seen in the ginseng-treated group compared to placebo. However, no change was seen in HbA1c levels with ginseng. Although there is some evidence from the above studies showing that ginseng lowers blood glucose, well-designed, randomized, and controlled trials evaluating its effects are still lacking. However, the widespread use of ginseng as an herbal remedy also warrants more rigorous investigation to assess its efficacy and safety.

26.3.4 GARLIC

Allium sativum (garlic) is a popular spice for cooking and is one of the first recorded herbal remedies that has a long history of traditional medicinal use in many countries. Scientific reports on the antidiabetic potential of garlic are available for the last 80 years. The use of garlic as a folk medicine for diabetes has been reported in Asia, Europe, and Africa (Rivlin 2006). Garlic contains allicin, an antibiotic, and phytoncide, an antifungal. In addition, garlic is also rich in sulfur-containing (e.g., alliin) and nonsulphur-containing compounds (e.g., allixin), which are mostly responsible for its biological activities (Keusgen 1997; Calvey et al. 1998).

An increasing number of animal studies have demonstrated the antidiabetic potential of garlic (Liu et al. 2007; Kook et al. 2009). Earliest experimental studies of the extracts of garlic have shown lowering of blood glucose and improved oral glucose tolerance in both normal and diabetic animal models (Jain and Vyas 1975; Swanston-Flatt et al. 1990). The active garlic compound allicin was also shown to lower fasting blood glucose, improve oral glucose tolerance, and improve tissue glucose uptake in rabbits with mild, but not severe, alloxan-induced diabetes (Mathew and Augusti 1973). In later studies, the hypoglycemic effect of garlic on fasting blood glucose has also been shown in diabetic animals treated with fresh garlic (Chang and Johnson 1980), with garlic oil (Farva et al. 1986; Anwar and Meki 2003; Liu et al. 2005), and with aqueous (El-Demerdash et al. 2005) and ethanolic (Eidi et al. 2006) extracts of garlic.

Although garlic has long been believed and experimentally demonstrated to possess a hypoglycemic effect, no well-controlled clinical trials of the hypoglycemic effect of garlic in diabetes patients have been reported, with the exception of a pilot study carried out in Thailand, which found no significant effects of garlic on glycemic control. Large-scale RCT studies with diabetic patients are needed to confirm the usefulness of garlic in the treatment and prevention of diabetes.

26.3.5 PRICKLY PEAR

Opuntia streptacantha (prickly pear) is traditionally used in Mexico to treat T2D and digestive disorders (Ibanez-Camacho and Roman-Ramos 1979; Ibanez-Camacho et al. 1983). So far, very little or no research has been conducted on the chemical composition of *Opuntia streptacantha*. A recent report shows the presence of (4-hydroxy)-phenyl acetic acid in this species (Andrade-Cetto and Wiedenfeld 2011). However, compounds such as 3-methoxytyramine, candicine, hordenine, *N*-methyltyramine, tyramine, betanin, and indicaxanthin were reported in other species of *Opuntia*.

Experimental studies in animal models of diabetes and in diabetic patients demonstrated hypoglycemic effect of prickly pear which was attributed to the decrease in intestinal glucose absorption by the high fiber and pectin content present in the extracts (Frati et al. 1990, 1991; Alarcon-Aguilar et al. 2003). A recent study confirmed the antihyperglycemic effect in maltose-loaded streptozotocin diabetic rats and showed that the effect is independent of the fiber or mucilage content (Andrade-Cetto and Wiedenfeld 2011). Data available on human studies are limited and no new studies are reported in recent times. In the study conducted by Frati-Munari et al. (1988), the hypoglycemic effect of pricky pear was evaluated in 29 T2D patients divided into three groups. Serum glucose and insulin were significantly reduced in the pricy pear-treated group compared to the control group.

26.3.6 GINGER

Zingiber officinale (ginger), a well-known food spice, has been used traditionally in a wide variety of ailments (Afzal et al. 2001). The major chemical constituents of ginger rhizome are classified into: (i) essential volatile oils and (ii) nonvolatile pungent compounds (Govindarajan 1982a,b). The volatile oil components in ginger consist mainly of sesquiterpene hydrocarbons, such as zingeberene (35%), curcumene (18%), and farnesene (10%), with lesser amounts of β-bisabolene and β-sesquiphellandrene. A smaller percentage of diterpenes such as galanalactone and at least

40 different monoterpenoids are present in ginger. The nonvolatile compounds of ginger include the gingerols, shogaols, paradols, and zingerone responsible for its "hot" sensation in the mouth (Govindarajan 1982a,b). The gingerols were identified as the major active components in the fresh rhizome (Jolad et al. 2004). In addition, the shogaols, the dehydrated form of the gingerols, are the predominant pungent constituents in dried ginger (Bao et al. 2010).

In laboratory experiments, ethanolic extract of ginger has been shown to reduce plasma lipid profiles in cholesterol-fed hyperlipidemic rabbits (Verma et al. 2004) and in streptozotocin-induced diabetic rats (Bhandari et al. 2005) and was also found to inhibit low-density lipoprotein (LDL) oxidation in atherosclerotic, apolipoprotein E-deficient mice (Fuhrman et al. 2000). A low to moderate, but significant, blood glucose lowering effect of the juice of ginger was observed in both normal and diabetic animals (Akhani, et al. 2004). The ethanolic extract has also been shown to produce significant reduction of blood glucose in normal rabbits (Mascolo et al. 1989) and rats (Ojewole 2006) and in alloxan (Kar et al. 2003) and streptozotocin-induced (Al-Amin et al. 2006) diabetic rats. Recent studies in our laboratory showed that a standardized extract of ginger protected the development of metabolic syndrome and T2D in high-fat-diet-fed rats (Nammi et al. 2009). We have also shown that ginger increases LDL receptors and decreases HMG-CoA reductase in the liver and attributed to the cholesterol-lowering actions of ginger (Nammi et al. 2010).

Although over 100 clinical studies on ginger have been documented for nausea and vomiting, very limited human studies have been conducted for its safety and efficacy in diabetes. In a double-blind placebo-controlled trial, Alizadeh-Navaei et al. (2008) have studied the effect of ginger powder on lipid levels in hyperlipidemic patients. The treatment group ($n = 45$) and the control group ($n = 40$) received ginger capsules or placebo capsules, respectively, for 45 days at a dose of 3 g/day. The results indicate a significant reduction in triglyceride, cholesterol, LDL, and very-low-density lipoprotein (VLDL) in the ginger group compared to the placebo group.

26.4   HERBAL MEDICINE RESEARCH AND DEVELOPMENT STRATEGIES

There has been significant progress in herbal medicine research worldwide owing to the increased public interest, availability of technology, and scientific expertise in this field. Compared to synthetic pharmaceutical medicines, herbal medicines have much more complex chemical profiles. In some traditional medicine systems such as TCM, patients are generally treated with a multiherbal formulation, which adds another level of complexity to their chemical compositions.

Preliminary evidence exists to support the capacity of these complex mixtures of bioactive components to enhance therapeutic efficacy by facilitating synergistic action and/or ameliorating/preventing potential side effects (Kroll and Cordes 2006; Wagner and Ulrich-Merzenich 2009). For example, clinical studies in healthy volunteers demonstrate the cognitive effects of a ginkgo–ginseng combination far outweighed those of either extract alone suggesting the possibilities of synergistic interactions between the extracts (Kennedy et al. 2001; Scholey and Kennedy 2002). Synergistic effects can occur in many ways, including, for example, where constituents from herbal extracts interact with one another to improve their solubility and hence the bioavailability (Wagner and Ulrich-Merzenich 2009). Furthermore, constituents of complex herbal extracts can affect multiple biological targets, which, at least in theory, make them ideal therapies for disorders such as diabetes, metabolic syndrome, and dementia which often have multifactorial/multisystem pathophysiological components (Jia et al. 2004).

Current research in herbal medicines involves a multifaceted approach, combining phytochemical, pharmacological, and molecular techniques. However, numerous challenges are encountered, including the variability of the plant materials, unknown active components, difficulties in quality control, lack of safety evaluation, the selection and implementation of appropriate high-throughput screening bioassays, unclear mechanism of action, and the scale-up of active compounds.

The current drug discovery approach for pharmaceutical medicine typically involves screening and identification of drug candidatures from various sources. This will be followed by chemical separation and/or synthesis, bioassay-based characterization of pharmacokinetic and pharmacodynamic properties, and establishment of toxicity profile. The clinical efficacy and safety will eventually be validated through randomized clinical trials. Herbal medicines, however, have a very complex chemical profile and pharmacological behaviors. The current pharmaceutical approach is perhaps less meaningful and inadequate for herbal medicine research. As such, several new research paradigms have been proposed by various authors. For example, Fonnebo et al. (2007) have suggested that the conventional pharmacological approach be inverted. Traditional herbal medicine is often experience based and self-evident through many years of clinical use. Focusing first and foremost on clinical practice will guide us to questions that are relevant to the practitioners and patients. Only when "effectiveness" has been established through clinical practice does it make sense to break the treatment down into its component parts, and then, using a placebo-controlled trial, determine which of the components are active (Fonnebo et al. 2007). Safety is often assumed through historical usage. But toxic dosage level and safety parameters should nonetheless be established using modern toxicological methods. This model demands redistribution of limited research resources away from the present labor-intensive pharmacological study of individual components of herbs and large-scale RCT-style study of effectiveness, efficacy, and mechanisms in favor of research at the case-study and clinical front-end. This will help reduce costs and time in the validation and development of herbal medicine products. Successful implementation of the model will require research designs, such as whole systems research and pragmatic trials (Verhoef et al. 2005), capable of sustained methodological rigor as well as clinical relevance.

Australian Therapeutic Goods Administration (TGA) has developed regulatory policies to address the unique nature of herbal medicines. The centerpiece of this is a risk-based, two-tier regulatory system splitting herbal medicines into two different categories—namely listed herbal medicines and registered herbal medicines to safeguard the health and well-being of herbal medicine consumers. The listed herbal medicines, which account for almost all herbal products currently on the market, are of low risk and do not require evaluation of efficacy of individual products. The safety profiles of these medicines can be established through providing evidence of a long history of traditional use and/or toxicological studies. Registered herbal medicines, on the other hand, are higher risk and are therefore subject to rigorous scientific evaluations of their chemical, pharmacological, and toxicological properties. The clinical efficacy will also need to be established through robust clinical trials. Similar regulatory models also exist in the United States (through US Food and Drug Administration—FDA), Europe (through the European Agency for the Evaluation of Medicinal Products—EMEA), Canada, Malaysia, and other selected jurisdictions. These regulatory systems demand a greater level of scientific evidence for the "registered" herbal medicine category and encourage herbal medicine developers and manufacturers to employ advanced scientific methods and tools to develop higher level herbal medicine products with a greater marketing edge.

26.5   SAFETY ISSUES RELATING TO USE OF HERBAL MEDICINE

Although herbal medicines are often considered safe when compared to their conventional pharmaceutical counterparts, harmful effects associated with their uses do occur. These effects are not limited to the direct toxicity of herbs. The concomitant use of herbal medicines with pharmaceutical medications has the potential of reducing the effectiveness or increasing the potency of the therapies. The quality of herbal medicine products is also of major concern. Contamination of herbal medicines with microorganisms, heavy metals, and pesticides can cause severe health concerns to their users.

26.5.1   Herbal Medicine Toxicity and Adverse Effects

Similar to pharmaceutical medicines, bioactive components of herbal medicines can cause predictable (type A) and idiosyncratic (type B) adverse reactions. The former is caused by the extension of the pharmacological effects of the herb and therefore are often predictable and dose dependent. For example, ginseng can exert effects on multiple body systems causing insomnia, diarrhea, headache, tremor, and skin eruptions. Bitter melon is considered to be safe at low doses, but it can cause abdominal pain and diarrhea at high doses. Other documented adverse effects of bitter melon include hypoglycemic coma and convulsions in children, reduced fertility, and headaches (Basch et al. 2003). Further, the abortifacient activity of raw bitter melon raises doubts regarding the safety of its consumption during pregnancy (Chan et al. 1986).

Idiosyncratic adverse reactions of herbal medicines usually happen in a small portion of patients and their occurrence is often unpredictable. The mechanisms of action for idiosyncratic reactions are poorly understood but they are suggested to be associated with genetic anomalies. Idiosyncratic adverse reactions often carry more severe consequences when occurring, causing significant morbidity or death. For example, royal jelly (regarded as part of Chinese herbal medicine) has been responsible for multiple deaths in Australia (Bensoussan and Myers 1996).

26.5.2   OTHER FACTORS AFFECTING SAFETY OF HERBAL MEDICINE

Besides the factors directly relating to the properties of herbs discussed above, there are also a range of extrinsic factors that could potentially contribute to the safety of herbal medicine use (Drew and Myers 1997). These include

- Misidentification and substitution of herbs due to the complex and confusing nomenclature of herbs used (botanic name, pharmaceutical name, scientific name, and common English name)
- Lack of standardization of herbal products because of the region and seasons where plants are sourced
- Contamination of herbs and herbal products with heavy metals, pesticides, and microorganisms in cultivation, and in the storage, transport, and manufacturing process
- Adulteration due to intentional or unintentional addition of pharmaceutical products in herbal preparations
- Incorrect preparation methods or dosages of herbs used by patients
- Inappropriate labeling/advertising by herbal manufacturers/companies

26.5.3   HERB–DRUG INTERACTIONS

An Australian study reported that approximately half of the CM therapy (including herbal medicine) users indicated that they also took conventional pharmaceutical medicines on the same day (MacLennan et al. 2006). Many of these patients are elderly and they are likely to suffer from multiple comorbidities and therefore use multiple long-term medications (Bin and Kiat 2011). The likelihood of interference of herbal medicines with prescribed medicines is increased leading to either increased potency or decreased effectiveness of their comedications. The herb–drug interactions may potentially prove life threatening when the pharmaceutical medications affected have a narrow therapeutic window (e.g., warfarin, digoxin, and hypoglycemic agents).

The prevalence of herb–drug interactions are unknown and is often believed to be underreported. The reasons for underreporting may include the failure of patients to reveal their herbal use to their medical practitioners, rigorous preclinical and clinical assessments of herbal medicine not being required by regulatory bodies, poorly designed clinical trials failing to provide vital herb–drug interactions information, and the lack of surveillance and reporting systems for herb–drug interactions (Hu et al. 2005).

Preclinical and clinical evidence exists to support the occurrence of herb–drug interactions. Some evidence is indirectly based on an understanding of the mechanism of these medicines while others come directly from clinical observation and/or clinical trials. For example, ginger has fibrinolytic activity and therefore it is assumed that patients taking anticoagulants such as warfarin need to be cautioned due to potential additive effect. Some potentially serious herb–drug interactions highlighted by the Australian TGA include interactions between gingko and warfarin causing bleeding and interactions between St John's wort and cyclosporin and oral contraceptives causing reduction in plasma concentration of these medicines (TGA 2005). It is also suggested that St John's wort may cause serotonin syndrome when used with selective serotonin re-uptake inhibitors (SSRIs) or tramadol (TGA 2005).

26.6 CONCLUSION

The use of CM is growing, with herbal medicine usage demonstrating one of the greatest relative increases. However, a significant gap exists between the level of consumer belief and use and the level of scientific evidence that support that use. This is reflected by the fact that since the introduction of the two-tier regulatory system for herbal medicine in Australia more than 20 years ago, there has only been very limited success of the herbal medicine industry gaining *Registered* status for their herbal medicine products.

While the current herbal medicine regulatory systems have created tremendous opportunities for the industry to develop higher-level herbal medicine products, the pathway and strategies to achieve this goal remains difficult and ambiguous. One way forward for capitalizing these opportunities is through engaging serious scientific research in support of claims and in fulfilling the evidence requirements for a *Registered* herbal medicine. The quality of herbal medicine products remains a major concern for public, regulatory authorities, and herbal medicine industry. Ideally, more emphasis should be placed on developing a *field-to-clinic* approach, which requires rigorous control in every aspect of the herbal medicine manufacturing and development process. This starts with the application of Good Agriculture Practice (GAP) principles in farming and raw material control, storage, and transport to minimize impurities, heavy metals, and pesticide contamination; Good Manufacturer Practice (GMP) which will help ensure the quality of finished herbal medicine products during manufacturing; and Good Clinical Practice (GCP) which will guide the conduct of clinical research and clinical practice of herbal medicine to ensure highest standards of health care outcomes.

Between 70% and 80% of the population of developed countries choose to use some form of CM and do so without knowledge of how cost effectively their health dollar is being spent (WHO 2008). The consequences of the paucity of an understanding of the cost effectiveness of herbal medicine and CM are manifold. CM is available to only those that can afford it, and health care bodies and governments may be missing out on considerable savings of scarce health resource dollars. The recent advancement in the development of tools for converting the costs of herbal interventions into monetary terms has strongly promoted research interest in this field (Doran et al. 2010).

Last but not least, one should not forget/ignore the traditional understanding of the therapeutic principles underpinning herbal medicine (e.g., individualization and holistic approach) in some sophisticated medical systems. These medical systems have played and will continue to play a crucial role in health maintenance and disease management throughout many parts of the world (especially Asia). This ancient wisdom is a source of medicine for the future.

REFERENCES

Afzal, M., D. Al-Hadidi, M. Menon, J. Pesek, and M. S. Dhami. 2001. Ginger: An ethnomedical, chemical and pharmacological review. *Drug Metabol Drug Interact* 18(3–4): 159–190.

Ahmad, N., M. R. Hassan, H. Halder, and K. S. Bennoor. 1999. Effect of *Momordica charantia* (Karolla) extracts on fasting and postprandial serum glucose levels in NIDDM patients. *Bangladesh Med Res Counc Bull* 25(1): 11–13.

Ahmed, I., E. Adeghate, E. Cummings, A. K. Sharma, and J. Singh. 2004. Beneficial effects and mechanism of action of *Momordica charantia* juice in the treatment of streptozotocin-induced diabetes mellitus in rat. *Mol Cell Biochem* 261(1–2): 63–70.

Ahmed, I., E. Adeghate, A. K. Sharma, D. J. Pallot, and J. Singh. 1998. Effects of *Momordica charantia* fruit juice on islet morphology in the pancreas of the streptozotocin-diabetic rat. *Diabetes Res Clin Pract* 40(3): 145–151.

Ajabnoor, M. A., and A. K. Tilmisany. 1988. Effect of *Trigonella foenum graceum* on blood glucose levels in normal and alloxan-diabetic mice. *J Ethnopharmacol* 22(1): 45–49.

Akhani, S. P., S. L. Vishwakarma, and R. K. Goyal. 2004. Anti-diabetic activity of *Zingiber officinale* in streptozotocin-induced type I diabetic rats. *J Pharm Pharmacol* 56(1): 101–105.

Al-Amin, Z. M., M. Thomson, K. K. Al-Qattan, R. Peltonen-Shalaby, and M. Ali. 2006. Anti-diabetic and hypolipidaemic properties of ginger (*Zingiber officinale*) in streptozotocin-induced diabetic rats. *Br J Nutr* 96(4): 660–666.

Alarcon-Aguilar, F. J., A. Valdes-Arzate, S. Xolalpa-Molina, T. Banderas-Dorantes, M. Jimenez-Estrada, E. Hernandez-Galicia, and R. Roman-Ramos. 2003. Hypoglycemic activity of two polysaccharides isolated from *Opuntia ficus-indica* and *O. streptacantha*. *Proc West Pharmacol Soc* 46: 139–142.

Ali, L., A. K. Azad Khan, Z. Hassan, M. Mosihuzzaman, N. Nahar, T. Nasreen, M. Nur-e-Alam, and B. Rokeya. 1995. Characterization of the hypoglycemic effects of *Trigonella foenum graecum* seed. *Planta Med* 61(4): 358–360.

Ali, L., A. K. Khan, M. I. Mamun, M. Mosihuzzaman, N. Nahar, M. Nur-e-Alam, and B. Rokeya. 1993. Studies on hypoglycemic effects of fruit pulp, seed, and whole plant of *Momordica charantia* on normal and diabetic model rats. *Planta Med* 59(5): 408–412.

Alizadeh-Navaei, R., F. Roozbeh, M. Saravi, M. Pouramir, F. Jalali, and A. A. Moghadamnia. 2008. Investigation of the effect of ginger on the lipid levels. A double blind controlled clinical trial. *Saudi Med J* 29(9): 1280–1284.

American Diabetes Association. 2008. Economic costs of diabetes in the U.S. in 2007. *Diabetes Care* 31: 596–615.

Andrade-Cetto, A. and H. Wiedenfeld. 2011. Anti-hyperglycemic effect of *Opuntia streptacantha* Lem. *J Ethnopharmacol* 133(2): 940–943.

Anwar, M. M. and A. R. Meki. 2003. Oxidative stress in streptozotocin-induced diabetic rats: Effects of garlic oil and melatonin. *Comp Biochem Physiol A Mol Integr Physiol* 135(4): 539–547.

Attele, A. S., J. A. Wu, and C. S. Yuan. 1999. Ginseng pharmacology: Multiple constituents and multiple actions. *Biochem Pharmacol* 58(11): 1685–1693.

Attele, A. S., Y. P. Zhou, J. T. Xie, J. A. Wu, L. Zhang, L. Dey, W. Pugh, P. A. Rue, K. S. Polonsky, and C. S. Yuan. 2002. Antidiabetic effects of *Panax ginseng* berry extract and the identification of an effective component. *Diabetes* 51(6): 1851–1858.

Baek, N. I., D. S. Kim, Y. H. Lee, J. D. Park, C. B. Lee, and S. I. Kim. 1996. Ginsenoside Rh4, a genuine dammarane glycoside from Korean red ginseng. *Planta Med* 62(1): 86–87.

Baldwa, V. S., C. M. Bhandari, A. Pangaria, and R. K. Goyal. 1977. Clinical trial in patients with diabetes mellitus of an insulin-like compound obtained from plant source. *Ups J Med Sci* 82(1): 39–41.

Bao, L., A. Deng, Z. Li, G. Du, and H. Qin. 2010. Chemical constituents of rhizomes of *Zingiber officinale*. *Zhongguo Zhong Yao Za Zhi* 35(5): 598–601.

Basch, E., S. Gabardi, and C. Ulbricht. 2003. Bitter melon (*Momordica charantia*): A review of efficacy and safety. *Am J Health Syst Pharm* 60(4): 356–359.

Bensoussan, A. and S. Myers. 1996. *Towards a Safer Choice: The Practice of Traditional Chinese Medicine in Australia*. Macarthur: UWS.

Bhandari, U., R. Kanojia, and K. K. Pillai. 2005. Effect of ethanolic extract of *Zingiber officinale* on dyslipidaemia in diabetic rats. *J Ethnopharmacol* 97(2): 227–230.

Bin, Y. S. and H. Kiat. 2011. Prevalence of dietary supplement use in patients with proven or suspected cardiovascular disease. *Evid Based Complement Altern Med* 2011: 1–12.

Broca, C., R. Gross, P. Petit, Y. Sauvaire, M. Manteghetti, M. Tournier, P. Masiello, R. Gomis, and G. Ribes. 1999. 4-Hydroxyisoleucine: Experimental evidence of its insulinotropic and antidiabetic properties. *Am J Physiol* 277(4 Pt 1): E617–E623.

Burke, A., K. Ginzburg, K. Collie, D. Trachtenberg, and M. Muhammad. 2005. Exploring the role of complementary and alternative medicine in public health practice and training. *J Altern Complement Med* 11(5): 931–936.

Calvey, E. M., K. D. White, J. E. Matusik, D. Sha, and E. Block. 1998. Allium chemistry: Identification of organosulfur compounds in ramp (*Allium tricoccum*) homogenates. *Phytochemistry* 49(2): 359–364.

Chan, W. Y., P. P. Tam, H. L. Choi, T. B. Ng, and H. W. Yeung. 1986. Effects of momorcharins on the mouse embryo at the early organogenesis stage. *Contraception* 34(5): 537–544.

Chang, C. I., C. R. Chen, Y. W. Liao, H. L. Cheng, Y. C. Chen, and C. H. Chou. 2006. Cucurbitane-type triterpenoids from *Momordica charantia*. *J Nat Prod* 69(8): 1168–1171.

Chang, M. L. and M. A. Johnson. 1980. Effect of garlic on carbohydrate metabolism and lipid synthesis in rats. *J Nutr* 110(5): 931–936.

Chen, Q., L. L. Chan, and E. T. Li. 2003. Bitter melon (*Momordica charantia*) reduces adiposity, lowers serum insulin and normalizes glucose tolerance in rats fed a high fat diet. *J Nutr* 133(4): 1088–1093.

Chen, Q. and E. T. Li. 2005. Reduced adiposity in bitter melon (*Momordica charantia*) fed rats is associated with lower tissue triglyceride and higher plasma catecholamines. *Br J Nutr* 93(5): 747–754.

Chen, L. Y., H. Zhou, and Y. B. Jau. 2007. TCM syndrome categorization on IGT [Tang nai liang di jian de zhong yi bian zheng fen xing]. *Chin J Basic Med Tradit Chin Med* 13(3): 223–224.

Cheng, H. L., H. K. Huang, C. I. Chang, C. P. Tsai, and C. H. Chou. 2008. A cell-based screening identifies compounds from the stem of *Momordica charantia* that overcome insulin resistance and activate AMP-activated protein kinase. *J Agric Food Chem* 56(16): 6835–6843.

Choate, C. 1999. Modern medicine and traditional Chinese medicine: Diabetes mellitus (Part Two). *J Chin Med* 59: 5–12.

Chuang, C. Y., C. Hsu, C. Y. Chao, Y. S. Wein, Y. H. Kuo, and C. J. Huang. 2006. Fractionation and identification of 9c, 11t, 13t-conjugated linolenic acid as an activator of PPARalpha in bitter gourd (*Momordica charantia* L.). *J Biomed Sci* 13(6): 763–772.

Colagiuri, S., R. Colagiuri, B. Conway, P. Davey, and D. Grainger. 2003. *DiabCost Australia: Assessing the Burden of Type 2 Diabetes in Australia*: The Australian Centre for Diabetes Strategies; Diabetes Australia.

Cummings, E., H. S. Hundal, H. Wackerhage, M. Hope, M. Belle, E. Adeghate, and J. Singh. 2004. *Momordica charantia* fruit juice stimulates glucose and amino acid uptakes in L6 myotubes. *Mol Cell Biochem* 261(1–2): 99–104.

Dai, F. F. 2005. Clinical observation on the intervention of 32 cases of impaired glucose with Ketangling granule [Ke tang ling ke li gan yu zhi liao tang nai liang jian di 32 li lin chuang guan cha]. *Jiangsu Journal of Traditional Chinese Medicine [Jiang Su Zhong Yu Yao]* 26(11): 24.

Diabetes Prevention Program Research Group. 2009. 10-year follow-up of diabetes incidence and weight loss in the Diabetes Prevention Program Outcomes Study. *Lancet* 374(9702): 1677–1686.

Doran, C., D. Chang, H. Kiat, and A. Bensoussan. 2010. Review of economic methods used in complementary medicine. *J Altern Complement Med* 16: 1–5.

Drew, A. K. and S. P. Myers. 1997. Safety issues in herbal medicines: implications for the health professions. *Med J Aust* 166: 538–541.

Eidi, A., M. Eidi, and E. Esmaeili. 2006. Antidiabetic effect of garlic (*Allium sativum* L.) in normal and streptozotocin-induced diabetic rats. *Phytomedicine* 13(9–10): 624–629.

El-Demerdash, F. M., M. I. Yousef, and N. I. El-Naga. 2005. Biochemical study on the hypoglycemic effects of onion and garlic in alloxan-induced diabetic rats. *Food Chem Toxicol* 43(1): 57–63.

Fan, G. J., G. B. Luo, and M. L. Qin. 2004. Effect of jiangtang bushen recipe in intervention treatment of patients with impaired glucose tolerance [article in Chinese]. *Zhongguo Zhong Xi Yi Jie He Za Zhi* 24(4): 317–320.

Fang, Z. H. 2007. Observation of the effectiveness of Dan zhi jiang tang capsules for IGT [Dan Zhi Jiang Tang Nang Gan Yu Pu Tao Tang Nai Liang Di Jian Liao Xiao Guan Cha]. *Journal of Emergency Traditional Chinese Medicine [Zhong Guo Zhong Yi Ji Zheng]* 16: 402–404.

Farva, D., I. A. Goji, P. K. Joseph, and K. T. Augusti. 1986. Effects of garlic oil on streptozotocin-diabetic rats maintained on normal and high fat diets. *Indian J Biochem Biophys* 23(1): 24–27.

Fernandes, N. P., C. V. Lagishetty, V. S. Panda, and S. R. Naik. 2007. An experimental evaluation of the antidiabetic and antilipidemic properties of a standardized *Momordica charantia* fruit extract. *BMC Complement Altern Med* 7: 29.

Fonnebo, V., S. Grimsgaard, H. Walach, C. Ritenbaugh, A. Norheim, and H. MacPherson. 2007. Researching complementary and alternative treatments—The gatekeepers are not at home. *BMC Med Res Methodol* 7(1): 7.

Frati-Munari, A. C., B. E. Gordillo, P. Altamirano, and C. R. Ariza. 1988. Hypoglycemic effect of *Opuntia streptacantha* Lemaire in NIDDM. *Diabetes Care* 11(1): 63–66.

Frati, A. C., B. E. Gordillo, P. Altamirano, C. R. Ariza, R. Cortes-Franco, and A. Chavez-Negrete. 1990. Acute hypoglycemic effect of *Opuntia streptacantha* Lemaire in NIDDM. *Diabetes Care* 13(4): 455–456.

Frati, A. C., N. Xilotl Diaz, P. Altamirano, R. Ariza, and R. Lopez-Ledesma. 1991. The effect of two sequential doses of *Opuntia streptacantha* upon glycemia. *Arch Invest Med (Mex)* 22(3–4): 333–336.

Fuhrman, B., M. Rosenblat, T. Hayek, R. Coleman, and M. Aviram. 2000. Ginger extract consumption reduces plasma cholesterol, inhibits LDL oxidation and attenuates development of atherosclerosis in atherosclerotic, apolipoprotein E-deficient mice. *J Nutr* 130(5): 1124–1131.

Govindarajan, V. S. 1982a. Ginger—Chemistry, technology, and quality evaluation: Part 1. *Crit Rev Food Sci Nutr* 17(1): 1–96.

Govindarajan, V. S. 1982b. Ginger—Chemistry, technology, and quality evaluation: Part 2. *Crit Rev Food Sci Nutr* 17(3): 189–258.

Grant, S., A. Bensoussan, D. Chang, H. Kiat, N. Klupp, and J. Liu. 2009. Chinese herbal medicines for people with impaired glucose tolerance or impaired fasting blood glucose. *Cochrane Database Syst Rev* (4). Art No.: CD006690. DOI: 10.1002/14651858.CD006690.pub2.

Grover, J. K., and S. P. Yadav. 2004. Pharmacological actions and potential uses of *Momordica charantia*: A review. *J Ethnopharmacol* 93(1): 123–132.

Gupta, A., R. Gupta, and B. Lal. 2001. Effect of Trigonella foenum-graecum (fenugreek) seeds on glycaemic control and insulin resistance in type 2 diabetes mellitus: A double blind placebo controlled study. *J Assoc Physicians India* 49: 1057–1061.

Gupta, D., J. Raju, and N. Z. Baquer. 1999. Modulation of some gluconeogenic enzyme activities in diabetic rat liver and kidney: Effect of antidiabetic compounds. *Indian J Exp Biol* 37(2): 196–199.

Hao, A. Z., Z. F. Liu, and Y. Cui. 2004. Therapeutic effect of Xiaoke Huayu tablet on impaired glucose tolerance [Xiao ke hua yu pian gan yu zhi liao tang nai liang jian di de lin chuang guan cha]. *Medical Journal of Chinese People's Liberation Army [Jie Fang Jun Yi Xue Za Zhi]* 29(11): 993–994.

Hasegawa, H., J. H. Sung, S. Matsumiya, and M. Uchiyama. 1996. Main ginseng saponin metabolites formed by intestinal bacteria. *Planta Med* 62(5): 453–457.

Hu, Z., X. Yang, P. C. L. Ho, S. Y. Chan, P. W. S. H. Heng, E. Chan, W, Duan. H. L. Koh, and S. Zhou. 2005. Herb-drug interactions: A literature review. *Drug* 65(9): 1239–1282.

Huang, J. X. 2003. Thirty-three cases of IGT with Chinese herbs [Zhong yao zhi liao tang nai liang jian di 33 li]. *J Pract Tradit Chin Med* 19(8): 411

Husain, J., I. J. Tickle, and S. P. Wood. 1994. Crystal structure of momordin, a type I ribosome inactivating protein from the seeds of *Momordica charantia*. *FEBS Lett* 342(2): 154–158.

Ibanez-Camacho, R., M. Meckes-Lozoya, and V. Mellado-Campos. 1983. The hypoglucemic effect of *Opuntia streptacantha* studied in different animal experimental models. *J Ethnopharmacol* 7(2): 175–181.

Ibanez-Camacho, R., and R. Roman-Ramos. 1979. Hypoglycemic effect of *Opuntia* cactus. *Arch Invest Med (Mex)* 10(4): 223–230.

International Diabetes Federation. 2008. *Diabetes Atlas*. In International Diabetes Federation (Eds.). Available from http://www.eatlas.idf.org/.

Jain, R. C., and C. R. Vyas. 1975. Garlic in alloxan-induced diabetic rabbits. *Am J Clin Nutr* 28(7): 684–685.

Jia, W., W. Cao, Y. Yan, J. Wang, Z. Xu, W. Zheng, and P. Xiao. 2004. The rediscovery of ancient Chinese herbal formulas. *Phytother Res* 18: 681–686.

John, A. J., R. Cherian, H. S. Subhash, and A. M. Cherian. 2003. Evaluation of the efficacy of bitter gourd (*Momordica charantia*) as an oral hypoglycemic agent—A randomized controlled clinical trial. *Indian J Physiol Pharmacol* 47(3): 363–365.

Jolad, S. D., R. C. Lantz, A. M. Solyom, G. J. Chen, R. B. Bates, and B. N. Timmermann. 2004. Fresh organically grown ginger (*Zingiber officinale*): Composition and effects on LPS-induced PGE2 production. *Phytochemistry* 65(13): 1937–1954.

Kar, A., B. K. Choudhary, and N. G. Bandyopadhyay. 2003. Comparative evaluation of hypoglycaemic activity of some Indian medicinal plants in alloxan diabetic rats. *J Ethnopharmacol* 84(1): 105–108.

Kennedy, D. O., A. B. Scholey, and K. A. Wesnes. 2001. Differential, dose dependent changes in cognitive performance following acute administration of a *Ginkgo biloba/Panax ginseng* combination to healthy young volunteers. *Nutr Neurosci* 4: 399–412.

Keusgen, M. 1997. TLC analysis of *Allium sativum* constituents. *Planta Med* 63(1): 93–94.

Khosla, P., D. D. Gupta, and R. K. Nagpal. 1995. Effect of *Trigonella foenum graecum* (Fenugreek) on blood glucose in normal and diabetic rats. *Indian J Physiol Pharmacol* 39(2): 173–174.

Kook, S., G. H. Kim, and K. Choi. 2009. The antidiabetic effect of onion and garlic in experimental diabetic rats: Meta-analysis. *J Med Food* 12(3): 552–560.

Kroll, U. and C. Cordes. 2006. Pharmaceutical prerequisites for a multi-target therapy. *Phytomedicine* 13: 12–19.

Kumar, G. S., A. K. Shetty, and P. V. Salimath. 2008. Modulatory effect of bitter gourd (*Momordica charantia* LINN.) on alterations in kidney heparan sulfate in streptozotocin-induced diabetic rats. *J Ethnopharmacol* 115(2): 276–283.

Kumar Shetty, A., G. Suresh Kumar, and P. Veerayya Salimath. 2005. Bitter gourd (*Momordica charantia*) modulates activities of intestinal and renal disaccharidases in streptozotocin-induced diabetic rats. *Mol Nutr Food Res* 49(8): 791–796.

Leatherdale, B. A., R. K. Panesar, G. Singh, T. W. Atkins, C. J. Bailey, and A. H. Bignell. 1981. Improvement in glucose tolerance due to *Momordica charantia* (karela). *Br Med J (Clin Res Ed)* 282(6279): 1823–1824.

Leung, L., R. Birtwhistle, J. Kotecha, S. Hannah, and S. Cuthbertson. 2009. Anti-diabetic and hypoglycaemic effects of *Momordica charantia* (bitter melon): A mini review. *Br J Nutr* 102(12): 1703–1708.

Li, H. B., Z. X. Xu, L. F. Ling, and Z. H. Hu. 2002. The interference of glucose tolerance reduction by qi-benefiting [Yi qi jian pi fang dui yuan fa xing gao xue ya]. *New Journal of Traditional Chinese Medicine [Xin Zhong Yi]* 34(11): 35–36.

Li, C. P., B. Xie, J. Huang, H. B. Li, and Q. M. Li. 2004. Clinical observation of the effect of Qimai jingtang yin on impaired glucose tolerance [Qi mai jiang tang yin dui tang nai liang di jian gan yu lin chuang liao xiao guan cha]. *Journal of Sichuan Traditional Chinese Medicine [Si Chuan Zhong Yi]*, 22(10): 32–33.

Li, S. L., X. T. Feng, C. B. Qin, and G. B. Lou. 2006. The recent studies, development and outlook on IGT and TCM *[Tang nai liang di jian de zhong yi yao yan jiu jin kuang yu zhan wang]*. *Central China Medicine Magazine* 30(5): 437–438.

Lian, J. 2004. The pattern discrimination and treatment of 60 cases of increased glucose tolerance. *Zhe Jiang Zhong Yi Za Zhi* 12: 521.

Lind, B. K., W. E. Lafferty, D. E. Grembowski, and P. K. Diehr. 2006. Complementary and alternative provider use by insured patients with diabetes in Washington State. *J Altern Complement Med* 12(1): 71–77.

Liu, C. T., H. Hse, C. K. Lii, P. S. Chen, and L. Y. Sheen. 2005. Effects of garlic oil and diallyl trisulfide on glycemic control in diabetic rats. *Eur J Pharmacol* 516(2): 165–173.

Liu, W. T., X. Liu, X. Lian, F. Zhu, and Y. Zhou. 2008. The current situation of Traditional Chinese Medicine intervention in IGT. *Medical Recapitulate* 14(11): 1693–1695.

Liu, D., S. Pu, S. Qian, and J. Zhang. 2011. Chemical constituents of Chinese red ginseng. *Zhongguo Zhong Yao Za Zhi* 36(4): 462–464.

Liu, C. T., L. Y. Sheen, and C. K. Lii. 2007. Does garlic have a role as an antidiabetic agent? *Mol Nutr Food Res* 51(11): 1353–1364.

Liu, C. X. and P. G. Xiao. 1992. Recent advances on ginseng research in China. *J Ethnopharmacol* 36(1): 27–38.

Lu, R. H., Y. B. Gao, and X. H. Yang. 1999. *A Summary of TCM Diagnosis and Treatment of Diabetes Mellitus*. Beijing: China Medico-Pharmaceutical Sciences and Technology Publishing House.

Luo, G. B., S. L. Li, A. H. Tang, and M. L. Jia. 2005. Clinical observation on the intervention of impaired glucose tolerance with the qi and yin deficiency [Du qi yin liang xu xing tang nai liang di jian zhe gan yu zhi liao de lin chuang guan cha]. *Chinese Journal of Basic Medicine in Tradtional Chinese Medicine [Zhong Guo Zhong Yu Ji Chu Yi Xue Za Zhi]* 11(11): 845–846.

Madar, Z., R. Abel, S. Samish, and J. Arad. 1988. Glucose-lowering effect of fenugreek in non-insulin dependent diabetics. *Eur J Clin Nutr* 42(1): 51–54.

Mascolo, N., R. Jain, S. C. Jain, and F. Capasso. 1989. Ethnopharmacologic investigation of ginger (*Zingiber officinale*). *J Ethnopharmacol* 27(1–2): 129–140.

Mathew, P. T., and K. T. Augusti. 1973. Studies on the effect of allicin (diallyl disulphide-oxide) on alloxan diabetes. I. Hypoglycaemic action and enhancement of serum insulin effect and glycogen synthesis. *Indian J Biochem Biophys* 10(3): 209–212.

Matsuur, H., C. Asakawa, M. Kurimoto, and J. Mizutani. 2002. Alpha-glucosidase inhibitor from the seeds of balsam pear (*Momordica charantia*) and the fruit bodies of *Grifola frondosa*. *Biosci Biotechnol Biochem* 66(7): 1576–1578.

Max, B. 1992. This and that: The essential pharmacology of herbs and spices. *Trends Pharmacol Sci* 13(1): 15–20.

McHughes, M. and B. N. Timmermann. 2005. A review of the use of CAM therapy and the sources of accurate and reliable information. *J Manag Care Pharm* 11(8): 695–703.

MacLennan, A. H., S. P. Myers, and A. W. Taylor. 2006. The continuing use of complementary and alternative medicine in South Australia: Costs and beliefs in 2004. *Med J Aust* 184: 27–31.

Mishkinsky, J., B. Joseph, and F. G. Sulman. 1967. Hypoglycaemic effect of trigonelline. *Lancet* 2(7529): 1311–1312.

Miura, T., C. Itoh, N. Iwamoto, M. Kato, M. Kawai, S. R. Park, and I. Suzuki. 2001. Hypoglycemic activity of the fruit of the *Momordica charantia* in type 2 diabetic mice. *J Nutr Sci Vitaminol (Tokyo)* 47(5): 340–344.

Murakami, T., A. Emoto, H. Matsuda, and M. Yoshikawa. 2001. Medicinal foodstuffs. XXI. Structures of new cucurbitane-type triterpene glycosides, goyaglycosides-a, -b, -c, -d, -e, -f, -g, and -h, and new oleanane-type triterpene saponins, goyasaponins I, II, and III, from the fresh fruit of Japanese *Momordica charantia* L. *Chem Pharm Bull (Tokyo)* 49(1): 54–63.

Nammi, S., M. S. Kim, N. S. Gavande, G. Q. Li, and B. D. Roufogalis. 2010. Regulation of low-density lipoprotein receptor and 3-hydroxy-3-methylglutaryl coenzyme A reductase expression by *Zingiber officinale* in the liver of high-fat diet-fed rats. *Basic Clin Pharmacol Toxicol* 106(5): 389–395.

Nammi, S., S. Sreemantula, and B. D. Roufogalis. 2009. Protective effects of ethanolic extract of *Zingiber officinale* rhizome on the development of metabolic syndrome in high-fat diet-fed rats. *Basic Clin Pharmacol Toxicol* 104(5): 366–373.

Ojewole, J. A. 2006. Analgesic, antiinflammatory and hypoglycaemic effects of ethanol extract of *Zingiber officinale* (Roscoe) rhizomes (Zingiberaceae) in mice and rats. *Phytother Res* 20(9): 764–772.

Ooi, C. P., Z. Yassin, and T. A. Hamid. 2010. *Momordica charantia* for type 2 diabetes mellitus. *Cochrane Database Syst Rev* (2): CD007845.

Parkash, A., T. B. Ng, and W. W. Tso. 2002. Purification and characterization of charantin, a napin-like ribosome-inactivating peptide from bitter gourd (*Momordica charantia*) seeds. *J Pept Res* 59(5): 197–202.

Qu, L. X. 2002. Clinical observation on the treatment of abnormal glucose tolerance by tang ping san [Tang ping san zhi liao tang nai liang yi chang de lin chuang guan cha]. *Zhe Jiang Zhong Yi Za Zhi* 12(1): 32.

Raghuram, T. C., R. D. Sharma, and B. Sivakumar. 1996. Effect of fenugreek seeds on intravenous glucose disposition in non-insulin dependent diabetic patients. *Phytother Res* 8: 83–86.

Raju, J., D. Gupta, A. R. Rao, P. K. Yadava, and N. Z. Baquer. 2001. Trigonellafoenum graecum (fenugreek) seed powder improves glucose homeostasis in alloxan diabetic rat tissues by reversing the altered glycolytic, gluconeogenic and lipogenic enzymes. *Mol Cell Biochem* 224(1–2): 45–51.

Rathi, S. S., J. K. Grover, and V. Vats. 2002. The effect of *Momordica charantia* and Mucuna pruriens in experimental diabetes and their effect on key metabolic enzymes involved in carbohydrate metabolism. *Phytother Res* 16(3): 236–43.

Ribes, G., Y. Sauvaire, C. Da Costa, J. C. Baccou, and M. M. Loubatieres-Mariani. 1986. Antidiabetic effects of subfractions from fenugreek seeds in diabetic dogs. *Proc Soc Exp Biol Med* 182(2): 159–166.

Rivlin, R. S. 2006. Is garlic alternative medicine? *J Nutr* 136(3 Suppl): 713S–715S.

Riyad, M. A., S. A. Abdul-Salam, and S. S. Mohammad. 1988. Effect of fenugreek and lupine seeds on the development of experimental diabetes in rats. *Planta Med* 54(4): 286–290.

Roglic, G. and N. Unwin. 2010. Mortality attributable to diabetes: Estimates for the year 2010. *Diab Res Clin Pract* 87(1): 15–19.

Rotshteyn, Y. and S. W. Zito. 2004. Application of modified *in vitro* screening procedure for identifying herbals possessing sulfonylurea-like activity. *J Ethnopharmacol* 93(2–3): 337–344.

Satyanarayana, S., G. S. Sarma, A. Ramesh, K. Sushruta, and N. srinivas. 2003. Evaluation of herbal preparations for hypoglycemic activity in normal and diabetic rabbits. *Pharm Biol* 41: 466–472.

Sauvaire, Y., P. Petit, C. Broca, M. Manteghetti, Y. Baissac, J. Fernandez-Alvarez, R. Gross, et al. 1998. 4-Hydroxyisoleucine: A novel amino acid potentiator of insulin secretion. *Diabetes* 47(2): 206–210.

Schoenberg, N. E., E. P. Stoller, C. S. Kart, A. Perzynski, and E. E. Chapleski. 2004. Complementary and alternative medicine use among a multiethnic sample of older adults with diabetes. *J Altern Complement Med* 10(6): 1061–1066.

Scholey, A. and D. O. Kennedy. 2002. Acute, dose-dependent cognitive effects of *Ginkgo biloba, Panax ginseng* and their combination in healthy young volunteers: Differential interactions with cognitive demand. *Human Psychopharmacol: Clin Exp* 17: 35–44.

Sharma, R. D., T. C. Raghuram, and N. S. Rao. 1990. Effect of fenugreek seeds on blood glucose and serum lipids in type I diabetes. *Eur J Clin Nutr* 44(4): 301–306.

Shibib, B. A., L. A. Khan, and R. Rahman. 1993. Hypoglycaemic activity of Coccinia indica and *Momordica charantia* in diabetic rats: Depression of the hepatic gluconeogenic enzymes glucose-6-phosphatase and fructose-1,6-bisphosphatase and elevation of both liver and red-cell shunt enzyme glucose-6-phosphate dehydrogenase. *Biochem J* 292(Pt 1): 267–270.

Shih, C. C., C. H. Lin, and W. L. Lin. 2008. Effects of *Momordica charantia* on insulin resistance and visceral obesity in mice on high-fat diet. *Diabetes Res Clin Pract* 81(2): 134–143.

Shih, C. C., C. H. Lin, W. L. Lin, and J. B. Wu. 2009. *Momordica charantia* extract on insulin resistance and the skeletal muscle GLUT4 protein in fructose-fed rats. *J Ethnopharmacol* 123(1): 82–90.

Singh, N. and M. Gupta. 2007. Regeneration of beta cells in islets of Langerhans of pancreas of alloxan diabetic rats by acetone extract of *Momordica charantia* (Linn.) (bitter gourd) fruits. *Indian J Exp Biol* 45(12): 1055–1062.

Song, X. 2007. Current status of research on Chinese medicine for impaired glucose tolerance (Chinese). *Gansu J TCM* 20(5): 88–91.

Sotaniemi, E. A., E. Haapakoski, and A. Rautio. 1995. Ginseng therapy in non-insulin-dependent diabetic patients. *Diabetes Care* 18(10): 1373–1375.

Srivastava, Y., H. Venkatakrishna-Bhatt, Y. Verma, and A. S. Prem. 1987. Retardation of retinopathy by *Momordica charantia* L. (bitter gourd) fruit extract in alloxan diabetic rats. *Indian J Exp Biol* 25(8): 571–572.

Sun, Y. 2005. Tonifying-qi nurishing-yin strengthening-kidney method for IGT in 40 cases [Yiqi yangyin bushen fa zhi liao tang nai liang di jian 40 li]. *Journal of Practical Traditional Chinese Internal Medicine [Shi Yong Zhong Yi Nei Ke Za Zhi]* 19(6): 567.

Swanston-Flatt, S. K., C. Day, C. J. Bailey, and P. R. Flatt. 1990. Traditional plant treatments for diabetes. Studies in normal and streptozotocin diabetic mice. *Diabetologia* 33(8): 462–464.

Tachikawa, E., K. Kudo, K. Harada, T. Kashimoto, Y. Miyate, A. Kakizaki, and E. Takahashi. 1999. Effects of ginseng saponins on responses induced by various receptor stimuli. *Eur J Pharmacol* 369(1): 23–32.

Tang, Q. Z., Z. S. Liao, M. J. Feng, X. L. Yao, Z. Z. Zhu, and M. Liu. 2007. The clinical study of Jianpi zishen huo xue (stengthen the spleen, nourish the kidney and activate the blood) method for IGT in 38 cases [Jian pi zi shen hup xue fa gan yu tang nai liang di jian 38 li lin chuang yan jiu]. *Journal of New Chinese Medicine [Xin Zhong Yi]* 39(9): 88–90.

TGA Adverse. 2005. Drug Reactions Advisory Committee (ADRAC). *Australian Adverse Drug Reactions Bulletin*. 24(1) http://www.tga.gov.au/hp/aadrb-0502.htm#a1.

Tongia, A., S. K. Tongia, and M. Dave. 2004. Phytochemical determination and extraction of *Momordica charantia* fruit and its hypoglycemic potentiation of oral hypoglycemic drugs in diabetes mellitus (NIDDM). *Indian J Physiol Pharmacol* 48(2): 241–244.

Uebanso, T., H. Arai, Y. Taketani, M. Fukaya, H. Yamamoto, A. Mizuno, K. Uryu, T. Hada, and E. Takeda. 2007. Extracts of *Momordica charantia* suppress postprandial hyperglycemia in rats. *J Nutr Sci Vitaminol (Tokyo)* 53(6): 482–488.

Verhoef, M. J., G. Lewith, C. Ritenbaugh, H. Boon, S. Fleishman, and A. Leis. 2005. Complementary and alternative medicine whole systems research: Beyond identification of inadequacies of the RCT. *Complement Ther Med* 13(3): 206–212.

Verma, S. K., M. Singh, P. Jain, and A. Bordia. 2004. Protective effect of ginger, *Zingiber officinale* Rosc on experimental atherosclerosis in rabbits. *Indian J Exp Biol* 42(7): 736–738.

Vuksan, V., M. K. Sung, J. L. Sievenpiper, P. M. Stavro, A. L. Jenkins, K. Di Buono, K. S. Lee, et al. 2008. Korean red ginseng (Panax ginseng) improves glucose and insulin regulation in well-controlled, type 2 diabetes: Results of a randomized, double-blind, placebo-controlled study of efficacy and safety. *Nutr Metab Cardiovasc Dis* 18(1): 46–56.

Wagner, H. and G. Ulrich-Merzenich. 2009. Synergy research: Approaching a new generation of phytopharmaceuticals. *Phytomedicine* 16: 97–110.

Waki, I., H. Kyo, M. Yasuda, and M. Kimura. 1982. Effects of a hypoglycemic component of ginseng radix on insulin biosynthesis in normal and diabetic animals. *J Pharmacobiodyn* 5(8): 547–554.

Wang, D. H., W. F. Liu, M. H. Xi, and H. Zhang. 1999. Analysis of the effectiveness of soothing-liver clearing-heat and promoting-blood circulation expelling-stagnation method for II DM in 120 cases [Shugan qin-gre huoxue huoyu fa zhi liao II xing tang niao bing 120 li liao xiao fen xi]. *Tianjin Journal of Traditional Chinese Medicine [Tianjin Zhongyi]* 16(2): 15–17.

Wang, Y. F. 2008. Observation of Shenqi Dihuang Tang intervention for blood and lipids in patients with IGT [Shenqi Dihuang Tang Dui tang nai liang jian di huan zhe xue tang, xue zhi de gan yu guan cha]. *Hebei Journal of Traditional Chinese Medicine [Hebei Zhong Yi]* 30(5): 473–474.

Wei, A., F. Sun, and J. Long. 2001. Effects of Xiaoke Yuye on Patients with Impaired Glucose Tolerance [Xiao ke yu ye shi liao tang nai liang jian tui lin chuang yan jiu]. *Journal of Shandong University of TCM* 25(4): 259–260.

World Health Organisation. 2005. National policy on traditional medicine and regulation of herbal medicines: Report of a WHO Global Survey. Geneva: World Health Organisation.

World Health Organisation. 2008. *World Health Organization. Diabetes Fact Sheet. 2008*. Retrieved from Available at: http://www.who.int/mediacentre/factsheets/fs312/en/.

Wu, S. 2004. Incapability of Spleen to disperse essence and its relation with IGT. *China J Tradit Chin Med Pharm* 19(8): 463–465.

Xie, H., S. Huang, H. Deng, Z. Wu, and A. Ji. 1998. [Study on chemical components of *Momordica charantia*]. *Zhong Yao Cai* 21(9): 458–459.

Xie, J. T., S. McHendale, and C. S. Yuan. 2005. Ginseng and diabetes. *Am J Chin Med* 33(3): 397–404.

Yang, B., W. X. Wang, W. Huo, H. Q. Min, D. X. Liu, and Z. He. 2004. Clinical observation of intervention of tangkangyin decoction on patients with impaired glucose tolerance [Tang kang yin gan yu zhi liao tang nai liang di jian lin chuang guan cha]. *Hebei Journal of Traditional Chinese Medicine [He Bei Zhong Yi]* 26(12): 893–895.

Yeh, G. Y., D. M. Eisenberg, R. B. Davis, and R. S. Phillips. 2002. Use of complementary and alternative medicine among persons with diabetes mellitus: Results of a national survey. *Am J Public Health* 92(10): 1648–1652.

Yeh, G. Y., D. M. Eisenberg, T. J. Kaptchuk, and R. S. Phillips. 2003. Systematic review of herbs and dietary supplements for glycemic control in diabetes. *Diabetes Care* 26(4): 1277–1294.

Yibchok-anun, S., S. Adisakwattana, C. Y. Yao, P. Sangvanich, S. Roengsumran, and W. H. Hsu. 2006. Slow acting protein extract from fruit pulp of *Momordica charantia* with insulin secretagogue and insulinomimetic activities. *Biol Pharm Bull* 29(6): 1126–1131.

Yin, B. 2007. The clinical observation of jin qi jiang tang for IGT in 41 cases [Jin qi jiang tang pian gan yu zhi liao IGT 41 li lin chuang guan cha]. *Journal of Practical Diabetology [Shi Yong Tang Niao Bing Za Zhi]* 2(3): 35.

Yuan, Y. R., Y. N. He, J. P. Xiong, and Z. X. Xia. 1999. Three-dimensional structure of beta-momorcharin at 2.55 A resolution. *Acta Crystallogr D Biol Crystallogr* 55(Pt 6): 1144–1151.

Zeng, Y. H., C. F. Wang, Y. S. Huang, Y. L. Rong, Y. F. Zhang, H. Z. Yang, B. K. Zhou, and S. X. Lao. 2000. Combination of Chinese traditional and western medicine in preventing and treating glucose tolerance abnormality and mild diabetes [Zhong xi yi jie he fang zhi tang nai liang yi chang ji qing xing tang niao bing liao xiao guan cha]. *Zhongguo Zhong Xi Yi Jie He Za Zhi* 8(4): 196–198.

Zia, T., S. N. Hasnain, and S. K. Hasan. 2001. Evaluation of the oral hypoglycaemic effect of Trigonella foenum-graecum L. (methi) in normal mice. *J Ethnopharmacol* 75(2–3): 191–195.

Zhou, Z. N. 2001. Observation of curative effect of self-prepared Huaqi jiangtang decoction on impaired glucose tolerance [Zi yi hua qi jiang tang fang yu tang nai liang yi chang liao xiao guan cha]. *Guangxi Journal of Traditional Chinese Medicine [Guang Xi Zhong Yi Yao]* 24(6): 13–15.

Section VI

Market to Innovative Products

27 Drivers and Barriers for Marketing Innovative Functional Food Products

Ruth D'Souza

CONTENTS

Since the 1990s we have been witnessing the blurring of boundaries between two industries—food and pharmaceuticals—which have led to the emergence of an interindustry segment, namely, nutraceuticals and functional foods. This convergence has created a multibillion dollar industry worldwide. Value propositions, technologies, markets, and demand structures have converged as consumers try to fulfill varied needs in the same transaction. Compounded with this is the fact that major metabolic disorders are not being addressed with an aim to cure. Instead, nutritional correction has now come to play a major role in these disorders.

Food and beverage makers have long fortified their products with vitamins and other nutrients in order to enhance the health benefits of the products. Changing consumer demands and demographics compounded by advances in food and medical science are fuelling growth in the functional foods market. Owing to advances in nutrition science and food manufacturing, the industry is now moving from identifying and correcting nutritional deficiencies to creating foods that promote optimal health and wellness as well as reduce the risk of chronic disease. Emerging healthcare trends, including personalized medicine, nanotechnology, greater incentives to reduce medical costs, and focus on prevention, will expand the potential of this segment.

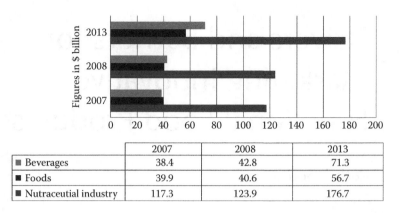

	2007	2008	2013
■ Beverages	38.4	42.8	71.3
■ Foods	39.9	40.6	56.7
■ Nutraceutial industry	117.3	123.9	176.7

FIGURE 27.1 Nutraceutical market. (Adapted from Nutraceuticals: Global Markets and Processing Technologies, *BCC Research*, July 2011.)

Figure 27.1 shows the share of the nutraceutical market in 2007 and 2008 as well as the estimated share in 2013.

As seen in Figure 27.1, the global market for nutraceutical products increased from $117.3 billion in 2007 to an estimated $123.9 billion in 2008. It should reach $176.7 billion in 2013, a compound annual growth rate (CAGR) of 7.4%. The nutraceutical foods industry, which comprises foods and beverages, currently has the largest share of the market and was worth $39.9 billion in 2007 and $40.6 billion in 2008; it is expected to reach $56.7 billion in 2013, at a CAGR of 6.9%. Nutraceutical beverages alone generated $38.4 billion in 2007 and an estimated $42.8 billion in 2008. According to a report published by BCC research, this segment is expected to dominate the market in 2013 with revenues of $71.3 billion, with a CAGR of 10.8%. Yet, food and beverage companies are facing greater challenges than ever before, striving to deliver sales and profit goals in the current competitive and complex marketplace. To deliver sustainable profitability, companies must boost innovation efficiency, translate productivity into dollars, manage business complexity, and ensure regulatory compliance.

27.1 INNOVATION AND THE FUNCTIONAL FOOD INDUSTRY

Businesses innovate to meet unmet needs of the customer and to sustain competitiveness. In a bid to remain competitive, companies are arriving at the conclusion that continuous innovation needs to be at the core. Innovation and introduction of augmented and future products will be one of the critical determinants of the economic success of businesses that wish to respond to changing customer demands, create new markets, and remain competitive in the long run.

Beginning with humble initiatives to improve public health, the functional foods industry has come a long way. Vitamin B enriched flour was introduced in the 1940s to combat pellagra; iodine fortified salt substantially decreased incidences of goiter; and vitamin D enriched milk virtually eliminated rickets. Originating in Japan about 20 years ago, companies are creating and marketing functional foods or nutrient rich products aimed at consumers who seek to prevent the onset of disease by actively seeking products that enhance health beyond basic nutritional needs. Some examples of nutraceuticals in functional foods include probiotics (microorganisms that provide digestive benefits), omega-3 (fish oil) extracts, and phytonutrients (found in plants such as soy beans, blueberries, and grapes).

Innovation in this emerging industry is shifting from the traditional emphasis on improving product quality and performance to a new level of customer centricity; it is moving away from being "market-driven" toward being "market-driving." Marketing innovators are taking major steps to drive the market by launching breakthrough products to replace incremental products and new product platforms to replace customary new products.

Foods and beverages fortified with pharmaceutical-like ingredients have hit the market. Benecol spreads, which also contain plant sterols; Kellogg's Smart Start cereals, enriched with antioxidants or soy protein; Wonder Bread with added folic acid; Yakult, a probiotic drink; Dannon's DanActive, a drink that contains 10 times the culture found in traditional yogurt and that claims to "strengthen your body's natural defenses"; Logic Juice 4 Joints, a fruit drink with glucosamine and chondroitin that may ease arthritis and joint pain; and Omega eggs, from chickens fed a diet rich in omega-3 fatty acids, which are believed to reduce the risk of heart disease are some of the innovative functional foods and beverages that have been launched.

27.2 DRIVERS OF MARKETING INNOVATIVE FUNCTIONAL FOODS

Changing trends in population demography, consumer affluence, increased education, life expectancy, and improved healthcare have given rise to a changing diet and health-conscious consumer clientele.

27.2.1 INCREASING HEALTH CONSCIOUSNESS

Increasing health consciousness has been one of the most important stimulating factors for the rapid global growth of the nutraceutical and functional food industry. Modern-day consumers are more aware of health risks and lifestyle-induced diseases and are seeking to take up a more proactive role in managing their health. Health consciousness combined with economic prosperity and an increased access to information through education, the Internet, and media coverage has fuelled a rapidly growing self-healthcare movement. The consumer recognizes that foods play a primary role in disease prevention and that health risks can be reduced by pursuing a healthier lifestyle. Consumer knowledge of the relationship between diet and health is increasing thanks to medical research which has been instrumental in strengthening the link between specific food components and specific health risks. In addition to eliminating harmful foods from their diet, consumers are also adding specific foods to benefit from their healthful benefits.

Consumer demand for functional foods will only increase as scientists gain a better understanding of the links among nutrition, normal body function, and disease. Scientists are working to identify new bioactive substances present in foods, establishing ideal levels, and gaining a better understanding of the role and optimum levels of traditional nutrients for specific segments of the population. Understanding the role of nutrients at the molecular level will result in even more specific recommendations for different population subgroups considering age, sex, health goals, lifestyle, and genetic disposition. Greater health awareness coupled with the potential for premium pricing will fuel growth in the functional foods market.

27.2.2 AGE OF THE POPULATION

Different age groups have different functional food preferences and needs. An examination of the age distribution of a country's population can suggest which types of functional foods may become more popular.

When marketing foods, it is important to keep in mind the consumer's age, which often provides a window into their buying habits. For example, baby boomers as a whole are trying to defy aging and want to get the most for their money when shopping. In recognition of their limited mortality, the baby-boomer birth cohort will focus on foods that will help them manage the vast array of age-related maladies that this group faces. Gen X consumers are media savvy and individualistic. Convenience means everything and they are willing to pay a premium for what they perceive as value added to a product. Organic food would be a case in point because they value the fact that it is free of chemicals and hormones.

Food manufacturers and marketers need to decide whether it is potentially more profitable to go after a small percentage of a large market through mass marketing or a large percentage of a smaller market by tailoring the product and the message to meet the needs of a specific demographic.

27.2.3 ESCALATING HEALTHCARE COSTS

Healthcare costs are escalating exponentially all over the world, forcing many consumers to seek out more cost-effective alternatives to those being provided by traditional forms of high-cost, professional, and structured medicine. Many costly and disabling conditions such as cardiovascular diseases, cancer, diabetes, and chronic respiratory diseases are linked by common preventable risk factors. Prolonged tobacco use, unhealthy nutrition, physical inactivity, and excessive alcohol intake are major causes and risk factors for these conditions.

A poor diet and lack of exercise can lead to metabolic syndrome, which is a combination of high blood pressure, blood fats, and blood sugar. Reducing the risk for disease by adding certain foods to the diet and eliminating excess saturated fat, cholesterol, and sodium can reduce the need for medical intervention. Eating more dietary fiber and less cholesterol can reduce the risk for heart disease and stroke. Dietary fiber may also combat the onset of cancer. Adding more calcium to the diet can improve bone density and reduce the effects of osteoporosis. Eating fish rich in omega-3 fatty acids, such as tuna and salmon, can improve cholesterol numbers. Hypertension can be prevented by decreasing sodium in the diet. Adding iron-rich foods, such as black beans, spinach, or red meat, decreases the risk of anemia.

27.2.4 ADVANCES IN RESEARCH AND TECHNOLOGY

Advances in the areas of food technology, food biochemistry, and the nutritional sciences (including nutritional genomics) are providing consumers with access to fresh and often supplemented produce with recognizable health benefits that were previously unavailable. New methods being used by the functional food industry to isolate, characterize, extract, and purify nutraceuticals from bacterial, plant, and animal sources are resulting in decreased costs to the industry and providing new options for the use of functional food products. Nanotechnology is a new frontier and will be a key source of innovation in the food industry, particularly in food formulation, processing, packaging, storage, and quality.

27.2.5 EVIDENCE BASED CLAIMS

Scientific evidence to support nutritional and medicinal claims being made within the functional food and nutraceutical industry are being increasingly demanded. There has been considerable discussion regarding the need for better characterization of functional foods and food products as well as the need for clinical trials demonstrating medicinal claims, and better labeling of products whose active agents may vary considerably in concentration due to genotypic variation, response to environment, and/or processing during preparation of a product.

As scientific studies reveal new discoveries with potential health benefits, more consumer support, credibility, and demand for functional foods and nutraceuticals will be generated, resulting in a marketplace with considerable potential for growth and many new opportunities.

27.2.6 EXPANSION OF THE GLOBAL MARKETPLACE

Better communications and transport for marketable goods is resulting in a more accessible global marketplace and an increase in international business opportunities. This, coupled with increased recognition for proprietary patented products, is resulting in a more business-friendly environment for expansion of the industry.

27.2.7 ATTRACTIVE MARKET OPPORTUNITY

Emerging technologies in food processing are leading to new methods for stabilizing ingredients, optimizing texture, and improving product taste. Premium pricing potential is attracting food and beverage companies to the market. Conventional foods face volatile margins as commodity prices fluctuate and competition intensifies. Margins on functional foods, on the other hand, tend to be consistently higher. Although these products typically require greater initial R&D and the ingredient costs are high, price premiums may reach 30% or higher, depending on the product.

27.3 BARRIERS TO SUCCESS

Even though the opportunities are vast, the challenges to successfully marketing functional foods are significant. The industry is highly competitive and maintaining consumer brand loyalty is emerging as a critical yet complex issue owing to the growing similarity among products and formulations.

27.3.1 REGULATORY FRAMEWORK

Most countries lack a suitable regulatory category for functional food products, which makes market development much more complicated. A clear regulatory system for production, sales, certification, and advertising of functional foods, together with consistent enforcement are critical factors in building consumer trust in functional foods. A credible system can also help to provide a level-playing field that fosters competition and encourages innovation.

27.3.2 UNDERLYING SCIENCE: ESTABLISHING CLAIMS AND EVIDENCE

The development and marketing of functional foods require significant research efforts because most markets require scientific evidence and proof of functionality. Even though certain foods may have been used for a long time for health-enhancement purposes, the definitive scientific support for claims as a functional product is often lacking. This involves identification of functional compounds and assessment of their physiological effect, taking into account bioavailability in humans and potential changes during processing and food preparation and clinical trials on product efficacy in order to gain approval for health-enhancing marketing claims. This research requires time, financing, and skilled labor, especially for products intended for export markets. Lastly, innovation and research capacity is required to screen local biodiversity to uncover potential new sources for functional foods. This is also a management culture challenge for researchers because the best results can be obtained through partnerships between formal science institutions and indigenous communities.

27.3.3 ADDRESSING CONSUMER INSIGHTS AND SCEPTICISM

Capturing consumer needs and incorporating them into products is a key driving force not only to create the next blockbuster, but also to successfully compete in the market. Taste is the top priority for consumers and one that cannot be compromised. Indeed, it is a challenge to incorporate function and nutrition without negatively affecting taste.

Consumer scepticism is another aspect that should be taken into consideration. Products are pushed to an often skeptical customer group and fail to neutralize the perceived risks associated with the new product.

Consumers may easily understand the concept of a functional yogurt and the role of helpful bacteria that traditional yogurts already contain. However, other functional products may be less intuitive to consumers, and consequently, customers may question the purpose of the product. Clearly communicating the benefits of the product and educating consumers will be a challenge for the marketer.

While there is a tidal wave of information, there is also an increasing degree of confusion about nutrition and micronutrition. There are too many contradictory messages pertaining to which foods are healthy or unhealthy, leading to concerns about incomplete knowledge, which is a relatively common and potentially significant problem.

27.3.4 FOOD SAFETY

Ensuring product safety is critical for consumer confidence and brand protection. Retailers and regulatory bodies are concerned about supplier quality and are enforcing new policies around product and raw material traceability in order to protect the public.

27.3.5 COMPETITION

Incorporating global development is necessary to help combat competition across the globe and with private label brands and niche vendors. Sustainability is emerging as a source of differentiation, competitive advantage, and profitability, from both a corporate and product standpoint. Supporting a fast-paced new product development environment with condensed time-to-market and time-to-profit metrics are essential for ensuring competitive advantage and locking in significant profit margins.

27.3.6 COST REDUCTION

Bringing products to the market at a lower cost is the main focus in a recession, as prices of commodities are set by what the market can tolerate. Meanwhile, costs are on the rise for both raw materials and compliance. Finding the right balance that maximizes value while minimizing costs is integral to managing growing supply chains, product proliferation, merged operations, reorganizations and government mandates.

27.4 CONCLUSION

The last few decades have witnessed a drastic change worldwide in consumers' attitudes toward food products. Food products are no longer being seen simply as a means for survival and pleasure. Many other factors and barriers affect consumers' decisions in selecting food products, thus wielding substantial power in influencing the food industry's decisions in producing and developing new food products.

Food safety, health, and environmental issues are a few of the reasons that motivate consumers to adopt new innovative food products—organic, private label, genetically modified, or functional—as part of their consumption.

Cost-effective organic food that consistently delivers nutritional standards for various genetic and metabolic differentiated races will demand a totally different research model than that presently followed by the manufacturing mindset. There is a growing need to identify the science of nutritional epidemiology and food consumption habits. The culture and science of eating will have to change for the better if humanity has to go beyond its obsession from longevity to quality of life lived.

The functional foods market holds numerous possibilities, but also a number of challenges.

BIBLIOGRAPHY

Basu, S. K., Thomas, J. E., and Acharya, S. N. 2007, Prospects for global nutraceuticals and functional foods markets—A Canadian perspective. *Australian Journal of Basic and Applied Sciences* 1(4), 637–649.

Belem, M. A. F. 1999, *Trends in Food Science & Technology, Application of Biotechnology in the Product Development of Nutraceuticals in Canada*, Elsevier, Canada, Vol. 10, pp. 101–106.

Childs, N. M. 2006. Marketing and regulatory issues for functional foods and nutraceuticals, *Handbook of Nutraceuticals, and Functional Foods*, 2nd edition, Wildman, R. (ed.), CRC Press, Boca Raton, FL, pp. 503–516.

Dillard, C. J. and German, B. J. 2000, Phytochemicals: Nutraceuticals and human health, *Journal of the Science of Food and Agriculture* 80(12), 1744–1756.

Drouin, A. and Gosselin, A. 2002, *Canadian Technological Roadmap on Functional Foods and Nutraceuticals*, KPMG, Canada, pp. 1, 7, 11, 24.

Hasler, C. M. 2000, *The Changing Face of Functional Foods, Functional Foods for Health Program*, University of Illinois, Urbana, USA.

Nutraceuticals: Global Markets and Processing Technologies, *BCC Research*, July 2011.

28 Marketing, PR, Advertising, and Media for Brand Building of Innovative Foods and Nutritional Products

M.G. Parameswaran

CONTENTS

In a focus group research held in the Indian metropolis of Kolkata, a woman came up with an interesting answer when asked "What is nutrition?" She said, "Nutrition is food taken on time, less spicy, easy to digest." When probed, the group responded that "Nutrition is not the same for everyone, it is different for different people."

The above interaction is possibly symptomatic of the level of knowledge that exists in developing markets like India among the consumers about nutrition. In fact, leading text books on marketing speak of nutrition primarily from the context of nutritional labeling (Kotler and Keller 2006).

This chapter addresses the challenges that face marketers when they develop and attempt to market innovative nutritional products to consumers whose understanding of nutrition is at best very basic. We will first examine what we mean by nutritional products, then review the international scenario with respect to nutritional products, then move to the challenges consumers face while selecting nutritional products, and finally look at methodologies that could be used to help consumers overcome the inertia to try and use innovative nutritional products.

28.1 DEFINING NUTRITIONAL PRODUCTS

Nutritional products have been with us for ages and as some experts point out it has become fashionable for traditional foods to get reinvented as "all-natural nutritional foods" (Mellentin 2009)—so products such as oats, almonds, cranberry juice, pomegranate, and even wheat grass have all got on to the nutritional brand wagon.

When we talk of nutritional products, we are looking at four types of products:

1. *Traditional products fortified with nutrition:* These products could be biscuits with added fiber or oats, breakfast cereals with additional iron, or fruit juices with added vitamins. Often, these products are part of a normal diet and marketers attempt to add value through additional nutritional ingredients.
2. *Nutritional supplements:* These groups of products are not part of a normal diet but will have to be consumed separately—cod liver oil capsules for children, calcium supplements for women, evening primrose oil for women, multivitamins for men and women, and so on.
3. *Dietary supplements:* These products have been developed to be added to the normal diet to make it nutrition-wise complete. Products such as oats breakfast mix, rice for diabetics, milk food drinks for children and adults, and specially created breakfast cereals would be part of this group.
4. *Nutraceuticals:* These are the new-generation nutritional supplements, and products such as probiotic drinks and capsules with new ingredients such as Omega3 would all form a part of this group.

The four categories listed above are by no means mutually exclusive. But the degree of difficulty varies with each type. The fifth type of products are those that contain less of some perceived harmful ingredient, such as low-fat milk, sugar-free ice cream, or low-sodium salt. The last class of products works on the consumer psyche of "less is better," though it is not sure if these products could be called nutritional just because they contain less of an ingredient such as sugar, fat, or sodium.

The degree of difficulty in marketing various types of nutritional products is not the same. Though the tools used for communicating the benefits may be somewhat similar, the emphasis may be dramatically different as will be examined later.

28.2 NUTRITIONAL INFORMATION AND CONSUMERS

The 1990 Nutrition Labelling and Education Act (NLEA) dramatically changed the labeling of nutritional products in the United States (Balasubramanian and Cole 2002). In fact, all marketing text books today devote a section on the NLEA and its impact on packaging and consumer behavior (Kotler and Keller 2006).

This landmark U.S. legislation was followed to some degree by governments across the world with similar rules passed in several countries. In India, nutritional labeling and labeling of the food products as "vegetarian" or "nonvegetarian" became mandatory in the last decade. But has this labeling led to a dramatic change in consumer behavior? Has this led to a dramatic increase in the sales of more nutritional products?

One of the earliest studies on nutritional information use (Moorman 1990), done before the NLEA law was passed, is indicative of what was to come. Moorman points out that consumers find that the consequences associated with negatively perceived nutrients (e.g., sugar and sodium) are more relevant than those associated with positive nutrients such as vitamins and minerals.

Studies done in the United States a decade after the NLEA was passed (Baltas 2001; Balasubramanian and Cole 2002) point toward both dimensions—a greater impact on negative labeling and some beneficial impact in positive nutritional labeling.

Baltas (2001) points out that their study found that the effect of nutritional information does matter in product choice decisions.

Their study indicates three broad guidelines toward nutritional labeling: (1) since consumers use nutritional information in the brand choice process, advertising claims should be justifiable by on-pack nutrition data. (2) Consumer response to nutrition information is not homogeneous (as our group in Kolkata pointed out); hence, marketers should take into account nutrition needs and preferences of specific target consumers. (3) Finally, marketers should identify relationships between heterogeneous attribute evaluation and media habits of consumers.

Balasubramanian and Cole's (2002) research indicate that one beneficial impact of NLEA was that food manufacturers were forced to respond with nutrition improvements: adding positive nutrients to the existing brands and deleting negative nutrients in brand extensions. But they too conclude that consumers rely more on negative than positive attributes. They point toward four broad themes: consumer's search for nutrition information is driven by their perception of the category; consumers who are desirous of weight loss may limit attention to a few negative nutrition attributes; consumers generally distrust information such as serving size and hard-to-verify nutrition claims, and finally food shoppers see themselves as purchasing agents balancing the budget, taste, and nutrition needs of the family. We will use the last observation later to develop a decision module and trade-off diagram that the consumer mentally goes through when accosted with new nutritional products.

The study done in the EU to understand the impact of the new European regulation on health-related claims indicates that there is little to expect from the new regulation on food advertisement claims and their impact on consumer understanding of nutrition (Brennan et al. 2008).

This quick review of published reports indicates that consumers are yet to fully comprehend the nutritional claims made by brands. While manufacturers tend to obfuscate claims, there seems to be some clarity in consumers' minds on the importance of watching out for negative ingredients, not so much on looking for positive nutrition.

These findings pose a huge challenge to marketers who are looking at introducing innovative nutritional brands in the market to ride the so-called health wave sweeping the world.

28.3   CONSUMER DECISION JOURNEY AND NUTRITIONAL PRODUCTS

Consumer awareness of nutritional needs and fortified nutritional products is growing by the day (Raterman 2008). Modern diets are deficient in fiber and it has been reported that Europeans and Americans only consume 30% of the recommended daily intake (Mellentin 2009). Top-selling U.S. supplements such as multivitamins ($4 billion), calcium ($1 billion), and vitamin B ($1 billion) have all grown to become very large markets. Even as far back as 1978, reports indicated that 77% of the consumers interviewed indicated that they were more interested in nutrition than a few years ago (Food Product Development 1978). When asked about deciding the family food diet, the trade-off was across budget constraints (41%), weight watching (35%), nutrient content (17%), and unsure factors (7%). In 1978, only 24% were considered very well informed, 63% fairly well informed, and 13% were not well informed about nutritional information.

Reports show that developed countries such as the United States are experiencing a crisis in childhood obesity; obesity rates have been doubling over the last three decades among preschool (ages 2–5) children and have tripled among children 6–11 years of age (Moore and Rideout 2007). While pointing out that advertising messages aimed at children through computer games rarely have any educational value, Lee et al. (2009) also observes that the U.S. food, beverage, and restaurant industries spend $1.6 billion annually to promote their products to children and adolescents, out of the total advertisement spend of $10 billion.

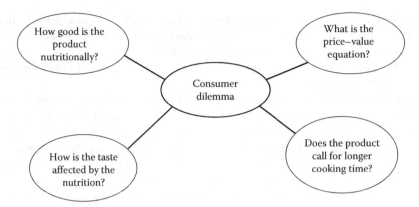

FIGURE 28.1 Consumer dilemma.

Consumer dilemma (Figure 28.1) while trying to adopt modern nutritional products arises out of the various benefits that they have to balance while planning the family's food basket.

28.3.1 INFORMATION ON NUTRITION

The Consumers' first dilemma stems from their lack of information and comprehension of the various nutritional needs of the human body and the food brands/products that provide them. Consumers in Kolkata when probed mentioned that nutrition meant proteins, minerals, and vitamins, and although some of them claim to get their knowledge from health magazines, none of them could explain what role these nutrients play in the growth, development, or maintenance of the human body. International research shows that consumers could articulate "negative nutrition" (fat, sugar, and sodium) and "positive nutrition" (vitamin, proteins, and minerals). They expressed their views as "nutrition for kids is for growth" and "nutrition for adults is for maintenance." The consumers claimed that nutritional labels are useful; however, they could not articulate what they really learnt from them.

28.3.2 TASTE PREFERENCES

Women are clear that taste cannot be sacrificed, especially when it comes to children. The Kolkata women even went on to say that without sugar food is not food. But be that as it may, taste is a key dimension on which food is weighed; if it is nutritious, is it also less tasty? Products that are high in protein such as soy meal chunks have often suffered from a poor taste halo. Similarly, unsweetened fruit juices are also seen as less tasty.

There is an inherent fear in consuming packaged food brands in developing markets such as India where vegetable and fish/meat products are bought on a daily basis, because of concerns regarding freshness and additives—consumer inertia is further heightened due to suspicion of taste attributes.

28.3.3 TIME FOR PREPARATION

More nutritious products often require a greater time for preparation—this is true of fresh fruits, vegetables, and so on. There is a perception for packaged products, that if the preparation time is less, they are not very nutritious.

Nutritious products have to overcome the twin issue of time taken for preparation and building conviction on nutritional claims.

28.3.4 VALUE PARADIGM

Finally, the clinching argument is the price–value equation as seen by the consumer. Food budgets still account for a large part of the monthly household budgets, especially in developing countries. When it comes to various food items, products such as milk, vegetables, meat, and fish do take up the largest share. The householder is often trading down or trading up depending on the price movements of food products—reducing consumption of fish/meat or selective use of cheaper vegetables is a common practice. Atul Sinha, vice president of New Product Development, Britannia Industries India, points out that, in India, there is still very little societal permission to use packaged foods, and when this is coupled with the rigidity of food habits and tastes in the country and the cost–value paradigm, the challenge is quite formidable.

To summarize, the consumer is balancing these four dimensions when they look at new nutritional brands. The challenge that marketers face is to get consumers to know enough about the nutritional benefits, understand the price paradigm, and convince them that there is no sacrifice on the taste or time.

Marketers will be successful with all their new innovative products if they can get consumers to understand the nutrition information and offer a perfect price–value equation without upsetting the time or taste dimension.

Often, the challenge is that not all these conditions can be fulfilled through product innovations and therefore marketers will have to use methods of communication to help the consumers' address these dilemmas.

28.4   CONNECTING WITH THE CONSUMERS

Mellentin (2009) points out that over the last 15 years, functional foods that have succeeded have done so by becoming an "expert brand." Brands such as Kellogg's Special K (the world's biggest weight management brand with $1 billion in sales) or DanoneActiva (helps improve digestive transit time) have all gained from an expert aura.

Mellentin (2009) clearly states that functional foods cannot become mass market from day one. They have to chart their journey by first focusing on the segments that consider health to be a critical part of their lifestyle. The four-step process he suggests are: focus on being an expert brand with one benefit, offer a benefit that the consumer can quickly feel, support through marketing education, and focus on the niche of the more health-conscious consumer.

These findings also hark back to the suggestions made by Balasubramanian and Cole (2002) on how consumers' search and use information on nutrition based on their readiness to accept new claims.

As Rimi Obra-Ratwatte, senior nutritionist at Kellogg observes, "we're cash rich, time poor generation and people are looking for quick and easy but enjoyable way to take nutrients ... we have to engage them with scientific platform but not by talking about intricacies of satiety ..."

28.5   BRIDGING THE GAP: ADDRESSING THE DILEMMAS

The first consumer dilemma is regarding the nutritional information. This can be addressed through a multiplicity of actions by the marketer:

- Information through packs
  - Consumers look for information on packs and though they may not fully comprehend all that is said, they do find it useful.
  - Nutritional products can also consider adding additional information through booklets along with packs.

- Information through intermediaries
  - Nutritional products cannot underestimate the power of the doctor or the healthcare worker—especially of products which are started after a health incident such as pregnancy or an ailment. Using the doctor as a conduit for nutritional message is both useful and critical.
  - Chemists and healthcare workers can also be an important information provider—not to be ignored in the information loop.

The second consumer dilemma on taste can be addressed through *intensive sampling*. Numerous marketers of nutritional products in India swear by the importance of sampling, be it for ready-to-serve soups, fruit juices, or value-added biscuits (Hindustan Times 2011). Nothing beats the taste hurdle than an intense sampling plan. Aniruddha Narasimhan, category director, health and wellness in the Indian biscuit major Britannia, observes "we see sampling as a route to build new categories and innovations. It helps where there is a barrier to purchase" (Hindustan Times 2011). Shreejit Mishra of Hindustan Unilever concurs saying, "we want to be winner in foods. This category is all about sampling." In fact, the Danone India spokesperson indicated that they expect to devote 30% of the marketing budgets to sampling.

The third hurdle is about *time*, especially in urban metros where the affluent householder is very time starved. The challenge of time is especially key in products that take time for preparation. Here, sampling will help in spreading the word about how difficult or easy the preparation time that is needed. Further mass communication and especially television and audiovisual media will help give a demonstration in front of the consumer. In the last 5 years, the growth of Indian malls has helped brands in demonstrating the ease of preparation in front of customers. Brands such as Act II popcorn and Quaker Oats have attempted to demonstrate the ease of preparation across thousands of locations, in front of potential consumers.

The fourth hurdle is of the *price–value equation*. Here, the dilemma is addressed only if the first three have been sufficiently handled. Trial-size economy packs can help the consumer make an entry into this category and lower the entry barrier. Similarly, larger-sized economy packs can help consumers stay on with the brand. The consumers will be ready to pay the premium if they see value. Often, price is quoted as an excuse because the consumer is not convinced about the value of the new product. The price–value equation is a critical dimension to address in developing markets. Marketers are well advised even while developing brands to keep an eye on the final consumer price and look at ways of value engineering through innovative packaging, manufacturing, and logistics (Figure 28.2).

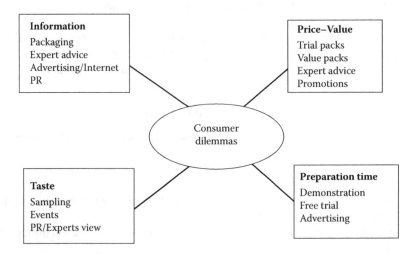

FIGURE 28.2   Addressing consumer dilemmas.

28.6   MARKETING COMMUNICATION: MULTIPLE ROLES TO BE PLAYED

28.6.1   Setting the Context

Innovative nutritional brands have a story to tell to consumers and hence will have to be adhered to as high-involvement products (Parameswaran 2009). In this context, the tone and manner of the communication, be it in the print medium or in the television medium, should stay consistent with the brand. As Mellentin (2009) has indicated, if the brand has to be presented as an "expert," its marketing communication should also sound "expert."

Nutrition is a complicated subject and consumers have only a partial knowledge of what is good for them and what is not so good. Hence, communication needs to be rich in information content but spoken in a consumer-friendly language—not to scare them away but to befriend them.

Though innovative nutritional brands will call for rational messaging, it is necessary to remember that the most persuasive messages have both rationality and emotionality embedded in them.

28.6.2   Role of Doctor Promotion

Innovative nutritional brands should endeavor to befriend the medical community. The success of Nestle in India can be traced to their strong relationships with the medical community (Sangameswaran 2011). It is also important to get the medical practitioners to know the science behind the brand while clearly signaling symptoms that warrant the use of the brand. It is also important to have a doctor on the side of the brand lest the doctor asks the patient to stop using a nutritional aid.

Many nutritional brand marketers tend to ignore the medical route. Enlisting a doctor in the marketing process is worthy of consideration in countries such as India, where a doctor is available for consultation almost within walking distance (especially in the bigger cities). Experienced professionals tell us how easy it is to get the doctor on the same side as the brand.

Literature, detailing aids, and liberal sampling need to be used to work with doctors and nurses on both the rational and emotional level.

The availability of freelance medical detailing forces in countries such as India opens up this avenue for marketers who do not have medical representatives on their rolls.

28.6.3   Role of PR

Consumers, especially the early adopters of innovative nutritional products, are voracious consumers of information. It is therefore important to get the right stories in the media about the product. Brands such as Yakult have used celebrities to get into media in India. Other brands have used nutritionists and even culinary experts. Addressing the PR angle requires appearance in the right places such as in mainline newspapers and magazines. Specially commissioned articles, interviews with nutrition experts, reports of studies conducted, and visits to manufacturing plants or testing sites are ways of making the story news-worthy.

The growth of the television medium and the increase in specialist channels on health, wellness, and food have given a great many opportunities to keep the consumer well informed about the product innovations.

28.6.4   Role of the Internet

Consumers who are innovators and early adopters are also heavy users of the World Wide Web for nutritional information. It is therefore a must for the brand to have a strong presence on the net. The digital presence could have the following dimensions to it:

- Website that provides all the information with a feature to address consumer queries
- Presence in key healthcare websites

- Presence in social media through interactive channels
- Search engine optimization and key work marketing
- Mobile marketing and information sharing through mobile

The use of the digital medium opens up a new cost-effective way to establish a one-to-one dialog with the consumer, by creating forums and enlisting brand evangelists.

Social media monitoring can help brands identify the most influential voices in the net, and help befriend them by providing them with all the information and product samples they may need.

The Internet if used wisely can help a great deal in creating a strong positive word-of-mouth among the early adopter community.

28.6.5   ROLE OF MASS MEDIA ADVERTISING

Innovative nutritional brands have to use mass media with a lot of caution. It is easy to create a television commercial and put a million dollars behind it over a 1 month period, but that may not do the trick, unless all other elements are in place!

The role of print even while using mass media can be significantly different from that of television. Although nothing can come close to the mass reach of television in markets such as India, the impact of television will be many times multiplied if print can play a complimentary role.

It has been observed over the last decade that nutritional brands in India can greatly benefit from an authority support—from either a medical practitioner or a medical association. If the relative lack of knowledge of consumers about nutrition is factored in, the presence of an authority figure plays a huge role in overcoming credibility issues.

Using mass media will also have to be dove-tailed to the geographic and demographic segmentation possibilities. In a vast country such as India, there are opportunities to do a pressure test in one market before making a campaign national. This can help reduce risk and also help fine tune the messages before putting big money behind campaigns.

28.6.6   ROLE OF RETAIL: SHOPPER MARKETING

A number of purchase decisions get made at the final point of purchase. The growth of organized retail in developing markets such as India has given innovative nutritional brands an added opportunity to address the consumers at the final battle ground, the retail counter. Brands have used retail presence to drive trial and increase consumption. Retail can also help brands generate trial, provide free sampling opportunity, and even provide an opportunity to do a one-on-one messaging about the benefits of the brand.

28.6.7   ROLE OF PROMOTIONS

Innovative nutritional products will also have to use several sales promotion methods such as free sampling. Sampling the product could be done through stand-alone sampling at retail outlets or at housing colonies. Another way of sampling could be as an "add-on" product to a fast-moving brand (e.g., probiotic curd along with milk), or along with magazines (e.g., green tea with women's magazine). Brands have used consumer promotions and other engagement methods in addition to sampling to involve the consumer (Choudhury 2001).

If we are to look at the Indian market scenario, over the last two decades, several innovative nutritional brands have been able to gain traction through astute use of marketing. Sundrop, one of the early pioneers of sunflower oil, become a large cooking oil brand (Parameswaran 2001); Tropicana overcame the hurdle of an unsweetened taste by focusing on the taste of good health (Parameswaran and Medh 2011); Complan became a large health beverage expanding the category from just being seen as a milk additive (Mazumdar 2007); Farex created a weaning foods category by targeting mothers and clinicians (Sengupta 1990); and Horlicks went beyond just a beverage to biscuits (Choudhury 2001).

There are several other successful brands in India such as Revital (multivitamin), Saffola (oil and fortified flour), Sunfeast (fortified biscuits), Nestle (low-fat milk and other products), Amul (probiotic ice cream), and so on (Fernandez 2006, Gupta 2009, Jacob 2010, Pinto 2011). However, the market is yet to be fully tapped given the high consumer inertia.

28.7   SUMMARY

Nutrition is a very potent word. At the top end of the demographic pyramid, the concern is about cutting out bad nutrition and providing good nutrition. At the bottom of the pyramid, the challenge is to provide affordable nutrition. No wonder this is a key concern area for CEOs of large companies.

Vinita Bali, MD, Britannia Industries India, observes very astutely "… focus is on our cause of nutrition and malnutrition amongst children. As many as 47% of children in India under the age of five are undernourished." "Similarly at the other end one out of five people in urban India miss breakfast completely every day, while up to 15% have an inadequate one" (Roy and Hecter 2011).

Nitin Paranjpe, MD, Hindustan Unilever India, observes that "the reality is that less than five percent of the foods opportunities has got converted" (Joshi 2011).

Companies such as Nestle India are working on nutrition awareness programs in association with universities such as Punjab Agricultural University (PAU), Ludhiana National Dairy Research Institute, Karnal, Haryana; University of Mysore, Karnataka; and the GB Pant University of Agriculture and Technology, Pantnagar, Uttarkhand (Sangameswaran 2011).

There are tremendous opportunities for brands to offer nutritional solutions to consumers. The opportunities exists at multiple levels, at the top of the pyramid for products such as probiotic ice cream (Amul), at the middle for products such as fortified fruit juices (Real), and at the bottom for enriched products such as biscuits and flour.

The marketer's challenge is to help consumers get through the four dilemmas:

- What will this additional nutrition do for me?
- How will the taste be affected?
- How will the preparation time be affected?
- What is the price–value I can see in this brand?

By using the various elements of the marketing mix, by using various types of marketing communication aids, and most importantly by understanding the consumer behavior dynamics, brands can endeavor to chart new territories and build mega nutritional brands in the future.

ACKNOWLEDGMENT

The author would like to acknowledge the inputs received from colleagues at Draftfcb-Ulka Advertising India and seasoned marketing professionals such as Atul Sinha (Britannia Industries).

REFERENCES

Balasubramanian, S.K. and Cole, C. 2002, Consumer's search and use of nutrition information: The challenge and promise of the nutrition labelling and education act, *Journal of Marketing*, 65, 112–127.
Baltas, G. 2001, The effects of nutrition information on consumer choice, *Journal of Advertising Research*, April–March, 57–63.
Brennan, R., Czarneka, B., Dahl, S., Eagle, L., and Mourouti, O. 2008, Regulation of nutrition and health claims in advertising, *Journal of Advertising Research*, March, pp. 57–70.
Business Standard 2009, Britannia Extends Health Offering, December 31.

Choudhury, P. 2001, *Successful Branding*, Hyderabad: Universities Press, pp. 15–19.

Fernandez, I. 2006, Beverages for 'Health and Wellness' in the Indian Market, *Frost & Sullivan Report*, October 24.

Food Product Development 1978, Consumer Study Unveils Emergence of New Nutrition Concepts, August, pp. 80–82.

Gupta, S.D. 2009, Green to Gold, *Business Standard*, February 21.

Hindustan Times 2011, Surround Sampling, February 21.

Jacob, S. 2010, Training ladies to promote products, *Economic Times*, August 31.

Joshi, P. 2011, On the front foot, *Business Standard*, February 21.

Kotler, P. and Keller, K.L. 2006, *Marketing Management*, 12th edition, New Delhi: Pearson Education.

Lee, M., Choi, Y., Quillan, E.T., and Cole, R.T. 2009, Playing with food: Content analysis of food advergames, *The Journal of Consumer Affairs*, 43(1), 129–154.

Mazumdar, R. 2007, *Product Management in India*, New Delhi: Prentice-Hall, pp. 245–247.

Mellentin, J. 2009, A future for functional foods, *Nutriceutical World*, November, 35–40.

Moore, E.S. and Rideout, V.J. 2007, The online marketing of food to children: Is it just fun and games, *Journal of Public Policy and Marketing*, 26(2), 202–220.

Moorman, C. 1990, The effects of stimulus and consumer characteristics on the utilization of nutrition information, *Journal of Consumer Research*, 17, 362–374.

Parameswaran, M.G. 2001. *FCB-Ulka Brand Building Advertising Concepts & Cases*, New Delhi: Tata McGraw Hill, pp. 25–34.

Parameswaran, M.G. 2009, *Ride The Change—A Perspective in the Changing Indian Consumer Market and Marketing*, New Delhi: Tata McGraw Hill, pp. 25–35.

Parameswaran, M.G. and Medh, K. 2011, *Draftfcb-Ulka Brand Building Advertising, Concepts & Cases Case Book II*, New Delhi: Tata McGraw Hill, pp. 41–48.

Pinto, V.S. 2011, Marico Whets Its Appetite for Foods, *Business Standard*, February 25.

Raterman, K.V. 2008, Vitamins and Minerals: New Wonder Nutrients, *Functional Ingredients*, December, pp. 20–21.

Roy, S. and Hecter, D. 2011, Miss Fixit, *Financial Express*, February 25.

Sangameswaran, P. 2011, Treading the fire line, *Business World*, February 7.

Sengupta, S. 1990, *Brand Positioning—Strategies for Competitive Advantage*, New Delhi, Tata McGraw Hill, New Delhi, pp. 103–106.

29 Financial Implications of Innovations

Girish P. Jakhotiya

CONTENTS

29.1 PREAMBLE

The word "innovation" in a general sense implies a positive probability of "betterment" (AIMA 1996, Peters 1999, Porus 2009). Therefore, the financial implications of innovations are to be viewed and reviewed both strategically and operationally. The "strategic view" refers to the long-term sustainability of the financial (or commercial) viability of an innovation. The "operational view" is about the convenience in the use (and conduct) of innovation and its relevant cost–benefit analysis. The financial implications of innovation are to be systematically viewed considering the entire process of innovation (or its value chain). We should also remember that the financial implications may vary based on the "type of innovation" conducted. For example, the innovation may be by design (i.e., through a well-planned, elaborate process) or by instinct (i.e., by a chance, promoted through an environment that nurtures the practice of attempting innovation) or by adaptation (i.e., imitating and altering an idea marginally to suit one's requirement) or by a trial-and-error method (i.e., right and wrong experimentations conducted with an element of calculated risk). Each type of innovation has its own process or value chain, impact, and the sustenance of such impact. Therefore, the financial implications could be very different.

Predicting the financial implications of innovations attempted and used by "design" is relatively simpler compared with the other types of innovations. A well-planned process of innovation creates a reasonable scope for projecting the investment (i.e., capital expenditure) to be made in such an attempt, its recurring cost and recurring benefit, the incremental capital expenditure to be incurred for "innovating the impact of innovation," and the organizational cost to be incurred to sustain a culture of innovation and institutionalizing it. There could be a difference between projecting the financial implications of an innovation attempted for "commercial purpose" and the innovation carried out for "social benefit." Normally the "earning model" of a socially relevant innovation could be suboptimal or complex because the price charged to the beneficiary could be a very subjective and complex issue. For a commercial innovation, the commercial expectations of both the provider of innovation and the customer of innovation are reasonably predictable. Therefore, a financier would show pragmatic interest in a project driven by commercial and predictable results. Hence, innovation of an "applied" nature is preferred by the funding agencies compared with an innovation which is aimed at long-term or fundamental improvisation. Of course, investors in innovation very often try to balance their "funding portfolio" between these two types as the financial gain from a successful conduct of long-term innovation could be phenomenal.

29.2 INNOVATION PROCESS AND THE FINANCIAL IMPLICATIONS

To understand the financial implications of innovations, we should briefly appreciate the "process of innovation." This appreciation is a must to differentiate the "risk and uncertainty" involved in attempting innovation. Further, if the process is carried out for the benefit of masses or it is conducted for improvising a product of "perfect competition" (under which the pricing is a very sensitive issue), then the financial implications could be based more on market uncertainty or on sociopolitical uncertainty. For example, funding a research project on organic or inorganic processes of cultivation in countries such as India or China would be very sociopolitically sensitive. The outcome of such a project shall be viewed as "social goods" and not so much as a commercially saleable product. On the other hand, a research on food habits and improvising the life cycle impact of food intake in an advanced country such as the United States could be relatively less sensitive on the sociopolitical parameters but it could be very complex in a perfect market condition on the parameter of its commercial sustainability.

The process of innovation (not from the laboratory point of view but from the market and financing view point) may be defined as follows (Jakhotiya, 2000):

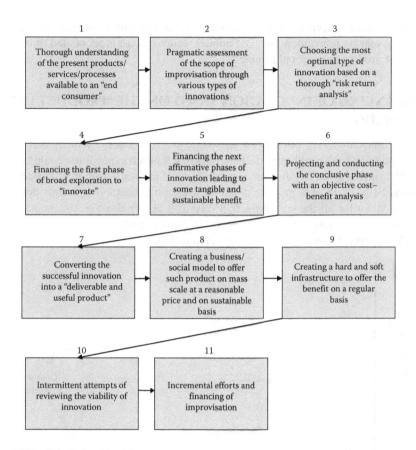

1	2	3
Thorough understanding of the present products/services/processes available to an "end consumer"	Pragmatic assessment of the scope of improvisation through various types of innovations	Choosing the most optimal type of innovation based on a thorough "risk return analysis"

4	5	6
Financing the first phase of broad exploration to "innovate"	Financing the next affirmative phases of innovation leading to some tangible and sustainable benefit	Projecting and conducting the conclusive phase with an objective cost–benefit analysis

7	8	9
Converting the successful innovation into a "deliverable and useful product"	Creating a business/social model to offer such product on mass scale at a reasonable price and on sustainable basis	Creating a hard and soft infrastructure to offer the benefit on a regular basis

10	11
Intermittent attempts of reviewing the viability of innovation	Incremental efforts and financing of improvisation

The above "generic" explanation of the entire value chain of innovation should facilitate our easy understanding of the financial implications of innovations. The "Risk–Uncertainty Assessment" and its resulting interpretation for a funding agency may be broadly presented as follows (using the above genetic explanation of the process of innovation):

Phase of the Innovation Process	1	2 and 3	4	5	6	7–11
Risk or uncertainty	Uncertainty	Not applicable	Uncertainty	Risk	Low risk	Low risk
Funding preference	Venture finance	Not applicable	Venture finance	Participative finance	Equity finance	Equity plus debt finance
Cost of funding	Very high	Not applicable	High	Moderate	Variable	Fixed plus variable

We shall discuss the "funding options" with different business and earning models in the later part of this chapter. "Innovation through adaptation" is a practical reality of today. Even genetically modified seeds, food grains, vegetables, and fruits are subjected to the "test of adaptation." Financial implications of this "very low risk adaptation" are reasonably practicable. As stated earlier, the earning model of these projects of adaptation could not be so "deterministic" as the "adapted versions" are difficult to price. Hence financing the actual execution of "innovation based on adaptation" depends more on the "original innovation" and its cost–benefit analysis.

Innovation through the trial-and-error method is always subjected to a policy framework of defining "acceptable risk" and therefore to "available funding budget." Ironically, small doses of "operational innovation" go through the routine method of trial and error and they are routinely funded through small capital budgets. A trial-and-error approach to innovation becomes the culture of the organization. Such an innovation is not limited to a single function or product. Therefore, quite a few world-class corporations devotionally spend a certain percentage of their gross or net revenue every year on innovation. Such an annual recurring cost is accounted through the normal mechanism of product costing and pricing.

29.3 FINANCING OF INNOVATION BASED ON THE "PRODUCT LIFE CYCLE" CONCEPT

Spending on innovation very often is not decided entrepreneurially by many corporations worldwide. A scientific and reasonable approach at providing for such expenditure could be the "life cycle concept." The entire capital funding and recurring cost of innovation are to be spread over a reasonably predicted life cycle of a product. Such an accounting method and cash flow management become convenient for all the stakeholders involved. It also makes the "financing of innovation" viable and hence acceptable to the shareholders (Jakhotiya, 2000).

A broad "life cycle financing" may be presented as follows:

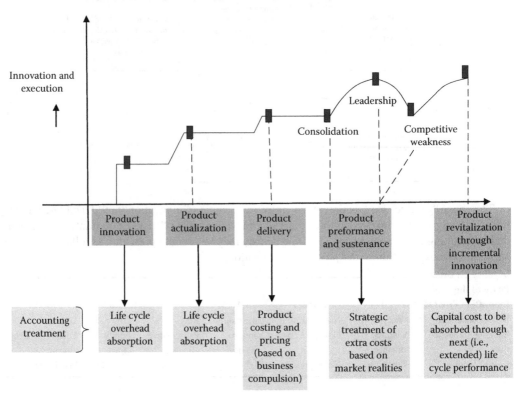

Innovators should present their "projected efforts" with clarity on the life cycle to the financiers. This would make it easy for the financiers to take appropriate decisions. The life cycle approach also facilitates the designing of various financial and operational models along with the "fiscal management", if the innovation is to be supported by the government. The fiscal side of funding the innovation is very critical as it seriously impacts on the costing and pricing of the "innovated" product.

29.4 STRATEGIC FINANCIAL IMPLICATIONS OF INNOVATIONS

It is well known that for a business enterprise, an organization or even the economy of a country to survive and grow, constant innovation is required. Hence, the financial implications of innovations should be viewed strategically. Following are the strategic dimensions (Jakhotiya, 2010):

1. Competitive advantage of a country or corporation depends on perpetual innovations. They offer newer competitive advantages and therefore, any cost incurred on them should be treated as an investment rather than expenditure.

2. Innovations create greater scope for better use of public resources. A nation's natural resources can be used more productively if the "process of use & purpose of use" are constantly innovated.

3. Investment in innovations creates strong intangible assets for a business enterprise. Such intangibles strengthen the balance sheet and increase the financial strength in a competitive market. An organization that nurtures innovation as a culture always enjoys greater bargaining power while working on joint ventures and partnerships.

4. Financing agencies should expect a long-term return on investment (ROI) from the workable life cycle of an innovation. Such an ROI could be suitably extrapolated to suit the innovator and the financier. Financing agencies should view investment in innovations as a strategic or a very long-term benefit. They may also combine short-term or applied innovation with long-term or fundamental innovation to mitigate the risk of their investment portfolio.

5. The fundamental implications of innovations also include matching of cash flows, tax concessions, business performance (in the case of commercial innovations), subsidization (in the case of social innovations), royalties based on the ownership of patents, and other commercial and legal compliances. Interestingly, these implications may vary from country to country depending on the economic models followed and the purchasing power of the "end users."

6. Innovations in the basic sectors such as food, health care, medical tourism, and food tourism should offer considerable bargaining power to a country. In a global economy, a participating country can explore and exploit "economic advantage" if it offers innovative products to the global customers. Hence, financing the innovations in the basic sectors should be treated as national investment. A country should impress the global financiers with its sovereign guarantee of innovations. This would require a good amount of "financial engineering" for designing suitable financial models.

29.5 LONG-TERM RETURN ON INVESTMENT FOR THE FINANCIERS OF INNOVATIONS

As stated earlier, the inventor and the financier will have to create a win–win situation for each other. This would depend on a reasonable long-term ROI which should be acceptable to both the parties. This ROI should be adjusted for all the possible risks associated with every phase of the process of innovation. An adjusted ROI may be computed keeping in mind the "time value of money." An illustration of such an ROI may be presented as follows:

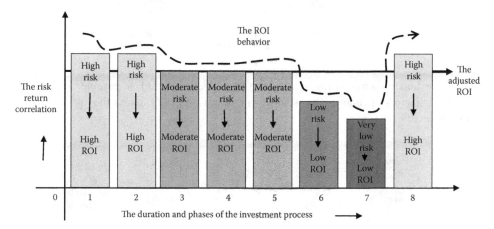

The adjusted ROI shall depend on a fine combination of the interdependent variables such as amount of funding, duration of funding, risk involved, and cost of capital incurred by the financier. Each variable will have its due weightage depending on the type of innovation. As stated earlier, a lower rate of ROI could be fixed if a government (or the innovating organization) offers absolute security of financier's funds, liquidity, timely and adequate payment of returns, and so on. Of course, the universal truth of "high risk—high return" is also applicable here. The financier may also be offered a "combined ROI" for financing a combination of innovation projects. Here, a low-risk project should compensate for a high-risk project. This should also promote a captive relationship between the innovator and the financier (Jakhotiya and Jakhotiya, 2010).

Another pragmatic adjustment in the ROI fixation may be based on a realistic combination of variable and fixed portions of the ROI. The financier may be offered an assured minimum rate of ROI and an extra incentive (i.e., extra ROI) based on the success of the innovation project. The success of the innovation project will have to be carefully defined by a few suitable parameters with their respective weightages. This "dual" arrangement may be illustrated as follows:

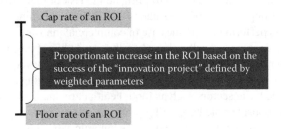

The financier may decide about the expected ROI considering the four dimensions (or value deciders) of an innovation as follows:

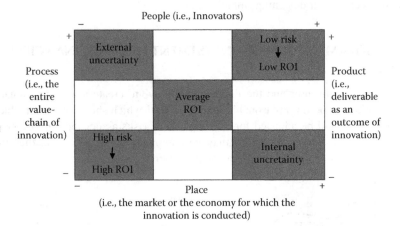

The above four dimensions together decide "the price expected or payable" by the end-user. Hence, the financiers of innovations would (very often) ruthlessly assess the "price payable" and target for their ROI:

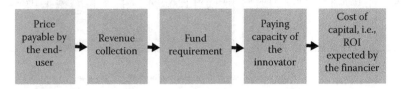

In the case of socially-relevant innovations in the field of food and health care, the financiers may club their "low ROI expectation" with other benefits from the participating government. For example, if a financing agency is invited to finance two projects—one based on innovation and the other a routine one, then the agency would expect tangible and intangible benefits from the routine project. This is mainly to create a situation of cross subsidization.

29.6 FINANCING MODELS OF INNOVATIONS

The financing models of innovations are mainly defined by either the purpose or period or process of innovation. Innovation of genetically modified food grains or basic methods of medication should offer "perpetual benefits to masses." Hence, the financing model here should depend on the "perpetuity concept." In a few cases, the end beneficiaries may like to participate in the financing agreement. A long-drawn innovation project may require "consortium funding" or "take away" concept of funding. Very focused innovation projects may be funded through the concept of "structured finance." A few financiers may prefer to fund the innovations taking unlimited risks for unlimited returns. So there are various permutations and combinations of the financing of innovations suited to the innovators and the financiers (from presentations done by Dr. Girish Jakhotiya to clients). A few the important features are discussed here.

29.6.1 EQUITY MODEL

The financier prefers to invest in the project as a "co-owner," by equally sharing the risk and returns associated with the projects. Normally a financier would look at a project that should offer long-term and sustainable returns for investing funds through the "equity" route. Some financiers opt for this approach as they would want to monitor the process of innovation. Some also finance through this route to co-own the "intellectual property rights" emerging out of such innovation. Innovation projects carried out with a "Public Private Partnership" (PPP) are mostly funded through this model. The government and the private enterprise are equal "equity partners" in a PPP.

29.6.2 TAKEAWAY FINANCE MODEL

This model is most suitable for those financiers who want to participate in a specific phase of the long-drawn value chain of the innovation project with a specific combination of risk return. For example, an ambitious venture financier may be ready for the first phase of "primary exploration" of innovation. This phase is full of uncertainty. A venturer would park his fund at this phase for a very high rate of return. After the project is reasonably successful, the venture financier may withdraw his funds and he is replaced by regular financiers. The regular financiers are satisfied with a moderate rate of return as they are ready to take moderate risk. Once the "innovation phases" are completed and the innovation is now executed through "deliverable products," the financiers of the "moderate risk phase" also may be partially or fully replaced by ordinary investors. These ordinary investors are averse to any risk and therefore invest in the tangible, determined results with lower expectation on the rate of returns. Normally, these are small investors who are interested in innovation funding bonds which offer them risk-free rate of returns.

The "take way" financing is the journey of the financiers from one milestone of innovation to the other. Each financier enters and exits the project based on his appetite for risk and return. The challenge here is about "timely and adequate" replacement of a financier which should guarantee a smooth flow of funding.

29.6.3 CONSORTIUM MODEL

Different financing agencies come together and form a consortium to fund a mega innovation project. The members in the consortium participate in the entire project with different intentions, for example, a banker may participate to fulfil his obligation of "priority sector lending," a microfinance agency may participate to support the innovation and own it in the interest of thousands of unwary beneficiaries, while another banker may participate just because additional liquid funds are available and is satisfied with a moderate rate of returns.

A serious consortium of financiers may choose a suitable innovation project very carefully and its members would bring in funds proportionately based on their investment needs. They may jointly decide on an average rate of return on their total investment based on their individual rates of cost of capital. A simple example may be given as follows:

Member of the Consortium	% Contribution in Funding the Innovation (A)	Factor of Risk Perceived (B)	Member's Own Cost of Sourcing Funds (%) (C)	Risk Weighted ROI Expected from the Project (%) (C × B)	Absolute Amount of Return Expected from the Project [A × (C × B)]
A	20	1.2	7	8.4	1.68
B	25	1.0	9	9.0	2.25
C	30	1.3	8	10.4	3.12
D	25	1.1	9	9.9	2.48
Total	100				9.53

The average rate of return thus should be 9.53% (i.e., 9.53 on 100). The "risk factor" used in this illustration is a combined expression of various risks perceived by a financier.

29.6.4 STRUCTURED FINANCE MODEL

The innovator and the financier come together and structure a financing deal based on their requirements. While doing so, they try to match the mutual needs of cash flows (i.e., liquidity), paying capacity (i.e., profitability), fiscal factors (i.e., tax planning, subsidy claims, etc.), portfolio need (i.e., financier's investment mix), leveraging (i.e., strength of the innovating organization), and so on. The model may be presented as follows:

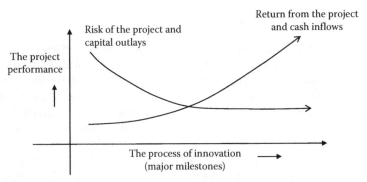

29.6.5 PUBLIC FINANCE MODEL

Innovation leading to the successful making of "public goods" may be funded by the public through "Innovation Bonds." A government may raise funds from public institutions (like Pension & Provident Funds) and the public who have a fair interest in the proposed innovation. Such "public finance" may flow through different types of voluntary and compulsory methods:

1. People at large may be compelled to pay an "innovation cess" over and above their normal tax liability.
2. Public may be issued "small size bonds" with a long-term maturity (the maturity period may be equated with the "positive returns duration" of an innovation project).

3. Those who would specifically benefit from the end results of the innovation project may pay their "beneficiary fees" in advance. This should recover a major portion of the capital outlay in the initial phase of the project.
4. The beneficiaries may be classified between the rich and the poor. The rich should pay for the poor through a higher rate of beneficiary fees.

29.6.6 REUSE FINANCE MODEL

Innovations for social benefit, carried out by the rich countries, may be offered to the poor countries at a considerably subsidized price. Having exploited maximum benefits and recovered majority portion of their capital outlay, the rich countries should offer their innovations to the poor countries at an appropriate price acceptable to both. Thus, the "Re-Use Finance Model" may be participated by a group of poor countries so that the cost is shared. The model may be alternatively used by the poor countries without offering any cash flows. They may facilitate the future projects on innovation to be conducted by the rich countries by offering them natural infrastructure. Of course, a suitable "valuation model" has to be evolved to decide an exchange ratio between the rich country's innovations and the poor country's environmental support.

29.6.7 ENTREPRENEURIAL FINANCE MODEL

The participants in an innovation project (i.e., the vendors, the employees, the bankers, the regulators, the innovators, etc.) may act as stakeholders and finance the project with an entrepreneurial interest. The employees and the innovators may finance their "equity participation" in this model through subsidized borrowings. A progressive government too can arrange such funds at lower rate of interest. As the entrepreneurs are also the "end beneficiaries," they would use the funds more carefully.

This model could be extended to the innovation on public goods and services also. In a few progressive countries, farmer associations and cooperative societies participate in agricultural innovations collectively. Likewise, the distributors and retailers of a pharmaceutical corporation may participate in their principal's innovation projects. The teachers in a school or college may also be the stakeholders of an innovation project.

The challenge in this model is of defining the ownership of "intellectual property rights." "Collective ownership of patents" should be the acceptable solution here.

29.6.8 PAY-PER-USE MODEL

This is a well-tested financing model which recovers the entire cost of innovation from the beneficiaries over a longer period of time. The initial investment may be made through PPP by various financiers. Here, the government is a major shareholder. The future cash flows of revenue generated are hypothecated to the present financiers. Such a hypothecation may be done through securitization of the future receivables. The institutional and individual users of the innovation should pay at "differential rates." The "pay-per-use" may also depend on the commercial or social use of the innovation. In quite a few progressive countries, the royalty payable for the use of pharmaceutical patents (both process and product) is decided differently for different end-users. A dual-royalty system is used for cross subsidization.

29.6.9 SPECIAL PURPOSE VEHICLE MODEL

A few organizations such as corporations and research agencies may come together and form a special purpose vehicle (SPV) to carry out projects on innovations. They would contribute funds to the SPV in a certain ratio. The partners of the SPV reap the benefit of a successful innovation over a period of time and own the patent jointly in the name of the SPV. Some countries also may form an SPV to conduct innovations in the field of food and medical care. The SPV mostly functions as an "Innovation Centre." It should have its own separate balance sheet and income statement. Any failure in the projects should be restricted to this balance sheet so that the balance sheets of the partnering corporations are not affected. Such isolation would encourage increasing number of organizations to participate in innovation projects. The SPV may also recover its cost by renting out its successful innovations to other customers for a certain reasonable amount of royalty.

29.6.10   INNOVATION FUND MODEL

A few corporations (or countries) may create an innovation fund by contributing to it regularly. Such contribution may be a certain percentage of their "gross revenue." The fund may sponsor innovation projects at universities and research institutions. The teachers and researchers may be given pragmatic targets for innovations of "applied nature." They may be encouraged through special incentives constituted by the innovation fund. In some cases, the researchers and the innovation fund may jointly own the intellectual property rights of the project.

A large organization may build its own internal innovation fund which would promote small- and medium-sized innovation projects undertaken in its various departments and business divisions. Such an organization may source "low-cost funds" from international financial institutions through a mutually beneficial contract.

29.6.11   COOPERATIVE FUND MODEL

A business organization may conduct innovations in the field of agriculture and textiles by inviting the farmers and small textile manufacturers. Here, the organizational structure shall be based on the principle of cooperation. This should avoid the dominance of one single partner who may contribute major portion of the finances required.

In this model, the farmers may contribute to the innovations project operationally by conducting the trial runs on their agricultural land. Thus, they would also be practically exposed to the process of innovation. With this concept, a federation or chamber or association of small and medium business enterprises may finance innovations projects perpetually through the "Cooperative Model" by involving its members. A bigger "Cooperative Federation" of the farmers' association and big "fast moving consumer good" (FMCG) corporations should be able to finance bigger innovation projects leading to fundamental research and long-term advantages. Here again, the principle of cooperation would avoid the dominance of one single partner.

29.6.12   CONVERTIBLE BOND MODEL

Small investors (i.e., the public) may invest in "innovation projects" of a corporation by subscribing to its special bonds. The initial rate of return on this bond would be "interest payable at a lower rate." Once the innovation project gets completed successfully, the same bond may be converted into "equity" (i.e., an equity share) of the corporation. This convertible bond should be an attractive investment proposition for a small investor who looks forward to sharing the fruits of innovation in the long run with an assured rate of return in the short run. This arrangement may be presented as follows:

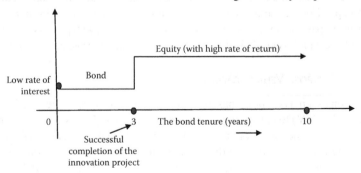

29.6.13 SEED FINANCING MODEL

Quite a few universities and research institutions conduct primary levels of innovation with reasonable success. They do not continue further for want of resources. The financing agencies or bigger corporations may scout for such "seed innovations" and acquire them after reasonable assessment. The challenge here is with regard to the valuation of such seed innovation. Instead of a onetime valuation and reward, the seed innovator and the acquirer may enter into a long-term agreement of "revenue sharing" and "joint ownership of intellectual property rights."

The seed (or incomplete but promising) innovations are found plenty in the sectors of agriculture, horticulture, basic medicine, basic livelihood or infrastructure, basic logistics, and so on. A suitable administrative structure may be evolved to search, select, and support such "seed innovations" financially. A few seed innovators too can come together and form a cooperative society for collective financing and process management.

29.7 MONITORING MECHANISM OF THE FINANCING OF INNOVATIONS

Both the innovator and the financier need to monitor the use of funds being apportioned to an innovation project carefully. This monitoring mechanism would require minute detailing of the major phases of the innovation process. Such detailing should facilitate the preparation of performance (or activity) budget and financial budget of the project. Activity-wise targets should at least be approximately defined. The budget should define a few "warning signals" also. These should alert the innovator about any wasteful use of funds. The mechanism should also spell out a pragmatic deadline for the completion of the project. A reasonable cutoff point should be defined as to when the innovator should abandon or alter the project. If the financiers are assured of the productive and proper use of their funds, they may overlook genuine failures.

The monitoring mechanism of the financing of innovations may slightly vary from one financing model to the other. A broad common structure may be suggested as follows:

ABC Innovation Project

Name of the project: _____

Primary purpose of the project: _____

Secondary purposes of the project: _____

Approximate duration: _____

Expected approximate outcome: _____

Financing model: _____

Target sheet: _____

Sr. No.	Phase-Wise Monitoring Parameters*	Targets (a)				Actual (b)			Variances (a − b)			Reasons and Remedial Actions
		Result	Time	Cost		Result	Time	Cost	Result	Time	Cost	
				Capital	Revenue							

* The monitoring parameters shall be mostly of technical nature. These are to be defined by the innovators. The financier should study and approve these parameters and respective targeted values.

The above target sheet should be supported by the following Cash flow statement (to be approved by the financier):

Type of Cash Flow*	Phases of the Innovation Project										Total
	1	2	3	4	5	6	7	8	9	10	
Capital Revenue											
Total											

* Capital cash flow is supposed to be spent on the long-term assets such as premises, machines, equipments, vehicles, furniture etc. required to conduct the innovations. Revenue cash flows are to be spent on routine expenses such as salaries, consumables, energy, and other overheads.

29.8 ACCOUNTING TREATMENT OF THE COST OF INNOVATIONS

The International Accounting Standards (IAS) are reasonably applicable to all types of costs of innovations carried out in various sectors. Yet, there could be an amount of subjectivity in the accounting treatment based on the purpose of innovation, longevity of the innovation process, its benefits, and the financing model. A few major accounting treatments may be described as follows.

29.8.1 CAPITALIZATION OF THE COST OF INNOVATION

A successful innovation becomes an "intangible asset" (e.g., patent, copyright, etc.). Therefore, the entire cost incurred on such successful project is normally "accumulated" in the name of the intangible assets and shown in the balance sheet. Further accounting treatment is as per the accounting standard on "intangible assets."

29.8.2 AMORTIZATION OF THE ACCUMULATED COST OF UNSUCCESSFUL INNOVATION

Such accumulated cost may be amortized over a period of few years depending on the capacity of the innovator to amortize it every year. Normally, the amortization is done without burdening the annual income statement too much.

29.8.3 ANNUAL (OR ROUTINE) ACCOUNTING OR ABSORPTION OF THE RECURRING (OR STANDARD) COSTS OF ONGOING EFFORTS OF INNOVATION

In an organization where "innovation" is a culture and a certain percentage of gross revenue is provided to conduct innovations, the annual expenses are charged to the respective year's income statement.

29.8.4 SETOFF AGAINST THE INNOVATION FUND

All annual expenses of innovations may be set off against a specially created innovation fund. Such an arrangement does not affect the organization's annual income statement.

29.9 CONCLUSION

Financial implications of innovations should be systematically addressed so that they do not adversely impact on the very purpose and process of innovation. Financial implications can be reasonably projected to the advantage of both—the innovator and the financier. Different types of innovations and their respective beneficiaries would decide the choice of suitable financing models. Financial implications are to be monitored carefully for the ultimate success of an innovation project. Any innovation, social or commercial, should be financially viable so that the final price charged to the end user is appropriate. Precious public resources can be effectively used for socially useful innovations if financial discipline is observed.

REFERENCES

Jakhotiya, G. 2000. *Strategic Financial Management* (3rd enlarged & revised edition), Vikas Publishing House, New Delhi, India.

Jakhotiya, G. 2010. *Aggregate Growth through Networking & Innovation, a Management Model.* Patent pending under Indian Patents Act.

Jakhotiya, G. and Jakhotiya, M. 2010. *Finance Made Simple.* Jakhotiya & Associates, Mumbai, India. All India Management Association (AIMA), 1996. *Innovation—Strategy for Corporate Renaissance.* Excel Books, New Delhi, India.

Peters, T. 1999. *The Circle of Innovation.* Vintage Books, New York, USA.

Porus, M. 2009. *Making Breakthrough Innovation Happen.* IBD, India.

30 Market-Focused Innovation in Food and Nutrition

R.B. Smarta

CONTENTS

30.1 INTRODUCTION

Adam and Eve did not have to worry too much about food. According to the Bible (Genesis 2:9), the Garden of Eden freely contained "every tree that is pleasant to the sight, and good for food." Then, because Eve tasted the apple, the ground was cursed so that it would yield food only with hard labor.

Ever since, the search for food has dominated our existence. But what is food and why is it so necessary for human existence?

In addition to enjoying food because it tastes good, human beings require food for three purposes:

1. *Energy:* Food is the fuel (calories) that is required to perform external work and to simply allow the heart, lungs, and all other organs to function.
2. *Building blocks:* Food contains raw materials (e.g., vitamins, enzymes, and some minerals) that the body needs to produce blood, skin, bones, hair, and internal organs. The human body is constantly replacing and renewing every cell on a daily to monthly basis.
3. *Catalysts:* Chemical compounds (e.g., vitamins, enzymes, and some minerals) are necessary to facilitate the chemical reactions that convert food into energy.

30.2   EVOLVING UNDERSTANDING OF FOOD

The human body is rather specialized (as organisms go) in its dietary needs. A plant can survive on just carbon dioxide, water, and certain inorganic ions. Some microorganisms likewise get along without any organic food; they are called "autotrophic" (self-growing), which means that they can grow in environments that contain no other living thing. The bread mold *Neurospora* begins to get a little more complicated: in addition to inorganic substances, it needs to have sugar and the vitamin biotin. As forms of life increase in complexity, they seem to become more dependent on their diet in order to obtain the organic building blocks necessary for building living tissue. The reason for this increasing dependence on diet is simply that they have lost some of the enzymes that primitive organisms possess.

A plant has a complete supply of enzymes required for making all the necessary amino acids, proteins, fats, and carbohydrates from inorganic materials. *Neurospora* has all the enzymes except for one or more of those needed to make sugar and biotin. By the time we get to human beings, we find that they lack the enzymes required to make many of the amino acids, vitamins, and various other necessities, and thus human beings must obtain these ready-made through food.

In the 1930s, the American nutritionist William C. Rose discovered the essential amino acid threonine. In the 1940s, Rose turned his attention to man's requirement for amino acids. He persuaded graduate students to submit to controlled diets in which a mixture of amino acids was the only source of nitrogen. In 1948, he announced that the adult male required only eight amino acids in the diet: phenylalanine, leucine, isoleucine, methionine, valine, lysine, tryptophan, and threonine. Since arginine and histidine, which are indispensable to the rat, are dispensable in the human diet, it would seem that in this respect man is less specialized than the rat or indeed any other mammal that has been tested in detail.

It was the English physician William Prout (the same Prout who was a century ahead of his time in suggesting that all elements were built from hydrogen) who first suggested that organic foods could be divided into three types of substances, later named as carbohydrates, fats, and proteins. The chemists and biologists of the nineteenth century, notably Justus von Liebig of Germany, gradually worked out the nutritive properties of these foods.

The Food and Nutrition Board of the National Research Council in its 1953 chart of recommendations suggested that the minimum requirement for adults is 1 g of protein per kg of body weight per day, which amounts to a little more than two ounces for the average grown man.

Human beings require food for energy every few hours and specific foods that function as building blocks and catalysts on a daily or semidaily basis. Our bodies are biologically programmed to immediately sense when energy is needed—we experience hunger pangs, a signal that the body needs food. Unfortunately, we usually become aware of missing building blocks or catalysts only when we become ill from nutrient deficiencies. Our bodies are also biologically programmed to seek out foods containing the highest amounts of energy; it is for this reason that foods containing sugar and fat, which are high in calorific value, taste the best. This has led to the creation of a successful platform for food businesses; in fact, successful exploitation of our biological programming by entrepreneurs and commercial providers of food is the major cause of obesity and ill health in the developed world today.

With regard to diet, there are three major problems worldwide today:

1. We eat too much.
2. Most people are not getting the minimum amounts of building blocks and/or catalysts that our bodies need.
3. Some sections of the population do not have food to eat.

The availability and type of food consumed, the cooking technique adopted, the lifestyle of the people, and dietary habits have all created challenges related to nutrition.

30.3   NUTRITION TRANSITION

All over the world, traditional cooking has undergone enormous changes.

The increasing pace of life, extensive use of technology, and the availability of a wide array of packaged, readymade foods have changed basic food habits, which were mainly dependent on crops and the seasons.

As a result of this transition in lifestyle, people have become conscious about health, but on the other hand have made a transition in their food habits, timing, and nutrition content! This phenomenon is referred to as nutrition transition (NT). The major implications of NT can be observed in a majority of people through obesity, an imbalance in nutrition which leads to many diseases.

The writing is on the wall regarding the unhealthy shifts in food consumption, and this situation needs to be checked and reversed immediately. Awareness and education need to be used extensively to counter the proliferation of NT, which has only led to degenerative and lifestyle diseases. The most susceptible people are those from the lower and middle classes in less affluent countries. Their regular intake of cheap, energy-intense, and nutrient-deficient food has led to a paradoxical situation of undernutrition (low on micronutrients and fiber) and overnutrition (high on salt, sugar, fats, etc.). This simultaneous double burden of under- and overnutrition has led to an epidemic of obesity and adult-onset diabetes. Healthcare costs to assuage the situation are steep and hence serious steps need to be taken to prevent the problem from snowballing any further.

30.4   CHANGE IN PERCEPTION OF CUSTOMERS

A major section of the world population suffers from nutritional imbalances, which indirectly affect the country's growth. Because of lifestyle changes and changing eating patterns, people today are not able to balance the recommended dietary allowance for various nutrients.

Generally, consumers consider traditional foods such as rice, wheat, bread, vegetables, and eggs to be safe. With an increase in awareness along with increased malnutrition (undernutrition as well as overnutrition), consumers have wisely started correlating nutrients to specific disease conditions. This increasing awareness has led to the emergence of a new industry of nutrient-specific products either mixed in food (functional foods) or in the form of a tablet/pill (supplements) to treat a particular disease.

In addition, consumers have started realizing the side effects of Western medicine, and their mindset has shifted from curative to corrective and preventive therapy. Consumers are thus developing a holistic approach to health, and food, diet, and nutrition have become the center of attraction for all stakeholders.

Consumers have also started focusing on the ingredients in food products as a solution to correct or prevent the unhealthy situation related to diet. It is predicted that by 2015, most mega-cities in the developing world will shift from a disease-centric to a prevention-centric medical model.

30.5   SHIFT TO INTEGRATED (HOLISTIC) MEDICINES FOR BETTER HEALTH

Integrated medicine is a new paradigm in health care that focuses on the "healthy individual," a synergy and deployment of the best aspects of diverse systems of medicine including modern medicine, Ayurveda, Homeopathy, Siddha, Unani, Yoga, and Naturopathy in the best interest of the patients and the community.

The increasing public demand for traditional medicines has led to considerable interest among policy-makers, health administrators, and medical doctors regarding the possibilities of bringing together traditional and modern medicine. Traditional medicine looks at health, disease, and causes of diseases in a different manner. The integration of traditional medicine with modern medicine may imply the incorporation of traditional medicine into the general health service system.

Surveys and other sources of evidence indicate that traditional medical practices are frequently utilized in the management of chronic diseases. Traditional medicine presents a low-cost alternative for rural and semiurban areas where modern medicine is inaccessible. An approach to harmonizing activities of modern and traditional medicine will promote a clearer understanding of the strengths and weaknesses of each and will encourage the provision of the best therapeutic option for patients.

30.6   NEW FOOD DEVELOPMENT

Owing to renewed focus on diet, which has changed due to NT, and the thrust on prevention of illness through the intake of the right food, new food development and innovation in food have become integral issues for society. This represents new opportunities for both science and business!

Food, whether natural or processed, has a great impact on our body. Processed foods have been altered from their natural state for reasons related to safety and convenience. We tend to think of such modified foods as bad, but it turns out that many processed foods are not unhealthy.

So, here we are with the marketers on one side and the customers on the other. Keen on developing new markets and introducing new products, marketers are employing a multitude of services and ideas to keep pushing their products and presence in the market. With technology and globalization working full time, the competition is extreme and the law of diminishing returns is repeatedly setting in and wasting critical resources. Expensive services and inputs are being pumped in, but the market, though burgeoning, is not exactly galloping.

30.7   NUTRITION INNOVATION-LED ECONOMY

In today's era of NT (i.e., increased consumption of unhealthy foods and increased prevalence of overweight in middle-to-low-income countries), changing perceptions and preferences of customers, and a shift toward integrated (holistic) medicines and a willingness to embrace a wide choice of foods to remain healthy, it has become very crucial to craft a customer value proposition focused on making people healthy.

There is a great historical irony at the heart of the current transformation in the choices of dietary preferences. The industry is being reshaped by technology in many ways, and is returning to the more vibrant, freewheeling ways of dealing with ailments. Until the early twentieth century, there was no technology in place for disseminating knowledge to a large number of people in a short span of time. Today, the world has shrunk owing to the leapfrogging development in technology in an array of disciplines. The Internet, which has been hailed as the innovation of the generation, has played a pivotal role in augmenting the world economy. It is an enabler with enormous power as it ensures that manufacturers are in constant proximity with the numerous suppliers and customers. Propelled by the proliferation of a multitude of technologies, the world is burgeoning with opportunity. However, many of the developed European countries and the United States have been mired in recession and are slowly emerging into a phase of growth. This is resulting in spiraling dominance of the Chinese and Indian economies, which have notched very impressive growth rates despite the economic gloom and turbulence around.

The heterogeneity of the global economy calls for a broader definition of innovation—one that distinguishes between "new to the world" innovation (creation and commercialization), "new to the market" knowledge (diffusion and absorption), and "explicit promotion of innovation to reduce poverty" (inclusive innovation). Thus, innovation should not be thought of as simply shifting focus toward the global technological frontier, but rather as improving practices across the entire economy. Thus, innovative activities would not be restricted to new products, but would also include innovations in processes and organizational or business models.

Creating the right environment for innovation would include drafting policies and setting up institutions and capabilities that support the creation and commercialization of new knowledge and the diffusion and absorption of existing knowledge, for both the formal and the informal sectors of the economy.

30.8 INSIDE-OUT APPROACH OF INNOVATION

The conventional approach of research and development (R&D) to markets involves discovery to development to availability of new food.

Companies typically see new product development as the first stage in generating and commercializing new products within the overall strategic process of the product life cycle. The approach involves idea generation, screening, business analysis, and then taking it to the markets.

Creation is inventive activity, often the result of formal R&D conducted by scientists and engineers. The key institutions involved in formal knowledge creation are public R&D laboratories, universities, private R&D centers, and enterprises. But not all knowledge creation is the result of formal R&D. It is often market- or application-based, driven by the innovator's understanding of what consumers want. Sometimes the invention comes from experiences with production or from informal trial and error. Sometimes it comes from serendipitous insight. Its origin raises a measurement problem because not all R&D results in inventions and not all inventions come from formal R&D.

Typically, two phases follow the transformation of a basic idea into an initial proposal format: proof of concept or initial prototyping and pilot demonstration. For some products (such as software), the first or "alpha" prototype is developed at a business customer location that agrees to be an alpha site because of the perceived value in being involved in testing rather than waiting to buy the product on the market. During this phase, the technical merit and commercial feasibility of the new idea or technology are explored. It is often at this phase that early-stage technology development (ESTD) grants and incubators are most helpful. Although there is no consensus on the definition of ESTD, it can be broadly defined as the stage at which "technology is reduced to industrial practice, when a production process is defined from which costs can be estimated and a market appropriate to the demonstrated performance specifications is identified and quantified" (Dutz 2007, p. 183) (Auerswald and Branscomb 2003). With proof of concept in hand, pilots are demonstrated and tested, with the development of second or "beta" versions of the prototype that allow early adopters to work out bugs and evaluate the commercialization potential of the idea. It is often at this second or pilot phase that seed and early-stage venture capital may start to become interested. After tweaks in the beta phase, the innovation is ready to reach the market.

30.9 OUTSIDE-IN APPROACH OF INNOVATION

The outside-in approach of innovation has a future-driven context that focuses on customer evolution, and the major drivers of innovation are lifestyles and trends and needs of customers (Figure 30.1).

The new approach of *Test → build capabilities → launch* to innovation would be the key to leverage market leadership and first mover's advantage; this approach involves first analyzing market trends and needs and then building competencies and capabilities to satisfy stakeholders' needs through the innovation platform.

30.10 OUTSIDE-IN PLATFORM

To create an innovation platform, it is essential to look at trends and to look at the gaps and work out what needs to be done to fill those gaps. The forces responsible for these trends include demographics, psychographics, and environmental changes.

To understand the way ahead, we need to scrutinize the marketing process.

Possibly the biggest failing of many companies is the unilateral decision and procedure they follow in trying to successfully place products in the market. Brainstorming sessions and rudimentary market research are carried out and product ideas are discussed. Democratic consensus may lead to a shortlisting and a further narrowing of a path of pursuit. A product may be conceived on

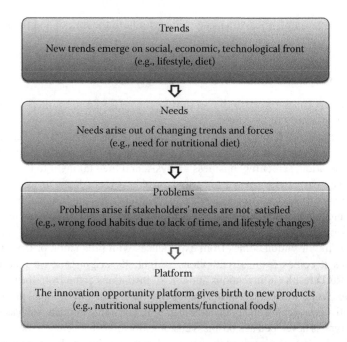

FIGURE 30.1   Outside-in approach.

the basis of market intelligence and exhaustive reports compiled by an enthusiastic marketing team. It is probably apparent that the customer is practically absent from the entire process, or contributes to it in a very peripheral way. Is it not strange that the customer, for whom the product is being developed, is not deeply involved in the process?

Very often, market research data and findings being used for product development are obsolete and redundant as the market trends have evolved. True, the path from mind to market is tediously long and convoluted. But that should give us a clue as to how to proceed. Make the customer the center of the process. Involve them intimately with every facet of the product. Familiarize them with every twist and turn in the entire product development process.

The customers have to move from being mere respondents to questions and a sounding board to being the actual developers of the product. If you are looking at infusing your product with a large measure of innovation, your customers must be the innovators. Their foresight and insights need to be carefully incorporated into the product. This close relationship with the customer brings a new dimension and meaning to the process of product *customization*.

The customer must be the alpha and omega of the process. The involvement and relationship with the customer should not be piecemeal or ad hoc. Very often customers are invited to react to a product; instead, they need to be proactive in conceiving and fine-tuning it through the entire process. It may take a little more or, in some cases, a lot more effort to introduce customers into the product development process in a 360 degree manner. But then, that is what innovation and going the extra mile is all about!

The following conceptual model of the outside-in innovation platform for foods has key elements, viz., the trends, stakeholders, platform, and forces (Figure 30.2).

Any product coming out of the outside-in innovation platform could either make competition redundant or it could be so superior as to surpass the competition. Obviously, to make this platform stronger, unarticulated needs of customers should be identified by continuously spotting changes that could affect future trends.

With regard to nutraceuticals and foods, these trends could originate from social and medical issues and could have economic, technological, and political dimensions. In addition, mapping

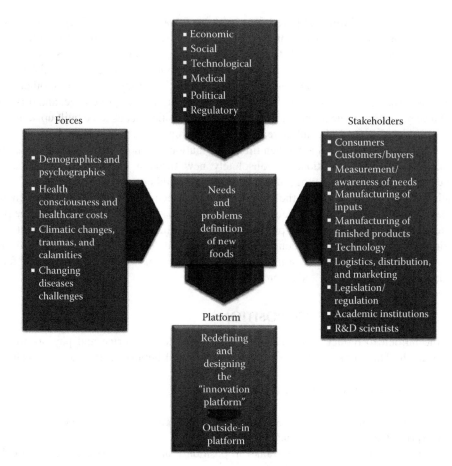

- Economic
- Social
- Technological
- Medical
- Political
- Regulatory

Forces

- Demographics and psychographics
- Health consciousness and healthcare costs
- Climatic changes, traumas, and calamities
- Changing diseases challenges

Needs and problems definition of new foods

Stakeholders

- Consumers
- Customers/buyers
- Measurement/ awareness of needs
- Manufacturing of inputs
- Manufacturing of finished products
- Technology
- Logistics, distribution, and marketing
- Legislation/ regulation
- Academic institutions
- R&D scientists

Platform

Redefining and designing the "innovation platform"

Outside-in platform

FIGURE 30.2 Outside-in "innovation platform" for foods. (Conceptual model by R.B. Smarta, Interlink knowledge cell_ interlink Insight Issue_ Innovation_ The new driving force_ Volume 1 No 3.)

regulatory trends would be equally important as the trend in technology involves going back to the root of genes, genetics, genomics, DNA analysis, and so on. Obviously, regulatory issues will be diverse and their definitions will change accordingly.

Mounting on this first layer of trends, industry must look at nutrieconomics. Changing disease challenges, health consciousness, and health costs provide enough insights on the needs of nutrieconomics. Obviously, it will be important to examine the profile of the customer and the forces acting on them. Hence, demographic psychographics, climate changes, traumas, and other noncontrollable forces need to be understood along with the bargaining power.

The third layer involves interfaces with all stakeholders. This third layer of interfaces and interests of all stakeholders will converge in the central frame of this particular platform.

Thus, according to the outside-in approach, innovation will start where there is a need or an unmet need. It may take a year or so to do the work and go to the market with this *outside-in innovation platform*.

30.11   CREATION OF A BUSINESS MODEL

While building a business model, we need to consider how the belief in our products, services, or ideas will be conveyed to potential buyers. In this regard, it is important to look at the core capabilities of the organization and the existing infrastructure. In the case of nutraceuticals and functional foods, the traditional structures and infrastructure are already available in every country.

However, the core capabilities required for plantation, processing, technology, and R&D, and a very good combination of academia and industry need to be properly chosen to develop the right product. An organization also needs to look at the partner network, as partners are required for actualizing and commercializing this innovation. If the product is similar to the existing ones, no configuration of value can be made and the product cannot be differentiated from other products; thus, it is important to make an offer to the customers, at the stage of preference, and this offer has to be of a very specific value proposition. This value proposition needs to be built up, and then that value proposition forms a link, and thereafter a relationship, with the customer. To make the product available to the customer at any given time, distribution channels are required. These distribution channels could be traditional or absolutely new through influencers. Sometimes, these influencers may have different types of channels, which could be nontraditional; these distribution channels can also be used to reach the target customers. Upcoming businesses, in particular, need to have a certain amount of cost structure and surplus so that the revenue streams can be properly characterized. In this case, a value proposition needs to be created. Unless you create a value proposition, there is no, let us say, identity of the business model because it does not need a regular stream and, similarly, it does not eat into any substantial surplus required for R&D and for developing new products, channels, and so on.

30.12 NEED FOR VALUE PROPOSITION

Under the burden to reduce costs, customers may just look at price and pay no attention to the sales pitch. Thus, one must help them recognize and believe in the superior value of the offerings.

Organizations would certainly need the following:

- The customer value proposition that defines the product(s) and/or the service offering(s) an enterprise delivers to its customers at a given price.
- The profit system or company value proposition that an enterprise employs to deliver economic value to its stakeholders.
- The key resources a company deploys to create value.
- The critical processes that guide and shape operations and how the company organizes and acts to create and deliver the value proposition to the customer and itself.

The example of amazon.com can be considered as a business model based on the *value proposition* concept:

Preparing content for the Web is dependent on patterns and brands. Readers of print and Web media differ in their consumption patterns. Print readers tend to read in a linear manner. Web surfers may interact with an article and read elements out of order, in a *nonlinear* or *branching* manner. Then, there are design issues. Some content specialists argue that vital information should remain "above the scroll" on all pages. And some suggested that matter be written in "chunks" delivered one page at a time.

As a result, the "chunks" strategy was adopted for content, and it was decided to repurpose print material into "chunks" such that each has a unique page. Each "chunk" is usually fewer than 150 words and text can be viewed on the screen without having to scroll and this is only one strategy—many sites do not use it!

Before publicly launching a site, it is not uncommon for a company to conduct "usability tests" with a test audience to determine whether the site is easy to navigate, which was done by Amazon (Figure 30.3).

The Amazon.com success story started with the evolution of a design and with personalization and automation. Today, Amazon.com is the world's largest e-commerce site.

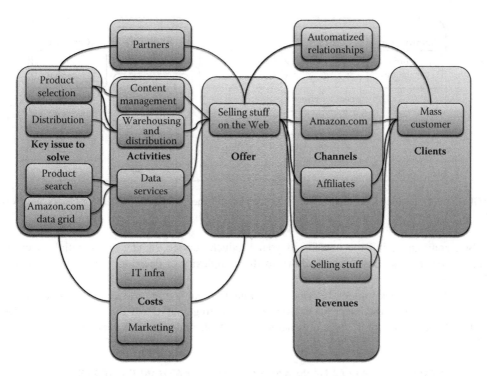

FIGURE 30.3 Customer value addition.

Amazon has over 35 e-commerce main product categories and hundreds of subcategories. Each category has at least one full-time editor. Some have several editors. Each editor is responsible for maintaining the front page of each "store" and subpages, including product detail pages. During the dot-com "boom," Amazon had hired aggressively as investor cash came in. It then got "bloated" and was described as inefficient site infrastructure. The company needed to streamline its content development strategy. This included a shift from an editor-created to a user-generated content model. With millions of products, Amazon.com needed help from the public to keep the pages up to date and filled with useful information and to provide "user-generated content." As a result of feedback, Amazon.com features contain reviews, listmania, "how-to" and buying guides, product manuals, customer images, ref-tags, discussion forums, and Wikis. In listmania, customers create their own lists and share them with others. Each item in the list is linked to a product; for example, Top 15 movies of 2005 by fattjoe37, Best Albums of 2006 by volantsolo, and "Awesome Books" by fantasyrules. Customers also create their own guides to share their expertise with others, such as how to set up a wireless home network or how to take a better picture with your digital camera.

Customers have indicated that they enjoy the "community" aspect of shopping. They trust the collective opinions of other shoppers more than that of the manufacturers. The "Amazon Review" has become a very powerful force in the industry and buying decisions are made for purchases both offline and online.

So, is a business model necessary?

Yes, a solid business model is necessary. Company must adopt "cutting edge" technology. It is important to learn that being first may not translate to success.

Similarly, key stakeholders in the content development teams must meet and agree on the "milestones." Each "milestone" is a mutually agreed upon "deliverable" in the product development cycle and deviation from the agreed-upon development is discouraged.

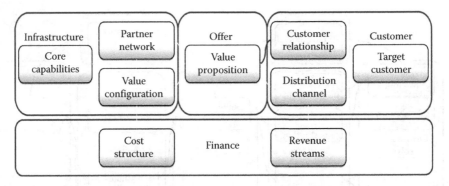

FIGURE 30.4   Value proposition model. (Adapted from Business Model Template/Alox Osterwalter/Nov 06.)

But, communicating the benefits of your product, service, or idea to potential buyers is the building block of success. It boils down to the complexity of decision making for the consumer (Figure 30.4).

The above business model describes the value an organization offers to various customers and portrays the capabilities and partners required for creating, marketing, and delivering this value and relationship capital with the goal of generating profitable and sustainable revenue streams.

30.13   COMMERCIALIZATION AND CUSTOMIZATION PROCESS

Innovation-led economy defines the innovation that distinguishes between creation, customization, commercialization and diffusion, and adoption of the same innovation.

The commercialization process starts with overlapping aspects of product innovation, marketing innovation, and the commercial process which is based on the Business Model.

Later on, the product stems toward acceptance and then it gets diffused in the market for better market share (Figure 30.5).

Commercialization is the process of bringing new innovations to market, that is, the market-based scaling-up of production from pilot to mass market that transforms new knowledge to wealth. Products are typically monetized either by licensing or selling the intellectual property, or by marketing and selling the product.

30.13.1   ADOPTION AND DIFFUSION FACTORS

30.13.1.1   Adopting Local Conditions

Technology often must be adapted to local conditions, for example, including local raw materials, special characteristics, or other idicsyncrasies such as local standards, climate, or power sources. It is important to have appropriate mechanisms with which to educate potential users about the benefits of the technology and the product. Education often involves more than providing technical information. Moverover, use of new technologies usually requires literacy and specialized training. Finally, beyond the specific skills, using new technology often requires access to complementary inputs and supporting industries and access to finance to purchase new equipment or inputs, or even to buy the technology license.

At the most basic level, a business model consists of four interlocking, interdependent components: Customer, technology, economy, and market. Technology is seen as one of the important drivers of increasing healthcare accessibility. The selection and adoption of appropriate technology often make a critical difference in the success of healthcare reform and reengineering, and it has the capability of revolutionizing the manner in which healthcare is delivered.

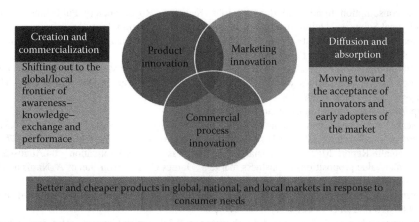

FIGURE 30.5 Adoption–diffusion process.

30.13.1.2 Customization with a Difference
The major characteristics that play a crucial role at the innovation platform are as follows:

- *Noticeability:* The extent to which the outcome of an innovation is visible to potential adopters.
- *Superiority:* The level to which the innovation is perceived to be superior to existing practice; in other words, it is the value created through the new product.
- *Compatibility:* The degree to which the innovation is perceived to be consistent with trends, perceived needs, and problems of stakeholders.
- *Practicability:* The scope to which the innovation can be experienced.
- *Complexity:* The extent to which an innovation is complicated to use or understand.

30.13.1.3 Marketing Infrastructure Development
For every business, it is important to either use the existing sales and marketing infrastructure to market the products or to develop a new way of making the products available at specific points. In the case of India and many other countries in which nutrition transformation has not taken place fully, the infrastructure for marketing nutraceuticals and new forms of foods is almost negligible, rendering it necessary to use the traditional setup.

30.13.1.4 Marketing Process Development
In order to make the marketing effective, each country needs to develop a common generic trading process and selling platform. On that platform, each company needs to develop different sales and marketing processes to capture market share or to develop a new market.

30.13.1.5 Awareness, Education, Exchange, and Performance
In order to popularize a particular brand or category, companies will have to make the targeted customers aware of the category and then develop campaigns to educate them about the positive aspects of the category. Once the customers are well educated and ready to accept the category as well as brands, the marketer will have to ensure that a smooth transaction and exchange takes place.

On repeating this process, a market can observe how a particular brand is performing.

BIBLIOGRAPHY

1. Barriers on market introduction of innovative products_ Wouter Tesink_ Faculty of Electrical Engineering, Mathematics and Computer Science University of Twente

2. Food consumption trends and drivers _John Kearney_ Royal Society Publishing_ Department of Biological Sciences_ Dublin Institute of Technology (DIT), Dublin, Eire
3. Unleashing India's innovation _Mark A. Dutz _ 2007 The International Bank for Reconstruction and Development / The World Bank_ Washington, DC 20433
4. Mastering innovation : Roadmap to sustainable value creation_ by Mr. Jatin DeSai_ The DeSai Group
5. Trends shaping tomorrow's world _ Mervin J. Cetron and Owen Davies _ Part Two_ The Futurist_ May<\#U2013>June 2008,
   http://www.lindenhoek.nl/downloads/files/trends.pdf
6. Describe and Improve your business model-1193048778204895-2_Slide No 12, 23,27,29,31
   http://www.scribd.com/doc/56988914/Describe-and-Improve-Your-Business-Model-1193048778204895-2
7. India Health Report 2012_Indicus Analytics & Business standard Publication _ 04 August,2012
8. Customer value propositions in business markets _ James C. Anderson, James A. Narus and Wouter Van Russan _ Harvard Business Review _ Mar 01, 2006.
9. Arvetica _ Competitive advantage business model design & Innovation_ slideshare_ Slide no 36,48,51,5 4,59,60,62,66,72,93,109,121,144
   http://www.slideshare.net/Alex.Osterwalder/business-model-design-and-innovation-for- competitive-advantage
10. http://www.businessmodelalchemist.com/ - 2012
11. Business model innovation _ Wikipedia_http://en.wikipedia.org/wiki/Business_model_innovation
12. Arvetica _ Business Model Template _ Brief Outline of Business Models _Nov 2006_ by Alexander Osterwalder_slideshare http://www.slideshare.net/Alex.Osterwalder/business-model-template
13. http://cognitrn.psych.indiana.edu/rgoldsto/complex/diffusion.ppt
14. The Six tastes—Our Guidemap to optimal nutrition—Review article
15. The Sattvic or Yogic Diet _ By Gary Gran, CYT, D.Ay_Archives Jan-Feb 2005
16. Interlink knowledge cell_ interlink Insight Issue_ Innovation_ The new driving force_ Volume 1 No 3

Section VII

Future Trends

31 Innovation in Food Tourism and Product Distribution

Timothy J. Lee, Tin-Chung Huang, and Kuan-Huei Lee

CONTENTS

31.1 INTRODUCTION

Gulati and Garino (2000) proposed that for traditional enterprises, e-commerce business models will improve their current value by using existing resources and merging them with a virtual market. Willcocks and Plant (2001) also suggested that strategic framework in e-commerce will offer enterprises the opportunities to think how to combine Internet resources to increase the penetration rate of the current market share. The strategies of the enterprises include technology, brand, service, and market (Hensmans, 2001). Amit and Zott (2001) pointed out the sources of value creation in an e-business are novelty, efficiency, lock-in, and complementarities. Figure 31.1 describes the corresponding relationships among them. Previous research related to novelty, efficiency, lock-in, and complementarities is shown in Figure 31.1.

Creating a successful food product in a market involves a large number of essential elements. Properly selecting and managing marketing channels is one such element. Various marketing channels have been popularized with the recent progress in modern technology. For instance, electronic commerce is being conducted for transactions in a wide variety of commodities throughout most of the world. Convenience stores, malls, and outlets have been part of 24-h marketing systems for a long time. The market distribution in Asian countries has experienced significant change and substantial growth over the past decades. For example, Japan has some unique features, such as many small family-owned food retail stores, complex wholesale channels, and an increasing number of online stores. However, the number of food retail establishments peaked in 1982 and then declined because of the recession in the early 2000s (Matsui et al., 2005). In Taiwan, convenience stores have become the most concentrated marketing channels of this decade, especially for the distribution of food and beverage commodities. Other food retail channels (e.g., chain stores) have also recently increased in their presence. These include drugstores, chophouses, tea, and coffee shops. Retail food souvenir (local specialty) shops in eastern Taiwan selling items such as moji rice cake, agar,

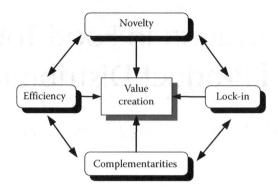

FIGURE 31.1 Value creation of e-commerce. (Adapted from Amit, R. and Zott, C. 2001. *Strategic Management Journal*, 22(6), 493–520.)

peeled chili, conserves, and cakes have rapidly expanded over the last decade. The retail store has become one of the most popular channels for promoting food products in Taiwan.

31.2 LITERATURE REVIEW

Matsui et al. (2005) predicted food retail density in relation to population density in Japan and China. They concluded that the decline in the number of retail stores in Japan was primarily because of the proliferation of car ownership and the expansion of the average dwelling size. This highlights the importance of inspecting the culture and customs that influence the trend in the development of marketing channels. It also inspires us to verify the relationship between a traders' channel density and their market share. Kannan (2001) found that the literature on e-commerce generally agrees that the Internet is an additional marketing channel. The Internet is considered to complement the traditional channels in some applications, act as a substitute in others, and in some cases generate new opportunities. The Internet is accepted as an easy instrument of transactional channels in modern society. Rylander et al. (1997) stress that the nature, scope, and consequences of commitment within marketing channels are resolved through the emergent rational commitment framework. They argue that the final outcome of increased commitment is improved channel structure quality. This argument demonstrates that market traders need constant adjustments in their marketing channel strategies with acute reactions.

After deploying marketing channels, market traders need to constantly create operational efficiency. The cooperative or competitive relationships among various channels have aroused scholars' interest. Geyskens et al. (1999) tested a conceptual model that compared economic and noneconomic satisfaction. The result of their meta-analysis indicates that conflict and satisfaction are developed first, followed by trust, whereas commitment to channel relationships only occurs in the long term. Therefore, market traders should coordinate the relationships among various channel members so that all members are satisfied. According to Zhuang et al. (2006), noncoercive power among channel members had a positive impact on the relationships. On the contrary, coercive power had a negative impact on a member's own power, even if the member was in a powerful position. Thus, maintaining the balance of power among channel members could construct an ideal cooperative atmosphere.

31.3 BACKGROUND OF FOOD SOUVENIR COMPANIES IN HUALIEN, TAIWAN

The entire food souvenir market in Taiwan in 2007 was U$100 million with consumption power. Their main products are traditional snacks such as rice cakes and vegetable pies that are made with unique local ingredients. These foods are popular with locals and tourists from different provinces

TABLE 31.1

Food Souvenir Products Producers in Hualien, Taiwan

Main Services/Enterprises	Huelan	Ebisu	Jota	Feng Shing	Yaji
Company website	Yes	Yes	Yes	Yes	No
Product delivery	Yes	Yes	Yes	Yes	Yes
Related to health	Yes	No	No	No	No
Confident suppliers	Yes	Yes	Yes	No	Yes

and countries as souvenir products. Most of them are sold either for immediate consumption or packaged for later. The market size of the food souvenir market in Hualien was approximately U\$2 million in 2007 (Economic Daily News, 2008).

The Hualien County is the largest county in Taiwan and is located on the mountainous eastern coast of Taiwan. The Hualien County is 4628 km^2 and has a population of approximately 350,000. It is the starting point of the Eastern Cross-Island Railway, and the finishing point of the Suao-Hualien Highway and the Central Cross-Island Highway. Four hundred years ago, Portuguese sailors passed through the East Coast of Taiwan and were fascinated by its beauty, calling it "Formosa." Of the total population in Hualien, 25% are aborigines (Hualien County Government, 2008). It is the most in-demand place to visit for national and international tourists in Taiwan. The Taroko National Park in Hualien is the best sightseeing destination in the country, although it is not the most frequently visited. It is considered the best tourist attraction with the highest satisfaction after visiting (Ministry of Transportation and Communication, 2008). The competitive environment for traditional indigenous product producers in Hualien scarcely calls for illustration. Table 31.1 shows the situations of five main food souvenir producers in Hualien, Taiwan. The study uses company websites, product delivery, relates to health, and confident suppliers as dimensions to measure the food souvenir product producers in Hualien.

In Table 31.2, the study uses price, time to market, market share, market segmentation, marketing channel, advantages in technology, key technologies application, and quality as dimensions to be weighed. After comparing Tables 31.1 and 31.2, these companies have room for improvement, though it cannot be proven that the introduction of a new e-commerce model will help to increase profitability immediately; however, it seems likely that these companies are competing at a unanimous level and should change their business model to become more competitive. The company that adopts the new e-commerce model will have "first mover" advantage over the rest of the competitors.

TABLE 31.2

Competitive Analysis of Food Souvenir Products Producers in Hualien, Taiwan

Items/Company	Huelan	Ebisu	Jota	Feng Shing	Yaji
Price	b	a	a	b	a
Time to market	c	a	b	a	c
Market share (%)	b	b	b	c	a
Market segmentation	a	b	c	c	c
Marketing channel	b	c	a	c	a
Advantages in technology	a	a	a	a	a
Key technologies application	a	a	a	a	a
Quality	a	a	c	a	b

Note: a, excellent; b, mediocre; c, poor.

31.4 MANAGERIAL IMPLEMENTATION OF THE BUSINESS MODEL

The commercialization of a business model in the project can be regarded as a profit-making procedure (Huang, 2005). For the application of a business model of e-commerce, Afuah and Tucci (2003) proposed nine models, such as the brokerage model, advertising model, intermediary model, merchant model, manufacturing model, and affiliate model, which are shown in Table 31.3.

31.4.1 INTRODUCTION STAGE

Because the policy of having 2 days off in 1 week is standard in Taiwan, the people's intentions for traveling are much higher. The national average for personal traveling is up to 109,340,000 times in 2004, accounting for a 6.8% growing rate compared with the previous year. The average number of national journeys by each person is 5.7 in the year 2004 (it was 5.39 in 2003). The total number of journeys estimated by the Taiwanese government for people traveling nationally is 109.34 million. If children under the age of 12 are included, the total number of travelers will be 131.55 million in the whole year.

With such a huge number of travelers, it would be a great opportunity for attracting the customer's attention to the purchase of food souvenir products and could activate the growth of the local industry. This turned out to be the starting motivation for this project to develop a new e-commerce model for the local food souvenir industry in Hualien, Taiwan. In addition, the authors expected that the outcome is going to change the management practice and the marketing channel in this industry and will educate consumers to understand the new business model with sufficient product information. By doing this, it may further increase the visitor's willingness to buy local food souvenir products with a greater efficiency. Therefore, the e-commerce business model in this project will cause the food souvenir manufacturers to innovate a new method for its store operations and supply chain management, for example, a virtual store and the Internet shopping without physical facilities.

31.4.2 INITIAL GROWTH STAGE

After attracting the consumer's eyes, a new wave of networks involves the rise of ethnicity, and several competitors will appear at the same time. At this stage, the main focus will be on efficiency to solve all the problems of the customers and the relative suppliers, and to increase the willingness for consumption. The authors suggest the organization of domestic and foreign Internet models and practices to reduce the time and cost that the customer uses to search for the products. Williamson (1983, 1985) proposes a transaction-cost theory about how to reduce unnecessary transaction costs to increase efficiency. The e-commerce business model in this stage can offer an efficient method for

TABLE 31.3
Stages of Complementation

Implication Stages	Dimensions	e-Commerce Business Models Theoretical Foundation	Models
Introduction stage	Novelty	Innovation theory	Advertising model Merchant model
Initial growth stage	Efficiency	Transaction cost economics	Brokerage model Intermediary model Manufacturing model
Final growth stage	Lock-in	Lock-in theory	Subscription model Utility model
Mature stage	Complementally	Resource-based viewpoint	Affiliate model Community model

reducing the searching costs for visitors when purchasing local food souvenir products. Meanwhile, the manufacturers could still use face-to-face selling channels to reach their customers.

31.4.3 FINAL GROWTH STAGE

At this stage, the customers will become interested in the products in the project. There are high switching costs that will then produce the so-called lock-in result (Press and Konstantinov, 2000). The business model for the e-commerce in the stage should avoid free enrollments; it is suggested that using membership subscriptions and fee-charging methods would generate appropriate returns for the enterprises.

31.4.4 MATURE STAGE

Customers will have sufficient knowledge to judge the services and be sensitive to price changes. At this stage, the business model of the e-commerce should focus on the establishment of complementary products as the core competence. In addition to the existing product or the service, the manufacturer would strengthen its core competence by outsourcing or establishing strategic alliances. The main consideration is to select partners in e-commerce using alliances or community models and to maintain the normal profit flow of the company.

31.5 DIFFERENCES BETWEEN OTHER BUSINESS MODELS

Food souvenir products are often bought by tourists. The sale amount is closely related to the number of tourism trips. We can also analyze the different channels that people use to receive messages. In general, most people receive travel information from friends, the electronic media, the print media, and the Internet. As shown in Figure 31.2, visitors use a traditional channel to buy the food souvenir products and the manufacturer provides its inventory by using a build-to-stock method.

Because of convenient transportation and the Internet network, customers do not have to go to a physical building. However, they can buy the food souvenir products through a website. The business model for the food souvenir products is indicated in Figure 31.3.

Although the aforementioned business models are convenient, there are still some potential problems, such as the long lead time for manufacturing, the high stock level of products and raw materials, and the complex ordering processes. In other words, the firms are unable to respond to the customer's real needs immediately and to reflect the efficiency that e-commerce could produce. The new e-commerce business model introduced in this project is revealed in Figure 31.4. It relies on the foundation of the aforementioned theories and coordinates with the present electronic database technology to establish a common network platform.

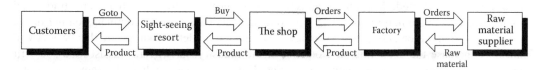

FIGURE 31.2 Business model in traditional indigenous stores in the past.

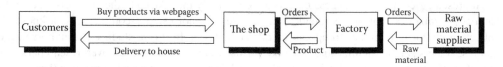

FIGURE 31.3 Business model in traditional indigenous products stores on the Internet.

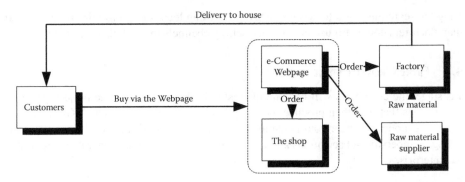

FIGURE 31.4   Business model in a traditional specialty goods shop in the project.

31.6   CONCLUSION: MAIN BENEFITS AND RESTRICTIONS IN THE BUSINESS MODEL

The model could be used not only by food souvenir product companies but also by all traditional industries. There are some benefits in this innovational e-commerce model. The obvious one is the amount of sales that will increase dramatically and the operational cost will be reduced at the same time (Ngai and Wat, 2002; Reiley and Spulber, 2000). The model will promote the sales volumes of all products to some extent and the marketing cost could be reduced by using the Internet network as the main sale channel. Moreover, the inventory will be reduced because of the make-to-order manufacturing. The manufacturer produces and provides its products according to the website purchase orders instead of building to stock; the inventory level could be decreased to a safe level.

However, there are some relevant facts to consider before running this business model. It is important to understand the visitor consumer behaviors toward purchasing food souvenir products. For instance, if visitors have a strong willingness to visit those tourist points to purchase these products, this point should be considered while introducing and designing the e-commerce purchasing channel. If visitors do not have a strong desire to purchase but are very concerned about the degree of the freshness of the products and have a strong intention of being at the point of purchase, the introduction of this new e-commerce business model will be questionable. The present economic environment is very positive for an e-commerce business development. This new way of doing business has influenced the industry at least in three aspects, lower costs, shorter time differences, and improved quality. From the consumption and organizational point of view, e-commerce has improved the mechanism of the market. From the economical point of view, the whole trading process has created a "multiple effect," the greater the scale of production, the higher is the economic power. Because cost has been reduced considerably and efficiency has been elevated, the profit margins for these enterprises are greater than in the traditional industries. This is the main reason why portfolio analysts have positive comments on the future growth of e-commerce enterprises. The new e-commerce model introduced by this project will not only increase the economic environment of the industry but will also assist food souvenir products producers to reach new volumes in sales. The authors believe that this innovative e-commerce model will change dramatically the business model of the traditional food producers in Taiwan.

At present, e-commerce business models are commonly introduced to the enterprises separately from the companies' business strategies. Enterprises are not using e-commerce as a knowledge collection platform to create strong and unique advantages. In future studies, the authors suggest that researchers should identify and integrate the above two subjects. Moreover, researchers could identify different e-commerce business models for different industries and implement these models according to each enterprise business strategy and developmental planning.

REFERENCES

Afuah, A. and Tucci, C. L. 2003. *Internet Business Models and Strategies: Text and Cases.* New York: McGraw-Hill.

Amit, R. and Zott, C. 2001. Value creation in e-business. *Strategic Management Journal*, 22(6), 493–520.

Economic Daily News. 2008. The Taiwanese Food Souvenir Market is Getting More Delicious. 12th of April, 2008, Page C1. Taipei, Taiwan.

Geyskens, I., Steenkamp, J. B., and Kumar, N. 1999. A meta-analysis of satisfaction in marketing channel relationships. *Journal of Marketing Research*, 36(2), 223–238.

Gulati, R. and Garino, J. 2000. Get the right mix of bricks and clicks. *Harvard Business Review*, 78(3), 107–114.

Hensmans, M. 2001. Clicks vs. bricks in the emerging online financial services industry. *Long Range Planning*, 34(2), 231–247.

Hualien County Government. 2008. Report of the Tourism Industry in Hualien. Hualien, Taiwan: Hualien County Government.

Huang, T. C. 2005. The study of e-commerce business model in knowledge management. In *2005 New Management Concept Academic Conference*, Taipei, Taiwan.

Kannan, P. K. 2001. Introduction to the special issues: Marketing in the e-channel. *International Journal of Electronic Commerce*, 5(3), 3–6.

Matsui, K., Lu, S., Nariu, T., and Yukimoto, T. 2005. Marketing channels and retail store density in East Asia. *Asian Economic Journal*, 19(4), 407–422.

Ministry of Transportation and Communication. 2008. Annual Survey Report on Visitors Expenditure and Trends in Taiwan in 2007. Taipei, Taiwan: Tourism Bureau, Ministry of Transportation and Communication.

Ngai, E. W. T. and Wat, F. K. T. 2002. A literature review and classification of electronic commerce research. *Information and Management*, 39(5), 415–429.

Press, V. and Konstantinov, J. 2000. Last man standing: A study on business-to-business e-markets. *Stockholm School of Economics*, 12, 38–64.

Reiley, L. D. and Spulber, D. F. 2000. Business-to-business electronic commerce. *Journal of Economic Perspectives*, 8, 84–98.

Rylander, D., Strutton, D., and Pelton, L. E. 1997. Toward a synthesized framework of relational commitment: Implications for marketing channel theory and practice. *Journal of Marketing Theory and Practice*, 5(2), 58–71.

Willcocks, L. P. and Plant, R. 2001. Pathways to e-business leadership: Getting from bricks and clicks. *MIT Sloan Management Review*, 42(3), 50–59.

Williamson, O. E. 1983. Credible commitments: Using hostages to support exchanges. *American Economic Review*, 73(4), 519–540.

Williamson, O. E. 1985. *The Economic Institutions of Capitalism.* New York: The Free Press.

Zhuang, G., Herndon Jr., N. C., and Zhou, N. 2006. Exercises of power in marketing channel dyads: Power advantage versus power disadvantage. *International Review of Retail, Distribution and Consumer Research*, 16(1), 1–22.

32 Regulations and Innovations Interphase

D.B. Anantha Narayana

CONTENTS

32.1 OBJECTIVES

The chapter looks at innovations and regulations, drawing the role of scientists and other players in innovations as well as the role of regulations and regulators. Coverage of various steps in taking innovations in healthy and functional foods to market, vis-à-vis existing and emerging regulations, and what it takes to bring in desired changes in regulations will form part of the chapter. Reforming regulations and factors that promote such reforms will be covered. In some places, possible examples or brief case studies are given.

32.2 INTRODUCTION

It is an accepted fact that the progress and prosperity of a country are linked to its people, earnings, and productivity. These are directly linked to the overall health of citizens of the nation. Each government hence has considerable interest in ensuring the health of its citizens through food, diet, availability of healthcare facilities, medicines, and other needs such as hygiene, sanitation, and clean drinking water. A fairly large industry hence exists to provide food as well as medicines. Nations put in place regulations to govern these areas primarily with a view to ensure safety of the food and medicines available in the country apart from overseeing quality, efficacy, and affordability.

Globally, over the last decade, major changes were observed in the way policy makers looked at food regulations. A paradigm shift is ongoing in food regulations—from preventing unsafe materials and foods usage, preventing mixing, adulteration, spoilage of foods, identifying unsafe products and people involved in putting such products in the market and punishing them to assessing and building of safety into foods, assessing risks involved and putting in place systems, processes, and peoples to manage the risk, and providing guidelines for operators in the food industry so that all the players in the industry comply with the guidelines by way of self-regulation. This shift toward the latter over a period of time has been triggered as a result of the realization among the regulators with regard to the huge cost involved in regulating this area by way of policing, sampling, testing, and prosecution which governments can ill afford.

1. Before the 1990s, the quantum of scientific information available through science on diet, exercise, nutrition, and health as well as role of medicines in disease were different than it is today. In the last two decades, growth in scientific studies and understanding as well as growth in information technology has increased consumer awareness in relation to the preventive role of food and diets for their health. Complete reliance on medicines alone to diagnose, treat, and provide relief in various disorders and diseases has changed and the need for medicines is felt for most serious conditions. In the early 1990s, the United States led this shift. It is understood that during 1991–1992 more than 150,000 citizens in the United States wrote to their senators or government[1] querying why everything they consume for their health and disease needs to be reviewed and approved by the US Food and Drug Administration (FDA), why they cannot have informed choice of using other than drugs approved by the US FDA to maintain and protect their health. A group of scientists and lawyers reviewed the issue and came up with a major reform in regulation which fundamentally recognizes that food itself can be medicine (recognizing the age-old adage, food-as medicine–medicine continuum). The resultant new regulations that were enacted in 1994 as "Dietary Supplements and Health Education Act—DSHEA."[2] DSHEA provided regulatory framework for defining dietary supplements, freeing such supplements from long and expensive premarket review and approval process by the FDA, providing guidelines for labeling and claims of health benefits that would be provided by a supplement as well as their marketing and offerings to public, providing guidelines on the nature, and extent of information on the supplement and their benefits to consumers, do's and don'ts for health education and informed choices, promotion, and clearly defined demarcation from medicines. This was the beginning of a major regulatory change resulting in quick and positive promotion of a highly innovative health supplement and functional foods industry.

The regulations covering all aspects of pharmaceuticals and medicines are highly regulated on a worldwide basis. For obvious reasons of ensuring complete knowledge on safety profile of medicines, understanding of risks (of safety and toxicity to consumers and patients), and efficacy, steps to manage the risks but get the desired efficacy and benefits to the patient. Pharmaceuticals hence are highly regulated with great clarity on scientific and technical information and data on the drug, the premises, equipment, process and personnel involved in manufacture, and the total chain till it reaches the patients are regulated. A fairly large amount of documentation is expected and demanded before any drug approved for marketing including permitting an approved drug to be imported to any country for marketing. Elaborate guidelines and documentation are required; inspection and audit of all stages are carried out in this process. This led to the development of a new category of scientists whose main expertise belongs to understanding the regulatory needs and preparing documentation in such detail and accuracy that would satisfy the regulator. Such personnel slowly became the bridge between R&D departments and business heads to support timely obtaining approval from regulators for introduction/marketing of drugs. Delays in getting approval in time would translate to financial loses as business declines. These experts with skills of reading the law and regulations and guidelines translating them to implementable SOP's, specifications, data, and help the R&D scientists to demonstrate through adequate and appropriate documentation, compliance to the requirements began to be called as regulatory experts. The whole area acquired the name as regulatory affairs. During these periods, regulations also existed for foods area covering foods prepared to serve in eateries, and processed and packaged foods that are transported and sold by the processed food industry. The latter involved a number of innovations to convert traditional foods and conventional foods to be manufactured on a large scale, packed in a way to stabilize them for much longer periods of storage so that they can be transported and will reach the consumer for use retaining its nutritional value, quality, and tastes. To achieve this, apart from packaging materials and technology use of different types and grades of additives, stabilizers, antioxidants, preservatives, colors, and flavors were needed, all of which had to be evaluated for safety. This involved lot of scientific data and long-term safety data and a review process. The stress on safety review and ensuring that safety is much higher than in the case of medicines as foods are consumed for a long period of time, and larger quantum and mostly consumed without any expert guidance compared with medicines. *Codex Alimentarius* has been involved in such a thorough review for safety of food additives for various categories.[3] Since most countries have regulations that define the categories of food and food formats and also publish list of permitted additives for each category with or without restrictions on levels of usage and labeling, innovators need to ensure compliance to these. It is to be recognized that unlike medicines no premarket approval of food products put in market by the processed food industry is required under regulations. However, compliance to overall categories, standards, additives permitted, labeling requirements, nutrition and health benefits, claims that can be made or cannot be made were to be complied with. In most countries and in most processed food organizations in the 1990s, this role was done by legally qualified persons manning the legal departments. Such legal experts not only reviewed the food formulations for these aspects but also liaised with regulators, fought cases of prosecution when they occurred, and dealt with noncompliance notices to ensure continuation of business and prevent loss.

2. However, in the last decade organizations are focused on growth and at the heart of growth are consumer-relevant innovations. The food industry began to push the agenda of innovations involving newer technologies, better products with greater shelf life, keeping qualities, providing dietary and dietary supplement products with specific health benefits, better taste, and appeal to fuel growth. The consumer pull for these have also been growing at a fast pace driven by changing lifestyles; packaged and convenience foods need to reduce the drudgery and time in preparing food yet providing taste and quality. The food industry naturally began looking for new processes, new technologies, and new additives to make innovations possible. However, this can be achieved only if the relevant regulations also changed at the same pace, which was a challenge to most regulators and governments. In this changing scenario, three distinct roles and expertise emerged to support and ensure that all innovations can be made within the ambit of law and change the law when required. These expertise have also spread to food and cosmetic industries and not just to the pharmaceutical industry and they are regulatory, legal, and external/corporate affairs. In order to appreciate these roles and the interface between regulations and innovations, here is a quote from a leading scientist who says

   - Problems are emotional.
   - Issues are technical.
   - Solutions are political.[4]

   Perhaps this quote summarizes the entire gamut of this area. Overall, innovations have a number of issues that are technical in nature (underpinning on science and technology related to the innovation) which need a political solution by way of amended, modified, and reformed regulations. To achieve the political solutions need, putting up a satisfactory case clearly identifying the issue and providing the technical and scientific background, proposed technical and scientific solutions, and propose a change in regulations to justify and satisfy the regulator. In many cases, a smart and intelligent scientist/technical person may be able to interpret the current regulation to give a go-ahead for the innovation without the need for any change in regulation. In some cases, minor amendments or major amendments to the existing regulations (like adding newer additives to the permitted list, permitting higher levels of usage than a lower currently, changing acceptable quality specifications, test methods and tolerance limits, permitting hitherto to unapproved processing technologies and packages, etc.) may be required for which a good dossier with all necessary and satisfactory scientific and technical data will need to be made and submitted to the relevant authorities. Dossier with such scientific and technical data will need to be provided to argue any challenges, show cause for noncompliance or regulatory actions are initiated. Obviously, such a job can be done by a technical/qualified person and this falls in a domain of regulatory affairs personnel who provide the information to either the legal or external affairs personnel.

Legal affairs expert would then help translate the technical dossiers into suitable legal language and draft the submissions, prepare strategies to get changes in regulations effected and provide defense to challenge noncompliance notices as well as defend the company's interest in judiciary. External affairs experts are specialized skills to strategize and effectively liaise with regulators including government officials and legislators to convince them for the need of change in regulations. In many firms, overlapping of this role in one or more individuals takes place but there is a need to recognize that each of these is clearly differentiated. It is fact that regulatory affairs are getting recognized in the food industry and more and more such experts are becoming part of the innovation teams.

Major roles of regulatory affairs expert
- Data mining/scientific literature survey
- Global regulatory literature survey
- Understanding/interpreting the above
- Support to innovation teams/clearances/guiding compliance
- Build relations with key opinion formers
- Perform risk assessment vis-à-vis current regulations
- Assist in risk management
- Prepare for initiating/facing challenges
- Preparing for representations for changes in regulations that block innovations
- Initiating dialogs/process for reforms in regulations

Major roles of legal affairs expert
- Interpreting current regulations
- Support innovations team for compliance/clearances/guiding
- Legal support to face official actions
- Legal support to face actions in courts/deal with senior officials
- Legal support to face challenges/initiate challenges
- Long-term strategy for compliance
- Legal support for actions against IPRs/counterfeiting/loss of business

Major roles of external affairs expert
- Build external relations with industry/trade bodies/officials
- Update legal/regulatory and innovations team on changing scenario
- Propose changes/reforms required in regulations and follow-up
- Create awareness on the industry's efforts and problems in implementing regulations
- Build forums and initiate awareness for IPR issues/counterfeiting

32.3   UNDERSTANDING/APPLICATION, CHANGING AND REFORMING THE REGULATIONS

The interface and steps involved in bringing innovations and making innovations that are compliant with the law are a continuous process of interaction between the innovating industry and the regulators not necessarily in that order. It is a common perception that industry initiates the need for change regulation that is not true in all the cases. DSHEA referred to a classic example of the regulator bringing in major change in regulations driven by consumers. Although not from the food industry, two more examples drive this point.

Example 1

All innovator pharmaceutical companies protected their innovated new drugs by way of IPR rights. The regulatory agency in the United States, namely the US FDA, was not able to give marketing authorization for the same molecule of active drug or its formulation to any manufacturer other than the innovator for a long time. The innovator not only had protection of product and market for the entire period of patent life but the brand of the drug also used to get protection as strict regulations existed before a pharmacist could switch brands. This was considered to have led to higher economics of the cost of medicines and thereby putting a higher load on expenses on drugs and healthcare management. Driven by the need to bring down the cost of healthcare management, a paradigm shift was thought of and the US government bringing a major change by way of Waxman–Hatch amendment[5] which permitted, under specific conditions, US FDA to approve generic versions of patented molecules/drugs to market after specified exclusivity period of a protected market of a first innovator. In this amendment, clear definitions of generic product and all other conditions for approval have been specified. The result was availability of generic drug formulations which are biologically and therapeutically equivalent to the innovators formulation but brought down cost by a high percentile lower to the innovators/brand formulation. This amendment has been in force for more than a decade now and is a history of "Regulations opening up and driving innovations to benefit the patients which also brought benefits to generic drug industry."

Example 2

Although unconnected to the food industry, the case of environmental laws becoming more and more stringent drove innovations. The shift to EURO II and later to EURO III levels of emissions and pollution from automobiles have led to innovations in automobile combustion and filters and a host of automobiles now meet the requirement. Initially when such laws were brought out, many complained, but eventually innovations built the business. In fact, now automobile makers proudly advertise the compliance and some of them "meeting even lower levels of pollutants/emissions than permitted."

The cycle of the various steps in this circle depicting "regulations and innovations interphase" is given thematically in Figure 32.1.

1. *Understanding applications*: For any innovator understanding, the current regulation is highly important; in fact, it is advisable to innovators that especially the scientists should keep up-to-date copies of regulation handy at their work place. Printed copies are handy and must be updated regularly and a process for the same should be in place. Accessing through the net may be a good idea but many sites may not have uploaded latest amendments. It is important to read the regulations carefully and understand them and their implications. Most regulations in many countries are written in English language which may be differing from the mother tongue of the user. It is best to read and interpret the regulation from both the technical/scientific and legal points of view point. The latter is equally important as punctuation marks in the sentence, explanatory notes/foot notes can legally mean something different than what a scientist may understand. What is not written in the regulation the way it is notified, unless specifically a restriction or prohibition is written, is equally important. Draft circulars, minutes of empowered scientific panels or task forces or expert committees, and clearances given by such committees may suit the scientists to go ahead and apply those changes, but from a legal point of view they are not yet enforced and will come with its own risks as one goes ahead to implement them in an innovation. In cases of doubt, it is best to prepare a carefully written note on the current regulation and ongoing discussions for change, timelines for change to getting to effect, and then take a decision on the innovation. Examples coming under this type of support to innovations could be

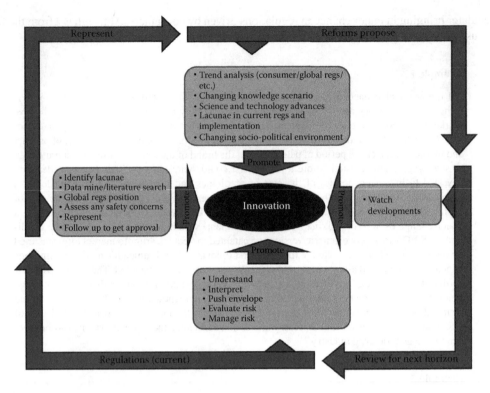

FIGURE 32.1   Regulations and innovations interphase.

approval of use of an additive at higher levels, approval of use of additives permitted in one category of food in another category of food, relaxation of lower or upper limits of tolerance for any quality-determinant test, approval for use of new processing technologies, or to provide for higher shelf life, if restricted fall into this category.

2. *Changing the regulation*: For all the examples cited in (a), if one wishes to get the regulations changed, it is important to propose those changes to the concerned departments supported with adequate justification, scientific data, opinions of leading scientists and key opinion formers, proof of support from regulations of other countries, data to remove any safety concerns, and inputs of how the change will benefit the consumer. It is best to submit such information after a personal hearing and discussions with the regulator and incorporating additional information to respond to any queries that the regulator brought up in the personal meeting. Submission of these data with a crisp and to-the-point covering letter providing an executive summary and highlighting the change in regulation restricted is important.

3. *Reforming regulations*: This is the toughest part and normally takes a long time, sometimes extending to many years. Reforms call for patient and sustained efforts, personnel and official interactions with not only the officials who are empowered to initiate reforms but also with political members of the legislature or senate or commissions. Often, reforms are aimed at changing the administrative and enforcing methodologies and processes, strategic change in the way regulation look at food products and processes, the way safety is assessed, regulated, and managed. The other aspect of reforms may extend in creating new categories shifting from restricted benefit claims to permitting bolder claims, permitting preapproved health benefit claims that border between food and drug into the food domain bringing certain categories of unrestricted food products to make them be given under medical or nutritionist advice. A Number of examples of creation of dietary supplements, nutraceuticals, food/health supplements, foods for specific health use, and functional foods fall into this category.

32.4 REFORMS SEEN IN THIS AREA SINCE 1994

32.4.1 TERMINOLOGIES AND DEFINITIONS

The term *functional foods* was first introduced in Japan in the mid-1980s and refers to processed foods containing ingredients that aid specific body functions, in addition to being nutritious. For defining functional foods, a variety of terminologies are used worldwide such as *nutraceuticals, dietary supplements, health supplements medifoods, vita foods*, and *fortified foods*. However, the term *functional foods* has become the predominant even though several organizations have attempted to differentiate this emerging food category. Health Canada, for instance, defines a *functional food* as "similar in appearance to a conventional food, consumed as part of the usual diet, with demonstrated physiological benefits, and/or to reduce the risk of chronic disease beyond basic nutritional functions" and a *nutraceutical* as "a product isolated or purified from foods that is generally sold in medicinal forms not usually associated with foods." In Korea, functional foods are defined as dietary supplements whose purpose is to supplement the normal diet and have to be marketed in measured doses, such as in pills and tablets. However, functional foods are generally considered as those foods that are intended to be consumed as part of the normal diet and that contain biologically active components which offer the potential of enhanced health or reduced risk of disease. According to this definition, unmodified whole foods such as fruits and vegetables represent the simplest form of a functional food. For example, broccoli, carrots, or tomatoes would be considered functional foods because they are rich in physiologically active components such as sulforaphane, β-carotene, and lycopene, respectively.

32.4.2 FUNCTIONAL FOOD REGULATIONS: INTERNATIONAL SCENARIO

Different countries have taken different approaches for defining food, drug, and dietary supplements.

In the United States, a dietary supplement as per DSHEA of the United States cannot make disease risk reduction claims unless approved and authorized from the FDA. Other functional claims do not need premarket approval. The law in the United States also requires such products to print a disclaimer on the label that "This statement has not been evaluated by the FDA. This product is not intended to diagnose, treat, cure, or prevent any disease."[6]

Japan permits a broader classification called Food with Health Claims (FHC) that refers to foods that comply with the specifications and standards established by the Ministry of Health, Labour and Welfare (MHLW) Japan and are labeled with certain nutritional or health functions. These foods are categorized into two groups, according to differences in purpose and function, that is, Food with Nutrient Claims (Standard Regulation System) and Food for Specified Health Uses (FOSHU—Individual Approval System). In order to sell a food as FOSHU, the assessment for the safety of the food and effectiveness of the function for health is required, and the claim must be approved by MHLW Japan. The prominent requirements for FOSHU approval include clearly proved effectiveness on the human body, absence of any safety issues, use of nutritionally appropriate ingredients, guarantee of compatibility with product specifications by the time of consumption, and established quality control methods. For giving the FOSHU approval MHLW Japan also consults Council on Pharmaceutical affairs and Food sanitation and Food Safety Commission for ascertaining the effectiveness and safety of the product, respectively. The products falling into "FOSHU" can bear health claims and even treatment claims as has been approved by the law.[7]

European Food Safety Authority (EFSA) has recently provided its scientific opinion/guidance on Nutrient Profiling and on Health Claim Authorization & Application. Nutrient profile refers to nutrient composition of the food and Nutrient Profiling refers to classification of foods for specific purposes based on their nutrient composition. European Union (EU) regulation 1924/2006 on Nutrition and Health Claims on Foods require foods or certain food categories to respect established nutrient profile in order to bear Nutrition and Health Claims. EFSA recommends a profile to be set for the combination of food in general across the categories, with some special cases to consider. In the opinion of panel, nutrients such as saturated fatty acids, sodium, dietary fiber, and unsaturated fatty acids are the ones whose intake does not comply with the recommended intake of EU, therefore such nutrients should be included in the nutrient profiling. EFSA stressed on the requirement of a database of energy and nutrients content of a range of foods on the EU market and thus classifying the food/food categories as eligible to bear nutrition claim, eligible to bear health claim, and ineligible to bear health claim. EFSA panel identified common important limitations for nutrient profiling as—inherent difficulty in applying the nutrient intake value for individual nutrients that are established for the overall diet; inability to take into account the changes in nutrient intake that occur during cooking or preparations including additions of fat, sugar, salt, and so on; inability to count on the habitual intake of the food or the pattern of consumption; and the lack of uniform data for food composition and consumption across the EU.[8]

EFSA opinion for Claim Authorization and Application are applicable to "disease risk reduction claim" and "for children's" claims (the latter is considered on a case-by-case basis as no explicit definition is available for such claim in European Commission regulation). EFSA opinion provides the direction that claims authorization document should comprise all data (in favor/nonfavor) both general or specific information and the same need to be submitted. Such application should give the information on physical and chemical nature, composition as well as stability and bioavailability of the food/constituent with which health benefit is associated; the wording of the health claim, any specified condition, target population, and so on needs to be proposed with the backup of scientific evidence of human intervention studies, human observational studies, other human studies, and nonhuman studies. A hierarchy has been suggested for the various scientific studies like in the case of human intervention studies it is randomized control trials (RCT) > other RCT (noncontrolled) > controlled, nonrandomized studies > other intervention studies. And in the case of human observational studies, that is, cohort studies > case–control studies > cross-sectional studies > other observational studies (e.g., case reports). In the case of cited studies, data should be comprehensive and peer reviewed, clearly defining the claimed effect and the associated biomarkers for measuring and validating the claimed effect. EFSA recommends not citing journal abstracts and articles published in newspapers, magazines, newsletters, or handouts that have not been peer reviewed. Finally, the health claim will be substantiated by taking into account the totality of the available scientific data.[9]

Regulators/scientific bodies like MHLW (Foods for FOSHU) in Japan and EFSA in EU provide more evolved regulation. Clearances for claims have been arrived based on careful scientific review of data available on benefits provided by substances or ingredients, with adequate and stringent review by regulatory authorities (see Table 32.1 for examples of 27 health benefit claims that are permitted for a FOSHU product, if the product contains the identified dietary ingredient in levels required).[10] These categories then offer clarity to both the manufacturers and the consumers. To the manufacturer—it is clear that if the product can be proven to contain the necessary food ingredient in levels which are required, then the product can make particular functional claim. To the consumer—it gives guarantee that the product contains necessary levels of the food/ingredient and if the product is taken as per directions, and for such periods as required, the consumer will get the health benefit.

Markets like the United States have measures to promote responsible nutrition and informed choices as against the tightly controlled FDA regime when it comes to drugs. In contrast, countries such as Japan, China, and Canada have more closely knit, protective regulatory approach with a view to protect citizens who are made of a mix of well and less literate. The governments in these countries have taken the need of performing the informed choice step and provide guidance to the consumers. Hence, in these countries the law adopts a strategy where regulators would take a step forward in providing the informed choice and justification of functional food claims.

32.4.3   FUNCTIONAL FOOD REGULATION: INDIAN SCENARIO[11]

India, while going by world opinion and scenario, rightly created the category titled as Functional Foods/Nutraceuticals/Foods for Special Dietary Uses/Health Supplements under the recently

TABLE 32.1

Health Claims Permitted by SFDA, China for Functional Foods

S. No.	Function	Target Population Group
1	Immunity enhancing	People with low immunity
2	Antioxidation	Middle-aged and aged people
3	Auxiliary memory improving	People need to improve memory
4	Manual fatigue relieving	People easy to fatigue
5	Weight losing	Fat and overweight people
6	Growth and development enhancing	Hypogenetic children
7	Anoxia tolerance enhancing	People under anoxic circumstances
8	Auxiliary protection from the irradiation hazard	People in contact with irradiation
9	Auxiliary blood lipid lowering	People with higher blood lipid content
10	Auxiliary blood sugar lowering	People with higher blood sugar content
11	Sleep improving	People with bad sleep
12	Malnourished anemia improving	People with malnourished anemia
13	Auxiliary protection from the chemical injury of liver	People in potential danger of chemical injury of liver
14	Lactation stimulating	Women in lactation
15	Eyesight fatigue relieving	People with easy-to-fatigue eyesight
16	Stimulating the lead expelling	People in contact with lead-polluted environment
17	Pharynx improving and clearing	People whose pharynx with discomfort
18	Auxiliary blood pressure lowering	People with higher blood pressure
19	Bone density increasing	Middle-aged and aged people
20	Intestinal microorganism regulating	People with inordinate intestinal functions
21	Digestion enhancing	Cacogastric people
22	Intestinal constipation purging	People with constipation
23	Auxiliary protection of stomach mucous membrane	People with light stomach mucous membrane injury
24	Acne dispelling	People with acne
25	Chloasma dispelling	People with chloasma
26	Skin moisture improving	People with dry skin
27	Skin lipid and oil improving	People whose skin lack of oil and lipid

promulgated Food Safety and Standards Act (FSSA) whereby the criteria for defining the category mentioned above include the following:

i. Foods specially formulated and processed to satisfy particular physical or physiological condition and/or specific diseases and disorders.
ii. The composition of such foods differs significantly from the composition of ordinary foods of comparable nature, if such ordinary food exists.
iii. Such foods may be formulated in the form of powders, granules, tablets, capsules, liquids, jelly, and other dosage forms but not parenterals, and are meant for oral administration.
iv. Only health benefit and promotional claims are allowed for such foods.
v. Such foods do not include drugs, Ayurveda or Unani medicines (AUM) and Ayurvedic proprietary medicine (APM) as defined by Indian Drugs & Cosmetics Act (D&C Act).

However, the strategy it seems to have adopted is similar to DSHEA (USA) which in turn linked to an open society where a consumer is left to make inform choices, whereas India is not at a free society and its citizens would have more benefited by an approach similar to that of Japan or EU, when it comes to functional food regulations.

32.4.4   FUNCTIONAL FOOD REGULATION IN INDIA: FUTURE WORK

Functional food regulations, being a new concept for eastern countries, are not so developed in these countries except for Japan.

The basic requirements for which rules are awaited in Indian regulations are as follows:

- Classification for functional foods and dietary supplements based on the intended target use
- Establishment of claims criteria
- Claims classification and authorization keeping in consideration the Indian nutritional need
- List of permitted health claims
- Adoption/reference of codex standards wherever suitable
- Integration of Indian traditional knowledge into the functional food regulatory concept with minimum interface of drugs

32.4.5   FUNCTIONAL FOOD REGULATION AND TRADITIONAL KNOWLEDGE

Many Asian countries are bestowed with different traditional systems such as Ayurveda in India and Sri Lanka, Chinese Traditional Medicine, Unani System of Medicine, and Nepalese traditional system of medicines. Ayurveda is a Sanskrit word derived from two roots, "ayu" and "ved," meaning science of life. It is known that there are four vedas (treatises) in India namely Rig Veda, Sama Veda, Yajur Veda, and Atharva Veda. Ayurveda is a part of these fourth vedas, and is considered as equivalent to a fifth veda, which includes detailed dissertations on philosophies of body, mind, spirit and senses, and health, and also describes diseases and methods for the treatment of the sick using mantras, herbs, and potions. Ayurvedic medicine is based on the principle that every individual person has a unique constitution that is related to energies within the body.[12]

Indian D&C Act 1940 defines Ayurvedic drugs and APM[*] and states that such medicines should be compliant with the recipes documented in 57 official texts recognized under the act. These are prepared as per recipes given in texts and standards for identity, purity, and strength as given in the editions of *Ayurvedic Pharmacopoeia of India* (API).[13] Also, with the introduction of *Indian Pharmacopeia* (IP) 2010[14] and an initiative to include herbal monographs in IP 2007, there appears to be a brighter future for traditional knowledge. Eighty-nine monographs for herbs used in India for centuries have already been included in IP 2010. In addition, for meeting the need of current industrial demand; herbal extracts and finished products (tablets, capsules, and dietary supplements) have been asked to give equivalent importance with that of crude herbal drugs; emphasis was also suggested for the process for the herbal extracts and finished products pharmacopoeia. Very likely, IP Botanical Reference Substance (BRS) as well as Phytochemical Reference Substance (PRS) will also be included in the pharmacopoeia. IP herbal monographs will be of only regulatory structure and are aimed in providing quality standards with as much as possible objectively accessible test methods. Inclusion of monograph in IP does not mean that the ingredient is approved as a drug/dietary supplement by the Indian government.[15] Ayurvedic treatises have a clear approach, for diet, diet as medicine, and medicines. It has recognized that the diet can be used as a food and as medicines under specific circumstances and thus functional foods were always a part of Indian culture. However, with the development of food technology over the centuries, functional foods became popular, though in a different manner and are primarily regulated under food law of the countries.

The Indian FSSA has sections that restrict AUM[†] (with specific mention as defined by Indian D&C Act 1940) to be marketed as functional food in India.[16] Regulators may have taken this route that all those formulations known in Ayurveda for preventive prophylactic or therapeutic use cannot

---

[*] Ayurvedic Proprietary medicines.
[†] Ayurveda, Unani medicines.

be marketed as functional food in India, for various reasons, including the much publicized policy of Indian government to promote the traditional medicines systems and their products coming from the Ayurveda, Unani, and Siddha systems and their products. This position would be counterproductive to prevent innovations of Ayurvedic knowledge/recipes with huge history of safe use as "food" to be made available to consumers as a supplement for maintaining health. The Indian regulations should be principled on the regulatory concept for functional food and "the intention of use" of functional food/food constituent to dictate the category to which it would fit. It would best be left to the marketer to decide under which regulations the product is marketed, as long as the concerned standards are adhered to.

Although one may wish to provide such products in traditional dosage forms and market them as traditional medicines, others may wish to provide them in modern formats including food formats (tea, biscuits, chocolates, soups, savories, etc.), which would otherwise not be allowed in the traditional medicines licensing systems. These two formats and marketing routes would have different ways of informing and influencing consumers to use the products.

An example for taking a decision on where a product fits is well explained in the US FDA's Guidance to Industry for Botanical Drugs (see Figure 32.2).[17]

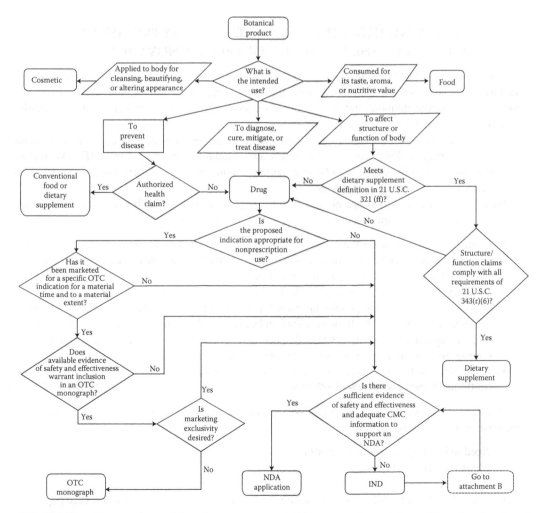

FIGURE 32.2 Schematic representation of the US approach for deciding the category of a plant-based ingredient.

However, such an approach cannot accommodate multicomponent herbal, medicinal plant-based ingredients or a combination of vitamins and minerals with botanicals, which may be expected to work on more than one target or one organ in the body simultaneously.

Another example which demonstrates the reform, is the change in regulation in many countries on the way vegetable oils used as cooking medium were regulated. In many countries, including India, in the 1990s, vegetable oils such as peanut, olive, corn, palm, and rice bran oils were allowed to be marketed as a single oil pack; it was a taboo and even declared as adulteration if anyone blended two oils in any proportion. Vegetable Oil Products (Control) Order, 1947 and Vegetable Oil Products (Standards of Quality) Order, 1975 regulations were applicable.[18] Supply of mixed oils driven by an objective to obtain higher profits by blending economic oil with costlier oil were seen as noncompliance and were defined as adulteration under these orders. However, a huge amount of emerging scientific information on nutrition value of vegetable oils, knowledge of proportions of unsaturated fatty acids (saturated fatty acid (SFA), poly-unsaturated fatty acid (PUFA), and mono unsaturated fatty acid (MUFA)), and their association with benefits to lipid profile and heart health poured in over the years. This led to major reforms in the regulations in the cooking medium and fat nutrition resulting in regulations that positively promoted blending of oils.[19] In fact, the American Heart Association has actually recommended blends[20] that are good for heart and general health.

32.5 INFLUENCING CREATION OF NEW REGULATORY PROVISIONS THAT OPEN UP THE POSSIBILITY OF LARGE INNOVATIONS

Most of the reforms that have emerged in the last decade and half globally are cases of the changing scenario of consumers wanting to move to maintain health, regulators wishing to move from the drug domain to the health domain, and sociopolitical domains changes brought out by many including industry and scientists.

One can see yet another such change in India with the proposed draft regulations that are being worked out to bring out Provisions in Food Safety and Standards Authority of India (FSSAI) regulations that would permit, under stipulated conditions, innovations of Ayurveda–Siddha–Unani—ingredients to be marketed as supplements.[21]

Such influencing processes are not easy, and do not occur overnight. It needs lots of patience; preparedness and many aspects play specific roles. Some of them are

- Is the proposed change good for overall industry or for any one sector/section or likely to exclude one sector/section—more so in developing countries where protection to medium- and small-scale industries is part of the policy?
- What are the safety/affordability implications?
- Who is making the proposal—an industry or scientific community or Civil Society representatives or trade body or necessitated because of the happenings in the market from existing regulations or Global change that needs the country's regulations to change, or is the change likely to create monopoly or is the change likely to create a trade barrier, and so on?
- Is the proposed change likely to alter drastically the bioavailability or not good for the traditionally processed materials?

One needs to prepare to open up regulations, and to create new markets. The dossiers justifications and case prepared do the following:

- Need to be crisp/focused/to the point.
- Think well before volunteering information.
- Executive summaries will be helpful.
- Make the reviewer's job easy by attaching all referenced material copies to the case papers. (Do not expect the reviewers/official to be able to data mine and see the supporting materials. Make their work easy and decision making will be faster.)

- In many cases, it may be good to even provide draft of the change in "the particular directive/provision/regulations clearly pointing out what is the present wording, and what terms/clauses to be changed to read what."
- While going for such meetings with officials be prepared to meet all exigencies—questions that may come up, responses that would be needed, make a "statement in one line what change is requested in what to making full presentations that has been prepared."
- "Brevity thy name is effectiveness" is the mantra for effective meetings with officials.
- It is best to submit the full representations after the personal hearing/meeting, by including queries raised and responses given.

32.6 EMERGING NEED FOR DEVELOPING SKILLS AND COMPETENCIES IN REGULATORY AFFAIRS PERSONNEL

There is thus an emerging need for developing personnel to operate and lead in regulatory affairs. Mapping the skills and competencies needed is the first step. A good scientist, who has an aptitude in legal matters, is the first criteria. Comprehension, analytical ability, ability to read in between the lines, efficient data mining, capability, good vocabulary and vocal presentation skills, and scientific writing skills are some of them. Knowledge of food technology/product developments/category, and so on can be the domain knowledge, but domain knowledge can be always given by training. Most of the regulatory affairs personnel in the foods and beverages field are "those who developed themselves due to their interest and passion to do such work," whereas in pharmaceutical industry they are taught many regulatory aspects systematically, including the auditing process.

32.7 SUMMARY

Functional food is an emerging area providing options for exploring the science of functional ingredients and thus the functional foods. Different terminologies such as functional foods, nutraceuticals, dietary supplements, and health supplements primarily refer to processed foods containing ingredients that aid specific body functions, in addition to being nutritious. Different countries have taken different approaches to regulate functional foods. Japan has developed a concept of FHC under which FOSHU are placed and a well-regulated mechanism for their categorization, approval for FOSHU seal, and claims substantiation is established governed by MHLW Japan. In the United States, the principle regulation for functional foods (Dietary Supplements) is under DSHEA, though Nutrition Labeling & Education Act (NLEA) also plays a significant role. Another well-regulated market for functional foods exists in EU whereby EFSA has provided its scientific opinion on nutrient profiling, claims authorization, and application procedure for functional foods. India being a new entry to functional food regulations is still in its infancy but with the introduction of recent new food law called FSSA, a separate category for functional foods has been created whereby AUM and APM formulations are explicitly excluded from the functional foods domain. It is likely that in future, Indian functional food regulations may include references from CODEX, EU regulation, Canada, the United States (DSHEA), and Japanese FOHSU system. If evaluated closely, the concept of functional food does not appear new to many of the Asian countries such as China, Japan, Malaysia, Nepal, and Pakistan where they have rich ancient knowledge of traditional therapeutic systems such as Ayurveda, Traditional Chinese Medicines, and so on and many of the food and nonfood functional ingredients have been recommended in these systems since ages. These traditional systems have defined approaches to use food as diet as well as "food as medicine," especially for maintaining health of a healthy individual. However, almost all the existing regulatory structure for functional foods does not give due consideration to the traditional knowledge, whereas these offer high potentials to come up with newer natural actives to deliver vitality. The regulatory structure for functional food regulations is not yet harmonized across the globe, and there is a need to understand the regulatory requirement of different countries. It is a fact that a single functional food may vary widely across countries; for example, a single product may be labeled and sold as Dietary Supplement in the United States, and as FOSHU in Japan, and as a Proprietary Food or an AUM or APM in India.

There is also a need to develop suitable strategies and structures to create regulatory affairs personnel who can guide taking the innovations effectively to market.

There is nothing like good or bad regulations, terms that many innovators use often. All regulations are aimed at protecting the consumers first, and then to promote innovations, make consumer friendly, convenient, enjoyable, effective, and useful products, which make the claims that are genuine and nonmisleading. To that extent, the regulators will always look at science and technology to guide them in making a decision. Most regulators are also open to change, but often they need to be convinced that it is good for all, and does not benefit only a few. It is for the scientists, industry, researchers, and innovators to justify any regulatory needs and changes demanded.

Unlike the common belief and accusations that regulations hinder innovations, "regulations actually drive innovations and in turn drive business." *It is what and how you see the regulations and how you work to shape them.*

REFERENCES

1. P.K. Dave, 1998; personal communication, Natures Formulary, USA.
2. US Food and Drug Administration; 2005; Guidance for Industry: A Dietary Supplement Labeling Guide; report available at http://vm.cfsan.fda.gov/~dms/dslg-toc.html.
3. http://www.codexalimentarius.net/web/index_en.jsp.
4. D. Dunkan, Unilever, Europe, in an internal meeting.
5. Drug Price Competition and Patent Term Restoration Act, Public Law 98-417, 1984 United States federal law.
6. R-US Food and Drug Administration; 2005; Guidance for Industry: A Dietary Supplement Labeling Guide; available at http://vm.cfsan.fda.gov/~dms/dslg-toc.html.
7. R-Website of Japanese Ministry of Health, Labor & Welfare; available at http://www/mhlw.go.jp/english/foodsafety/fhc/index.html; accessed on March 27, 2008.
8. EFSA; Scientific Opinion of the Panel on Dietetic Products, Nutrition and Allergies; 2008; The setting of nutrient profiles for Foods Bearing Nutrition & Health Claims Pursuant to Article 4 of the Regulation (EC No 1924/2006); *The EFSA Journal* 644, 1–44.
9. EFSA opinion of the Scientific Panel on Dietetic Products, Nutrition & Allergies; 2007; Scientific and Technical Guidance for the preparation and presentation of the application for authorization of a health claim; *The EFSA Journal* 530, 1–44.
10. Republic of China, SFDA website http://www.sda.gov.cn/eng/.
11. Food Safety and Standards Act, Government of India, 2006; available at http://www.fssai.gov.in/; Sec 22(1).
12. Drugs & Cosmetic Act, 1940, Government of India, Ministry of Health & Family Welfare; Sec 3(a) and G. Warrier and D. Gunawant, 1997; *The Complete Illustrated Guide to Ayurveda: The Ancient Healing Tradition*; Elements Books Limited, UK, 12–18.
13. Ayurvedic Pharmacopeia of India, Ministry of Health & Family Welfare, Government of India, 8 Volumes, latest vol. 8, 2011.
14. Indian Pharmacopeia, Ministry of Health & Family Welfare, Government of India, 2010; Vol. I Chapter—Notices 9–14., and section on herbs and herbal products.
15. Indian Pharmacopeia, Ministry of Health & Family Welfare, Government of India, 2010; Vol. I Chapter—Notices 9–14.
16. Food Safety and Standards Act, Government of India, 2006; available at http://www.fssai.gov.in/; Sec 22(1).
17. US FDA Guidance to Industry for use of botanical ingredients; available at http://www.fda.gov/cder/guidance/index.htm.

18. Vegetable Oil Products (Control) Order, 1947 and Vegetable Oil Products (Standards of Quality) Order, 1975, Government of India.
19. Blended Edible Vegetable Oils Grading and Marking Rules, Government of India Gazette Notification, GSR NO, vide G.S.R. 657(E); dated 29/10/91.
20. AHA Guidelines; available at http://www.lowfatlifestyle.com/lifestyle_diets/ahaguidelines.htm.
21. Draft Regulations on Functional Foods for Consultations, FICCI website http://cifti.org/working-groups.php.

33 Nano-Functional Foods
Nanotechnology, Nutritional Engineering, and Nutritionally Reductive Food Marketing

Gyorgy Scrinis and Kristen Lyons

CONTENTS

Over the past decade, a new range of nutrients and other food components have come to be celebrated for their claimed health benefits, such as omega-3 fats, vitamin D, plant sterols, antioxidants, and other bioactive compounds. Food manufacturers have responded by finding ways to add these newly fetishized nutrients to food products. This new wave of *nutritionally engineered foods* have come to be categorized as "functional foods," a designation that is in part intended to distinguish these products from earlier types of nutritionally engineered foods, such as fat-reduced and vitamin-fortified products. Proponents of functional foods claim that they offer more targeted health benefits, and are able to not merely restore nutrient balance in one's diet but to also deliver an "enhanced" state of health and optimized bodily functioning.

The development of this latest range of nutritionally engineered foods has in part been enabled by the development of new food-processing technologies, including new chemical technologies, biotechnologies, and most recently nanotechnologies. The addition of nano-scale nutrients and other food components, the use of nano-scale encapsulation techniques, and the nano-scale reformulation of food materials offers a range of new possibilities for manufacturing foods with altered nutrient profiles. This chapter outlines some of the applications of nanotechnology in the production of functional foods, and critically evaluates the nutrition and health claims of such nutritionally engineered food products.

33.1 DEFINING FUNCTIONAL FOODS: HEALTH CLAIMS, NUTRITIONAL ENGINEERING, AND FOOD PROCESSING

While the term "functional foods" has been in use since the early 1990s, it remains poorly defined (Scrinis 2008b, 2012). The widely quoted definition in the "European Consensus Document" prepared by the International Life Sciences Institute (ILSI) states:

A food can be regarded as "functional" if it is satisfactorily demonstrated to affect beneficially one or more target functions in the body, beyond adequate nutritional effects, in a way that is relevant to either an improved state of health and well-being and/or reduction of risk of disease (Diplock et al. 1999).

In their position paper on functional foods, the American Dietetic Association (ADA) argues that

... all foods as functional at some physiological level because they provide nutrients or other substances that furnish energy, sustain growth, or maintain/repair vital processes. However, functional foods move *beyond necessity* to provide *additional health benefits* that may reduce disease risk and/or promote optimal health (ADA 2009).

These and many other definitions have a number of common characteristics. They often refer to the "targeting" of particular bodily functions; to the "enhancement" of bodily health; and to the way these foods provide more than just "basic nutrients" (Doyon and Labrecque 2008).

Despite these attempts to offer precise and rigorous definitions, the distinction between functional foods and other foods—that is, nonfunctional, conventional, or everyday foods—is not very clearly drawn. For example, many definitions emphasize that functional foods are those that are claimed to enhance particular bodily processes or functions. However, with few exceptions, all foods contain at least one nutrient or component which can be claimed to benefit or enhance a particular bodily process or function. In this sense, all foods are "functional," thereby rendering the term meaningless. Even a sugary breakfast cereal containing added vitamin D could be claimed to be a functional food.

Although it is not always explicit, these definitions seem intended to favor the inclusion of foods whose nutrient profile has been deliberately modified or engineered in some way, rather than to unprocessed whole foods. Those definitions that emphasize the need to go "beyond" the mere provision of "basic nutrients," and to provide a "functional" dose of beneficial nutrients, are skewed toward such nutritionally engineered processed foods. Simply meeting one's adequate nutrient intake by eating a well-balanced whole-food diet does not—these definitions imply—provide the "additional health benefits" that functional foods are meant to confer, such as reduced disease risk.

Instead of attempting to define the intrinsic healthful properties of functional foods, a perhaps more accurate and less contentious definition of functional foods is those foods that are advertised with health claims (Katan and De Roos 2004; Nestle 2007). Whether or not these foods are "functional," they can be described as *functionally marketed foods*, in that they tend to either make direct health claims or else implied health claims via the use of nutrient-content claims (Scrinis 2008b). The ability to advertise nutrient-content and health claims drives much of the research and innovation associated with functional foods, and this in turn promotes the development of new techniques for modifying the nutrient profile and adding beneficial nutrients to foods.

33.2 NANO-ENGINEERED FOODS

Nanotechnologies are tools for manipulating and constructing materials and organisms at a scale of 100 nm or less, or at the level of molecules and atoms. In the realm of food processing and packaging, nanotechnologies create new possibilities for transforming foods, ingredients, and packaging materials at the nano-scale. There are a number of types of functional nanostructures that can be used "as building blocks to create novel structures and introduce new functionalities into foods" (Sekhon 2010: p.3). These include nanoliposomes, nano-emulsions, nanoparticles, and nanofibers. The three main categories of engineered nanomaterials found in food products are inorganic, surface functionalized materials, and organic engineered nanomaterials (Sekhon 2010).

These nano-scale materials may enhance the types of processing already being carried out at the molecular and cellular levels, and thereby facilitate the production of relatively cheap processed foods. They also enable the introduction or enhancement of particular properties of a food, such as its durability, taste, texture, or nutritional characteristics. Nano-food innovations may create the potential for a new round of productivity increases, efficiency gains, and cost savings. An example is the use of nano-sized food additives that accelerate the processing of industrial sausages and cured meats (Friends of the Earth 2008). Nanotechnologies may also enable new innovations in taste and texture in order to increase the palatability of processed food products. For example, a process for engineering ingredients by targeting specific taste receptors is being developed, which may minimize the bitter taste of some additives or reduce the quantities of additives required (Anonymous 2006).

The ability to manipulate foods at the nano-scale also provides new possibilities for engineering the nutrient profile and characteristics of foods. While there are already a range of techniques for introducing or removing nutrients and components into foods, there are a number of limitations with existing techniques. Some nutrients are not easily incorporated into foods; they may be sensitive to damage or deterioration, such as through exposure to oxygen, light, and temperature extremes or fluctuations or they may affect the color, smell, and taste of the food product (Robinson and Morrison 2009). Nanotechnology can be used to overcome some of these limitations, while also opening up new possibilities. This includes the fortification of foods with nano-scale nutrients and other food components that may enhance their bioavailability; the nano-encapsulation of food components added to foods; and the transformation of the nano-scale properties of foods to enable a reduction of supposedly "detrimental" nutrients such as fats or excess calories.

The reduction in size of existing nutrients and food components from the micro- to the nano-scale may enhance their bioavailability and rate of absorption into the body. In doing so, the use of nano-scale nutrients may either increase nutrient levels in the body for a given quantity of additives or else enable food companies to use less of these food components and to thereby achieve cost savings. A major area of research is in the use of nanomaterials as delivery mechanisms for nutrients, particularly in the form of nano-encapsulated nutrients. Micro-encapsulated nutrients are already being used in food products, but nano-encapsulation offers a number of advantages, such as improved tolerance, longer shelf-life, and more controlled and targeted delivery of nutrients within the body. Nano-encapsulated nutrients may be more easily dispersed within water-based products, and offer improved stability and bioavailability. For example, nano-encapsulated CoQ10 may offer a sevenfold increase in intestinal uptake when delivered via nano-dispersions, compared with traditional powder formulations (Sekhon 2010). Other applications are the nano-encapsulation of lipids to limit oxidation and nano-encapsulated fish oils to enhance the bioavailability, stability, and transparency of these oils (Sekhon 2010; Zimet and Livney 2009).

The use of nano-structured materials to modify the texture and taste of foods is another approach being harnessed by food manufacturers as a means of facilitating the nutritional modification of a food. One application is the development of low-fat ice creams, mayonnaise, and spreads with nano-structured food ingredients that are able to reproduce the creamy taste and texture of full-fat products (Chaudhry et al. 2008; Sekhon 2010).

The ability to manipulate food materials at the nano-scale may also enable the development of "smart" or "interactive" functional food products able to more precisely target or release nutrients in particular circumstances. Chen and Shahidi describe the promise of more personalized and targeted food products:

> ... advances in nanotechnology may lead to multifunctional nanoscale nutraceutical delivery systems that can simultaneously detect and recognize the appropriate location, analyze the local and global needs, decide whether or how much of the payload should be released and monitor the response for feedback (Chen and Shahidi 2006).

While it may be many years before such applications are realized and commercialized, such promises currently play a role in promoting of nano-food innovation. By generating such hopeful and futuristic visions, these promised applications are also a means for overcoming any emerging consumer concerns over the health and safety risks associated with the use of nano-scale ingredients in foods (Scrinis and Lyons 2010).

33.3 CLAIMED HEALTH BENEFITS AND POTENTIAL HEALTH RISKS OF NANO-FUNCTIONAL FOODS

Nano-engineered ingredients and foods can be understood as being highly processed, in that they involve processing and reconstituting foods and ingredients at the molecular level. Yet, by using these same techniques to tinker with the nutrient profile of foods, they are also able—within the terms of the dominant nutritional paradigm—to be positioned as healthful and health enhancing. They do so by essentially concealing or distracting attention from their technologically reconstituted character. The added nano-scale components may be applied to foods that are minimally processed, such as the addition of components to milk or plain yoghurt, or to refined-extracted food and beverages, such as orange juice. But they are just as likely to be applied to poor quality and highly processed foods and beverages, such as snack bars or sugary breakfast cereals.

As with all nutritionally engineered foods, the claimed health benefits of these kinds of nano-functional foods will in most cases be based on the assumption that adding or subtracting single nutrients or ingredients to foods will significantly enhance a consumers' health in some way. This *nutritionally reductive* understanding of the relationship between nutrients, foods, and health is a central feature of the *nutritionism paradigm* that has been dominant within nutrition science research, dietary guidelines, and food engineering and marketing practices (Scrinis 2008a). One characteristic of nutritionism is that individual nutrients, as well as individual foods, are *decontextualized*, in the sense of being taken out of the context of the foods and dietary patterns in which they are embedded. The reductive focus on, and interpretation of, single nutrients ignores the interactions and synergies that may occur between nutrients found within the matrix of whole foods (Jacobs and Tapsell 2007). The role of single nutrients, and of the single foods in which these nutrients are embedded, also tend to be *exaggerated*, in that these single nutrients and foods are claimed to have a significant role in changing health outcomes regardless of the broader eating patterns an individual consumes.

Food scientists and manufacturers take this reductive *understanding* of food a step further when they translate it into nutritionally engineered food products. When single nutrients are more or less arbitrarily added to a food, any claimed health benefits of this nutritional modification assumes that—as with nutritional supplements—these single nutrients act in isolation from the other nutrients and foods with which they are consumed. The use of nutrient-content claims and health claims on food labels is similarly based on the assumption that consuming more or less of single nutrients confers health benefits, with labeling regulations typically ignoring the nutrient profile or the overall quality of the foods in which they are embedded. Single nutrient claims may give a food product a "health halo" or enhanced nutritional aura that may conceal the quality of a product and its ingredients (Roe et al. 1999; Wansick 2006).

This reductive interpretation of the claimed beneficial or detrimental effects of a single nutrient has been most evident in the now-discredited low-fat campaign that dominated dietary guidelines in the 1980s and 1990s. Consuming low-fat or reduced-fat foods was promoted by nutrition experts as reducing the risk of heart disease, cancer, diabetes, and obesity. The science underpinning these claims was itself relatively flimsy (Willett 2009), yet it was translated into definitive and precise dietary guidance, such as the recommendation to reduce fat to below 30% of total calories. The food industry in turn easily exploited this reductive understanding of fat by successfully marketing any low-fat or reduced-fat food as inherently healthy, or at least healthier than their full-fat counterparts, regardless of the overall quality of the food.

The nano-engineering of the nutrient profile of foods is based upon, and reinforces, this nutritionally reductive scientific understanding and marketing of nutrients and food. Nanotechnology is at present largely being used to continue this engineering of single nutrients into and out of foods.

The significance of this technological innovation is in part that it greatly expands the possibilities of the type of nutrients with which foods are fortified, as well as the types of foods in which they are embedded. Nano-food applications also enable food manufacturers to better respond to the contemporary demand for more targeted and personalized diets and nutritional products.

The very techniques and materials that are used to confer these claimed health benefits are, however, also the subject of intense scientific and regulatory concerns regarding their safety. Both the type of materials being used to produce nano-engineered food components and additives, and the nano-scale of these food components may pose health risks. An FAO/WHO expert panel on nanotechnology and food concluded that the reduced size of nanomaterials "results in novel features that are determined by the high surface-to-volume ratio, which may also give rise to altered toxicity profiles" (FAO/WHO 2010). Yet, few nanoparticles have been evaluated for their potential toxicity (Das et al. 2009). Some engineered nanoparticles may increase the production of oxyradicals, and that may in turn "lead to inflammatory reactions and oxidative damage to the cell" (Tran and Chaudhry 2010). Nanoparticles may also have the ability to penetrate the gut wall and to cross natural barriers, such as the cellular, blood–brain, placenta, and blood–milk barriers (Tran and Chaudhry 2010). Pustzai and Bardocz note that there is evidence that nanoparticle-size titanium oxide and silicone dioxide are cytotoxic, yet they are already being added to food products and have GRAS (generally recognized as safe) approval by the U.S. Food and Drug Administration (Pustzai and Bardocz 2006).

Despite these health and safety concerns, and the paucity of studies examining their effects, a range of nano-scale materials may already be in use in food products (Friends of the Earth 2008). However, regulatory institutions around the world have been slow to address the new safety and regulatory challenges posed by nano-foods. At present, food regulation frameworks generally do not acknowledge the distinction between micro- and nano-scale food ingredients or additives, particularly in cases where they may have a similar molecular structure (Gergely et al. 2011). Despite the novel nature of nano-scale food components, in many cases, these food components may not fall within the regulation of "novel foods" that exist in countries and regions such as the European Union and Australia (Gergely et al. 2011).

At present it is not clear how many or what types of nano-foods—foods produced using nanotechnologies or containing engineered nano-scale ingredients—have been commercialized. A 2008 report by Friends of the Earth claimed that several hundred products containing nanoparticles in their ingredients or in packaging had already been commercialized around the world (Gergely et al. 2011). At present there is also an absence of labeling requirements for nano-foods, in the sense that the presence of engineered nanomaterials or nano-reconstituted ingredients does not need to be declared on the food label. The lack of a precise and shared definition of nanoparticles and materials would make labeling a challenge (Rollin et al. 2010).

33.4   FROM GM FOODS TO NANO-FOODS

The technological manipulation of food is now generally viewed by the public with suspicion. Healthy foods have become synonymous with whole foods and minimally processed foods. A problem for the nano-food industry is in convincing the public that nano-functional foods are both safe and health enhancing. Food companies seem willing to market the health benefits of nutritionally engineered foods, but less willing to disclose the use of nanotechnologies or nanomaterials in their production. However, this lack of disclosure may exacerbate public unease and mistrust of novel food technologies, as it has in the case of genetically modified foods.

A recurring theme in the nanotechnology and nano-food literature has been the need to "avoid the mistakes" and "learn the lessons" of the GM food controversy (David and Thompson 2008). The GM food controversy has been characterized by a strong and long-running opposition by consumer groups, farming groups, and environmental organizations in many countries. This opposition has been based on a range of concerns, including the health risks of consumption of GM foods, adverse environmental impacts of GM crops, and the corporate ownership and control of GM seeds (Schurman and Munro 2010). For the food industry and governments, "learning the lessons" may simply mean finding ways to prevent a similar recurrence of public opposition, rather than engaging with this range of concerns. Some civil society groups, such as Friends of the Earth Australia, have already called for a moratorium on the release of all products of nanotechnology, including nano-foods (Friends of the Earth 2008; Miller and Scrinis 2011).

With the development of nano-food ingredients and processing techniques still in its early stages, and the threat of public resistance and bad publicity, many large food companies, such as McDonald's and Kraft, have taken the extraordinary step of making public announcements that they are not currently using the products of nanotechnology in their foods or food packaging (Kraft 2011; McDonald's 2011). It is a sign of the success of the anti-GM foods campaign that companies are now extremely cautious when it comes to adopting potentially controversial, "risky," or unpopular technological innovations (Blay-Palmer 2008). The marketing success of nano-functional foods can not yet be taken for granted. It may depend on the building of trust in the safety of nano-scale engineering of foods and food components, backed by a rigorous safety testing, regulatory, and food labeling regime. But it will also rely on the continued dominance and uncritical acceptance of a nutritionally reductive understanding of the health benefits of nutritionally engineered foods.

REFERENCES

American Dietetic Association (ADA). 2009. Position of the American Dietetic Association: Functional foods. *Journal of the American Dietetic Association*, 109(4), 735–46.

Anonymous. 2006. Flavor firm uses nanotechnology for new ingredient solutions, *Food Navigator*, www.foodnavigator-usa.com/news/ng.asp?n-flavor-firm-uses, accessed 27 March 2009.

Blay-Palmer, A. 2008, *Food Fears: From Industrial to Sustainable Food Systems* (Hampshire: Ashgate).

Chaudhry, Q. et al. 2008, Applications and implications of nanotechnologies for the food sector, *Food Additives and Contaminants*, 25(3), 215–8.

Chen, H. and Shahidi, F. 2006, Nanotechnology in nutraceuticals and functional foods, *Food Technology*, March, 30–6.

Das, M., Saxena, N., and Dwivedi, P. 2009, Emerging trends of nanoparticles application in food technology: Safety paradigms, *Nanotoxicology*, 3(1), 10–8.

David, K. and Thompson, P. (eds.) 2008, *What Can Nanotechnology Learn from Biotechnology? Social and Ethical Lessons for Nanoscience from the Debate over Agri-Food Biotechnology and GMOs* (Burlington, MA: Academic Press).

Diplock, A.T., Aggett, P.J., Ashwell, M. et al. 1999, Scientific concepts of functional foods in Europe: Concensus document, *British Journal of Nutrition*, 81(4), S1–S27.

Doyon, M. and Labrecque, J. 2008, Functional foods: A conceptual definition, *British Food Journal*, 110(11), 1133–49.

FAO/WHO. 2010, *FAO/WHO Expert Meeting on the Application of Nanotechnologies in the Food and Agriculture Sectors: Potential Food Safety Implications: Meeting Report* (Rome: FAO/WHO).

Friends of the Earth. 2008, *Out of the Laboratory and on to Our Plates: Nanotechnology in Food and Agriculture* (Friends of the Earth, Australia).

Gergely, A., Chaudhry, Q., and Bowman, B.A. 2011, Regulatory perspectives on nanotechnologies in foods and contact materials, in G. Hodge, D. Bowman, and A. Maynard (eds.), *International Handbook on Regulating Nanotechnologies* (Cheltenham, UK: Edward Elgar).

Jacobs, D. and Tapsell, L. 2007, Food, not nutrients, is the fundamental unit in nutrition, *Nutrition Reviews*, 65(10), 439–50.

Katan, M.B. and De Roos, N. 2004, Promises and problems of functional foods, *Critical Reviews in Food Science and Nutrition*, 44, 369–77.

Kraft. 2011, http://www.kraftfoodscompany.com/deliciousworld/food-safety-quality/nanotech.aspx.

McDonald's. 2011, http://www.aboutmcdonalds.com/mcd/csr/about/sustainable_supply/product_safety/anti-biotics_and_animal_cloning.html.

Miller, G. and Scrinis, G. 2011, The role of NGOs in governing nanotechnologies: Challenging the "benefits versus risks" framing of nanotech innovation, in G. Hodge, B.A. Bowman, and A. Maynard (eds.), *International Handbook on Regulating Nanotechnologies* (Cheltenham, UK: Edward Elgar).

Nestle, M. 2007, *Food Politics: How the Food Industry Influences Nutrition and Health* (2nd edn.; Berkeley: University of California Press).

Pustzai, A. and Bardocz, S. 2006, The future of nanotechnology in food science and nutrition: Can science predict its safety?, in G. Hunt and M. Mehta (eds.), *Nanotechnology Risk, Ethics and Law* (London: Earthscan).

Robinson, D. and Morrison, M. 2009, *Nanotechnology Developments for the Agrifood Sector—Report of the ObservatoryNANO* (www.observatorynano.eu).

Roe, B., Levy, A., and Derby, B. 1999, The impact of health claims on consumer serach and product evaluation outcomes: Results from FDA experimental data, *Journal of Public Policy & Marketing*, 18(1), 89–105.

Rollin, F., Kennedy, J., and Wills, J. 2010, Consumers and new food technologies, *Trends in Food Science and Technology*, 22(2–3), 99–111.

Schurman, R. and Munro, W. 2010, *Fighting for the Future of Food: Activists versus Agribusiness in the Struggle over Biotechnology* (London: University of Minnesota Press).

Scrinis, G. 2008a, On the ideology of nutritionism, *Gastronomica*, 8(1), 39–48.

Scrinis, G. 2008b, Functional foods or functionally-marketed foods: A critique of, and alternatives to, the category of functional foods, *Public Health Nutrition*, 11(5), 541–5.

Scrinis, G. 2012. Nutritionism and functional foods, in D. Kaplan, (ed.), *The Philosophy of Food* (Berkeley: University of California Press), pp. 269–91.

Scrinis, G. and Lyons, K. 2010, Nanotechnology and the techno-corporate agri-food paradigm, in G. Lawrence, K. Lyons, and T. Wallington (eds.), *Food Security, Nutrition and Sustainability* (London: Earthscan), pp. 252–70.

Sekhon, B. 2010, Food nanotechnology—An overview, *Nanotechnology, Science and Applications*, 3, 1–15.

Tran, L. and Chaudhry, Q. 2010, Engineered nanoparticles and food: An assessment of exposure and hazard, in Q. Chaudhry, L. Castle, and R. Watkins (eds.), *Nanotechnologies in Food* (Cambridge, UK: Royal Society of Chemistry).

Wansick, B. 2006, *Mindless Eating: Why We Eat More than We Think* (New York: Bantam Books).

Willett, W.C. 2009, Nutrition recommendations for the general population: Where is the science?, in C.S. Mantzoros (ed.), *Nutrition and Metabolism: Underlying Mechanisms and Clinical Consequences* (Totowa, New Jersey: Humana Press).

Zimet, P. and Livney, Y. 2009, Beta-lactoglobulin and its nanocomplexes with pectin as vehicles for w-3 polynsaturated fatty acids, *Food Hydrocolloids*, 23, 1120–6.

34 Sustainability of Local Food Production

A Review on Energy and Environmental Perspectives

Sumita Ghosh

CONTENTS

34.1 INTRODUCTION

The world's food demand will continue to escalate substantially with the population growth of an additional 2.7 billion people by 2050 (UNEP 2009, p. 6), generating a significant pressure on our future food supply. In recent years, "food" has become a very important topic of debate and media discussions and has gained significant interests across multiple disciplines in research and practice. Consideration of food now extends to a wider domain and reflects human–nature relationships for improved sustainability. Food connects to social (equitable food access, community and household participation, good nutrition, and public health problems, e.g., obesity), cultural (traditional food growing and cuisine, food places, and eating experiences), environmental (impact of different diets, energy consumption, greenhouse gas emissions, spatial distributions of food outlets), and economic (financial investment, local economy, and employment generation) implications (Wolf et al. 2003; Heller and Keoleian 2003; Wallgren 2006; Daniels et al. 2008; Hartman Group 2008; Garnett 2011). The five main trends of global food consumption patterns are changed in diets, roles of retail shops and supermarkets for food, branding and advertising, growth of organic food sales, and eating out (Daniels et al. 2008). Fast food and slow food are two important areas of food cultures. While the fast food relates to the conventional food supply system, the slow food links to alternative or localized food production systems. "Globalization process has facilitated the distribution of food products to different parts of the world" and can also be seen "as a delocalization of food supply" (Wallgren 2006, p. 234). On the other hand, globalization has strengthened local food connections and has initiated the rise of food localism or supports for alternative food networks.

"Alternative food networks (AFNs) are commonly defined by attributes such as the spatial proximity between farmers and consumers, the existence of retail venues such as farmers markets, community-supported agriculture (CSA) and a commitment to sustainable food production and consumption" (Jarosz 2008, p. 231).

The key components of alternative food systems are short food supply chains (SFSCs), social embeddedness, quality of the produce, and defensive localism. The defensive localism argues for the greater importance of local compared to quality from ecological and environmental sustainability perspectives (Daniels et al. 2008). Localism could be defined as a phenomenon where people value traditional, healthy, and fresh local foods such as vegetables, meat, dairy, and so on that are organically produced in small farms, community, allotments, and home gardens within a region or nearby neighborhoods or in their own backyards. The consumers buy the products directly from the producers in the farmers' markets, box systems, and other outlets to assist in the local economic growth. The SFSC minimizes the number of nodes between primary production and final consumer, reduces food miles, and facilitates direct marketing and contacts between producers and consumers. Provision of local foods in cooperative stores, community food box schemes, local farmers markets, and others such as community-supported agriculture (CSA) could help in developing more sustainable food supply systems. Community-supported agriculture programs connect producers and consumers directly and develop a shorter food supply chain. Marsden et al. (2000) identified three types of local food supply chains. First, within a "spatially proximate" SFSC, the food products are sold through local outlets in the region and the consumer has higher local knowledge about the product supply chain (Marsden et al. 2000 as quoted in Daniels et al. 2008). Second, in "spatially extended" SFSCs, products are sold through the Internet located outside the region and the consumer may have limited knowledge of the area of production (Daniels et al. 2008, p. 161). Third, in "face-to-face" SFSCs, consumers directly purchase a product from the producer (Ilbery and Maye 2005, p. 334). In the first case, the consumers are aware about the processes in the food chain and therefore the sustainability of the food chain is high. This is comparatively less in the second case as the consumers are unaware of ecological and environmental costs of that production. In the third type, the direct communication helps to build and reconnect the producers to consumers. While the fast food relates to standardized and commercial food supply system, the slow food links to alternative or localized food production systems with shorter food supply chains. The social embeddedness of slow food as alternative food network incorporates vital economic qualities (e.g., price and market potential) and social relations that could significantly influence sustainable behavior and practices (Ilbery and Maye 2005, p. 334).

Community gardens, home or domestic gardens, and allotment gardens as small local food-producing spaces are intrinsically linked to alternative or localized sustainable food systems. A National Gardening Association, USA (2009) survey report indicates that 58% of the households grow their own food to get better-tasting food, 54% to save food expenditure, 51% for better quality, and 48% for safe food. Out of a total of 33 million households in the United States, 91% have food gardens at home; 5% share gardens with friends, neighbors, and family; and 3% have gardening spaces in community gardens (National Gardening Association 2009). Community gardens are generally defined as cooperative enterprises which can provide the space, resources, and low investment opportunities for people to grow food locally, develop social networks, initiate community education, create sustainability awareness, provide recreation, and improve public health and local environmental qualities (Lawson 2005; Australian City Farms and Community Gardens Network 2011). Land ownerships in community gardens could vary from local authority public land (often as part of a park), to semiprivate land, like school grounds, to private community gardens such as those run by churches and community organizations, and land areas are leased to people for food production. Allotments are very similar to community gardens, but land is held either by a local authority or by government organizations. Small areas of land are leased to people as allotment holders for local food production. In Germany, the government leased 200–400 m^2 of garden plots as allotments to the people (Drescher 2001). A home or domestic garden is commonly defined as a space other than a dwelling in a residential parcel or subdivision (Smith et al. 2005; Loram et al. 2008). The home gardens differ from community gardens in terms of their ownership, mode of operation, land cover patterns, and social performance (Ghosh 2010).

Vegetables are important parts of our daily diet. The World Health Organization (WHO) recommends a daily intake of five servings of vegetables for getting adequate nutrition (WHO 2003). In Australia, the Commonwealth Scientific and Industrial Research Organisation's (CSIRO) "Total Wellbeing Diet" suggests a daily intake of 400 g or 4–5 servings of vegetables from four groups: starchy (e.g., potato); orange yellow (e.g., carrots and pumpkin); dark green leafy (e.g., cabbage, spinach, and broccoli), and other vegetables (e.g., peas, green beans, lettuce, and zucchini) (CSIRO 2011). Nutrition obtained from vegetables as a part of daily diet has clear links to improved public health. Inadequate consumption of vegetables could lead to cardiovascular diseases, micronutrient deficiencies, hypertension, anemia, premature delivery, low birth weight, obesity, diabetes, and cerebrovascular disease, and lowers the risk of some cancers by 30–40% (WHO 1990 and WCRF 1997 as quoted in Pederson and Robertson 2001).

A Ministry of Health survey in New Zealand (1999) analyzed some of the difficulties in eating vegetables as an important part of the diet. Out of all the survey participants, 18% of the surveyed males and 16% of the females cited the reason for not eating vegetables being that they did not always have vegetables available at home. Out of all the difficulties considered for this survey, 12% of the males and 9% of the females reported the difficulties of storing vegetables for a long time (Ministry of Health, New Zealand 1999). The vegetables that are produced in the backyards are easily available and could be eaten fresh after picking them from the gardens. Heim et al. (2011) conducted a pilot study on four to sixth grade children (using a parental reporting method through pre-post surveys) to understand the interventions of "The Delicious and Nutritious Garden" in their home food environments in south eastern Minnesota in the United States. Almost 99% of the parents reported that the children enjoyed the food-growing activities very much and engaged themselves very well in planting and growing fruits and vegetables in the gardens. The participation promoted positive attitudes in children to eat fresh and nutritious fruits and vegetables in their daily diets that were grown by them in their gardens (Heim et al. 2011). The WHO and Food and Agriculture Organization of the United Nations (FAO) are collaboratively developing a fruit and vegetable promotion initiative. In this program, part of the objectives are to promote a complete supply chain focus, possible small-scale food production, and improve access to fresh food and vegetables (WHO 2003).

This chapter aims to analyze and synthesize research focusing on community and home gardens as local food production sites to identify their potential for improved sustainability performance and barriers to sustainable local food production and supply. As vegetables are very important in the daily diet and one of the most common household produce, this chapter also focuses on exploring environmental sustainability perspectives of growing vegetables in community and home gardens. It does not include discussions on fruit, meat, and dairy production in these local food production sites and also does not include discussions on commercially produced vegetables in larger agricultural farms. This chapter reviews the present potential of human settlements to accommodate local food production. This review offers an alternative perspective that seeks to comprehend whether human settlements could be retrofitted with on-site provisions for growing their own food for households in the future.

34.2 BARRIERS TO SUSTAINABLE LOCAL FOOD PRODUCTION AND SUPPLY

34.2.1 POPULATION GROWTH AND LAND AVAILABILITY

Population growth and land availability are two important factors that will significantly impact the food demand and production in the future. By 2030, two-thirds of the world's population will be living in urban areas (Population Reference Bureau 2011). Urbanization will be one of the important reasons for the loss of productive land. Wolf et al. (2003) calculated that with the application of a "high external input system of agriculture," in 2050, 55% of the present global agricultural land area would be able to support the future food demand. The remaining 45% of the total land could be utilized for biomass production. But with a "low external input system of agriculture," the total agricultural land area available at a global scale would be required for future food production and no land area would be available for biomass production (Wolf et al. 2003). In the United States, between 1982 and 1992, the total conversion of high-quality farm land to urban or built-up land was 18.5 ha every hour. On the other hand, a significant amount of underutilized land areas are locked in the millions of private outdoor garden spaces, smaller urban spaces, allotments and vacant plots in cities, suburbs, and towns of the world. If these land areas are put to productive use, they could generate a considerable amount of daily food for people, improving food self-sufficiency in the future. The different densities of urban development patterns will also have significant effect on the availability of spaces for growing food as individual and community gardens. These potentials are discussed in the later sections of this chapter. But even if the land is available, specifically in the dense inner cities, there are some issues such as soil contamination and land ownership patterns that could alter the possibilities of local food production.

34.2.2 SOIL CONTAMINATION

Soil contamination in urban areas is a great threat to local food production. Generally, in inner cities, the limited land areas available are mainly brownfield areas. These areas have been previously subjected to other land uses, such as an industrial site, a fuel station, or a mechanical workshop, which have created possibilities for contamination of the land by fuel, chemicals (e.g., pesticides), heavy metals (including lead, zinc, copper, etc.), and other solid and industrial wastes. Local food grown on these sites could absorb these toxic materials from the soil and could impact significantly on the health of those people eating the produce. Although there are different bioremediation methods that can be applied to restore the contaminated land, it is expensive and there is an uncertainty about the success of the remediation methods (Heinegg et al. 2002). This further limits the abilities of the people to appropriately utilize limited inner city land areas for food production.

34.2.3 LAND OWNERSHIP

Land tenure or land ownership also plays a vital role in food production for the cities. With the population growth, the demand for land escalates and the tenure patterns in the cities will have to change to adapt to rising immense challenges and conflicts. As explained later in this chapter, the prospects of biofuel production could impact on the land ownership patterns considerably across the globe and could create immense pressures on future food production. A home garden provides a total flexibility for growing food as land is held under individual ownership, but depends on personal motivations of the household members. Although a community garden is generally held under a collective ownership, it could provide a better opportunity for community food growing. The FAO identifies that "... for long term improvement, land tenure arrangements for urban food production can be addressed in a land policy that recognizes and provides for urban agriculture" (FAO 2011a: 1). This highlights the significance of the protection of productive land in urban areas of the world. This should be provided through urban planning instruments such as zoning and regulations. The land tenure should be restructured and managed through retrospective tools such as spatial imagery for sustainable development. This FAO study also recommends developing regulations for rooftop gardens and the establishment of individual and collective garden spaces for food growing (FAO 2011a).

34.2.4 Biofuels and Food Production

To reduce fossil fuel use and greenhouse gas emissions, biofuels as a component of sustainable renewable energy mix for the future have gained considerable attention. There is an ongoing debate that increasing trends of acquisition of land for producing energy crops or biofuels could create significant shortages of land for food production (The World Bank 2011; Friends of the Earth, Europe 2010; Horst and Vermeylen 2011). The proponents argue that the energy crops facilitate the use of marginal lands and they are only a small part of the total agricultural production. Horst and Vermeylen (2011) highlighted that social impacts of domestic production of biofuel in developed countries are minimal and NGOs undermine ethical aspects of biofuels to a considerable extent. The sustainability implications of this "green" fuel, such as in reducing carbon emissions, need to be considered in policy planning (Horst and Vermeylen 2011).

According to a World Bank (2011) report, in 2008, the total estimated land area for biofuel production was 36 million hectares and by 2030, the total land conversion for biofuel production would range between 18 and 44 million hectares in different countries. The biofuel crops such as soybean, rapeseed, palm oil, and others would hold the major shares of the key commodities grown on these land areas and would mainly affect sub-Saharan Africa, Latin America, the Caribbean region, and Southeast Asia (The World Bank 2011). Friends of the Earth, Europe (2010) reports similar results. The future demand for biofuel production in Europe is a major driver for "land grabbing" for biofuel production across 11 countries in Africa. This study shows that around 5 million hectares representing one-third of the land sold or acquired in Africa is likely to be used for biofuel production. This would use the fertile food-growing farm land for biofuel production and could create a global-scale problem of land availability for food production. The various systems of property rights in different countries would affect the land ownership patterns in different ways. All these would create conflicts in land ownership patterns between overseas investors and local communities. The influence of biofuel crop production on land use change would extend beyond the boundary of an individual country, creating global impact zones and other critical problems linked to food production. In developing countries mainly, where households produce food for sustenance and livelihoods, with the diminishing availability of farm lands for food production, home and community gardens provide opportunities for growing at least some of their daily food requirements. Good public policy will be essential to optimize the benefits of biofuel production and to achieve meaningful energy efficiency and sustainability targets such as reducing greenhouse gas emissions, protecting biodiversity, and managing food security (Tilman et al. 2009, p. 271).

34.2.5 Food Waste

In rich countries, a significant part of the food that people buy gets wasted as a part of common lifestyle pattern (Waste Resources Action Programme 2009). The total amount of food wasted at home and at food outlets is almost 26% of the total edible food available for consumption (Heller and Keoleian 2003). A United Nations study revealed that one-third of the food produced globally is lost or wasted (Provost 2011) and reducing food losses will have significant impacts in developing countries to improve their food security and livelihoods (FAO 2011b). The *Sydney Morning Herald* newspaper (October 9, 2009), based on a University of Western Sydney research study, reported that householders in Sydney waste more than $600 million worth of fresh food produce annually. This value is almost equivalent to the total income of the farmers in the Sydney metropolitan basin. Sydney residents spent one-third of the total household food expenditure in eating out (Jopson 2009). NSW householders waste 800,000 tonnes of food annually which is equal to 38% of the garbage bin waste, $2.5 billion worth of food per year, and $1000 waste per household. Including business, the total annual food wastage in NSW amounts to over 1.1 million tonnes of food and is higher in the higher income categories (NSW Government 2011). The comparison of food wastage at the regional and state levels in Australia establishes the significance of this issue and the need to reduce food wastage.

The Waste and Resources Action Programme (WRAP) in the United Kingdom estimated that over two-thirds or 68.8% of a total of 566,000 tonnes of food waste produced in Scottish households with costs equivalent to nearly £1 billion pounds in a year at 2008 prices could be avoided with proper planning and management for storage and use. The top five food groups that are thrown away for the reason that they are not used in time include bakery items, fresh vegetables and salads, dairy items (including milk), fresh fruit, and meat and fish. Out of these five items, 38,000 tonnes of fresh vegetables worth £67 million and 28,000 tonnes of fresh fruits worth £54 million are thrown away annually (WRAP 2009). Garnett (2007) had found an interesting connection between wastage and refrigeration of food.

Garnett (2007) distinguished between "reducing refrigeration energy use" and "reducing refrigeration dependence." The former could be achieved using improved technologies and management practices. The latter requires change in lifestyles and food choices such as depending less on food such as meat and dairy which requires prolonged refrigeration.

The household food waste as organic waste goes to landfill sites generating landfill gas such as methane. In order to tackle the growing issue of household food wastage, the NSW government in partnership with North Sydney Council formulated a "Love Food Hate Waste" program. Other partners in this program are Woolworths, one of the large supermarket chains, Australian Food and Grocery Council, and the Local Government and Shires Associations of NSW. This program emphasizes the need for planning weekly meals, considering serving sizes, checking the fridge before preparing shopping lists, using leftover foods, and appropriate storages for effective utilization (NSW Government 2011). It will be important to develop a sustainable behavioral pattern. Comparatively, the food grown on individual, community, and allotment gardens are seasonal and flows through a relatively shorter food chain; therefore, the chances of food waste are greatly reduced. The food grown in backyards could be consumed within the house and in this case, the producer transforms into a consumer. Thus, more transparent relations and connections are generated between food, producer, and consumer (Kneafsey et al. 2008) which can contribute immensely toward better sustainability performance.

34.2.6 WATER AND FERTILIZER

Availability of water as a resource is vital for local food production. The Metropolitan Water Plan (MWP) 2006 for Sydney outdoor and indoor water demand categorizes water uses in the home and shows that 23% of all household consumption of water is used for lawns and gardening (New South Wales Government 2006, p. 68). During the growing season, the water requirements for vegetable gardens in Mississippi, USA is about 1 in. or 2.5 cm of water per week or 630 gallons per 1000 sq. ft. (Mississippi State University 2010). This water is usually sourced through rain water, gray water harvesting, or irrigation, and the potential for supplying water also varies with the different rainfall patterns in different climatic regions of the earth. Using effective watering systems such as drip irrigation system and gray water (e.g., from kitchen) could also reduce the overall water usage (Straw 2009). It is also possible to harvest adequate water from alternative sources, such as rain water. Ghosh and Head (2009) in a study two traditional and contemporary residential areas in Australian suburbs and found that using harvested rain water from the building roofs and storing them in rain tanks for garden uses could help to achieve 63–135% self-sufficiency in supplying water demand at a neighborhood level. Social research has identified that people adapt to informal water gathering practices such as the "bucket in the shower" (Head and Muir 2007b) to save water for use in the garden which may include water savings for food production. Water savings for vegetable growing is achievable, knowing the critical watering periods for different types of vegetables and mulching. Planting in blocks instead of rows and knowing soil types on which the vegetables are grown could be very useful (Straw 2009).

Fertilizers such as nitrogen (N), phosphorus (P), and potassium (K), or others supply important micronutrients for food production and their reserves in the earth are finite too (Dawson and Hilton 2011). Most fertilizers are used in commercial food production. As community and home gardens focus on producing food using organic fertilizers obtained through composting methods, the discussions on barriers of nonavailability of commercial fertilizers such as phosphorus and others in food production are not included in this chapter.

The barriers to producing and supplying local food in future are interconnected and significant areas of overlap exist. The land tenure relates to changing land ownership patterns by land grabbing for biofuel production across the globe, affecting land availability for future food production. On the contrary, biofuel production is likely to assist in cleaner energy fuel for transport, reducing transport emissions. Food waste is linked to energy use and GHG emissions from landfill sites and food security issues. It will be essential to explore and evaluate these interlinkages comprehensively to understand and to determine strategies for overcoming the barriers to local food production for sustainability.

34.3 LOCAL FOOD PRODUCTION IN HUMAN SETTLEMENTS

34.3.1 LOCAL FOOD AND SPATIAL SCALE

Local food production will play a vital role in feeding our future communities in town, cities, and remote areas. Geographies of scale play an important role in understanding spatial distribution of food networks and systems. Peters et al. (2009) identified a "foodshed" as that extent of a geographic area from which a population gets its all food supply. "The food shed concept reconstructs the geography of food systems by compelling social and political decisions on food to be orientated within specific delineated spaces" (Feagon 2007, p. 26). The food shed concept links to local food very well as it analyzes the connections between producers and the consumers in a local food supply chain. Research has identified the potential extent of the influence zone or food shed of a local food system. A survey by the Hartman Group (2008) in the United States reveals that consumers' understanding of buying local food could extend the geographic boundary of local food production sources for people up to a 100 miles distance and links to consumers' "diverse connotations depending on place, culture and lifestyle" (Hartman Group 2008). These consumers included 50% of the respondents of all consumers surveyed (Hartman Group 2008). Koc (1999) identifies that a wider food system view could effectively analyze multilayered interconnections in terms of social, economic, environmental, health, power, access, and equity at different spatial scales (e.g., household, neighborhood, municipal, regional, national, and global).

Recently, there are increasing examples of applications of Geographic Information Systems (GIS) in understanding spatial distributions of fast food outlets and Internet or web mapping in estimating local productive capacities in different countries and neighborhoods. A good access to healthy food outlets within a catchment area selling food at lower prices for low-income communities is significantly important for the better health in communities (NSW Government 2009). A study by Kwate et al. (2009) using GIS spatially mapped distributions of fast food outlets in New York, USA reveals that socioeconomic variables correlate with fast food density patterns. Locating high-energy fast food retailers, especially in the poorer communities, increases the rates of obesity immensely. "Your Food Environment Atlas" developed by the United States Department of Agriculture (USDA) and Economic Research Service provides a geospatial tool for mapping various social, economic, health, access, physical activity, taxes, insecurity, and other relevant variables linked to household food as indicators of food environments across various states in the United States. Local food as one of the mapping themes included mapping further subcategories such as numbers, percentages, and per capita direct sales from local farms (2007), total and per 1000 population numbers of farmers markets (2009, 2010), total vegetables and per 1000 population harvested (2007), and farm to school program data (USDA and Economic Research Service 2011). In

Melbourne, Australia, Victorian Eco Innovation Lab (VEIL) (2011) has created an online VEIL Food Map that records data on quantity and different types of local food produced within Melbourne in a database for informed policy making and spatially represents the data at neighborhood and city scales. These upcoming applications of online mapping using GIS in local food research will generate meaningful platforms for visualizing current and potential future local food production and distribution patterns and will generate significant community and individual awareness for growing food sustainably.

34.3.2 LOCAL FOOD PRODUCTION IN FEEDING CITIES: A REVIEW

Growing food in human settlements is not a new concept and is a very common activity as evidences support. In 1999, London could produce approximately 232,000 tonnes of fruit and vegetables from allotment gardens and it was calculated using a productive capacity of land at 10.7 tonnes per hectare (Garnett 1999). This would supply 18% of their daily intake considering WHO recommendations for five portions of daily intake of fruits and vegetables (Garnett 1999). An Ipsos-Reid poll in 2002 on behalf of City Farmer, Canada's Office of Urban Agriculture, found that in the Greater Vancouver area, 44% of people live in households that produce some of their own food locally (City Farmer 2002). Home-produced food made up 28% of the income of the residents in cities of the former Soviet Republic of Georgia. In Romania that increased from 25% to 37% between 1989 and 1994 and 47% of urban residents of Bulgaria were self-reliant in fruit and vegetables (Pederson and Robertson 2001). Singapore produces around 25% of its locally consumed vegetables while in China, Shanghai produces 60% and Hong Kong produces 45% of their vegetables within the city boundaries (RUAF Foundation 2011). In Havana, Cuba, 90% of the fresh produce consumed is grown in and around the city (Companioni et al. 2002).

The FAO recently (June 10, 2011) reported that FAO's urban horticulture program conducted in the five main cities of the Democratic Republic of Congo has helped urban growers produce annually a total of 330,000 tonnes of vegetables equivalent to a market value of over $400 million dollars. This program has generated 28.6 kg of vegetables annually for each city dweller, increased individual daily intake of micronutrients by eating greens, created 60,000 jobs, supplied fresh nutritional food to 11.5 million people, and thus improved enormously the food security issues in Congo (FAO 2011c). Pederson and Robertson (2001) informs that in 1997, Poland produced 500,000 tonnes of vegetables and fruits, one-sixth of the national consumption, in 8000 council gardens. Currently, over 26,000 gardens cover 2439 ha in Havana, producing 25,000 tonnes of local food annually, and 40% of households are involved in urban agriculture (Kisner 2008). Cuba had met the goal of having more than 15 houses self-sufficient in household food production in every settlement in 2002. Using unique gardening practices such as organopónicos or raised bed containers filled with nutrient-rich compost on poor soil or asphalt in urban settings, intense vegetable production has been achieved. In Cuba, by 2003, farmers had converted over 300,000 backyard patios to gardens and is expected to rise to half a million in the future (Kisner 2008) (Table 34.1).

Research shows that the residential garden spaces are the largest single land use type in an urban area. Mapping land use using GIS shows that 36% of the total urban area in Dunedin, New Zealand (Mathieu et al. 2007:179) and approximately 33% of the urban area with a mean area of 151 m^2 per garden of the city of Sheffield, UK (Gaston et al. 2005) are used as domestic residential garden spaces. Garden sizes are important as larger gardens support a variety of land covers, therefore larger areas of vegetable patches than the smaller-size gardens (Smith et al. 2005). Local food production has environmental benefits of improving soil stability, infiltration capacity and biodiversity, stormwater management, and reducing urban heat island effects in dense urban areas (Ghosh et al. 2008). In 2009, the median area of food garden was 96 sq. ft. per household in the United States (National Gardening Association, USA 2009). An Australian Bureau of Statistics (ABS) survey on home production of food in 1992 estimated that the Australian backyard grew on average 70.4 kg vegetables (ABS 1992). Ho's 48 m^2 demonstration vegetable garden in Mangere, Auckland grew

TABLE 34.1
Community Food Growing Spaces—Some Examples

Location	Management, Descriptions, and Outcomes
Seattle, Washington	P-Patch Community Garden Program
	In total 60 community gardens, 1900 plots on 12 acres of land, cultivated by 4600 gardeners
	Out of 60 gardens, three CSA programs and public housing residents use 19 community gardens. In 2000, the CSA generated $30,000 in produce sales from 150 subscribers, supplied vegetables to 40 growers' household and each family received $500 for the year
Portland, Oregon	Parks and Recreation Department, Portland
	30 community gardens with 3000 people participation
	47 public school gardens, 11 farmers markets
	19 CSA's programs for job training
	A 13-acre site for public school students for education program in Portland State University, community gardens grow over half million dollars of produce each year
Toronto, Ontario, Canada	Department of Parks and Recreation
	Annex Organics provides funding for new community gardens
	More than 100 community gardens, 3000 plots on 4500 participants
	Number of gardens increased from 50 to 122 gardens between 1991 and 2001
	6–10 new gardens per year
Montreal, Qubec, Canada	CSA network, more than 100 community gardens, more than 8000 plots, more than 10,000 gardener, 77 peri urban farms
	Collective gardens for food security
Vancouver, Canada	18 gardens, 950 plots, 16–24 school gardens
	More than 1500 gardeners
Waterloo, Canada	25 community gardens with a total of 679 plots, 38% of Waterloo residents grow some part of their own food locally
Berlin, Germany	934 allotment gardens contain 77,526 small plots covering a land area of ~3064 ha, small 200–400 m² garden plots for food production
Auckland Region, New Zealand	23 community gardens, managed by community groups and local councils
Melbourne, Australia	17 community gardens
Sydney, Australia	23 community gardens, Sydney Metropolitan area, sizes from very small with a few square meters to over 60 m²

Sources: Adapted from Kaethler T. M., 2006. *Growing Space: The Potential for Urban Agriculture in the City of Vancouver, Canada:* School of Community and Regional Planning, University of British Columbia; Australian City Farm and Communities Garden Network, 2011; Bartolomei, L., Judd, B., and Thompson, S. 2003. *A Bountiful Harvest: Community Gardens and Neighbourhood Renewal in Waterloo.* Sydney: University of New South Wales; Drescher A. W. 2001. The German Allotment Gardens—A Model for Poverty Alleviation and Food Security in Southern African Cities? *Proceedings of the Sub-Regional Expert Meeting on Urban Horticulture,* Stellenbosch, South Africa, January 15–19, 2001, FAO/University of Stellenbosch; Senate Department for Urban Development, Germany. 2011. Allotment gardens: Data and facts. http://www.stadtentwicklung.berlin.de/umwelt/stadtgruen/kleingaerten/en/daten_fakten/index.shtml (accessed on June 15, 2011); Ecomatters Environmental Trust. 2011. Community gardens in the Auckland region. http://ecomatters.org.nz/community/community-gardens-in-the-auckland-region (accessed on June 12, 2011).

285.2 kg of vegetables from December 1999 to December 2000 annually (Ho 2001). Under the Biodiversity in Urban Gardens in Sheffield (BUGS) project, a total sample of 267 domestic rear gardens in five U.K. cities (Belfast (North Ireland), Cardiff (Wales), Edinburgh (Scotland), Leicester (England), and Oxford (England)) revealed that 20.2% of all land use types in rear gardens were vegetable patches (Loram et al. 2008). A study on backyards in Australia (Sydney, Wollongong, and Alice Springs) found that vegetables and/or herbs were grown in 52% of the 265 backyards studied

(Head and Muir 2007a, p. 90). Kortright's (2007) interviews with 125 residents and gardeners in Toronto in two contrasting neighborhoods revealed that in these 23 home gardens, 27 different types of vegetables and 16 types of herbs were grown. Tomatoes were one of the most common vegetables grown in 87% of the gardens (Kortright 2007). Within a multicultural landscape, cultural identities are reflected in growing traditional and culturally appropriate fruits and vegetables as food in backyards (Head and Muir 2007a).

Media reports support the growing interests of people in local food production. An article in the *New York Times* (June 11, 2008) indicates that Garden Writers Association's annual national consumer telephone survey for a period of 5 years identified that vegetables contribute as one of the main shares of garden expenses (Burros 2008). This is further supported by two horticulture companies, W. Atlee Burpee Company and Harris Seeds in the United States, whose sales of vegetable and herb seeds and plants are up by 40% in 2007, which is double the annual growth in the last 5 years. The Harris Seeds noted that vegetables such as peppers, tomatoes, and kitchen herbs which could be grown on smaller urban spaces and containers had the maximum increases in sales. A similar trend was also noticed by the D. Landreth Seed Company. Barbara Melera, the coowner of the company, identified these vegetables as "survival vegetables: peas, beans, corn, beets, carrots, broccoli, kale, spinach, and the lettuces" (Burros 2008).

Rooftop gardens are becoming common as alternative food-growing spaces in cities. In northern Singapore, approximately one-fifth of the total and equal to 212 ha of rooftop areas of apartment and commercial buildings using inorganic hydroponics produce 39,000 tonnes of fresh vegetables annually (Wilson 2005). Another example, at Trent University, Canada, is a vegetable garden on the roof area of the Environmental Sciences building that grows vegetables and supplies them to university restaurants (Blyth and Menagh 2006). Although detailed discussions on roof gardens is beyond the scope of this chapter, these emerging growing spaces for food in human settlements could contribute positively toward improved sustainability.

Due to increasing food prices and also other associated environmental and social factors, there is a significant increase in numbers of households growing their own food, especially vegetables in home and community gardens. A total of 34% of all U.S. households surveyed agreed that the current recession worked as a motivation for growing their own food (National Gardening Association, USA 2009). In 2008, 36 million U.S. households were growing their fruits and vegetables, which is likely to increase by 19% to 43 million households in 2009. It is estimated five million U.S. households would be very interested to have garden spaces in a community garden close to home in the future (National Gardening Association, USA 2009). In a peak oil situation, the current oil reserves of the earth will not be able to supply the fossil fuel demand for transport; hence the options for transporting food from different parts of the world become very limited. Under this circumstance, the future communities would essentially need to become self-sufficient in sourcing food that is being produced within that region. This would replace the present longer food supply chains with much shorter food supply chains and the length of the journey of the food from the farm to the plate would reduce. This would lower the household carbon footprints, improve public health with local supply of fresh produce, increase food accessibility, and promote better social interactions (Winklerprins 2002; Ghosh et al. 2008). The community and home gardens as important sites of sustainable local food production in urban and suburban landscapes could contribute meaningfully in achieving household self-sufficiency and food sustainability in the future.

34.4   LOCAL FOOD AND SUSTAINABILITY

In 1987, the United Nations World Commission on Environment and Development (WCED) or the Brundtland Commission in "Our Common Future" defined "sustainable development" as "... that development that meets the needs of today's generation without compromising the ability of the future generations to meet their own needs" (WECD 1987, p. 43). Agenda 21 is considered as a blueprint of sustainability as it addresses current and future challenges, represents global cooperation and consensus, and provides a framework for promotion of sustainable development (United Nations 2011). While Local Agenda 21 (LA21) sets the context for implementing Agenda 21 at a local level, Local Action 21 further strengthens Local Agenda 21 (LA21) into actions (United Nations 2011).

The system of food production currently is in transition and is influenced by a paradigm shift that highlights the importance of a well-maintained sustainable system over a longer time period (Heller and Keoleian 2003).

"A just and sustainable food system is defined as one in which food production; processing, distribution and consumption are integrated to enhance the environmental, economic, social and nutritional health of a community" (Heller and Keoleian 2003, p. 16).

Within an agro food system, the connections of the food supply chain is important and "the food chain as a whole is the ultimate framework for a scrutiny of sustainability" (Cobb et al. 1999, p. 209 as quoted in Ilbery and Maye 2005). Ilbery and Maye (2005) conducted an analysis on the sustainability of a number of different food supply chains of small and medium enterprises (SMEs) in the Scottish/English borders following Sustain's food sustainability criteria. The results indicate that there is an overlap between conventional and alternative food systems, and hybrid food systems are being generated. Growing vegetables in community and home gardens initiates an informal and alternative production method generating environmentally sustainable food resource (Gaynor 2006). Growing food locally in home and community gardens is important, and positively links to "thinking globally and acting locally" and aligns well with the overall goals of Local Agenda 21 and Local Action 21 (Ghosh et al. 2008).

34.4.1 FOOD ENERGY DEMAND

The dietary energy consumption per person may be defined as the daily quantity of food required to support daily energy demand for an individual or person in a population and is expressed in energy units such as kcal per day (FAO 2010). The FAO data indicates that dietary energy consumption in New Zealand was 3150 kcal per person per day for the period 2003–2005 (FAO 2010). In Australia, average daily per capita food energy demand is 2150 kcal (Haug et al. 2007, p. 674). The FAO estimates dietary energy consumption for different countries depending on the amount of food available for human consumption. Total food demand is relative and could vary depending on food consumption patterns, food availability, personal choices, and sociocultural influences in different countries (FAO 2010). However, the actual food consumption values taking account of food wastage and losses during storage, in preparation, and during cooking may be lower than the dietary energy consumption values based on food availability.

Considering global population sizes in 1990 and 1998, Wolf et al. (2003) calculated three (low, medium, and high) food demand scenarios in grain equivalents for 2050. These diets consider daily caloric intake and daily protein requirements, and differ in composition and expressed in "grain equivalents" for easy comparison (Wolf et al. 2003). "Grain equivalents" is a unit of measure in dry weight in grains and equal values could be calculated for various food items such as cereals, wheat, vegetables, dairy, and meat for different types of diets. They found that a "moderate" conventional diet is nearly 1.8 times and the "affluent" diet is 3.2 times the impact of a vegetarian diet. Pimentel and Pimentel (2003) findings similarly show that a meat-based diet requires higher amounts of land, water, and energy resources to generate than a lactoovovegetarian diet. In a lactoovovegetarian diet, the meat and fish are replaced and their equivalent calories are obtained by increasing eating of other foods.

34.4.2 FOOD MILES AND GREENHOUSE GAS EMISSIONS FROM LOCAL FOOD

Food miles relate to the transport emissions generated by the transportation distances travelled by different food commodities to reach from production sites to the plate and have increased significantly over the years (Halweil 2002; Cairns 2005). Halweil (2002) estimated that a meal sourced through standard food supply system requires 4–17 times more petrol consumption than the meal that comes from local and regional food production sites (Halweil 2002). In the United Kingdom, car trips for food and other household items constitute 40% of all shopping trips. The average numbers of trips for food is 122 per person per year compared to nonfood trips that are only 96 per person per year between 1998 and 2000 (Cairns 2005). In the United Kingdom, 12% of the nation's fuel consumption is food related and is spent on packaging and transporting food (Garnett 1997). In New Zealand, for food transport, 10.5 MJ per kg food per person per day is required. Considering its total population of 3.6 million in 1996, New Zealand would require 39,000 GJ per day for transporting food (Pritchard and Vale 1999:2).

Wallgren (2006) studied 21 producers in Farmers Owned Market at Sodermalm in Sweden to compare transport energy use of local and conventional food distribution systems. The Farmers-Owned Market collected data on the distance traveled from the farm to the marketplace, the fuel consumption per 100 km, vehicle efficiency, and the total quantity of products sold and quantified "energy use per kilogram of sold product." The "transport energy intensity" used as a measure of food transport energy is defined as the energy used to transport 1 kg of the product to the market. The "transport energy intensity" specifically for fruits and vegetables is lower for Farmers-Owned Market (0.2–1.8 MJ/kg) compared with a conventional food distribution system (2.8–7.7 MJ/kg) in Sweden. These values for conventional system could increase up to 50 MJ/kg when the values for airfreights were added. The values also vary between the four different types of products, breads/flours, vegetables/fruits, preserved/honey, and meat/cheese in two different food distribution systems.

Coley et al. (2009) compared carbon emissions in two case studies on food miles: large-scale mass food distribution vegetable box system and customer's travel to an organic farm shop. It considered standard emission factors of diesel, natural gas, and electricity, measured values in only CO_2 units, and excluded soil and animal CO_2 emissions. This research highlighted that if a customer travels more than 7.4 km in the round trip to purchase organic vegetables, then the CO_2 emissions are larger than doorstep food delivery system. This study argues that buying local produce may not lower carbon emissions to contribute effectively to food sustainability. Using "carbon emission per unit of produce over the transport chain" could provide better sustainability measurement than using the concept of food miles in isolation. It is considered, however, much wider than simple fuel use in food transport and should include influence of other factors such as social justice, biodiversity and landscape, and local economies at across cross-disciplinary levels (Coley et al. 2009).

Food accounts between 15% and 28% of all GHG emissions in developed countries (Garnett 2011). The total annual carbon emissions added from the Australian vegetable industry are about 1,047,008 tonnes of CO_2-equivalent (O'Halloran et al. 2008). If all foods are grown within 100 km farm-to-plate travel distance, a 96% reduction in emissions is possible in current food transport emissions in New Zealand (Pritchard and Vale 1999, p. 2). Garnett (2011) argued that producing meat and dairy food could be highly GHG intensive. The rising demand for meat and dairy food coupled with future population growth could outweigh new technological improvements and innovations. This study identified low-GHG food behaviors considering high-, medium-, and low-priority areas. Most of the action areas are targeted to medium-priority behaviors and include actions such as reducing food wastage, eating seasonal food, accepting variability of supply and quality, cooking in an energy-efficient way for more than one person and reducing consumption of food with low nutritional values (e.g., tea and coffee). Eating fewer meat and dairy products and well-balanced healthy food are in high-priority behaviors while using pedestrian modes for travel for shopping is in the low priority (Garnett 2011). Therefore, it is more important to adapt to sustainable food behavior that would allow secured future food supply and would limit energy consumption and emissions within the carrying capacity of earth.

WRAP in the United Kingdom calculated that 3.8 tonnes of CO_2 equivalent emissions are generated from 1 tonne of food waste (Foodwise 2012). Using these values of CO_2 equivalent emissions of food waste, it is calculated that 3,040,000 tonnes of CO_2 equivalent emissions could be generated annually only from household food waste in Sydney in Australia. Local food when consumed daily reduces food waste, does not require prolonged refrigeration and storage, and subsequently could reduce overall food demand. Thus, food produced locally could increase energy efficiency and reduce overall GHG emissions.

Connecting local food production sites to local selling outlets at spatial locations that are easily accessible for community is highly important for providing fresh, healthy, and nutritional food and shortening the overall length of the food supply chain. Sustain (alliance for better food and farming) (http://www.sustainweb.org/) is an environmental campaigning group established in 1999 that represents over 1000 national public interest groups at the international, national, and local levels. The project "Sustainable Food Chains" focuses on sustainable provision and addresses three policy arenas: local food economies, food miles, and public procurements (Daniels et al. 2008). Out of eight, Sustain's four "sustainable food" criteria emphasize the impacts of spatial locations on energy use in the whole of the food chain, importance of healthy food, environmentally beneficial production systems, and better understanding to food-fostering education and knowledge for appropriate food choices (Daniels et al. 2008). If the complex processes of food production, distribution, and consumption are sustainably contained within the geographical boundary of a food shed catchment area, it could provide better energy and environmental solutions. This could improve access and affordability of the low-income residents to eat healthy food regularly if the food is available at comparatively lower prices at the local outlets. These food retail outlets also act as unique sources to provide sustainability education and to generate community awareness. The programs such as "New Seasons Market" in Portland, Oregon, USA showcase how building relationships between local producers such as farmers, fishermen, and customers is really useful (Strategic Alliance for Healthy Food and Activity Environments 2011). "NorthWest Initiative's Food Systems Project" in Lansing, Michigan and "People's Grocery," a food justice group in California, are working toward addressing challenges to improve access to healthy and affordable food communities using innovative strategies (Strategic Alliance for Healthy Food and Activity Environments 2011). "FoodRoutes Network" and "Community Involved in Sustaining Agriculture (CISA)" have produced toolkits for providing harvesting supports for individuals and organizations to promote locally grown food production through a multimedia marketing campaign and includes useful market research information, evaluation tools, and resources (FoodRoutes 2011). In Toronto, Annex Organics, a nonprofit organization runs various local food-growing and distribution programs for improved community access to affordable and nutritious food (Lazarus 2011). All these approaches will strengthen economically viable long-term local food systems.

34.4.3 Local Food and Energy

Energy consumption at various stages of a food system, production, processing, packaging, distribution, and disposal, together could account for a considerable share of energy at the national scale. Life cycle energy may be defined as the total direct and indirect energy required in the production, operation, disposal, and other associated activities over the life cycle of a system. Through a life cycle approach, multilayered linkages of social, economic, and environmental domains can be well understood as it provides a systematic framework for studying the entire spectrum of production to consumption and widens the system boundary (Heller and Keoleian 2003; Edward-Jones 2008). Life cycle energy consumption studies of the conventional U.S. food system have revealed the energy consumption at different stages of the food production and supply chains (Heller and Keoleian 2003; Murray 2005). The total percentages of life cycle food energy expenditures at various stages according to one of these studies are

* Agricultural production (21%)
* Food transport (14%)
* Processing (16%)

- Packaging (7%)
- Food retailing (4%)
- Restaurants and caterers (7%)
- Home refrigeration and preparation (32%) (Murray 2005)

The embodied energy is different from the life cycle energy as it includes only the "upstream" or "frontend" component and does not include the energy required for operation and disposal (Department of the Environment, Water, Heritage and the Arts 2010). Approximately 7.3 units of fossil energy are required primarily to produce one unit of food energy in the United States (Heller and Keoleian 2003, p. 1033).

"The data from Treloar and Fay show an annual figure for the total embodied energy of food and drink in Australia of 42 GJ per person, which can be compared to the recommended average dietary energy requirement of 4.2 GJ per year" (Pritchard and Vale 1999:3).

According to the figures from Pritchard and Vale, the total embodied energy content of food could be almost 10 times the total average dietary energy requirements. The embodied energy of food can be very large when grown off site as it includes food production, processing, transport, storage, and delivery. In contrast, vegetable production in home gardens uses minimal fossil fuel, fertilizers, and pesticides and is normally without the processing needs of commercial vegetable production and therefore reduces household ecological footprints, enhancing sustainability. Any amount of vegetables or food grown locally lowers the embodied energy content of that food as the transport and other needs are greatly reduced.

Wackernagel and Rees (1996) developed ecological footprint as a land-based measure or indicators of sustainability. The "Ecological Footprint" considers that a finite productive land area or water area is needed to generate the energy consumption, material demand, and waste discharge of a human population or economy. Ecological footprint can estimate the amount of biologically productive land and water available per person on the planet that will be needed to sustain human consumption pattern of a population or economy. It provides an equivalent value in land area global hectares (gha) per person (Wackernagel and Rees 1996). The "ecological footprint" has already been applied as one of the comprehensive and effective sustainability measurement method at local, national, and global scales in different parts of the world. Cowell and Parkinson (2003) adopted land area and energy use values as indicators of local food production in the United Kingdom which could link very well to ecological footprint concept and analysis. As the earth's land area has limited resources, this could be used effectively to estimate the food demands of an increasing population in the future. The selection of these two factors as indicators of food production and consumption is justified as they are the two critical attributes of local food production (Cowell and Parkinson 2003).

How much vegetables (in energy units) could be produced locally? A very limited research has been done in this field, estimating the amount of local production of vegetables in home and community gardens and their equivalent energy values in the daily diets for the households. Some studies address these issues for specific regions of the world. Allen (1999) estimated that in the Auckland Region, New Zealand, vegetables that could be produced from a 35 m² garden plot amount to 102.2 kg per 4 months (Allen 1999 quoted in Chhima 2001:149–150) and the total equivalent energy content is 19,921 kcal. This study indicates that out of the total weight of vegetables produced, only a portion of that vegetables are edible for supplying daily food energy demand after discarding the nonedible parts of the produce and varies with the type of vegetables. Assuming no further wastage from vegetables, it is estimated that the edible energy available from the vegetables is 59,763 kcal or 0.25 GJ per year. In general, approximately 1708 kcal of energy from vegetables could be produced per square meter of garden annually (Chhima 2001:150). The New Zealand Nutrition Taskforce (1991) guidelines recommend 3+ servings of vegetables per day in New Zealand (Ministry of Health 1999: 5). Then, a 35 m² vegetable garden is able to produce approximately only 43% of the vegetable requirements (except the embodied energy content) per capita per year (Ghosh 2004). According to

Canada's *Food Guide to Healthy Eating*, the recommendation for vegetables is 3.75 servings per day (British Columbia Ministry of Agriculture and Lands 2011) but in reality, considering actual production, an average Canadian in the British Columbia region could get only 2.91 servings per day (British Columbia Ministry of Agriculture and Lands 2011). The home-grown production of vegetables in British Columbia is estimated to be equal to 1.6 million kilograms. These home-grown vegetables could supply up to 43% of the total annual dietary food energy required from vegetables. This percentage value is very similar to the value that Ghosh (2004) calculated based on data from Allen's study (1999) for a single home vegetable garden of 35 m² at a much smaller spatial scale in Auckland, New Zealand.

In a research study using GIS, the amount of productive land area available for local food production was calculated after subtracting the total land cover areas in buildings and ancillary structures, trees and shrubs, and roads and pathways from the total site area (Figure 34.1). A total of five residential neighborhood case studies at varying physical densities (low, medium, and high) were selected from Auckland, New Zealand (Ghosh 2004; Ghosh et al. 2008). Based on Chhima (2001) and Allen's (1999) research, the energy production from home-grown vegetables (excluding the embodied energy content) is calculated to be equal to 0.007 GJ/m² or 70 GJ/ha annually in Auckland (Ghosh 2004). Vegetables constitute 10% of the total diet in New Zealand (MAF 1995) and requirements per capita are assumed to be equal to 0.58 GJ. The total food energy demand for vegetables is calculated in GJ at a neighborhood level. Based on available productive land areas, the total on-site vegetable production possible at that neighborhood is

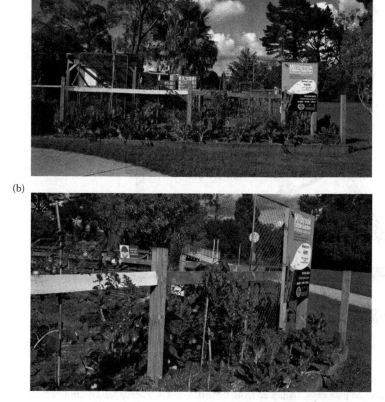

FIGURE 34.1 (a) Millbrook edible garden for people, Henderson, Waitekere City, New Zealand. (b) Common vegetables grown in Millbrook. (Photos by Sumita Ghosh.)

calculated and then the surplus or deficit energy values in producing vegetables on site are also calculated. A GIS-based model for estimating the sustainability potential of growing vegetables in energy and land area units was developed for different residential neighborhoods. This research uses the ecological footprint conversion method to convert estimated energy demand, available energy, and surplus and deficit energy into a household land area measure land area equivalents (LEQ) (ha/household/year), including embodied energy contents of vegetables. It calculates a land-for-energy ratio based on Wackernagel and Rees (1996) and is equal to an average value for New Zealand equal to 135 GJ per hectare (Ghosh 2004; Ghosh et al. 2008) (Figure 34.2).

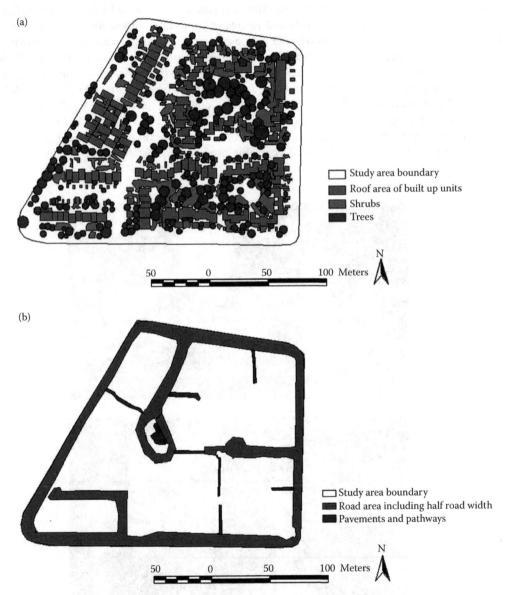

FIGURE 34.2 High-density residential case study in Auckland, New Zealand. (a) Trees, shrubs, and buildings. (b) Roads and pathways. (Adapted from Ghosh, S. 2004. *Simple Sustainability Indicators for Residential Areas of Auckland, New Zealand*. PhD thesis. School of Architecture and Planning, The University of Auckland, New Zealand.)

- The LEQ of total annual household *demand* for vegetables is defined as the household's share of land area in hectares required for growing the total demand for vegetables in an off-site location.
- The LEQ of total *available* annual household vegetables is defined as the household's share of on-site available productive land areas for growing vegetables in hectares.
- The LEQ of total annual household *deficit* or *surplus* for vegetables is the household's share of off-site land area required to generate the remaining part of the total demand for vegetables (Ghosh et al. 2008).

The results indicated that the lower- and medium-density neighborhoods are more self-sufficient and are generating on site surplus amount of vegetables compared to their food demand (Figure 34.3). Positive values of percentages indicate surplus while negative values represent deficits. Out of the five New Zealand case studies, on average, two low-density neighborhoods (Low density 1–10 households/ha and Low density 2–14 households/ha) could generate between 30% and 51% surplus demand of vegetables. One of the medium-density neighbourhood (Medium density 1–18 households/ha) could produce surplus up to 21% while the other neighborhood (Medium density 2–21 households/ha) with 10% deficit and the high density (29 households/ha) with 36% deficit in supplying demand. These two case studies of medium-density neighborhoods are different depending on the on-site available productive land areas. The placement and size of the dwelling, solar orientation or solar access on the plot for vegetable production, subdivision, or plot size, and household size become important in growing vegetable demand for the household.

Following on from this research, this methodology has been applied to "traditional" with older houses and "modern" or contemporary with new and larger houses in Australian suburban neighborhoods (Ghosh and Head 2009). This study tested for both case studies in the first scenario the potential of converting 50% of the total available lawn spaces into productive land areas after keeping aside a minimum of 20 m^2 as mandatory private open space area for each subdivision or parcel as specified by local planning authorities. By utilizing only 50% of the available lawn areas in the gardens, annual household local food (vegetable) production potential of the "traditional" was significantly higher and was equal to 836 kg of vegetables per household while the same for the "modern" is 731 kg of vegetables per household. In the second scenario, an additional 50% of available lawn areas were allocated to vegetable production in addition to the first scenario. The "traditional" neighborhood potential had nearly increased by 34% to 1119 kg per household. On the other hand,

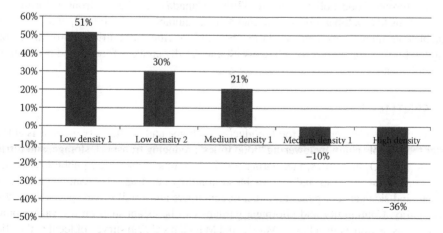

■ Percentage of surplus/deficit vegetable production to total vegetable demand

FIGURE 34.3 Percentage of surplus/deficit vegetable production to total vegetable demand. (Calculated based on data from Ghosh, S. 2004. *Simple Sustainability Indicators for Residential Areas of Auckland, New Zealand*. PhD thesis. School of Architecture and Planning, The University of Auckland, New Zealand.)

as the "modern" with large houses and swimming pools had limited lawn areas to offer for food production, vegetable production capacity remained the same (Ghosh and Head 2009). This study indicates that there are potential land areas available for local food production within the residential areas which could be effectively put to productive use for food.

Today's busy life may not motivate many individuals to make commitments to growing their own food. It is possible if initiatives are undertaken by local authorities to create programs and policies that would help to utilize these land banks for food production by allowing sharing schemes. Blake and Cloutier-Fisher's research (2009) uniquely focused on exploring the benefits and challenges of sharing home or backyard garden spaces and the feasibility of developing partnerships. Due to rapid urbanization, the availability of community gardens becomes limited, as so, this backyard sharing project is seen as alternative option. Results show that it could promote physical activity, psychosocial well-being, and social connectedness between the partners. WinklerPrins (2002) showed that house-lot gardens in Santarém, Pará, Brazil could restore social balances and cohesion through product exchange and could effectively link the urban to the rural.

Local food and sustainable behavior are interconnected as food consumption patterns are shaped by attitudes, cultural practices, lifestyle patterns, and habits. As mentioned in this chapter, Garnett (2011) developed high-, medium-, and low-priority behaviors for reducing GHG emissions. The Department for Environment, Food and Rural Affairs (Defra)'s (2008) report on proenvironmental behavior provides information on evidences on peoples' values, attitudes, and behaviors; categorizes different behavioral patterns into various groups; and identifies potential for behavior change across these different groups. The behavior change areas identified in this report that link to food are reducing food waste, purchasing locally grown seasonal food, using food labels to understand certified foods, and eating foods that have lower environmental impacts (Defra 2008). Also, Garnett (2011) focuses on the similar areas for behavior change. It is interesting to note that these critical areas also need consideration from energy and environment perspectives and signifies the connections between sustainability of food and behavior change.

Local food production policies for community gardens are being formulated by local governments in cities and towns all over the globe, although policies on home gardens are not that common to date. In 1998, Berkeley, California, authorities formulated policies to identify long-term gardening sites and similarly Seattle's 1994 Comprehensive Plan aimed to increase the numbers of community gardens (Wekerle 2002). Auckland City Council, New Zealand and City of Sydney, Australia have already formulated their community gardens policies (Auckland Council 2011, City of Sydney 2011). The Toronto Food Policy Council (TFPC), Canada is in the forefront of formulating food policy and aims to develop a food system that fosters equitable access to food, nutrition, health, and sustainable community development (TFPC 2011). More cities are putting significant emphasis on making food policy for improved public health and for the uptake of local food production within human settlements.

34.5 SYNTHESIS

As reviewed in this chapter, local food production in home and community gardens is able to build a shorter food supply chain by lowering "food miles"; reducing transport, storage, and refrigeration energy use and CO_2 emissions; facilitating physical exercise; improving public health; and could foster critical social networks and sustainable community building. Food can be grown at home in front, rear, and side garden spaces and also in containers and small urban spaces depending upon the availability. Community and allotment gardens can be established on the vacant plots in the inner city areas as well as in suburbs. Martin and Marsden's (1999) survey of local authorities in the United Kingdom emphasized the vital significance of small spaces, such as underused and vacant areas of lands, backyards, and container gardening, for food growing. This could establish and promote a sustainable land use system and could improve household and community food security at different spatial levels. The energy or land equivalent values of amount of produce in these local food production sites could be developed as measures or indicators of self-reliance or self-sufficiency of communities in generating their own food. The urban and suburban neighborhoods could be revitalized with sustainable food and edible landscapes, improved amenity, quality of life, social connectivity, and a new thriving local economy.

34.5.1 KEY TRENDS

The key research trends in understanding sustainability of local food production include the following areas:

- LCA analysis of energy consumption and improvement potential in various stages of a food supply chain
- Comparison of transport emissions of large-scale food versus small-scale food distribution systems
- Energy requirements of producing food for different diets (e.g., vegetarian and meat based)
- Food waste
- Development of local food models for estimating the sustainability potential of growing food in home gardens
- Public health and access (considering socioeconomic variables) issues of growing local foods
- Developing new technologies and food policies for local food production in urban spaces
- Exploring alternative places for local food production (e.g., rooftop gardens, vertical walls) in cities
- Potential for creating a new local economy and employment generation
- Social connectedness, household engagement, and community participation
- Food security issues of growing local food in developed and developing countries

Home gardens are a less explored area of research compared to community gardens. The research on community gardens focuses mainly on vital social capabilities of community gardens to promote sustainability. A limited research has been conducted on energy and emission perspectives of community and home gardens in quantitative terms. Detailed accounting of fruits or vegetables produced in community and home gardens is rarely documented. In some cases, the amount of vegetables produced and the corresponding economic values are recorded. There is very limited research that has recorded the edible portions of the vegetables that were included in the daily food requirements of people. Therefore, the calculations for actual energy potential of these vegetables and connecting this to actual food demand and nutritional values of home-grown food are very difficult to estimate. Also, there exist a number of other research gaps. The production of vegetables is influenced by climate, rainfall patterns, soil characteristics, and personal motivation. It is also not known how much human labor is involved in the process of food production and participation rates. The fossil fuel emissions from transport in making trips to purchase seeds and other essential materials for growing vegetables should be included to estimate the true cost of home gardening. Therefore, some studies question the sustainability of growing local food (DeWeerdt 2011). But it is to be noted that a holistic local food production system would also include different subsystems such as small-scale farms, organic farms, community, home and roof gardens, and others embedded in the overall supply chain. It may be possible that community and home gardens could provide a "niche" to supply sufficient vegetables for household food demand if they used appropriate gardening practices, and they would be able to display excellent sustainability performances. Therefore, future research should assess the capabilities of these subsystems appropriately from energy and environmental perspectives.

34.5.2 FUTURE RESEARCH DIRECTIONS

The energy and environmental implications of growing vegetables as local food in home and community gardens would require focus on the following key future research areas:

- Identification of potential future local food production sites, their spatial distributions, and extent of utilization
- Spatial connectivity of local food production sites and retail outlets and energy flow analysis
- Sustainability performance of various subsystems in a local food supply chain
- Analysis of life cycle energy (LCA) and embodied energy contents of locally produced vegetables
- Community and household participation in growing local food
- Adaptation capabilities of individuals and communities toward sustainable behavior change for food
- Identification of varying local food perspectives and possible case-specific solutions for developed and developing countries
- Appropriate training and guidelines for growing food efficiently in their own gardens
- Innovative solutions and policy development for relocalization of food
- Establishment of best-practice local food production examples as powerful change agents for future food sustainability
- Development of a resilient local food system to withstand impacts of climate change

Food at the "post farm gate stage" has multiple options for achieving improved energy efficiency by using renewable energy, such as solar, biomass, and clean fuels, and reducing resource use through recycling and reuse (Garnett 2011). Further exploratory analysis of the concepts of food miles and of local food systems using case studies and evidence-based research will be able to identify the sustainability parameters that could make meaningful contributions (Coley et al. 2009). A food-shed concept could work as a tool to provide better understanding of flow within a food system and for developing a sustainable framework for the future (Peters et al. 2008, pp. 1–2). It will be beneficial to develop an integrated conceptual sustainability framework for local food production for the community and home gardens in the future. The entire local food production and distribution systems, including that in community and home gardens, are susceptible to unpredictable pressures of extreme weather events and natural disasters (e.g., flood, earthquake, tsunami, and volcanic eruption) some of which could become more frequent in the future. It is essential to understand the critical factors vital for adapting to climate change. The local food system should be resilient to withstand all these challenges and adapt extremely well with changing faces of a dynamic environment to generate a resource-efficient future.

Local food production is a vast and complex area incorporating multidisciplinary fields of science, social science, economics, urban planning and policy, geography, health, and others. It will be necessary to understand the interlinkages in order to comprehend the combined sustainability performance of a local food system. Connecting social, economic, and scientific research to policy and appropriate implementation strategies for community and home gardens will be essential for success. Developing collaborative partnerships between government institutions, private companies, nonprofit organizations, and communities will provide foundations for initiating the local food production. An integrated approach to link local food, energy and environment dimensions, strategic directions, sustainability regulations, local innovations, and political commitments will be fundamental to address future challenges of sustainable local food production.

34.6 CONCLUSIONS

In the face of the world's increasing food demand coupled with population growth, examining the vegetable production potential of community and home gardens offers us a small window of possibilities for addressing issues of sustainable food in the future such as food security and energy efficiency, and reducing environmental impacts of emissions and pollution. The community and home gardens as alternative food networks (AFN) are currently part of a greater global food movement. These local production sites show significant potential and promise for household self-reliance and are coming up noticeably in different parts of the world. The increases in sales of vegetable seeds, growing numbers of gardens in different cities and towns, and peoples' shifting motivations to growing food for combating with increasing food prices establish these facts very well. Within the escalating problems of soil contamination, decreasing availability of productive land, conflicts of land tenure, land grabbing for biofuel production in developing countries, and water scarcity, these small pockets of productive land areas in home and community gardens bring some hope for an innovative food future for humanity.

Vegetable production in these local food production sites reduces transport emissions by reducing garden-to-plate distance enormously, food wastage, and storage. It facilitates direct contacts between the producer and the consumer, enhancing sustainability awareness and knowledge; strengthens social connectedness; and supports localism. Land availability and ownership patterns are important in obtaining a growing space in community gardens. As the land is held under individual ownerships in home gardens, the flexibilities for translating a motivation into reality for growing own food are significantly high. Data on food wastage alerts us about the amount of food produced that goes to landfill as organic waste, producing methane which is 21 times heavier than carbon dioxide, as result of lifestyle patterns. If this food is not wasted, it could improve the global level of food insecurity and sustainability. Vegetables are only a small part of the total diet but their importance cannot be ignored as they link to better health, nutrition, and disease prevention measures. Creating interests among children about growing vegetables in school vegetable gardens, home and community gardens, and other relevant urban, suburban, and rural food production areas will equip the future communities with the knowledge and skills for facing food challenges in a well-prepared manner. It will be important to generate community awareness not only about healthy and local food growing, but also on the importance of appropriate eating patterns and behavior for achieving sustainable food futures. A greater focus on local food production will also create passion for understanding human and nature relations in a resource-constrained future and thus making this planet sustainable for a long-term period.

ACKNOWLEDGMENTS

The author would like to acknowledge the support of all who have provided help for this research. The author would also like to thank anonymous referees for their valuable comments.

REFERENCES

Allen, L. 1999. *Gardening for Kitchen*. B. Arch. thesis Elective Study. School of Architecture. University of Auckland, New Zealand.

Auckland Council. 2011. *Community Gardens Policy*. Auckland, New Zealand. http://www.aucklandcity.govt.nz/council/documents/gardenpolicy/default.asp (accessed on April 30, 2011).

Australian Bureau of Statistics (ABS). 1992. *Home Production of Selected Foodstuffs*. Australia. Canberra: Australian Bureau of Statistics.

Australian City Farms and Community Gardens Network. 2011. Community gardening: Growing food growing community. http://communitygarden.org.au/wp-content/uploads/2009/08/community_gardening.pdf (accessed on February 10, 2011).

Bartolomei, L., Judd, B., and Thompson, S. 2003. *A Bountiful Harvest: Community Gardens and Neighbourhood Renewal in Waterloo*. Sydney: University of New South Wales.

Blake, A., and Cloutier-Fisher, D. 2009. Backyard bounty: Exploring the benefits and challenges of backyard garden sharing projects. *Local Environment* 14(9):797–807.

B.C. Ministry of Agriculture and Lands. 2011. *B.C.'s Food Self-Reliance, Can B.C.'s Farmers Feed Our Growing Population?* British Columbia, Canada. http://www.agf.gov.bc.ca/resmgmt/Food_Self_Reliance/BCFoodSelfReliance_Report.pdf (accessed on June 18, 2011).

Burros, M. 2008. Banking on gardening. *The New York Times*. June 11, 2008.

Blyth, A., and Menagh, L. 2006. *From Rooftop to Restaurant—A University Cafe Fed by a Rooftop Garden*. City Farmer, Canada's Office of Urban Agriculture. http://www.cityfarmer.org/TrentRoof.html (accessed on March 20, 2011).

Cairns, S. 2005. Delivering supermarket shopping: More or less traffic? *Transport Reviews* 25:51–84.

Chhima, D. 2001. *Sustainable Development and Compact Urban Form*. Masters thesis. The University of Auckland, New Zealand.

City Farmer. 2002. City dwellers are growing food in surprising numbers! Canada's Office of Urban Agriculture. http://www.cityfarmer.org/40percent.html (accessed on January 21, 2011)

City of Sydney. 2011. Community gardens policy. http://www.cityofsydney.nsw.gov.au/Residents/ParksAndLeisure/CommunityGardens/CommunityGardensPolicy.asp (accessed on May 29, 2011).

Cobb, D., Dolman, P., and O'Riordan, T. 1999. Interpretations of sustainable agriculture in the UK. *Progress in Human Geography* 23: 209–235.

Coley, D., Howard, M., and Winter, M. 2009. Local food, food miles and carbon emissions: A comparison of farm shop and mass distribution approaches. *Food Policy* 34:150–155.

Common Wealth Scientific and Industrial Research Organisation (CSIRO). 2011. *Fruit and Vegetables and the Total Wellbeing Diet*. Australia: CSIRO. http://www.csiro.au/resources/ps22z.html (accessed March 12, 2011).

Companioni, N. Y. O., Hernandez, E., Paez, and Murphy C. 2002. The growth of urban agriculture. In *Sustainable Agriculture and Resistance: Transforming Food Production in Cuba*, ed. F. Funes, L. García, M. Bourque, N. Peréz, and P. Rosset. pp. 72–89. Oakland, CA: Food First Books.

Cowell S. J., and Parkinson, S. 2003. Localisation of UK food production: An analysis using land area and energy as indicators. *Agriculture, Ecosystems and Environment* 94:221–236.

Daniels, P., Bradshaw, M., Shaw, D., and Sidaway, J. 2008. *An Introduction to Human Geography*. 3rd edition. England: Pearson Education Limited.

Dawson, C. J., and Hilton, J. 2011. Fertiliser availability in a resource-limited world: Production and recycling of nitrogen and phosphorus. *Food Policy* 36:14–22.

Department of the Environment, Water, Heritage and the Arts. 2010. *Chapter 5.2: Embodied Energy in Your Home Technical Manual*. http://www.yourhome.gov.au/technical/pubs/fs52.pdf, (accessed on February 12, 2011).

Department for Environment, Food and Rural Affairs (Defra). 2008. *Promoting Pro-Environmental Behaviours*. UK: Department of Environment, Food and Rural Affairs. http://archive.defra.gov.uk/evidence/social/behaviour/documents/behaviours-jan08-report.pdf (accessed on May 20, 2011).

DeWeerdt, S. 2011. Is Local Food Better? World Watch Magazine, May/June, Volume 22: 3. http://www.worldwatch.org/node/6064 (accessed on September 29, 2011).

Drescher A. W. 2001. The German Allotment Gardens—A Model for Poverty Alleviation and Food Security in Southern African Cities? *Proceedings of the Sub-Regional Expert Meeting on Urban Horticulture*, Stellenbosch, South Africa, January 15–19, 2001, FAO/University of Stellenbosch.

Edwards-Jones, G., Canals, L.M., Hounsome, N., Truninger, M., Koerber, G., Hounsome, B., Cross, P. et al. 2008. Testing the assertion that local food is best: The challenges of an evidence-based approach. *Trends in Food Science & Technology* 19: 265–274.

Ecomatters Environmental Trust. 2011. Community gardens in the Auckland region. http://ecomatters.org.nz/community/community-gardens-in-the-auckland-region (accessed on June 12, 2011).

Feagon, R. 2007. The place of food: Mapping out the "local" in local food systems. *Progress in Human Geography* 31(1):23–42.

Friends of the Earth, Africa and Friends of the Earth, Europe. 2010. *The Scale and Impact of Land Grabbing for Agrofuels*. Friends of the Earth, Europe.

Food and Agriculture Organization of the United Nations (FAO). 2010. Food security statistics: Food consumption—Nutrients—Dietary energy, protein and fat. http://www.fao.org/economic/ess/food-security-statistics/en/ (accessed February 5, 2010).

Food Security in Southern African Cities? *Proceedings of the Sub-Regional Expert Meeting on Urban Horticulture*, Stellenbosch, South Africa, January 15–19, 2001, FAO/University of Stellenbosch, 2001.

Food and Agricultural Organisation of United Nations (FAO). 2011a. Food for cities: Land tenure and food production. FAO Factsheet. ftp://ftp.fao.org/docrep/fao/011/ak003e/ak003e11.pdf (accessed on June 11, 2011).

Food Agriculture Organisation of the United Nations (FAO). 2011b. Global food losses and food waste: Extent, causes and prevention. http://www.fao.org/docrep/014/mb060e/mb060e00.pdf (accessed on June 15, 2012).

Food Agriculture Organisation of the United Nations (FAO). 2011c.Urban horticulture in DRC reaps $400min for small growers: City malnutrition drops as more affordable fruits and vegetables available. http://www.fao.org/news/story/en/item/79813/icode/ (accessed on June 10, 2011).

FoodRoutes Network. 2011. Buy local toolkit. http://www.foodroutes.org/bl_toolkit.jsp (accessed on June 8, 2011).

Foodwise. 2011. Fast facts. http://foodwise.com.au/did-you-know/fast-facts.aspx (accessed on June 15, 2012).

Garnett, T. 1997. Digging for change: The potential of urban food production. *Urban Nature Magazine* 3(2):62–65.

Garnett, T. 1999. *CityHarvest: The Feasibility of Growing More Food in London.* Sustain: The alliance for better food and farming. A National Food Alliance Publication.

Garnett, T. 2007. Food refrigeration: What is the contribution to greenhouse gas emissions and how might emissions be reduced? Food Climate Research Network, University of Surrey, UK.

Garnett, T. 2011. Where are the best opportunities for reducing greenhouse gas emissions in the food system (including the food chain)? *Food Policy* 36:23–32.

Gaston, K. J., Warren, P. H., Thompson, K., and Smith, R. M. 2005. Urban domestic gardens (IV): The extent of the resource and associated features. *Biodiversity and Conservation* 14:3327–3349.

Gaynor, A. 2006. *Harvest of the Suburbs: An Environmental History of Growing Food in Australian Cities.* Crawley, WA: University of Western Australia Press.

Ghosh, S. 2010. Sustainability potential of suburban gardens: Review and new directions. *Australasian Journal of Environmental Management* 17:49–59.

Ghosh, S., and Head, L. 2009. Retrofitting suburban garden: Morphologies and some elements of sustainability potential of two Australian residential suburbs compared. *Australian Geographer* 40(3):319–346.

Ghosh, S., Vale, R. J. D., and Vale. B. A. 2008. Local food production in home gardens: Measuring onsite sustainability potential of residential development. *International Journal of Environment and Sustainable Development (IJESD)* 7(4):430–451.

Ghosh, S. 2004. *Simple Sustainability Indicators for Residential Areas of Auckland, New Zealand.* PhD thesis. School of Architecture and Planning, The University of Auckland, New Zealand.

Hartman Group. 2008. Consumer Understanding of Buying Local. http://www.hartman-group.com/hartbeat/2008-02-27 (accessed on March 20, 2011).

Halweil, B. 2002. *Home Grown: The Case for Local Food in a Global Market.* World Watch Paper 163. World Watch Institute.

Haug, A., Brand-Miller, J. C., Christoperson, O. A., McArthur, J., Fayet, F., and Truswell, S. 2007. A food "lifeboat": Food nutrition considerations in the event of a pandemic or other catastrophe. *Medical Journal of Australia* 187(11/12):674–676.

Heller, M. C., and Keoleian, G. A. 2003. Assessing the sustainability of the US food system: A life cycle perspective. *Agricultural Systems* 76(3):1007–1041.

Head, L., and Muir, P. 2007a. *Backyard.* New South Wales, Australia: University of Wollongong Press.

Head, L., and Muir, P. 2007b. Changing cultures of water in eastern Australian backyard Gardens. *Social and Cultural Geography* 8(6):889–905.

Heim, S., Bauer, K. W., Stang J., and Ireland, M. 2011. Can a community-based intervention improve the home food environment? Parental perspectives of the influence of the delicious and nutritious garden. *Journal of Nutrition Education and Behavior* 43(2):130–134.

Heinegg A., Maragos, P., Mason, E., Rabinowicz, J., Straccini, G., and Walsh, H. 2002. *Soil Contamination and Urban Agriculture, A Practical Guide to Soil Contamination Issues for Individuals and Groups.* Montreal, Quebec, Canada: McGill School of Environment, McGill University.

Ho, S. 2001. *Urban Food Growing and the Sustainability of Cities.* Master thesis. The University of Auckland, New Zealand.

Horst, D. V. D., and Vermeylen, S. 2011. Spatial scale and social impacts of biofuel production. *Biomass and Bioenergy* 35(6):2435–2443.

Ilbery, B., and Maye, D. 2005. Food supply chains and sustainability: Evidence from specialist food producers in the Scottish/English borders. *Land Use Policy* 22:331–344.

Jarosz, L. 2008. The city in the country: Growing alternative food networks in metropolitan areas. *Journal of Rural Studies* 24:231–244.

Jopson, D. 2009. Sydney's $1b rubbish bin. *The Sydney Morning Herald*, October 9, 2009. http://www.smh.com.au/national/sydneys-1b-rubbish-bin-20091008-goz8.html#ixzz1OwdrSVmx (accessed on March 20, 2011).

Kaethler T. M., 2006. *Growing Space: The Potential for Urban Agriculture in the City of Vancouver,* Canada: School of Community and Regional Planning, University of British Columbia.

Kisner, C. 2008. *Green Roofs for Urban Food Security and Environmental Sustainability: Urban Agriculture Case Study: Havana, Cuba.* Washington DC, USA: Climate Change Institute. http://www.climate.org/topics/international-action/urban-agriculture/havana.htm (accessed on 11 February, 2010).

Kneafsey, M., Cox, R., Holloway, L., Venn, L., and Dowler, E. 2008. *Reconnecting Consumers, Producers and Food: Exploring Alternatives*. New York: Berg Publishers.

Koc, M. 1999. *For Hunger-Proof Cities: Sustainable Urban Food Systems*. Ottawa, ON, Canada: IDRC Books.

Kortright, R. 2007. *Edible Backyards: Residential Land Use for Food Production in Toronto*. Master of Arts thesis. University of Toronto, Canada.

Kwate, N. O. A., Yau, C. Y., Loh, J. M., and Williams, D. 2009. Inequality in obesigenic environments: Fast food density in New York City. *Health & Place* 15(1):364–373.

Lawson, L. J. 2005. *City Bountiful: A Century of Community Gardening in America*. Berkeley: University of California Press.

Loram, A., Warren, P. H., and Gaston, K. J. 2008. Urban domestic gardens (XIV): The characteristics of gardens in five cities. *Environmental Management* 42(3):361–376.

Lazarus, C. 2011. Innovation and experimentation: Annex organics/field to table, Toronto, Ontario. http://www.newvillage.net/Journal/Issue2/2annexorganics.html (accessed on May 25, 2011).

Martin, R., and Marsden, T. 1999. Food for urban spaces: The development of urban food production in England and Wales. *International Planning Studies* 4:389–419.

Marsden, T., Banks, J., and Bristow, G. 2000. Food supply chain approaches: Exploring their role in rural development. *Sociologia Ruralis* 40: 424–438.

Mathieu, R., Freeman, C., and Aryal, J. 2007. Mapping private gardens in urban areas using object-oriented techniques and very resolution satellite imagery. *Landscape and Urban Planning* 81:179–192.

Ministry for Agriculture and Fisheries (MAF), New Zealand. 1995. *The National Food Survey 1993*. Wellington, New Zealand: MAF.

Ministry of Health, New Zealand. 1999. *NZ Food: NZ People, Key Results of the 1997 National Nutrition Survey*. Wellington, New Zealand: Ministry of Health.

Mississippi State University. 2010. Vegetable gardening in Mississippi. http://msucares.com/lawn/garden/vegetables/watering/index.html (accessed on February 22, 2011).

Murray, D. 2005. *Oil and Food: A Rising Security Challenge, Plan B Updates*, May 9, 2005. Earth Policy Institute.http://www.earth-policy.org/index.php?/plan_b_updates/2005/update48 (accessed on February 5, 2010).

National Gardening Association (NGA). 2009. *The Impact of Home and Community Gardening in America*. South Burlington, VT, USA: National Gardening Association Inc.

New South Wales Government (NSW). 2011. *North Sydney Council Partners with NSW Government to Reduce Food Waste. Media Release* April 15, 2011. Sydney, Australia. http://www.environment.nsw.gov.au/media/DecMedia11041501.htm (accessed on May 20, 2011).

New South Wales Government (NSW). 2009. *Healthy Urban Development Checklist, A Guide for Health Services When Commenting on Development Policies, Plans and Proposals*. Sydney, Australia: NSW Health.

New South Wales Government (NSW). 2006. *2006 Chapter 6: Reducing Demand. Water for Life in Metropolitan Water Plan*, pp. 51–76. Sydney, Australia.

O'Halloran, N., Fisher, P., and Rab, A. 2008. *Preliminary Estimation of the Carbon Footprint of the Australian Vegetable Industry*. Discussion paper 4. Vegetable Industry CarbonFootprint Scoping Study. Sydney, Australia: Horticulture Australia Ltd.

Pederson, R. M., and Robertson, A. 2001. Food policies are essential for healthy cities. *Urban Agriculture Magazine* 3:9–10.

Peters, C. J., Bills, N. L., Wilkins, J. L., and Fick, G. W. 2009. Foodshed analysis and its relevance to sustainability. *Renewable Agriculture and Food Systems* 24(1):1–7.

Population Reference Bureau. 2011. *World Population Highlights 2007: Urbanization*. Washington DC, USA: Population Reference Bureau. http://www.prb.org/Articles/2007/623Urbanization.aspx (accessed on February 24, 2011).

Pimentel, D., and Pimentel, M. 2003. Sustainability of meat-based and plant-based diets and the environment. *American Journal of Clinical Nutrition* 78(3):660–663.

Pritchard, M., and Vale, R. 1999. How to save yourself (possibly the world) on 20 minutes a day. *Proceedings of the 6th Conference of the Sustainable Energy Forum, Threshold 2000, Can Our Cities Become Sustainable?* 23–25 June, 1999, Latest version 2003. Auckland, New Zealand.

Provost, C. 2011. One-third of the world's food goes to waste, says FAO. May 12, 2011. http://www.guardian.co.uk/global-development/2011/may/12/food-waste-fao-report-security-poor (accessed on May 28, 2011).

Resource Centre on Urban Agriculture and Food Security (RUAF) Foundation. 2011. Fact sheet on urban agriculture. Presence and output of urban agriculture. *Urban Agriculture Magazine*, Special edition. http://urbanag.pbworks.com/f/RUAF+urban+ag+fact+sheet.pdf (accessed on March 20, 2011).

Senate Department for Urban Development, Germany. 2011. Allotment gardens: Data and facts. http://www.stadtentwicklung.berlin.de/umwelt/stadtgruen/kleingaerten/en/daten_fakten/index.shtml (accessed on June 15, 2011).

Smith, R. M., Gaston, K. J., Warren, P. H., and Thompson, K. 2005. Urban domestic gardens (V): Relationships between landcover composition, housing and landscape. *Landscape Ecology* 20:235–253.

Straw, R. A., 2009. *Irrigating the Home Garden, Horticulturist, Southwest Virginia Agricultural Research and Extension Center.* Virginia Tech. USA. http://pubs.ext.vt.edu/426/426–322/426–322.html (accessed on January 11, 2011).

Strategic Alliance for Healthy Food and Activity Environments. 2011. Community Food Environment.http://www.eatbettermovemore.org/sa/enact/neighborhood/localfood.php (accessed on June 15, 2011).

The World Bank. 2011. *Rising Global Interest in Farmland: Can It Yield Sustainable and Equitable Benefits?* Washington D.C., USA: The World Bank.

Tilman, D., Socolow, R., Foley, J. A., Hill J., Larson, E., Lynd, L., Pacala, S. et al. 2009. Beneficial biofuels—The food, energy, and environment trilemma. *Science* 35:270–271.

Toronto Food Policy Council (TFPC). 2011. *Food Policy.* Toronto, Ontario, Canada. http://www.toronto.ca/health/tfpc_index.htm (accessed on March 20, 2011).

United Nations Environment Programme (UNEP). 2009. The environmental food crisis–The environment's role in averting future food crises. A UNEP rapid response assessment. Nellemann, C., MacDevette, M., Manders, T., Eickhout, B., Svihus, B., Prins, A. G., Kaltenborn, B. P. (Eds). United Nations Environment Programme: GRID—Arendal, Norway.

United Nations World Commission on Environment and Development (WCED). 1987. *Our Common Future.* The Brundtland Report. Oxford: Oxford University Press.

United Nations, 2011. Agenda 21. http://www.un.org/esa/dsd/agenda21/ (accessed on March 20, 2011).

United States Department of Agriculture (USDA) and Economic Research Service. 2011. Your food environment atlas. http://maps.ers.usda.gov/FoodAtlas/ (accessed on June 12, 2011).

Wackernagel, M., and Rees, W. 1996. *Our Ecological Footprint, Reducing Human Impact on Earth.* Gabriola Island, BC, Canada: New Society Publishers.

Wallgren, C. 2006. Local or global food markets: A comparison of energy use for transport. *Local Environment* 11(2):233–251.

Waste and Resources Action Programme (WRAP). 2009. Food waste in Scotland Final Report. WRAP Project EVA077-001. Banbury, U.K. http://www.wrap.org.uk/downloads/Food_waste_in_Scotland_FINAL_report_28_August_2009.93ffe07f.7550.pdf (accessed on June 12, 2011).

Wekerle, G. R. 2002. *Toronto's Official Plan from the Perspective of Community Gardening and Urban Agriculture.* Toronto, Canada. http://www.cityfarmer.org/torontoplan.html (accessed on April 4, 2011).

Wilson, G. 2005. *Singapore's New Business Opportunity: Food from the Roof.* City Farmer, Canada's Office of Urban Agriculture. http://www.cityfarmer.org/singaporeroof.html#singapore (accessed on January 15, 2011).

WinklerPrins, M. G. A. A. 2002. House-lot gardens in Santarém, Pará, Brazil: Linking rural with urban. *Urban Ecosystems* 6:43–65.

Wolf, J., Bindraban, P. S., Luijtenc, J. C., and Vleeshouwersa, L. M. 2003. Exploratory study on the land area required for global food supply and the potential global production of bioenergy. *Agricultural Systems* 76(8):41–861.

World Health Organisation (WHO). 2003. Fruit and vegetable promotion initiative./A Meeting Report/25-27/08/03. http://www.who.int/hpr/NPH/fruit_and_vegetables/fruit_and_vegetable_report.pdf (accessed on March 20, 2011).

Index

A

AA, *see* Arachidonic acid (AA)
AAFC, *see* Agriculture and Agri-Food Canada (AAFC)
AAS, *see* Atomic absorption and atomic emission (AAS)
ABS, *see* Australian Bureau of Statistics (ABS)
ACE, *see* Angiotensin-I converting enzyme (ACE)
Acid casein
    advantage, 374
    compositions, 373
    manufacturing processes, 373
    suspension, 374
Acid stress, 288–289
Acid whey powder, 377
Active ingredient, 186
Active packaging (AP), 219; *see also* Antimicrobial
        packaging; Intelligent packaging;
        Nanocomposite packaging
    absorbents types, 222
    absorbers, 219
    applications, 220–221
    bitter-tasting components, 222
    Ethicap, 222
    uses, 223
AD, *see* Alzheimer's disease (AD)
Adenosine diphosphate (ADP), 25, 34, 48
ADHD, *see* Attention-deficit hyperactivity disorder
        (ADHD)
Adoption–diffusion process, 519
ADP, *see* Adenosine diphosphate (ADP)
AFN, *see* Alternative food network (AFN)
Agri-food commodities, 137
Agricultural production, 126, 127
Agriculture and Agri-Food Canada (AAFC), 144
AI-2, *see* Autoinducer-2 (AI-2)
ALA, *see* α-linolenic acid (ALA)
Alginate, 277, 283
Allergenicity, 46
Allergic disorders, 404
α-LA, *see* α-lactalbumin (α-LA)
α-lactalbumin (α-LA), 364, 379
α-linolenic acid (ALA), 30
α-tocopherol, 22–23
Alternative food network (AFN), 556
Alzheimer's disease (AD), 424
American Society for Testing of Materials (ASTM), 225
Amino acids, 35
Amplification rDNA restriction analysis (ARDRA), 391
Amyloid-beta (Aβ), 424
Analysis of variance (ANOVA), 309
Angiotensin-I converting enzyme (ACE), 401
Animal products, 129
Anna—anna aushadhi—aushadhi continuum, 166
ANOVA, *see* Analysis of variance (ANOVA)
Antidiabetic effects, 337
Antimicrobial activity, 338

Antimicrobial packaging; *see also* Active packaging (AP);
        Intelligent packaging; Nanocomposite
        packaging
    antimicrobial agents, 225
    antimicrobial films, 224
    applications, 225
Antioxidants, 106, 337
Antioxidants and nutrients, 33
    arginine, 35
    capsaicin, 34
    carnosine and β-alanine, 35
    creatine, 34
    curcumin, 33
    glutamine, 36
    piperine, 33
    protein and amino acids, 35
    whey protein, 36
Antisolvent extraction, 347, 355
AP, *see* Active packaging (AP)
API, *see* Ayurvedic Pharmacopoeia of India (API)
APM, *see* Ayurvedic Proprietary medicines (APM)
ApoE4, *see* Apolipoprotein E (ApoE4)
Apolipoprotein E (ApoE4), 424
Arachidonic acid (AA), 426
ARDRA, *see* Amplification rDNA restriction analysis
        (ARDRA)
Arginine, 35
Arrhenius equation, 206
Artemisinin, 347
Ascorbic acid, 24, 194
Astaxanthin, 26, 355
ASTM, *see* American Society for Testing of Materials
        (ASTM)
Atomic absorption and atomic emission (AAS), 52
Attention-deficit hyperactivity disorder (ADHD), 426
    LCn-3PUFA, 427
    parameters, 427
    subjects and studies, 426, 427
    symptoms, 426
AUM, *see* Ayurveda, Unani medicines (AUM)
Australian Bureau of Statistics (ABS), 562
Autoinducer-2 (AI-2), 398
Axerophthol, *see* Retinol
Ayurceuticals
    fortune at bottom of, 175
    phytochemical paths to, 176
Ayurveda, 166–167, 540
Ayurveda, Unani medicines (AUM), 540
Ayurvedic Pharmacopoeia of India (API), 540
Ayurvedic Proprietary medicines (APM), 540
Aβ, *see* Amyloid-beta (Aβ)

B

BCAA, *see* Branched-chain amino acis (BCAA)
BDMC, *see* Bis-demethoxycurcumin (BDMC)

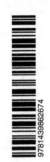